MCAT®

Biology Review

3rd Edition

The Staff of The Princeton Review

Penguin
Random
House

The Princeton Review
110 E. 42nd Street
New York, NY 10017

Published in the United States by Penguin Random House LLC, New York, and in Canada by Random House of Canada, a division of Penguin Random House Ltd., Toronto.

Terms of Service: The Princeton Review Online Companion Tools ["Student Tools"] for retail books are available for only the two most recent editions of that book. Student Tools may be activated only once per eligible book purchased, for a total of 24 months of access. Activation of Student Tools more than once per book is in direct violation of these Terms of Service and may result in discontinuation of access to Student Tools Services.

The material in this book is up-to-date at the time of publication. However, changes may have been instituted by the testing body in the test after this book was published.

If there are any important late-breaking developments, changes, or corrections to the materials in this book, we will post that information online in the Student Tools. Register your book and check your Student Tools to see if there are any updates posted there.

ISBN: 978-0-593-51623-2
ISSN: 2770-453X

The MCAT is a registered trademark of the Association of American Medical Colleges.

The Princeton Review is not affiliated with Princeton University.

Editor: Aaron Riccio
Production Artist: John Stecyk
Production Editor: Liz Dacey, Sarah Litt

Manufactured in China.

10 9 8 7 6 5 4 3 2

3rd Edition

For customer service, please contact **editorialsupport@review.com,** and be sure to include:

- full title of the book

- ISBN

- page number

CONTRIBUTORS

Daniel J. Pallin, M.D.
    Senior Author
Judene Wright, M.S., M.A.Ed.
    Senior Author

TPR MCAT Biology and Biochemistry Development Team:

Jessica Adams, Ph.D.
Britney McMurren, B.H.Sc., M.Sc.
Judene Wright, M.S., M.A.Ed., Senior Editor, Lead Developer
Sarah Woodruff, B.S., B.A.

Edited for Production by:

Judene Wright, M.S., M.A.Ed.
    National Content Director, MCAT Program, The Princeton Review

The TPR MCAT Biology and Biochemistry Team and Judene would like to thank the following people for their contributions to this book :

Kashif Anwar, M.D., M.M.S., John Bahling, M.D., Kristen Brunson, Ph.D., Phil Carpenter, Ph.D., Khawar Chaudry, B.S., Nita Chauhan, H.BSc, MSc, Dan Cho, M.P.H., Glenn E. Croston, Ph.D., Nathan Deal, M.D., Ian Denham, B.Sc., B.Ed., Joshua Dilworth, M.D., Ph.D., Annie Dude, Rob Fong, M.D., Ph.D., Chris Fortenbach, B.S., Kirsten Frank, Ph.D., Isabel L. Jackson, B.S., Erik Kildebeck, George Kyriazis, Ph.D., Ben Lee, Heather Liwanag, Ph.D., Travis MacKoy, B.S., Joey Mancuso, M.S., D.O., Evan Martow, BMSc, Brian Mikolasko, M.D., M.BA, Abhisehk Mohapatra, B.A., Christopher Moriates, M.D., Stephen L. Nelson, Jr., Ph.D., Rupal Patel, B.S., Mary Qiu, Ina C. Roy, M.D., Jayson Sack, M.D., M.S., Will Sanderson, Jeanine Seitz-Partridge, M.S., Oktay Shuminov, B.S., Andrew D. Snyder, M.D., Preston Swirnoff, Ph.D., M.S., Jenkang Tao, B.S., B.A., Rhead Uddin, Jia Wang.

PERIODIC TABLE OF THE ELEMENTS

1																	18
1 **H** 1.0	2												13	14	15	16	17	2 **He** 4.0
3 **Li** 6.9	4 **Be** 9.0												5 **B** 10.8	6 **C** 12.0	7 **N** 14.0	8 **O** 16.0	9 **F** 19.0	10 **Ne** 20.2
11 **Na** 23.0	12 **Mg** 24.3	3	4	5	6	7	8	9	10	11	12	13 **Al** 27.0	14 **Si** 28.1	15 **P** 31.0	16 **S** 32.1	17 **Cl** 35.5	18 **Ar** 39.9
19 **K** 39.1	20 **Ca** 40.1	21 **Sc** 45.0	22 **Ti** 47.9	23 **V** 50.9	24 **Cr** 52.0	25 **Mn** 54.9	26 **Fe** 55.8	27 **Co** 58.9	28 **Ni** 58.7	29 **Cu** 63.5	30 **Zn** 65.4	31 **Ga** 69.7	32 **Ge** 72.6	33 **As** 74.9	34 **Se** 79.0	35 **Br** 79.9	36 **Kr** 83.8
37 **Rb** 85.5	38 **Sr** 87.6	39 **Y** 88.9	40 **Zr** 91.2	41 **Nb** 92.9	42 **Mo** 95.9	43 **Tc** (98)	44 **Ru** 101.1	45 **Rh** 102.9	46 **Pd** 106.4	47 **Ag** 107.9	48 **Cd** 112.4	49 **In** 114.8	50 **Sn** 118.7	51 **Sb** 121.8	52 **Te** 127.6	53 **I** 126.9	54 **Xe** 131.3
55 **Cs** 132.9	56 **Ba** 137.3	57 ***La** 138.9	72 **Hf** 178.5	73 **Ta** 180.9	74 **W** 183.9	75 **Re** 186.2	76 **Os** 190.2	77 **Ir** 192.2	78 **Pt** 195.1	79 **Au** 197.0	80 **Hg** 200.6	81 **Tl** 204.4	82 **Pb** 207.2	83 **Bi** 209.0	84 **Po** (209)	85 **At** (210)	86 **Rn** (222)
87 **Fr** (223)	88 **Ra** (226)	89 **†Ac** (227)	104 **Rf** (267)	105 **Db** (268)	106 **Sg** (271)	107 **Bh** (270)	108 **Hs** (269)	109 **Mt** (278)	110 **Ds** (281)	111 **Rg** (282)	112 **Cn** (285)	113 **Nh** (286)	114 **Fl** (289)	115 **Mc** (289)	116 **Lv** (293)	117 **Ts** (294)	118 **Og** (294)

*Lanthanoids	58 **Ce** 140.1	59 **Pr** 140.9	60 **Nd** 144.2	61 **Pm** (145)	62 **Sm** 150.4	63 **Eu** 152.0	64 **Gd** 157.3	65 **Tb** 158.9	66 **Dy** 162.5	67 **Ho** 164.9	68 **Er** 167.3	69 **Tm** 168.9	70 **Yb** 173.0	71 **Lu** 175.0
†Actinoids	90 **Th** 232.0	91 **Pa** (231)	92 **U** 238.0	93 **Np** (237)	94 **Pu** (244)	95 **Am** (243)	96 **Cm** (247)	97 **Bk** (247)	98 **Cf** (251)	99 **Es** (252)	100 **Fm** (257)	101 **Md** (258)	102 **No** (259)	103 **Lr** (266)

CONTENTS

Get More **(Free)** Content
at **PrincetonReview.com/prep**

As easy as **1·2·3**

1 Go to PrincetonReview.com/prep or scan the **QR code** and enter the following ISBN for your book:
9780593516232

2 Answer a few simple questions to set up an exclusive Princeton Review account. *(If you already have one, you can just log in.)*

3 Enjoy access to your **FREE** content!

Once you've registered, you can...

- Take **3** full-length practice MCAT exams

- Find useful information about taking the MCAT and applying to medical school

- Check to see if there have been any corrections or updates to this edition

- Get our take on any recent or pending updates to the MCAT

Need to report a potential **content** issue?

Contact **EditorialSupport@review.com** and include:

- full title of the book
- ISBN
- page number

Need to report a **technical** issue?

Contact **TPRStudentTech@review.com** and provide:

- your full name
- email address used to register the book
- full book title and ISBN
- Operating system (Mac/PC) and browser (Chrome, Firefox, Safari, etc.)

Chapter 1
MCAT Basics

SO YOU WANT TO BE A DOCTOR

So...you want to be a doctor. If you're like most premeds, you've wanted to be a doctor since you were pretty young. When people asked you what you wanted to be when you grew up, you always answered "a doctor." You had toy medical kits, bandaged up your dog or cat, and played "hospital." You probably read your parents' home medical guides for fun.

When you got to high school you took the honors and AP classes. You studied hard, got straight A's (or at least really good grades!), and participated in extracurricular activities so you could get into a good college. And you succeeded!

At college you knew exactly what to do. You took your classes seriously, studied hard, and got a great GPA. You talked to your professors and hung out at office hours to get good letters of recommendation. You were a member of the premed society on campus, volunteered at hospitals, and shadowed doctors. All that's left to do now is get a good MCAT score.

Just the MCAT.

Just the most confidence-shattering, most demoralizing, longest, most brutal entrance exam for any graduate program. At about 7.5 hours (including breaks), the MCAT tops the list...even the closest runners up, the LSAT and GMAT, are only about 4 hours long. The MCAT tests significant science content knowledge along with the ability to think quickly, reason logically, and read comprehensively, all under the pressure of a timed exam.

The path to a good MCAT score is not as easy to see as the path to a good GPA or the path to a good letter of recommendation. The MCAT is less about what you know, and more about how to apply what you know...and how to apply it quickly to new situations. Because the path might not be so clear, you might be worried. That's why you picked up this book.

We promise to demystify the MCAT for you, with clear descriptions of the different sections, how the test is scored, and what the test experience is like. We will help you understand general test-taking techniques as well as provide you with specific techniques for each section. We will review the science content you need to know as well as give you strategies for the Critical Analysis and Reasoning Skills (CARS) section. We'll show you the path to a good MCAT score and help you walk the path.

After all...you want to be a doctor. And we want you to succeed.

WHAT IS THE MCAT...REALLY?

Most test-takers approach the MCAT as though it were a typical college science test, one in which facts and knowledge simply need to be regurgitated in order to do well. They study for the MCAT the same way they did for their college tests, by memorizing facts and details, formulas and equations. And when they get to the MCAT, they are surprised…and disappointed.

It's a myth that the MCAT is purely a content-knowledge test. If medical-school admission committees want to see what you know, all they have to do is look at your transcripts. What they really want to see is how you *think*, especially how you think under pressure. That's what your MCAT score will tell them.

The MCAT is really a test of your ability to apply basic knowledge to different, possibly new, situations. It's a test of your ability to reason out and evaluate arguments. Do you still need to know your science content? Absolutely. But not at the level that most test-takers think they need to know it. Furthermore, your science knowledge won't help you on the Critical Analysis and Reasoning Skills (CARS) section. So how do you study for a test like this?

You study for the science sections by reviewing the basics and then applying them to MCAT practice questions. You study for the CARS section by learning how to adapt your existing reading and analytical skills to the nature of the test. (More information about the CARS section can be found in *MCAT Critical Analysis and Reasoning Skills Review*.)

The book you are holding will review all the relevant MCAT Biology content you will need for the test, and a little bit more. It includes hundreds of questions designed to make you think about the material in a deeper way, along with full explanations to clarify the logical thought process needed to get to the answer. It also comes with access to three full-length online practice exams to further hone your skills. For more information on accessing those online exams, please refer to the "Get More (Free) Content" spread on pages x–xi.

MCAT NUTS AND BOLTS

Overview

The MCAT is a computer-based test (CBT) that is *not* adaptive. Adaptive tests base your next question on whether or not you've answered the current question correctly. The MCAT is *linear*, or *fixed-form*, meaning that the questions are in a predetermined order and do not change based on your answers. However, there are many versions of the test, so that on a given test day, different people will see different versions. The following table highlights the features of the MCAT exam.

Registration	Online via www.aamc.org. Begins as early as six months prior to test date; available up until week of test (subject to seat availability).
Testing Centers	Administered at small, secure, climate-controlled computer testing rooms.
Security	Photo ID with signature, electronic fingerprint, electronic signature verification, assigned seat.
Proctoring	None. Test administrator checks examinee in and assigns seat at computer. All testing instructions are given on the computer.
Frequency of Test	Many times per year distributed over January, April, May, June, July, August, and September.
Format	Exclusively computer-based. NOT an adaptive test.
Length of Test Day	7.5 hours
Breaks	Optional 10-minute breaks between sections, with a 30-minute break for lunch.
Section Names	1. Chemical and Physical Foundations of Biological Systems (Chem/Phys) 2. Critical Analysis and Reasoning Skills (CARS) 3. Biological and Biochemical Foundations of Living Systems (Bio/Biochem) 4. Psychological, Social, and Biological Foundations of Behavior (Psych/Soc)
Number of Questions and Timing	59 Chem/Phys questions, 95 minutes 53 CARS questions, 90 minutes 59 Bio/Biochem questions, 95 minutes 59 Psych/Soc questions, 95 minutes
Scoring	Test is scaled. Several forms per administration.
Allowed/ Not allowed	No timers/watches. Noise reduction headphones available. Noteboard booklet and wet-erase marker given at start of test and taken at end of test. Locker or secure area provided for personal items.
Results: Timing and Delivery	Approximately 30 days. Electronic scores only, available online through AAMC login. Examinees can print official score reports.
Maximum Number of Retakes	The test can be taken a maximum of three times in one year, four times over two years, and seven times over the lifetime of the examinee. An examinee can be registered for only one date at a time.

Registration

Registration for the exam is completed online at www.aamc.org/students/applying/mcat/reserving. The AAMC opens registration for a given test date at least two months in advance of the date, often earlier. It's a good idea to register well in advance of your desired test date to make sure that you get a seat.

Sections

There are four sections on the MCAT, all of which consist of multiple-choice questions:

Section	Concepts Tested	Number of Questions and Timing
Chemical and Physical Foundations of Biological Systems	Basic concepts in chemistry and physics, including biochemistry; scientific inquiry; reasoning; research and statistics skills.	59 questions in 95 minutes
Critical Analysis and Reasoning Skills	Critical analysis of information drawn from a wide range of social science and humanities disciplines.	53 questions in 90 minutes
Biological and Biochemical Foundations of Living Systems	Basic concepts in biology and biochemistry, scientific inquiry, reasoning, and research and statistics skills.	59 questions in 95 minutes
Psychological, Social, and Biological Foundations of Behavior	Basic concepts in psychology, sociology, and biology; research methods; and statistics.	59 questions in 95 minutes

Most questions on the MCAT (44 in the science sections, all 53 in the CARS section) are passage-based; the science sections have 10 passages each and the CARS section has 9. A passage consists of a few paragraphs of information on which several following questions are based. In the science sections, passages often include equations or reactions, tables, graphs, figures, and experiments to analyze. CARS passages come from literature in social sciences, humanities, ethics, philosophy, cultural studies, and population health, and they do not test content knowledge in any way.

Some questions in the science sections are freestanding questions (FSQs). These questions are independent of any passage information and appear in four groups of about three to four questions, interspersed throughout the passages. Fifteen of the questions in the science sections are freestanding, and the remainder are passage-based.

Each section on the MCAT is separated by either a 10-minute break or a 30-minute lunch break. We recommend that you take these breaks.

Section	Time
Test Center Check-In	Variable, can take up to 40 minutes if center is busy.
Tutorial	10 minutes
Chemical and Physical Foundations of Biological Systems	95 minutes
Break (optional)	10 minutes
Critical Analysis and Reasoning Skills	90 minutes
Lunch Break (optional)	30 minutes
Biological and Biochemical Foundations of Living Systems	95 minutes
Break (optional)	10 minutes
Psychological, Social, and Biological Foundations of Behavior	95 minutes
Void Option	5 minutes
Survey (optional)	5 minutes

The survey includes questions about your satisfaction with the overall MCAT experience, including registration, check-in, etc., as well as questions about how you prepared for the test.

Scoring

The MCAT is a scaled exam, meaning that your raw score will be converted into a scaled score that takes into account the difficulty of the questions. There is no guessing penalty. All sections are scored from 118–132, with a total scaled score range of 472–528. Because different versions of the test have varying levels of difficulty, the scale will be different from one exam to the next. Thus, there is no "magic number" of questions to get right in order to get a particular score. Plus, some of the questions on the test are considered "experimental" and do not count toward your score; they are just there to be evaluated for possible future inclusion in a test.

At the end of the test (after you complete the Psychological, Social, and Biological Foundations of Behavior section), you will be asked to choose one of the following two options, "I wish to have my MCAT exam scored" or "I wish to VOID my MCAT exam." You have five minutes to make a decision, and if you do not select one of the options in that time, the test will automatically be scored. If you choose the VOID option, your test will not be scored (you will not now, or ever, get a numerical score for this test), medical schools will not know you took the test, and no refunds will be granted. You cannot "unvoid" your scores at a later time.

So, what's a good score? The AAMC is centering the scale at 500 (i.e., 500 will be the 50th percentile), and recommends that application committees consider applicants near the center of the range. To be on the safe side, aim for a total score of around 510. Remember that if your GPA is on the low side, you'll need higher MCAT scores to compensate, and if you have a strong GPA, you can get away with lower MCAT scores. But the reality is that your chances of acceptance depend on a lot more than just your MCAT scores. It's a combination of your GPA, your MCAT scores, your undergraduate coursework, letters of recommendation, experience related to the medical field (such as volunteer work or research), extracurricular activities, your personal statement, etc. Medical schools are looking for a complete package, not just good scores and a good GPA.

GENERAL LAYOUT AND TEST-TAKING STRATEGIES

Layout of the Test

In each section of the test, the computer screen is divided vertically, with the passage on the left and the range of questions for that passage indicated above (e.g., "Passage 1 Questions 1–5"). The scroll bar for the passage text appears in the middle of the screen. Each question appears on the right, and you need to click "Next" to move to each subsequent question.

In the science sections, the freestanding questions are found in groups of 3–4, interspersed with the passages. The screen is still divided vertically; on the left is the statement "Questions [X–XX] do not refer to a passage and are independent of each other," and each question appears on the right as described above.

CBT Tools

There are a number of tools available on the test, including highlighting, strike-outs, the Flag for Review button, the Navigation and Review Screen buttons, the Periodic Table button, and of course, the noteboard booklet. All tools are available with both mouse control (buttons to click) or keyboard commands (Alt+ a letter). As everyone has different preferences, you should practice with both types of tools (mouse and keyboard) to see which is more comfortable for you personally. The following is a brief description of each tool.

1) **Highlighting:** This is done in the passage text (including table entries and some equations, but excluding figures and molecular structures), in the question stems, and in the answer choices (including Roman numerals). Select the words you wish to highlight (left-click and drag the cursor across the words), and in the upper left corner click the "Highlight" button to highlight the selected text yellow. Alternatively, press "Alt+H" to highlight the words. Highlighting can be removed by selecting the words again and in the upper left corner clicking the down arrow next to "Highlight." This will expand to show the "Remove Highlight" option; clicking this will remove the highlighting. Removing highlighting via the keyboard is cumbersome and is not recommended.

2) **Strike-outs:** This can be done on the answer choices, including Roman numeral statements, by selecting the text you want to strike out (left-click and drag the cursor across the text), then clicking the "Strikethrough" button in the upper left corner. Alternatively, press "Alt+S" to strikeout the words. The strike-out can be removed by repeating these actions. Figures or molecular structures cannot be struck out, however, the letter answer choice of those structures can.

3) **Flag for Review button:** This is available for each question and is found in the upper right corner. This allows you to flag the question as one you would like to review later if time permits. When clicked, the flag icon turns yellow. Click again to remove the flag. Alternatively, press "Alt+F."

4) **Navigation button:** This is found near the bottom of the screen and is only available on your first pass through the section. Clicking this button brings up a navigation table listing all questions and their statuses (unseen, incomplete, complete, flagged for review). You can also press "Alt+N" to bring up the screen. The questions can be sorted by their statuses, and clicking a question number takes you immediately to that question. Once you have reached the end of the section and viewed the Review screen (described below), the Navigation screen is no longer available.

5) **Review Screen button:** This button is found near the bottom of the screen after your first pass through the section, and when clicked, brings up a new screen showing all questions and their statuses (either incomplete, unseen, or flagged for review). Questions that are complete are assigned no additional status. You can then choose one of three options by clicking with the mouse or with keyboard shortcuts: Review All (Alt+A), Review Incomplete (Alt+I), or Review Flagged (Alt+R); alternatively, you can click a question number to go directly back to that question. You can also end the section from this screen.

6) **Periodic Table button:** Clicking this button will open a periodic table (or press "Alt+T"). Note that the periodic table is large, covering most of the screen. However, this window can be resized to see the questions and a portion of the periodic table at the same time. The table text will not decrease, but scroll bars will appear on the window so you can center the section of the table of interest in the window.

7) **Noteboard Booklet (Scratch Paper):** At the start of the test, you will be given a spiral-bound set of four laminated 8.5"×14" sheets of paper and a wet-erase black marker to use as scratch paper. You can request a clean noteboard booklet at any time during the test; your original booklet will be collected. The noteboard is only useful if it is kept organized; do not give in to the tendency to write on the first available open space! Good organization will be very helpful when/if you wish to review a question. Indicate the passage number, the range of questions for that passage, and a topic in a box near the top of your scratch work, and indicate the question you are working on in a circle to the left of the notes for that question. Draw a line under your scratch work when you change passages to keep the work separate. Do not erase or scribble over any previous work. If you do not think it is correct, draw one line through the work and start again. You may have already done some useful work without realizing it.

General Strategy for the Science Sections

Passages vs. FSQs in the Science Sections: What to Start With

Since the questions are displayed on separate screens, it is awkward and time consuming to click through all of the questions up front to find the FSQs. Therefore, go through the section on a first pass and decide whether to do the passage now or to save it for later, basing your decision on the passage text and the first question. Tackle the FSQs as you come upon them. More details are below.

Here is an outline of the procedure:

1) For each passage, write a heading on your noteboard with the passage number, the general topic, and its range of questions (e.g., "Passage 1, thermodynamics, Q 1–5" or "Passage 2, enzymes, Q 6–9"). The passage numbers do not currently appear in the Navigation or Review screens, thus having the question numbers on your noteboard will allow you to move through the section more efficiently.

2) Skim the text and rank the passage. If a passage is a "Now," complete it before moving on to the next passage (also see Attacking the Questions below). If it is a "Later" passage, first write "SKIPPED" in block letters under the passage heading on your noteboard and leave room for your work when you come back to complete that passage. (Note that the specific passages you skip will be unique to you; in the Bio/Biochem section, you might choose to do all Biology passages first, then come back for Biochemistry. Or in Chem/Phys you might choose to skip experiment-based or analytical passage. Know ahead of time what type of passage you are going to skip and follow your plan.)

3) Next, click on the "Navigation" button at the bottom to get to the Navigation screen. Click on the first question of the next passage; you'll be able to identify it because you know the range of questions from the passage you just skipped. This will take you to the next passage, where you will repeat steps 1–3.

4) Once you have completed the "Now" passages, go to the Review screen and click the first question for the first passage you skipped. Answer the questions, and continue going back to the Review screen and repeating this procedure for other passages you have skipped.

Attacking the Questions

As you work through the questions, if you encounter a particularly lengthy question, or a question that requires a lot of analysis, you may choose to skip it. This is a wise strategy because it ensures you will tackle all the easier questions first, the ones you are more likely to get right. If you choose to skip the question (or if you attempt it but get stuck), write down the question number on your noteboard, click the Flag for Review button to flag the question in the Review screen, and move on to the next question. At the end of the passage, click back through the set of questions to complete any that you skipped over the first time through, and make sure that you have filled in an answer for every question.

General Strategy for the CARS Section

Ranking and Ordering the Passages: What to Start With

Ranking: Since the questions are displayed on separate screens, it is awkward and time consuming to click through all of the questions before making a "Now, "Later," or "Killer" decision. Therefore, rank the passage and decide whether or not to do it on the first pass through the section based on the passage text, skimming the first 2–3 sentences.

Ordering: Because of the additional clicking through screens (or, use of the Review screen) that is required to navigate through the section, the "Two-Pass" system (completing the "Now" passages as you find them) is likely to be your most efficient approach. However, if you find that you are continuously making a lot of bad ranking decisions, it is still valid to experiment with the "Three-Pass" approach (ranking all nine passages up front before attempting your first "Now" passage).

Here is an outline of the basic Ranking and Ordering procedure to follow.

1) For each passage, write a heading on your noteboard with the passage number and its range of questions (e.g., "Passage 1 Q 1–7"). The passage numbers do not currently appear in the Navigation or Review screens, thus having the question numbers on your noteboard will allow you to move through the section more efficiently.

2) Skim the first 2–3 sentences and rank the passage. If the passage is a "Now," complete it before moving on to the next. If it is a "Later" or "Killer," first write either "Later" or "Killer" and "SKIPPED" in block letters under the passage heading on your noteboard and leave room for your work if you decide to come back and complete that passage. Then click through each question, flagging each one and filling in random guesses, until you get to the next passage.

3) Once you have completed the "Now" passages, come back for your second pass and complete the "Later" passages, leaving your random guesses in place for any "Killer" passages that you choose not to complete. Go to the Review screen and use your noteboard notes on the question numbers; click on the number of the first question for that passage to go back to that question and proceed from there. Alternatively, if you have consistently flagged all the questions for passages you skipped in your first pass you can use "Review Flagged" from the Review screen to find and complete your "Later" passages.

4) Regardless of how you choose to find your second pass passages, unflag each question after you complete it, so that you can continue to rely on the Review screen (and the "Review Flagged" function) to identify questions that you have not yet attempted.

Previewing the Questions

The formatting and functioning of the tools facilitates effective previewing. Having each question on a separate screen will encourage you to really focus on that question. Even more importantly, you can highlight in the question stem and in the answer choices.

Here is the basic procedure for previewing the questions:

1) Start with the first question, and if it has lead words referencing passage content, highlight them. You may also choose to jot them down on your noteboard. Once you reach and preview the last question for the set on that passage, THEN stay on that screen and work the passage (your highlighting appears and stays on every passage screen, and persists through the whole 90 minutes).

2) Once you have worked the passage and defined the Bottom Line—the main idea and tone of the entire passage—work **backward** from the last question to the first. If you skip over any questions as you go (see Attacking the Questions below), write down the question number on your noteboard. Then click **forward** through the set of questions, completing any that you skipped over the first time through. Once you reach and complete the last question for that passage, clicking "Next" will send you to the first question of the next passage. Working the questions from last to first the first time through the set will eliminate the need to click back through multiple screens to get to the first question immediately after previewing, and will also make it easier and more efficient to do the hardest questions last (see Attacking the Questions below).

3) Remember that previewing questions is a CARS-only technique. It is not efficient to preview questions in the science section.

Attacking the Questions

The question types and the procedure for actually attacking each type will be discussed later. However, it is still important **not** to attempt the hardest questions first (potentially getting stuck, wasting time, and discouraging yourself).

So, as you work the questions from last to first (see Previewing the Questions above), if you encounter a particularly difficult and/or lengthy question (or if you attempt a question but get stuck), write down the question number on your noteboard (you may also choose to Flag it) and move on backward to the next question. Then click **forward** through the set and complete any that you skipped over the first time through the set, unflagging any questions that you flagged that first time through and making sure that you have filled in an answer for every question.

Pacing Strategy for the MCAT

Since the MCAT is a timed test, you must keep an eye on the timer and adjust your pacing as necessary. It would be terrible to run out of time at the end only to discover that the last few questions could have been easily answered in just a few seconds each.

In the science sections you will have about one minute and thirty-five seconds (1:35) per question, and in the CARS section you will have about one minute and forty seconds (1:40) per question (not taking into account time reading the passage before answering the questions).

Section	# of Questions in Passage	Approximate Time (including reading the passage)
Chem/Phys, Bio/Biochem, and Psych/Soc	4	6.5 minutes
	5	8 minutes
	6	9.5 minutes
CARS	5	8.5 minutes
	6	10 minutes
	7	11.5 minutes

When starting a passage in the science sections, make note of how much time you will allot for it and the starting time on the timer. Jot down on your noteboard what the timer should say at the end of the passage. Then just keep an eye on it as you work through the questions. If you are near the end of the time for that passage, guess on any remaining questions, make some notes on your noteboard, Flag the questions, and move on. Come back to those questions if you have time.

For the CARS section, keep in mind that many people will maximize their score by *not* trying to complete every question or every passage in the section. A good strategy for test-takers who cannot achieve a high level of accuracy on all nine passages is to randomly guess on at least one passage in the section, and spend your time getting a high percentage of the other questions right. To complete all nine CARS passages, you have about ten minutes per passage. To complete eight of the nine, you have about 11 minutes per passage.

To help maximize your number of correct answer choices in any section, do the questions and passages within that section in the order *you* want to do them in.

Process of Elimination

Process of Elimination (POE) is probably the most useful technique you have to tackle MCAT questions. Since there is no guessing penalty, POE allows you to increase your probability of choosing the correct answer by eliminating those you are sure are wrong.

1) Strike out any choices that you are sure are incorrect or that do not address the issue raised in the question.
2) Jot down some notes to help clarify your thoughts if you return to the question.
3) Use the "Flag for Review" button to flag the question for review. (Note, however, that in the CARS section, you generally should not be returning to rethink questions once you have moved on to a new passage.)
4) Do not leave it blank! For the sciences, if you are not sure and you have already spent more than 60 seconds on that question, just pick one of the remaining choices. If you have time to review it at the end, you can always debate the remaining choices based on your previous notes. For CARS, if you have been through the choices two or three times, have re-read the question stem and gone back to the passage and you are still stuck, move on. Do the remaining questions for that passage, take one more look at the question you were stuck on, then pick an answer and move on for good.

5) Special Note: If three of the four answer choices have been eliminated, the remaining choice must be the correct answer. Don't waste time pondering *why* it is correct, just click it and move on. The MCAT doesn't care if you truly understand why it's the right answer, only that you have the right answer selected.

6) More subject-specific information on techniques will be presented in the next chapter.

Guessing

Remember, there is NO guessing penalty on the MCAT. NEVER leave a question blank!

QUESTION TYPES

In the science sections of the MCAT, the questions fall into one of three main categories.

1) Memory questions: These questions can be answered directly from prior knowledge and represent about 25 percent of the total number of questions.

2) Explicit questions: These questions are those for which the answer is explicitly stated in the passage. To answer them correctly, for example, may just require finding a definition, reading a graph, or making a simple connection. Explicit questions represent about 35 percent of the total number of questions.

3) Implicit questions: These questions require you to apply knowledge to a new situation; the answer is typically implied by the information in the passage. These questions often start "if…then…." (For example, "If we modify the experiment in the passage like this, then what result would we expect?") Implicit style questions make up about 40 percent of the total number of questions.

In the CARS section, the questions fall into four main categories:

1) Specific questions: These either ask you for facts from the passage (Retrieval questions) or require you to deduce what is most likely to be true based on the passage (Inference questions).

2) General questions: These ask you to summarize themes (Main Idea and Primary Purpose questions) or evaluate an author's opinion (Tone/Attitude questions).

3) Reasoning questions: These ask you to describe the purpose of, or the support provided for, a statement made in the passage (Structure questions) or to judge how well the author supports his or her argument (Evaluate questions).

4) Application questions: These ask you to apply new information from either the question stem itself (New Information questions) or from the answer choices (Strengthen, Weaken, and Analogy questions) to the passage.

More detail on question types and strategies can be found in Chapter 2.

TESTING TIPS

Before Test Day

- Take a trip to the test center at least a day or two before your actual test date so that you can easily find the building and room on test day. This will also allow you to gauge traffic and see if you need money for parking or anything like that. Knowing this type of information ahead of time will greatly reduce your stress on the day of your test.
- During the week before the test, adjust your sleeping schedule so that you are going to bed and getting up in the morning at the same times as on the day before and morning of the MCAT. Prioritize getting a reasonable amount of sleep during the last few nights before the test.
- Don't do any heavy studying the day before the test. This is not a test you can cram for! Your goal at this point is to rest and relax so that you can go into test day in a good physical and mental condition.
- Eat well. Try to avoid excessive caffeine and sugar. Ideally, in the weeks leading up to the actual test, you should experiment a little bit with foods and practice tests to see which foods give you the most endurance. Aim for steady blood sugar levels during the test: sports drinks, peanut-butter crackers, trail mix, etc. make good snacks for your breaks and lunch.

General Test Day Info and Tips

- On the day of the test, arrive at the test center at least a half hour prior to the start time of your test.
- Examinees will be checked in to the center in the order in which they arrive.
- You will be assigned a locker or secure area in which to put your personal items. Textbooks and study notes are not allowed, so there is no need to bring them with you to the test center.
- Your ID will be checked, a scan of your palm will be taken, and you will be asked to sign in.
- You will be given a noteboard booklet and a wet-erase marker, and the test center administrator will take you to the computer on which you will complete the test. You may not choose a computer; you must use the computer assigned to you.
- Nothing, not even your watch, is allowed at the computer station except your photo ID, your locker key (if provided), and a factory sealed packet of ear plugs.
- If you choose to leave the testing room at the breaks, you will have your palm scanned again, and you will have to sign in and out.
- You are allowed to access the items in your locker, except for notes and cell phones. (Check your test center's policy on cell phones ahead of time; some centers do not even allow them to be kept in your locker.)
- Don't forget to bring the snack foods and lunch you experimented with during your practice tests.
- At the end of the test, the test administrator will collect your noteboard and clean off your notes.
- Definitely take the breaks! Get up and walk around. It's a good way to clear your head between sections and get the blood (and oxygen!) flowing to your brain.
- Ask for a clean noteboard at the breaks if you want a fresh one.

Chapter 2
Biology Strategy
for the MCAT

2.1 SCIENCE SECTIONS OVERVIEW

There are three science sections on the MCAT:

- Chemical and Physical Foundations of Biological Systems
- Biological and Biochemical Foundations of Living Systems
- Psychological, Social, and Biological Foundations of Behavior

The Chemical and Physical Foundations of Biological Systems section (Chem/Phys) is the first section on the test. It includes questions from General Chemistry (about 30%), Physics (about 25%), Organic Chemistry (about 15%), Biochemistry (about 25%), and Biology (about 5%). Further, the questions often test chemical and physical concepts within a biological setting: for example, pressure and fluid flow in blood vessels. A solid grasp of math fundamentals is required (arithmetic, algebra, graphs, trigonometry, vectors, proportions, and logarithms); however, there are no calculus-based questions.

The Biological and Biochemical Foundations of Living Systems section (Bio/Biochem) is the third section on the test. Approximately 65% of the questions in this section come from biology, approximately 25% come from biochemistry, and approximately 10% come from Organic and General Chemistry. Math calculations are generally not required on this section of the test; however, a basic understanding of statistics as used in biological research is helpful.

The Psychological, Social, and Biological Foundations of Behavior section (Psych/Soc) is the fourth and final section on the test. About 65% of the questions will be drawn from Psychology (and about 5% of these will be Biological Psychology), about 30% from Sociology, and about 5% from Biology. As with the Bio/Biochem section, calculations are generally not required, however, a basic understanding of statistics as used in research is helpful.

Most of the questions in the science sections (44 of the 59) are passage-based, and each section has ten passages. Passages consist of a few paragraphs of information and include equations, reactions, graphs, figures, tables, experiments, and data. Four to six questions will be associated with each passage.

The remaining 25% of the questions (15 of 59) in each science section are freestanding questions (FSQs). These questions appear in approximately four groups interspersed between the passages. Each group contains three to four questions.

There are 95 minutes allotted to each of the science sections. This breaks down to approximately one minute and 35 seconds per question.

2.2 SCIENCE PASSAGE TYPES

The passages in the science sections fall into one of three main categories: Information and/or Situation Presentation, Experiment/Research Presentation, or Persuasive (or Scientific) Reasoning.

Information and/or Situation Presentation

These passages either present straightforward scientific information or they describe a particular event or occurrence. Generally, questions associated with these passages test basic science facts or ask you to predict outcomes given new variables or new information. Here is an example of an Information/Situation Presentation passage:

> Figure 1 shows a portion of the inner mechanism of a typical home smoke detector. It consists of a pair of capacitor plates which are charged by a 9-volt battery (not shown). The capacitor plates (electrodes) are connected to a sensor device, D; the resistor R denotes the internal resistance of the sensor. Normally, air acts as an insulator and no current would flow in the circuit shown. However, inside the smoke detector is a small sample of an artificially produced radioactive element, americium-241, which decays primarily by emitting alpha particles, with a half-life of approximately 430 years. The daughter nucleus of the decay has a half-life in excess of two million years and therefore poses virtually no biohazard.

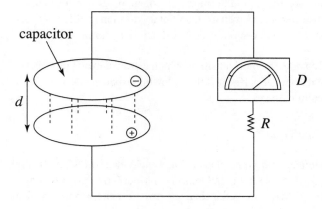

Figure 1   Smoke detector mechanism

> The decay products (alpha particles and gamma rays) from the ^{241}Am sample ionize air molecules between the plates and thus provide a conducting pathway which allows current to flow in the circuit shown in Figure 1. A steady-state current is quickly established and remains as long as the battery continues to maintain a 9-volt potential difference between its terminals. However, if smoke particles enter the space between the capacitor plates and thereby interrupt the flow, the current is reduced, and the sensor responds to this change by triggering

the alarm. (Furthermore, as the battery starts to "die out," the resulting drop in current is also detected to alert the homeowner to replace the battery.)

$$C = \varepsilon_0 \frac{A}{d}$$

Equation 1

where ε_0 is the universal permittivity constant, equal to 8.85 $\times 10^{-12}$ $C^2/(N\ m^2)$. Since the area A of each capacitor plate in the smoke detector is 20 cm^2 and the plates are separated by a distance d of 5 mm, the capacitance is 3.5×10^{-12} F = 3.5 pF.

Experiment/Research Presentation

These passages present the details of experiments and research procedures. They often include data tables and graphs. Generally, questions associated with these passages ask you to interpret data, draw conclusions, and make inferences. Here is an example of an Experiment/Research Presentation passage:

The development of sexual characteristics depends upon various factors, the most important of which are hormonal control, environmental stimuli, and the genetic makeup of the individual. The hormones that contribute to the development include the steroid hormones estrogen, progesterone, and testosterone, as well as the pituitary hormones FSH (follicle-stimulating hormone) and LH (luteinizing hormone).

To study the mechanism by which estrogen exerts its effects, a researcher performed the following experiments using cell culture assays.

Experiment 1:

Human embryonic placental mesenchyme (HEPM) cells were grown for 48 hours in Dulbecco's Modified Eagle Medium (DMEM), with media change every 12 hours. Upon confluent growth, cells were exposed to a 10 mg per mL solution of green fluorescent-labeled estrogen for 1 hour. Cells were rinsed with DMEM and observed under confocal fluorescent microscopy.

Experiment 2:

HEPM cells were grown to confluence as in Experiment 1. Cells were exposed to Pesticide A for 1 hour, followed by the 10 mg/mL solution of labeled estrogen, rinsed as in Experiment 1, and observed under confocal fluorescent microscopy.

Experiment 3:

Experiment 1 was repeated with Chinese Hamster Ovary (CHO) cells instead of HEPM cells.

Experiment 4:

CHO cells injected with cytoplasmic extracts of HEPM cells were grown to confluence, exposed to the 10 mg/mL solution of labeled estrogen for 1 hour, and observed under confocal fluorescent microscopy.

The results of these experiments are given in Table 1.

Table 1 Detection of Estrogen (+ indicates presence of Estrogen)

Experiment	Media	Cytoplasm	Nucleus
1	+	+	+
2	+	+	+
3	+	+	+
4	+	+	+

After observing the cells in each experiment, the researcher bathed the cells in a solution containing 10 mg per mL of a red fluorescent probe that binds specifically to the estrogen receptor only when its active site is occupied. After 1 hour, the cells were rinsed with DMEM and observed under confocal fluorescent microscopy. The results are presented in Table 2.

The researcher also repeated Experiment 2 using Pesticide B, an estrogen analog, instead of Pesticide A. Results from other researchers had shown that Pesticide B binds to the active site of the cytosolic estrogen receptor (with an affinity 10,000 times greater than that of estrogen) and causes increased transcription of mRNA.

Table 2 Observed Fluorescence and Estrogen Effects (G = green, R = red)

Experiment	Media	Cytoplasm	Nucleus	Estrogen effects observed?
1	G only	G and R	G and R	Yes
2	G only	G only	G only	No
3	G only	G only	G only	No
4	G only	G and R	G and R	Yes

Based on these results, the researcher determined that estrogen had no effect when not bound to a cytosolic, estrogen-specific receptor.

Persuasive (Scientific) Reasoning

These passages typically present a scientific phenomenon, along with a hypothesis that explains the phenomenon, and may include counterarguments as well. Questions associated with these passages ask you to evaluate the hypothesis or arguments. Persuasive Reasoning passages in the science sections of the MCAT tend to be less common than Information Presentation or Experiment-based passages. Here is an example of a Persuasive Reasoning passage:

Two theoretical chemists attempted to explain the observed trends of acidity by applying two interpretations of molecular orbital theory. Consider the pK_a values of some common acids listed along with the conjugate base:

acid	pK_a	conjugate base
H_2SO_4	< 0	HSO_4^-
H_2CrO_4	5.0	$HCrO_4^-$
H_2PO_4	2.1	$H_2PO_4^-$
HF	3.9	F^-
HOCl	7.8	ClO^-
HCN	9.5	CN^-
HIO_3	1.2	IO_3^-

Recall that acids with a $pK_a < 0$ are called strong acids, and those with a $pK_a > 0$ are called weak acids. The arguments of the chemists are given below.

Chemist #1:

"The acidity of a compound is proportional to the polarization of the H—X bond, where X is some nonmetal element. Complex acids, such as H_2SO_4, $HClO_4$, and HNO_3 are strong acids because the H—O bonding electrons are strongly drawn towards the oxygen. It is generally true that a covalent bond weakens as its polarization increases. Therefore, one can conclude that the strength of an acid is proportional to the number of electronegative atoms in that acid."

Chemist #2:

"The acidity of a compound is proportional to the number of stable resonance structures of that acid's conjugate base. H_2SO_4, $HClO_4$, and HNO_3 are all strong acids because their respective conjugate bases exhibit a high degree of resonance stabilization."

Mapping a Passage

"Mapping a passage" refers to the combination of on-screen highlighting and noteboard notes that you take while working through a passage. Typically, good things to highlight include the overall topic of a paragraph, unfamiliar terms, italicized terms, unusual terms, numerical values, hypothesis, and experimental results. Noteboard notes can be used to summarize the paragraphs and to jot down important facts and connections that are made when reading the passage. More details on passage mapping will be presented in Section 2.5.

2.3 SCIENCE QUESTION TYPES

Questions in the science sections are generally one of three main types: Memory, Explicit, or Implicit.

Memory Questions

These questions can be answered directly from prior knowledge, with no need to reference the passage or question text. Memory questions represent approximately 25 percent of the science questions on the MCAT. Usually, Memory questions are found as FSQs, but they can also be tucked into a passage. Here's an example of a Memory question:

Which of the following acetylating conditions will convert diethylamine into an amide at the fastest rate?

A) Acetic acid / HCl
B) Acetic anhydride
C) Acetyl chloride
D) Ethyl acetate

Explicit Questions

Explicit questions can be answered primarily with information from the passage, along with prior knowledge. They may require data retrieval, graph analysis, or making a simple connection. Explicit questions make up approximately 35–40 percent of the science questions on the MCAT; here's an example (taken from the Information/Situation Presentation passage):

The sensor device *D* shown in Figure 1 performs its function by acting as:

A) an ohmmeter.
B) a voltmeter.
C) a potentiometer.
D) an ammeter.

Implicit Questions

These questions require you to take information from the passage, combine it with your prior knowledge, apply it to a new situation, and come to some logical conclusion. They typically require more complex connections than do Explicit questions, and they may also require data retrieval, graph analysis, etc. Implicit questions usually require a solid understanding of the passage information. They make up approximately 35–40 percent of the science questions on the MCAT; here's an example (taken from the Experiment/Research Presentation passage):

If Experiment 2 were repeated, but this time exposing the cells first to Pesticide A and then to Pesticide B before exposing them to the green fluorescent-labeled estrogen and the red fluorescent probe, which of the following statements will most likely be true?

A) Pesticide A and Pesticide B bind to the same site on the estrogen receptor.
B) Estrogen effects would be observed.
C) Only green fluorescence would be observed.
D) Both green and red fluorescence would be observed.

The Rod of Asclepius

You may notice this Rod of Asclepius icon as you read through the book. In Greek mythology, the Rod of Asclepius is associated with healing and medicine; the symbol continues to be used today to represent medicine and healthcare. You won't see this on the actual MCAT, but we've used it here to call attention to medically related examples and questions.

2.4 BIOLOGY ON THE MCAT

Biology is by far the most information-dense section on the MCAT. MCAT Biology topics span six different semester-length courses (molecular biology, cell biology, microbiology, genetics, anatomy, and physiology). Further, the application of this material is potentially vast; passages can discuss anything from the details of some viral life cycle to the complexities of genetic studies, to the nuances of an unusual disease. Fortunately, biology is the subject that MCAT students typically find the most interesting, and the one they have the most background in. People who want to go to medical school have an inherent interest in biology; thus this subject, although vast, seems more manageable than all the others on the MCAT.

The science sections of the MCAT have 10 passages and 15 freestanding questions (FSQs). The Biological and Biochemical Foundations of Living Systems section (Bio/Biochem) is primarily biology (65%) and biochemistry (25%). The remaining 10% are General and Organic Chemistry questions. Further, Biology questions can show up in the Psychological, Social, and Biological Foundations of Behavior section (about 10%) and in the Chemical and Physical Foundations of Biological Systems section (about 5%). Note also that about 25% of the Chem/Phys section is Biochemistry, and frequently the passages and questions are biology-based.

2.5 TACKLING A BIOLOGY PASSAGE

Generally speaking, time is not an issue in the Bio/Biochem section of the MCAT. Because students have a stronger background in biology than in other subjects, the passages seem more understandable; in fact, readers sometimes find themselves getting caught up and interested in the passage. Often, students report having about 5 to 10 minutes "left over" after completing the section. This means that an additional minute or so can potentially be spent on each passage, thinking and understanding.

Passage Types as They Apply to Biology

Experiment/Research Presentation: Biology

This is the most common type of Biology passage. It typically presents the details behind an experiment along with data tables, graphs, and figures. Often these are the most difficult passages to deal with because they require an understanding of the reasoning behind the experiment, the logic to each step, and the ability to analyze the results and form conclusions. A basic understanding of biometry (basic statistics as they apply to biology and biology research) is necessary.

Information/Situation Presentation: Biology

This is the second most common type of Biology passage on the MCAT. These passages generally appear as one of two variants: either a basic concept with additional levels of detail included (for example, all the detail you ever wanted to know about the electron transport chain), or a novel concept with ties to basic information (for example, a rare demyelinating disease). Either way, Biology passages are notorious

2.5

for testing concepts in unusual contexts. The key to dealing with these passages is to, first, not become anxious about all the stuff you might not know, and second, figure out how the basics you do know apply to the new situation. For example, you might be presented with a passage that introduces hormones you never heard of or novel drugs to combat diseases you didn't know existed. First, don't panic. Second, look for how these new things fit into familiar categories: for example, "peptide vs. steroid" or "sympathetic antagonist." Then answer the questions with these basics in mind.

That said, you have to know your basics. This will increase your confidence in answering freestanding questions, as well as increase the speed with which to find the information in the passage. The astute MCAT student will never waste time staring at a question thinking, "Should I know this?" Instead, because she has a solid understanding of the necessary core knowledge, she'll say, "No, I am NOT expected to know this, and I am going to look for it in the passage."

Persuasive Reasoning: Biology

This is the least common passage type in Biology. It typically describes some biological phenomenon and then offers one or more theories to explain it. Questions in Persuasive Reasoning passages ask you to determine support for one of the theories, or present new evidence and ask which theory is now contradicted.

One last thought about Biology passages in general: because the array of topics is so vast, Biology passages often pull questions from multiple areas of biology into a single, general topic. Consider, for example, a passage on renal function. Question topics could include basics about the kidney, transmembrane transport, autonomic control, blood pressure, hormones, biochemical energy needs, or a genetics question about a rare kidney disease.

Reading a Biology Passage

Although tempting, try not to get bogged down reading all the little details in a passage. Again, because most premeds have an inherent interest in biology and the mechanisms behind disease, it's very easy to get lost in the science behind the passages. In spite of having that "extra" time, you don't want to use it all up reading what isn't necessary. Each passage type requires a slightly different style of reading.

Information/Situation Presentation passages require the least reading. These should be skimmed to get an idea of the location of information within the passage. These passages include a fair amount of detail that you might not need, so save the reading of these details until a question comes up about them. Then go back and read for the finer nuances.

Experiment/Research Presentation passages require the most reading. You are practically guaranteed to get questions that ask you about the details of the experiment, why a particular step was carried out, why the results are what they are, how to interpret the data, or how the results might change if a particular variable is altered. It's worth spending a little more time reading to understand the experiment. However, because there will be a fair number of questions unrelated to the experiment, you might consider answering these first and then going back for the experiment details.

Persuasive Argument passages are somewhere in the middle. You can skim them for location of information, but you also want to spend a little time reading the details of and thinking about the arguments presented. It is extremely likely that you will be asked a question about them.

Advanced Reading Skills

To improve your ability to read and glean information from a passage, you need to practice. Be critical when you read the content; watch for vague areas or holes in the passage that aren't explained clearly. Remember that information about new topics will be woven throughout the passage; you may need to piece together information from several paragraphs and a figure to get the whole picture.

After you've read, highlighted, and mapped a passage (more on this in a bit), stop and ask yourself the following questions:

- What was this passage about? What was the conclusion or main point?
- Was there a paragraph that was mostly background?
- Were there paragraphs or figures that seemed useless?
- What information was found in each paragraph? Why was that paragraph there?
- Are there any holes in the story?
- What extra information could I have pulled out of the passage? What inferences or conclusions could I make?
- If something unique was explained or mentioned, what might be its purpose?
- What am I *not* being told?
- Can I summarize the purpose and/or results of the experiment in a few sentences?
- Were there any comparisons in the passage?

This takes a while at first, but eventually it will become second nature and you'll start doing it as you read the passage. If you have a study group you are working with, consider doing this as an exercise with your study partners. Take turns asking and answering the questions above. Having to explain something to someone else not only solidifies your own knowledge, but helps you see where you might be weak.

Mapping a Biology Passage

Mapping a Biology passage is a combination of highlighting and noteboard notes that can help you organize and understand the passage information.

Resist the temptation to highlight everything! (Everyone has done this: You're reading a biology textbook with a highlighter, and then look back and realize that the whole page is yellow!) Restrict your highlighting to a few things:

- the main theme of a paragraph
- an unusual or unfamiliar term that is defined specifically for that passage (e.g., something that is italicized)
- statements that either support the main theme or contradict the main theme
- general topics of a list that appears in paragraph form within a passage
- relationships (how one thing changes relative to another thing)

The noteboards should be organized. Make sure the passage number appears at the top of your noteboard notes. For each paragraph, note "P1," "P2," etc., on the noteboard, and jot down a few notes about that paragraph. Try to translate biology jargon into your own words using everyday language (this is particularly useful for experiments). Also, make sure to note down simple relationships (e.g., the relationship between two variables).

Pay attention to equations, figures, and the like to see what type of information they deal with. Don't spend a lot of time analyzing at this point, but do jot down on your noteboard "Fig 1" and a brief summary of the data. Also, if you've discovered a list in the passage, note its topic and location down on your noteboard.

Let's take a look at how we might highlight and map a passage. Below is a passage on eye physiology.

The wall of the human eye is composed of three layers of tissue, an outer layer of tough connective tissue, a middle layer of darkly pigmented vascular tissue, and an inner layer of neural tissue. The outer layer is subdivided into the sclera, the white portion, and the cornea, the clear portion. The inner layer is more commonly known as the *retina* and contains several types of cells.

Figure 1   Retina Structure

The photoreceptors of the retina include rods and cones which respond to light under different circumstances. Rods are more sensitive to light but cannot distinguish color; cones are less sensitive to light overall, but can respond to different wavelengths. Response to light involves visual pigments, which in all cases consist of a light-absorbing molecule called *retinal* (derived from vitamin A) bound to a protein called *opsin*. The type of opsin in the visual pigment determines the wavelength specificity of the retinal. The specific visual pigment in rod cells is called *rhodopsin*.

Figure 2   The Two Forms of Retinal

In the absence of light, Na^+ channels in the membranes of rod cells are kept open by cGMP. The conformational change in retinal upon light absorption causes changes in opsin as well; this triggers a pathway by which phosphodiesterase (PDE) is activated. Active PDE converts cGMP to GMP, causing it to dissociate from the Na^+ channel and the channel to close. Until retinal regains its bent shape (helped by enzymes), the rod is unable to respond further to light.

2.5

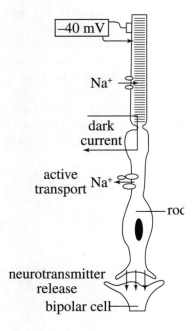

Figure 3 Rod Cell in Darkness

Visual defects can be caused by abnormal visual pigments or by misshapen eyeballs; for example, myopia (nearsightedness) is due to an eyeball that is too long, causing light rays from distant objects to focus in front of the retina so the image appears blurry.

Analysis and Passage Map

This passage is an Information Presentation passage and starts out with a paragraph about the structure of the eye and its layers. This is primarily a background paragraph and can be skimmed quickly, with a few words highlighted. Figure 1 shows the detail of the retina.

The second paragraph goes into more detail about the photoreceptors, and specifically compares the functions of rods and cones. There are few more italicized terms; this paragraph is presenting information that is beyond what you are expected to know about the eye for the MCAT. Figure 2 shows the conversion between the two forms of retinal.

The third paragraph presents details about rod cells, and in particular, points out a unique feature of rod cells: that their Na^+ channels are typically open in the absence of light. On stimulation by light, they close. This is unusual behavior in the nervous system, since it is the opposite of what typically occurs. Figure 3 confirms this, as the cell in darkness appears to be resting at −40 mV, 30 mV more positive than typical neurons rest at.

The final paragraph is a brief description of visual defects. Like paragraph 1, it only needs to be skimmed briefly. Here's what your passage map might look like:

P1 – 3 layers of eyeball, Fig 1 retina detail
P2 – photoreceptors
    rods no color, more sensitive
    cones less sensitive, respond to different colors
    details on vis pigments. Fig 2 convert retinal
P3 – rod function. WEIRD Na⁺ channels open in dark, close in light.
    depol in dark, hyperpol in light
P4 – visual defects

2.5

Let's take a look at a different passage. Below is an Experiment/Research Presentation passage.

The development of sexual characteristics depends upon various factors, the most important of which are hormonal control, environmental stimuli, and the genetic makeup of the individual. The hormones that contribute to the development include the steroid hormones estrogen, progesterone, and testosterone, as well as the pituitary hormones FSH (follicle-stimulating hormone) and LH (luteinizing hormone).

To study the mechanism by which estrogen exerts its effects, a researcher performed the following experiments using cell culture assays.

Experiment 1:

Human embryonic placental mesenchyme (HEPM) cells were grown for 48 hours in Dulbecco's Modified Eagle Medium (DMEM), with media change every 12 hours. Upon confluent growth, cells were exposed to a 10 mg per mL solution of green fluorescent-labeled estrogen for 1 hour. Cells were rinsed with DMEM and observed under confocal fluorescent microscopy.

Experiment 2:

HEPM cells were grown to confluence as in Experiment 1. Cells were exposed to Pesticide A for 1 hour, followed by the 10 mg/mL solution of labeled estrogen, rinsed as in Experiment 1, and observed under confocal fluorescent microscopy.

Experiment 3:

Experiment 1 was repeated with Chinese Hamster Ovary (CHO) cells instead of HEPM cells.

Experiment 4:

CHO cells injected with cytoplasmic extracts of HEPM cells were grown to confluence, exposed to the 10 mg/mL solution of labeled estrogen for 1 hour, and observed under confocal fluorescent microscopy.

The results of these experiments are given in Table 1.

Table 1 Detection of Estrogen
(+ indicates presence of estrogen)

Experiment	Media	Cytoplasm	Nucleus
1	+	+	+
2	+	+	+
3	+	+	+
4	+	+	+

After observing the cells in each experiment, the researcher bathed the cells in a solution containing 10 mg/mL of a red fluorescent probe that binds specifically to the estrogen receptor only when its active site is occupied. After 1 hour, the cells were rinsed with DMEM and observed under confocal fluorescent microscopy. The results are presented in Table 2.

The researcher also repeated Experiment 2 using Pesticide B, an estrogen analog, instead of Pesticide A. Results from other researchers had shown that Pesticide B binds to the active site of the cytosolic estrogen receptor (with an affinity 10,000 times greater than that of estrogen) and causes increased transcription of mRNA.

Table 2 Observed Fluorescence and Estrogen Effects
(G = green, R = red)

Experiment	Media	Cytoplasm	Nucleus	Estrogen effects observed?
1	G only	G and R	G and R	Yes
2	G only	G only	G only	No
3	G only	G only	G only	No
4	G only	G and R	G and R	Yes

Based on these results, the researcher determined that estrogen had no effect when not bound to a cytosolic, estrogen-specific receptor.

Analysis and Passage Map

This passage starts out with a very general background paragraph. Not much to do here, but it does tell us that estrogen is going to be the hormone of focus.

The next few paragraphs are short descriptions of four different experiments. These should be read to understand not only what's happening in each experiment but also what the differences in the experiments are. Note this on your noteboard.

Table 1 shows the results of the four experiments. It should jump out at you that estrogen is found everywhere; in other words, it is not restricted from any area of the cell.

After Table 1, the passage describes two modifications to the experiments. As with the original experiments, it's worth taking a little time to read and understand what's going on. The first big difference is that the researchers aren't just looking for the presence of estrogen, but also want to know when it's bound to its receptor. The second big difference is the testing of an estrogen analog, Pesticide B.

Table 2 shows the results of when estrogen is bound and when it isn't. These results could be combined with the experiment description results on your map:

> *P1 – hormones that contribute to development, estrogen*
> *E1 – HEPM cells exposed to estrogen, green + red = estrogen effects*
> *E2 – Pesticide A, green only, must inhibit binding of estrogen to recept.*
> *E3 – CHO cells, green only, no recept.*
> *E4 – CHO cells + HEPM cytoplasm, green + red, recept is in cytoplasm*
> *Table 1 – estrogen is not restricted from anywhere in the cell*
> *Further exp'ts – red probe for bound active site, and Pesticide B (estrogen analog w/higher affinity)*

One last thought about passages: Remember that, as with all sections on the MCAT, you can do the passages in the order *you* want to. There are no extra points for taking the test in order. Generally, passages will fall into one of four main subject groups:

- biochemistry
- other non-physiology
- physiology
- organic/general chemistry

Figure out which group you are most comfortable with, and do those passages first. (See Chapter 1 for general strategies for moving around in the sections efficiently.)

2.6 TACKLING THE QUESTIONS

Questions in the Biology section mimic the three typical questions of the science sections in general: Memory, Explicit, and Implicit.

Question Types as They Apply to Biology

Biology Memory Questions

Memory questions are exactly what they sound like: they test your knowledge of some specific fact or concept. While Memory questions are typically found as freestanding questions, they can also be tucked into a passage. These questions, aside from requiring memorization, do not generally cause problems for students because they are similar to the types of questions that appear on a typical college biology exam. Below is an example of a freestanding Memory question:

> Regarding embryogenesis, which of the following sequence of events is in correct order?
>
> A) Implantation—cleavage—gastrulation—neurulation—blastulation
> B) Blastulation—implantation—cleavage—neurulation—gastrulation
> C) Implantation—blastulation—gastrulation—cleavage—neurulation
> D) Cleavage—blastulation—implantation—gastrulation—neurulation

The correct answer to the question above is choice D. Here's another example. This question is from a passage:

> The genital organs of the *guevedoche* that develop at puberty are derivatives of the mesodermal germ layer. Which of the following is/are also derivatives of the mesodermal germ layer?
>
> I.   Skeletal muscle
> II. Liver
> III. Kidney
>
> A) I only
> B) II only
> C) I and III only
> D) II and III only

Note that this question includes an additional, unnecessary sentence at the beginning, but it is a Memory question all the same. You don't need to know anything about the *guevedoche* to answer the question, and the information in that first sentence does not help you in any way. The correct answer is choice C.

There is no specific "trick" to answering Memory questions; either you know the answer or you don't.

If you find that you are missing a fair number of Memory questions, it is a sure sign that you don't know the content well enough. Go back and review.

Biology Explicit Questions

True, pure Explicit questions are rare in the Biology section. A purely Explicit question can be answered only with information in the passage. Below is an example of a pure Explicit question taken from the eye passage above:

> The middle layer of the eyeball wall most likely contains:
>
> A) bipolar cells.
> B) photoreceptors.
> C) blood vessels.
> D) collagen fibers.

Referring back to the map for this passage, it indicates that information about the layers of the eyeball are in paragraph 1. It states that the middle layer is a "darkly pigmented vascular layer," meaning that it contains blood vessels. The correct answer is choice C.

However, more often in the biology section, Explicit questions are more of a blend of Explicit and Memory; they require not only retrieval of passage information, but also recall of some relevant fact. They usually do not require a lot of analysis or connections. Here's an example of the more common type of Explicit question:

> Pesticide A most likely functions as:
>
> A) an agonist.
> B) an inhibitor.
> C) a lipase.
> D) a receptor.

To answer this question, you first need to retrieve information from the passage about the effects of Pesticide A. From Table 2 we know that it prevents estrogen from binding to its receptor (and we noted this on our passage map). You also need to remember the definitions of the terms in the answer choices (agonists cause similar effects, inhibitors prevent effects, lipases break down lipids, and receptors bind ligands to cause effects). Based on our known definitions, choices A and D can be eliminated, and while Pesticide A could be functioning as a lipase that breaks down estrogen, "inhibitor" is a more accurate term (choice B is better than choice C and is the correct answer).

A final subgroup in the Explicit question category are graph interpretation questions. These fall into one of two types: those that ask you to take graphical information from the passage and convert it to a text answer, or those that take text from the passage and ask you to convert it to a graph. On the following page is an example of the latter type:

Which of the following graphs would best illustrate the binding of estrogen (E) to its receptor in the presence of its analog, Pesticide B?

From our passage map, we know that information about Pesticide B is found near the end of the passage, where it describes "further experiments." The passage states that Pesticide B functions as an estrogen analog that binds to the estrogen receptor with a much higher affinity than does estrogen. In other words, if Pesticide B is around, the receptor will preferentially bind it, and not estrogen. So as the concentration of Pesticide B rises, the amount of estrogen bound to the receptor should fall. This is shown in choice B.

If you find that you are missing Explicit questions, practice your passage mapping. Make sure you aren't missing the critical items in the passage that lead you to the right answer. Slow down a little; take an extra 15 to 30 seconds per passage to read or think about it more carefully.

Biology Implicit Questions

Implicit questions require the most thought. These require recall of not only biology information but also information gleaned from the passage and a more in-depth analysis of how the two relate. Implicit questions require more analysis and connections to be made than Explicit questions. Often they take the form "If...then...." Below is an example of a classic Implicit question, taken from the Experiment passage shown earlier.

If Experiment 2 were repeated, but this time exposing the cells first to Pesticide A and then to Pesticide B before exposing them to the green fluorescent-labeled estrogen and the red fluorescent probe, which of the following statements will most likely be true?

A) Pesticide A and Pesticide B bind to the same site on the estrogen receptor.
B) Estrogen effects would be observed.
C) Only green fluorescence would be observed.
D) Both green and red fluorescence would be observed.

To answer this question, conclusions have to be drawn from the experiments described in the passage, and new conclusions have to be predicted based on the new circumstance. Many more connections need to be made than when answering an Explicit question. From the passage, we need to figure out that Pesticide A is an inhibitor. We also have to figure out that it does not bind at the active site of the receptor (data from Table 2). We have to know what green fluorescence and red fluorescence imply. We have to draw on the information provided about Pesticide B to know that it is an analog and that it binds to the active site of the estrogen receptor. We have to combine all of this together and come to a logical conclusion: since Pesticide A is an inhibitor, it would prevent the binding of Pesticide B and thus prevent estrogen effects (choice B can be eliminated). If Pesticide B cannot bind, we would only see green fluorescence (choice D can be eliminated, and choice C is probably correct). Since Pesticide A by itself does not produce red fluorescence, it must not be binding at the active site, which is where Pesticide B binds, (choice A can be eliminated, and choice C is definitely correct).

2.6

Here's another example of an Implicit question, drawn from the same passage:

> When the researcher performed Experiment 2 using Pesticide B instead of Pesticide A, which of the following fluorescence and estrogen effects did the researcher most likely observe?
>
> A) *Media*: green and red
> *Cytoplasm*: green and red
> *Nucleus*: green and red
> *Estrogen effects*: no
>
> B) *Media*: green only
> *Cytoplasm*: green and red
> *Nucleus*: green and red
> *Estrogen effects*: no
>
> C) *Media*: green only
> *Cytoplasm*: green and red
> *Nucleus*: green and red
> *Estrogen effects*: yes
>
> D) *Media*: green only
> *Cytoplasm*: green and red
> *Nucleus*: green only
> *Estrogen effects*: no

To answer this question, we again must combine passage information with logical inference and working memory. Since red fluorescence indicates binding of the receptor, and since the receptor is never in the media, there can never be red fluorescence in the media (choice A can be eliminated). We know from the passage that Pesticide B binds at the active site of the receptor, and we know that the receptor is found in the cytoplasm. We also know from the passage that Pesticide B causes increased mRNA transcription, and we know from memory that to induce mRNA transcription, the receptor must move into the nucleus. Thus, red fluorescence must be observed in the nucleus as well (choice D can be eliminated). Since Pesticide B is defined as an "estrogen analog," and since we know from memory that analogs cause similar effects, it is likely that estrogen effects will be observed. The fact that increased mRNA transcription occurs supports this idea (choice B can be eliminated, and choice C is correct). Again, many more connections need to be made to answer Implicit questions; Process of Elimination is typically the best approach.

If you find that you are missing a lot of Implicit questions, first make sure that you are using POE aggressively. Second, go back and review the explanations for the correct answer to figure out where your logic went awry. Did you miss an important fact in the passage? Did you forget the relevant Biology content? Did you follow the logical train of thought to the right answer? Once you figure out where you made your mistake, you will know how to correct it.

2.7   SUMMARY OF THE APPROACH TO BIOLOGY

How to Map the Passage and Use the Noteboard

1) The passage should not be read like textbook material, with the intent of learning something from every sentence (science majors especially will be tempted to read this way). Passages should be read to get a feel for the type of questions that will follow and to get a general idea of the location of information within the passage.

2) Highlighting—Use this tool sparingly, or you will end up with a passage that is completely covered in yellow highlighter! Highlighting in a Biology passage should be used to draw attention to a few words that demonstrate one of the following:
    - the main theme of a paragraph
    - an unusual or unfamiliar term that is defined specifically for that passage (e.g., something that is italicized)
    - statements that either support the main theme or counteract the main theme
    - list topics (see below)
    - relationships

3) Pay brief attention to equations, figures, and experiments, noting only what information they deal with. Do not spend a lot of time analyzing at this point.

4) For each passage, start by noting the passage number, the general topic, and the range of questions on your noteboard. You can then work between your noteboard and the Review screen to easily get to the questions you want to (see Chapter 1).

5) For each paragraph, note "P1," "P2," etc. on the noteboard and jot down a few notes about that paragraph. Try to translate biology jargon into your own words using everyday language. Especially note down simple relationships (e.g., the relationship between two variables).

6) Lists—Whenever a list appears in paragraph form, jot down on the noteboard the paragraph and the general topic of the list. It will make returning to the passage more efficient and help to organize your thoughts.

7) The noteboard is only useful if it is kept organized! Make sure that your notes for each passage are clearly delineated and marked with the passage number and question range. This will allow you to easily read your notes when you come back to review a flagged question. Resist the temptation to write in the first available blank space as this makes it much more difficult to refer back to your work.

Biology Question Strategies

1) Remember that the content in Biology is vast, so don't panic if something seems completely unfamiliar. Understand the basic content well, find the basics in the unfamiliar topic, and apply them to the question.

2) Process of Elimination is paramount! The strikeout tool allows you to eliminate answer choices; this will improve your chances of guessing the correct answer if you are unable to narrow it down to one choice.

3) Answer the straightforward questions first (typically the memory questions). Leave questions that require analysis of experiments and graphs for later. Take the test in the order YOU want. Make sure to use your noteboard to indicate questions you skipped.

4) Make sure that the answer you choose actually answers the question and isn't just a true statement.

5) Try to avoid answer choices with extreme words such as "always," "never," etc. In biology, there is almost always an exception and answers are rarely black-and-white.

6) Roman numeral questions: Whenever possible, start by evaluating the Roman numeral item that shows up in exactly two answer choices. This allows you to quickly eliminate two wrong answer choices regardless of whether the item is true or false. Typically then, you will only have to assess one of the other Roman numeral items to determine the correct answer. Always work between the I-II-III items and the answer choices. Once an item is found to be true (or false), strike out answer choices which do not contain (or do contain) that item number. Make sure to strike out the actual Roman numeral item as well, and highlight those items that are true.

7) LEAST/EXCEPT/NOT questions: Don't get tricked by these questions that ask you to pick that answer that doesn't fit (the incorrect or false statement). Make sure to highlight the words "LEAST," "EXCEPT," or "NOT" in the question stem. It's often good to use your noteboard and write "A B C D" with a T or F next to each answer choice. The one that stands out as different is the correct answer!

8) Again, don't leave any question blank.

A Note About Flashcards

For most of the exams you've taken previously, flashcards were likely very helpful. This was because those exams mostly required you to regurgitate information, and flashcards are pretty good at helping you memorize facts. However, the most challenging aspect of the MCAT is not that it requires you to memorize the fine details of content knowledge, but that it requires you to apply your basic scientific knowledge to unfamiliar situations: flashcards alone may not help you there.

Flashcards can be beneficial if your basic content knowledge is deficient in some area. For example, if you don't know the hormones and their effects in the body, flashcards can certainly help you memorize these facts. Or, maybe you are unsure of the functions of the different brain regions. You might find that flashcards can help you memorize these. But unless you are trying to memorize basic facts in your personal weak areas, you are better off doing and analyzing practice passages than carrying around a stack of flashcards.

Chapter 3
Biologically Important
Molecules

The biological macromolecules are grouped into four classes of molecules that play important roles in cells and in organisms as a whole. All of them are polymers, strings of repeated units (monomers).

This chapter discusses the biomolecules from a biological perspective: what they are made of, how they are put together, and what their roles are in the body. These molecules are also discussed in *MCAT Biochemistry Review* in more detail, as well as in *MCAT Organic Chemistry Review* from an organic chemistry perspective: nomenclature, chirality, etc.

3.1 PROTEIN BUILDING BLOCKS

Proteins are biological macromolecules that act as enzymes, hormones, receptors, channels, transporters, antibodies, and support structures inside and outside cells. Proteins are composed of twenty different amino acids linked together in polymers. The composition and sequence of amino acids in the polypeptide chain is what makes each protein unique and able to fulfill its special role in the cell.

Amino Acid Structure and Nomenclature

Understanding the structure of amino acids is key to understanding both their chemistry and the chemistry of proteins. The generic formula for all twenty amino acids is shown below.

Figure 1 Generic Amino Acid Structure

All twenty amino acids share the same nitrogen-carbon-carbon backbone. The unique feature of each amino acid is its **side chain** (variable R-group), which gives it the physical and chemical properties that distinguish it from the other nineteen. Much more detail about amino acid structure, including their chemical properties, can be found in *MCAT Biochemistry Review*.

3.2 PROTEIN STRUCTURE

There are two common types of covalent bonds between amino acids in proteins: the **peptide bonds** that link amino acids together into polypeptide chains and **disulfide bridges** between cysteine R-groups.

The Peptide Bond

Polypeptides are formed by linking amino acids together in peptide bonds. A peptide bond is formed between the carboxyl group of one amino acid and the α-amino group of another amino acid with the loss of water. The figure below shows the formation of a dipeptide from the amino acids glycine and alanine.

Figure 2   Peptide Bond (Amide Bond) Formation

In a polypeptide chain, the N–C–C–N–C–C pattern formed from the amino acids is known as the **backbone** of the polypeptide. An individual amino acid is termed a **residue** when it is part of a polypeptide chain. The amino terminus is the first end made during polypeptide synthesis, and the carboxy terminus is made last. Hence, by convention, the amino-terminal residue is also always written first.

- In the oligopeptide Phe-Glu-Gly-Ser-Ala, which residue has a free α-amino group, and which residue has a free α-carboxyl group? (Refer to the beginning of the chapter for structures.)[1]

---

[1]   As stated above, the amino end is always written first. Therefore, the oligopeptide begins with an exposed Phe amino group and ends with an exposed Ala carboxyl; all the other backbone groups are hitched together in peptide bonds.

Hydrolysis of a protein by another protein is called **proteolysis** or **proteolytic cleavage**, and the protein that does the cutting is known as a **proteolytic enzyme** or **protease**. Proteolytic cleavage is a specific means of cleaving peptide bonds. Many enzymes only cleave the peptide bond adjacent to a specific amino acid. For example, the protease trypsin cleaves on the carboxyl side of the residues arginine and lysine, while chymotrypsin cleaves adjacent to hydrophobic residues such as phenylalanine. (Do *not* memorize these examples.)

Figure 3   Specificity of Protease Cleavage

- Based on the above, if the following peptide is cleaved by trypsin, what amino acid will be on the new N-terminus and how many fragments will result: Ala-Gly-Glu-Lys-Phe-Phe-Lys?[2]

The Disulfide Bond

Cysteine is an amino acid with a reactive thiol (sulfhydryl, SH) in its side chain. The thiol of one cysteine can react with the thiol of another cysteine to produce a covalent sulfur-sulfur bond known as a disulfide bond, as illustrated below. The cysteines forming a disulfide bond may be located in the same or different polypeptide chain(s). The disulfide bridge plays an important role in stabilizing tertiary protein structure; this will be discussed in the section on protein folding. Once a cysteine residue becomes disulfide-bonded to another cysteine residue, it is called *cystine* instead of cysteine.

Figure 4   Formation of the Disulfide Bond

---

[2]   Trypsin will cleave on the carboxyl side of the Lys residue, with Phe on the N-terminus of the new Phe-Phe-Lys fragment. There will be two fragments after trypsin cleavage: Phe-Phe-Lys and Ala-Gly-Glu-Lys.

Protein Structure in Three Dimensions

Each protein folds into a unique three-dimensional structure that is required for that protein to function properly. Improperly folded, or **denatured**, proteins are non-functional. There are four levels of protein folding that contribute to their final three-dimensional structure. Each level of structure is dependent upon a particular type of bond, as discussed in the following sections.

Denaturation is an important concept. It refers to the **disruption of a protein's shape without breaking peptide bonds**. Proteins are denatured by *urea* (which disrupts hydrogen bonding interactions), by *extremes of pH*, by extremes of *temperature,* and by *changes in salt concentration (tonicity)*.

Primary (1°) Structure: The Amino Acid Sequence

The simplest level of protein structure is the order of amino acids bonded to each other in the polypeptide chain. This linear ordering of amino acid residues is known as primary structure. Primary structure is the same as **sequence**. The bond which determines 1° structure is the peptide bond, simply because this is the bond that links one amino acid to the next in a polypeptide.

Secondary (2°) Structure: Hydrogen Bonds Between Backbone Groups

Secondary structure refers to the initial folding of a polypeptide chain into shapes stabilized by hydrogen bonds between backbone NH and CO groups. Certain motifs of secondary structure are found in most proteins. The two most common are the α-**helix** and the β-**pleated sheet**.

Figure 5 An α Helix

There are two types of β-sheets: one with adjacent polypeptide strands running in the *same* direction (**parallel** β-pleated sheet) and another in which the polypeptide strands run in *opposite* directions (**antiparallel** β-pleated sheet), as shown in Figure 6.

Figure 6   A β-Pleated Sheet

- If a single polypeptide folds once and forms a β-pleated sheet with itself, would this be a parallel or antiparallel β-pleated sheet?[3]

Tertiary (3°) Structure: Hydrophobic/Hydrophilic Interactions

The next level of protein folding, tertiary structure, concerns interactions between amino acid residues located more distantly from each other in the polypeptide chain. The folding of secondary structures such as α-helices into higher order tertiary structures is driven by interactions of R-groups with each other and with the solvent (water). Hydrophobic R-groups tend to fold into the interior of the protein, away from the solvent, and hydrophilic R-groups tend to be exposed to water on the surface of the protein (shown for the generic globular protein).

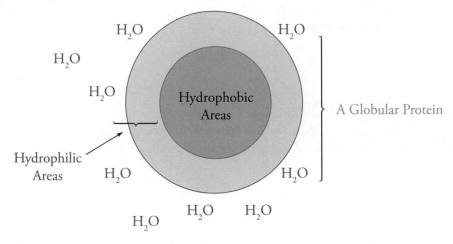

Figure 7   Folding of a Globular Protein in Aqueous Solution

---

[3] It would be antiparallel because one participant in the β-pleated sheet would have a C to N direction, while the other would be running N to C.

Under the right conditions, the forces driving hydrophobic avoidance of water and hydrogen bonding will fold a polypeptide spontaneously into the correct conformation, the lowest energy conformation.

- Which of the following may be considered an example of tertiary protein structure?[4]
    I. van der Waals interactions between two Phe R-groups located far apart on a polypeptide
    II. Hydrogen bonds between backbone amino and carboxyl groups
    III. Covalent disulfide bonds between cysteine residues located far apart on a polypeptide

Quaternary (4°) Structure: Various Bonds Between Separate Chains

The highest level of protein structure, quaternary structure, describes interactions between polypeptide subunits. A **subunit** is a single polypeptide chain that is part of a large complex containing many subunits (a **multisubunit complex**). The arrangement of subunits in a multisubunit complex is what we mean by quaternary structure. For example, mammalian RNA polymerase II contains twelve different subunits. The interactions between subunits are instrumental in protein function, as in the cooperative binding of oxygen by each of the four subunits of hemoglobin.

The forces stabilizing quaternary structure are generally the same as those involved in tertiary structure—non-covalent interactions, van der Waals forces, hydrogen bonds, disulfide bonds, and electrostatic interactions. It is key to understand, however, that there is one bond that may not be involved in quaternary structure—the peptide bond—because this bond defines sequence (1° structure).

- What is the difference between a disulfide bridge involved in quaternary structure and one involved in tertiary structure?[5]

3.3 CARBOHYDRATES

Carbohydrates can be broken down to CO_2 in a process called **oxidation**, which is also known as burning or combustion. Because this process releases large amounts of energy, carbohydrates generally serve as the principle energy source for cellular metabolism. Glucose in the form of the polymer cellulose is also the building block of wood and cotton.

Monosaccharides and Disaccharides

A single carbohydrate molecule is called a **monosaccharide** (meaning "single sweet unit"), also known as a **simple sugar**. Monosaccharides have the general chemical formula $C_nH_{2n}O_n$.

---

[4] **Item I is true:** this is a good example of 3° structure. Item II is false: this describes 2°, not 3°, structure. **Item III is true:** this describes the disulfide bridge, which is considered to be tertiary.

[5] Quaternary disulfides are bonds that form between chains that aren't linked by peptide bonds. Tertiary disulfides are bonds that form between residues in the same polypeptide.

Figure 8 Some Metabolically Important Monosaccharides

Two monosaccharides bonded together form a disaccharide, a few form an oligosaccharide, and many form a polysaccharide. The bond between two sugar molecules is called a **glycosidic linkage**. This is a covalent bond, formed in a dehydration reaction that requires enzymatic catalysis.

Figure 9 Disaccharides and the α- or β-Glycosidic Bond

Some common disaccharides you might see on the MCAT are sucrose (Glc-α-1,2-Fru), lactose (Gal-β-1,4-Glc), maltose (Glc-α-1,4-Glc), and cellobiose (Glc-β-1,4-Glc). However, you should NOT try to memorize these linkages.

Polymers made from these disaccharides form important biological macromolecules. Glycogen serves as an energy storage carbohydrate in animals and is composed of thousands of glucose units. Starch is the same as glycogen (except that the branches are a little different), and serves the same purpose in plants. Cellulose is a polymer of cellobiose; but note that cellobiose does not exist freely in nature. It exists only in its polymerized, cellulose form. The glycosidic bonds allow the polymer to assume a long, straight, fibrous shape. Wood and cotton are made of cellulose.

Figure 10   The Polysaccharide Glycogen

3.4   LIPIDS

Lipids are oily or fatty substances that play three physiological roles, summarized here and discussed below.

1)   In adipose cells, triglycerides (fats) store energy.
2)   In cellular membranes, phospholipids constitute a barrier between intracellular and extracellular environments.
3)   Cholesterol is a special lipid that serves as the building block for the hydrophobic steroid hormones.

The cardinal characteristic of the lipid is its **hydrophobicity**. *Hydrophobic* means "water-fearing." It is important to understand the significance of this. Since water is very polar, polar substances dissolve well in water; these are known as "water-loving," or **hydrophilic** substances. Carbon-carbon bonds and carbon-hydrogen bonds are nonpolar. Therefore, substances that contain only carbon and hydrogen will not dissolve well in water. Here are some examples: Table sugar dissolves well in water, but cooking oil floats in a layer above water or forms many tiny oil droplets when mixed with water. Cotton T-shirts become wet when exposed to water because they are made of glucose polymerized into cellulose; a nylon jacket does not become wet because it is composed of atoms covalently bound together in a nonpolar fashion. A synonym for hydrophobic is **lipophilic** (which means "lipid-loving"); a synonym for hydrophilic is **lipophobic**. We return to these concepts below.

Fatty Acid Structure

Fatty acids are composed of long unsubstituted alkanes that end in a carboxylic acid. The chain is typically 14 to 18 carbons long, and because they are synthesized two carbons at a time from acetate, only *even-numbered* fatty acids are made in human cells. A fatty acid with no carbon-carbon double bonds is said to be **saturated** with hydrogen because every carbon atom in the chain is covalently bound to the maximum number of hydrogens. **Unsaturated** fatty acids have one or more double bonds in the tail. These double bonds are almost always (Z) (or *cis*).

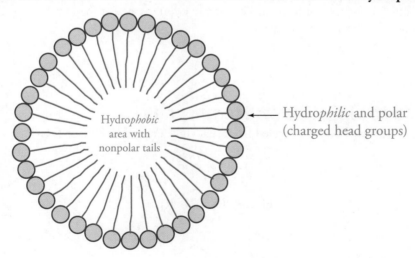

Figure 11   Fatty Acid Structure

- How does the shape of an unsaturated fatty acid differ from that of a saturated fatty acid?[6]
- If fatty acids are mixed into water, how are they likely to associate with each other?[7]

Figure 12 illustrates how free fatty acids interact in an aqueous solution; they form a structure called a **micelle**. The force that drives the tails into the center of the micelle is called the **hydrophobic interaction**.

Hydro*phobic* area with nonpolar tails

← Hydro*philic* and polar (charged head groups)

Figure 12   A Fatty Acid Micelle

---

[6]   An unsaturated fatty acid is bent, or "kinked," at the *cis* double bond.

[7]   The long hydrophobic chains will interact with each other to minimize contact with water, exposing the charged carboxyl group to the aqueous environment.

Triacylglycerols (TG)

The storage form of the fatty acid is fat. The technical name for fat is **triacylglycerol** or **triglyceride** (shown below). The triglyceride is composed of three fatty acids esterified to a glycerol molecule. Glycerol is a three-carbon triol with the formula $HOCH_2–CHOH–CH_2OH$. As you can see, it has three hydroxyl groups that can be esterified to fatty acids. It is necessary to store fatty acids in the relatively inert form of fat because free fatty acids are reactive chemicals.

Figure 13   A Triglyceride (Fat)

Lipases are enzymes that hydrolyze fats. Triacylglycerols are stored in fat cells as an energy source. Fats are more efficient energy storage molecules than carbohydrates for two reasons: packing and energy content.

1) **Packing:** Their hydrophobicity allows fats to pack together much more closely than carbohydrates. Carbohydrates carry a great amount of water-of-solvation (water molecules hydrogen-bonded to their hydroxyl groups).

2) **Energy content:** All packing considerations aside, fat molecules store much more energy than carbohydrates. In other words, regardless of what you dissolve it in, a fat has more energy carbon-for-carbon than a carbohydrate.

Introduction to Lipid Bilayer Membranes

Membrane lipids are **phospholipids** derived from diacylglycerol phosphate or DG-P.

Figure 14   A Phosphoglyceride (Diacylglycerol Phosphate, or DGP)

We saw above how fatty acids spontaneously form micelles. Phospholipids also minimize their interactions with water by forming an orderly structure—in this case, it is a **lipid bilayer** (below). Hydrophobic interactions drive the formation of the bilayer, and once formed, it is stabilized by van der Waals forces between the long tails.

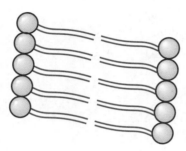

Figure 15   A Small Section of a Lipid Bilayer Membrane

- Would a saturated or an unsaturated fatty acid residue have more van der Waals interactions with neighboring alkyl chains in a bilayer membrane?[8]

A more precise way to give the answer to the question above is to say that double bonds (unsaturation) in phospholipid fatty acids *tend to increase membrane fluidity*. Unsaturation prevents the membrane from solidifying by disrupting the orderly packing of the hydrophobic lipid tails. The right amount of fluidity is essential for function. Decreasing the *length* of fatty acid tails also increases fluidity. The steroid **cholesterol** (discussed a bit later) is a third important modulator of membrane fluidity. At low temperatures, it increases fluidity in the same way as kinks in fatty acid tails; therefore, it is known as *membrane antifreeze*. At high temperatures, however, cholesterol attenuates (reduces) membrane fluidity. Don't ponder this paradox too long; just remember that cholesterol keeps fluidity at an *optimum level*. Remember, the structural determinants of membrane fluidity are: degree of saturation, tail length, and amount of cholesterol.

Terpenes

A terpene is a member of a broad class of compounds built from isoprene units (C_5H_8) with a general formula $(C_5H_8)_n$.

Figure 16   Isoprene Unit

---

[8]   The bent shape of the unsaturated fatty acid means that it doesn't fit in as well and has less contact with neighboring groups to form van der Waals interactions. Phospholipids composed of saturated fatty acids make the membrane more solid.

Terpenes may be linear or cyclic, and are classified by the number of isoprene units they contain. For example, monoterpenes consist of two isoprene units, sesquiterpenes consist of three, and diterpenes contain four.

limonene
$C_{10}H_{16}$
(a monoterpene)

humulene
$C_{15}H_{24}$
(a sesquiterpene)

taxadiene
$C_{20}H_{32}$
(a diterpene)

Figure 17   Terpene Structures

Squalene is a triterpene (made of six isoprene units) and a particularly important compound, as it is biosynthetically utilized in the manufacture of steroids. Squalene is also a component of earwax.

Figure 18   Squalene

Whereas a terpene is formally a simple hydrocarbon, there are a number of natural and synthetically derived species that are built from an isoprene skeleton and functionalized with other elements (O, N, S, etc.). These functionalized-terpenes are known as *terpenoids*. Vitamin A ($C_{20}H_{30}O$) is an example of a terpenoid.

Figure 19   Vitamin A

Steroids

Steroids are included here because of their hydrophobicity, and, hence, similarity to fats. Their structure is otherwise unique. All steroids have the basic tetracyclic ring system (see below) based on the structure of **cholesterol**.

As discussed earlier, the steroid cholesterol is an important component of the lipid bilayer. It is both obtained from the diet and synthesized in the liver. It is carried in the blood packaged with fats and proteins into **lipoproteins**. One type of lipoprotein has been implicated as the cause of atherosclerotic vascular disease, which refers to the build-up of cholesterol "plaques" on the inside of blood vessels.

Figure 20   Cholesterol-Derived Hormones

Steroid hormones are made from cholesterol. Two examples are **testosterone** (an androgen or male sex hormone) and **estradiol** (an estrogen or female sex hormone).

3.5 PHOSPHORUS-CONTAINING COMPOUNDS

Phosphoric acid is an *inorganic* acid (it does not contain carbon) with the potential to donate three protons. The pK_as for the three acid dissociation equilibria are 2.1, 7.2, and 12.4. Therefore, at physiological pH, phosphoric acid is significantly dissociated, existing largely in anionic form.

Figure 21   Phosphoric Acid Dissociation

Phosphate is also known as orthophosphate. Two orthophosphates bound together via an **anhydride linkage** form **pyrophosphate**. The P–O–P bond in pyrophosphate is an example of a **high-energy phosphate bond**. This name is derived from the fact that the hydrolysis of pyrophosphate is extremely favorable.

There are three reasons that phosphate anhydride bonds store so much energy:

1) When phosphates are linked together, their negative charges repel each other strongly.
2) Orthophosphate has more resonance forms and thus a lower free energy than linked phosphates.
3) Orthophosphate has a more favorable interaction with the biological solvent (water) than linked phosphates.

The details are not crucial. What is essential is that you fix the image in your mind of linked phosphates acting like compressed springs, just waiting to fly open and provide energy for an enzyme to catalyze a reaction.

Figure 22   The Hydrolysis of Pyrophosphate

Nucleotides

Nucleotides are the building blocks of nucleic acids (RNA and DNA). Each nucleotide contains a **ribose** (or **deoxyribose**) **sugar** group; a **purine** or **pyrimidine base** joined to carbon number one of the ribose ring; and one, two, or three **phosphate units** joined to carbon five of the ribose ring. The nucleotide **a**denosine **trip**hosphate (ATP) plays a central role in cellular metabolism in addition to being an RNA precursor. Significantly more information about the structure of the nucleic acids can be found in *MCAT Biochemistry Review*. More information on the function of the nucleic acids will be provided in Chapter 4 of this book.

ATP is the universal short-term energy storage molecule. Energy extracted from the oxidation of foodstuffs is immediately stored in the phosphoanhydride bonds of ATP. This energy will later be used to power cellular processes; it may also be used to synthesize glucose or fats, which are longer-term energy storage molecules. This applies to *all* living organisms, from bacteria to humans. Even some viruses carry ATP with them outside the host cell, though viruses cannot make their own ATP.

Figure 23   Adenosine Triphosphate (ATP)

Chapter 3 Summary

- Amino acids (AAs) consist of a tetrahedral α-carbon connected to an amino group, a carboxyl group, and a variable R-group, which determines the AA's properties.

- Proteins consist of amino acids linked by peptide bonds, which are very stable. The primary structure of a protein consists of its amino acid sequence.

- The secondary structure of proteins (α-helices and β-sheets) is formed through hydrogen-bonding interactions between atoms in the backbone of the molecule.

- The most stable tertiary protein structure generally places polar AAs on the exterior and non-polar AAs on the interior of the protein. This minimizes interactions between nonpolar AAs and water, while optimizing interactions between side chains inside the protein.

- Proteins have a variety of functions in the body including (but not limited to) enzymes, structural roles, hormones, receptors, channels, antibodies, transporters, etc.

- The monomer for a carbohydrate is a monosaccharide (simple sugar), with the molecular formula $C_nH_{2n}O_n$. The common monosaccharides are glucose, fructose, galactose, ribose, and deoxyribose.

- Two monosaccharides joined with a glycosidic linkage form a disaccharide. The common disaccharides are maltose, sucrose, and lactose. Mammals can digest α glycosidic linkages, but generally not β linkages.

- Polysaccharides consist of many monosaccharides linked together. Glycogen (animals) and starch (plants) are storage units for glucose and can be broken down for energy. Cellulose is also a glucose polymer, but the beta linkage prevents digestion. It forms wood and cotton.

- Lipids are found in several forms in the body, including triglycerides, phospholipids, cholesterol and steroids, and terpenes. Triglycerides and phospholipids are linear, while cholesterol and steroids have a ring structure.

- Lipids are hydrophobic. Triglycerides are used for energy storage, phospholipids form membranes, and cholesterol is the precursor to the steroid hormones.

- The building blocks of nucleic acids (DNA and RNA) are nucleotides, which are comprised of a pentose sugar, a purine or pyrimidine base, and 2-3 phosphate units.

CHAPTER 3 FREESTANDING PRACTICE QUESTIONS

1. Why is ATP known as a "high energy" structure at neutral pH?

A) It exhibits a large decrease in free energy when it undergoes hydrolytic reactions.
B) The phosphate ion released from ATP hydrolysis is very reactive.
C) It causes cellular processes to proceed at faster rates.
D) Adenine is the best energy storage molecule of all the nitrogenous bases.

2. Which of the following best describes the secondary structure of a protein?

A) Various folded polypeptide chains joining together to form a larger unit
B) The amino acid sequence of the chain
C) The polypeptide chain folding upon itself due to hydrophobic/hydrophilic interactions
D) Peptide bonds hydrogen-bonding to one another to create a sheet-like structure

3. Phenylketonuria (PKU) is an autosomal recessive disorder that results from a deficiency of the enzyme phenylalanine hydroxylase. This enzyme normally converts phenylalanine into tyrosine. PKU results in intellectual disability, growth retardation, fair skin, eczema, and a distinct musty body odor. Which of the following is most likely true?

A) Treatment should include a decrease in tyrosine in the diet.
B) The musty body odor is likely caused by a disorder in aromatic amino acid metabolism.
C) Patients with PKU should increase the amount of phenylalanine in their diet.
D) PKU can be acquired by consuming too much aspartame (an artificial sweetener that contains high levels of phenylalanine).

4. A genetic regulator is found to contain a lysine residue that is important for its binding to DNA. If a mutation were to occur such that a different amino acid replaces the lysine at that location, which of the following resulting amino acids would likely be the least harmful to its ability to bind DNA?

A) Glycine
B) Glutamate
C) Aspartate
D) Arginine

5. Increasing the amount of cholesterol in a plasma membrane would lead to an increase in:

A) membrane permeability.
B) atherosclerotic plaques.
C) membrane fluidity at low temperatures but a decrease in membrane fluidity at high temperatures.
D) membrane fluidity at high and low temperatures.

6. A human space explorer crash-lands on a planet where the native inhabitants are entirely unable to digest glycogen, but are able to digest cellulose. Consequently, they make their clothing out of glycogen-based material. The starving space explorer eats one of the native inhabitants' shirts and the natives are amazed. Based on this information, which of the following is/are true?

   I. The explorer can digest α-glycosidic linkages.
   II. The native inhabitants can digest α-glycosidic linkages.
   III. The native inhabitants can digest starch.

A) I only
B) I and III only
C) II and III only
D) I, II, and III

CHAPTER 3 PRACTICE PASSAGE

Photosynthesis is the process plants use to derive energy from sunlight and is associated with a cell's chloroplasts. The energy is used to produce carbohydrates from carbon dioxide and water. Photosynthesis involves light and dark phases. Figure 1 represents two initial steps associated with the light phase.

The light phase supplies the dark phase with NADPH and a high-energy substrate.

A researcher attempted to produce a photosynthetic system outside the living organism according to the following protocols:

- Chloroplasts were extracted from green leaves and ruptured, and their membranes were thereby exposed, then a solution of hexachloroplatinate ions carrying a charge of −2 was added.

- The structure of the composite was analyzed, and the amount of oxygen produced by the system was measured.

The researcher concluded that the ions were bound to the membrane's Photosystem 1 site by the attraction of opposite charges. The resulting composite is shown in Figure 2. It was found that the hexachloroplatinate-membrane composite was photosynthetically active.

Figure 1

Figure 2

1. In concluding that the hexachloroplatinate ions were bound to Photosystem 1 due to the attraction of opposite charges, the researchers apparently assumed that the structure of the membrane was:

A) determined solely by hydrophobic bonding.
B) positively charged.
C) covalently bound to the platinate.
D) negatively charged.

2. Figure 1 indicates that:

A) photoactivation of the chloroplast membrane results in the reduction of the anhydride-containing molecule $NADP^+$.
B) electrons are lost from Photosystem 1 through the conversion of NADPH to $NADP^+$, and are replaced by electrons from Photosystem 2.
C) there is a net gain of electrons by the system.
D) electrons are lost from Photosystem 1 through the conversion of $NADP^+$ to NADPH, but are not replaced by electrons from Photosystem 2.

3. If $NADP^+$ is fully hydrolyzed to its component bases, phosphates, and sugars, what type of monosaccharide would result?

A) A three-carbon triose
B) A hexose
C) A pentose
D) An α-D-glucose

4. If in a given cell the photosynthetic dark phase were artificially arrested while the light phase proceeded, the cell would most likely experience:

A) decreased levels of NADPH.
B) increased levels of NADPH.
C) increased levels of carbohydrate.
D) increased photoactivation of the chloroplast.

5. To determine the primary structure of the protein portion of Photosystem 1, a series of cleavage reactions was undertaken. To break apart the protein, the most logical action to take would be to:

A) decarboxylate free carboxyl groups.
B) hydrolyze peptide bonds.
C) repolymerize peptide bonds.
D) hydrolyze amide branch points.

6. A researcher examined a sample of the principal substance produced by the photosynthetic dark phase and concluded that he was working with a racemic mixture of glucose isomers. Which of the following experimental findings would be *inconsistent* with such a conclusion?

A) The sample is composed of carbon, hydrogen, and oxygen only.
B) The sample consists of an aldohexose.
C) The sample rotates the plane of polarized light to the left.
D) The sample is optically inactive.

SOLUTIONS TO CHAPTER 3 FREESTANDING PRACTICE QUESTIONS

1. **A** Choice A is the best answer because it directly addresses the energetics of ATP hydrolysis. Choice B discusses the reactivity of the released phosphate ion and not the structure of ATP itself, so it can be eliminated. Choice C can be eliminated because it describes the rate of cellular processes, not the energy of ATP. Choice D can be eliminated because the structure of adenine is not related to why ATP is a good energy storage molecule.

2. **D** The secondary structure of proteins is the initial folding of the polypeptide chain into α-helices or β-pleated sheets. Choice A can be eliminated because it describes the formation of a quaternary protein, choice B can be eliminated because it describes the primary protein structure, and choice C can be eliminated because it describes the tertiary protein structure.

3. **B** A defect in phenylalanine hydroxylase (or the THB cofactor) would result in a build-up of phenylalanine. This would lead to an excess of phenylalanine byproducts such as phenyl-acetate, phenyllactate, and phenylpyruvate, and a decrease in tyrosine. Therefore, patients with PKU should increase the amount of tyrosine in their diet (it becomes an essential amino acid in this condition; choice A is wrong), as well as eliminate phenylalanine from their diet (choice C is wrong). PKU is a genetically acquired disorder (autosomal recessive), as mentioned in the passage, and thus it is not acquired by consuming too much phenyl-alanine (choice D is wrong). It is true that phenylalanine and its derivatives are aromatic amino acids and that the high levels of these compounds lead to the distinct musty body odor (choice B is correct). Process of Elimination (POE) is probably the best method to use in answering this question since it is unclear (without prior knowledge of PKU) what the underlying mechanism of the body odor would be.

4. **D** While knowing the structures of the different amino acids is unlikely to be important for the MCAT, knowing which of the amino acids are basic (histidine, arginine, lysine) and which are acidic (glutamate, aspartate) is likely to be relevant. In this case, since lysine is basic (and therefore best at binding the negatively charged DNA), one can assume that a mutation resulting in another basic amino acid would cause the least change in its ability to bind DNA. Therefore, a mutation from lysine to arginine would cause the least harm (choice D is correct). A mutation from lysine to glutamate or aspartate (both acidic) would likely cause the most harm to its ability to bind DNA (choices B and C are wrong). Glycine is a neutral amino acid (choice A is wrong).

5. **C** Plasma membranes can be up to 50% composed of sterols. Sterols help stabilize the membrane at both spectrums of the temperature. At low temperatures, cholesterol increases fluidity because the ring structure of cholesterol does not allow for tight phospholipid tail packing. At high temperatures, cholesterol decreases membrane fluidity (the OH group of cholesterol prevents phospholipid dispersion; choice C is correct, and choice D is wrong). Cholesterol decreases the permeability of membranes by filling in the "holes" between the fatty acid tails (choice A is wrong). The formation of atherosclerotic plaques, while related to cholesterol, is due to high levels of blood cholesterol, not membrane cholesterol (choice B is wrong).

6. **A** Item I is true: humans can digest α-glycosidic linkages, such as those found in glycogen. If the natives' shirts are made of glycogen, the space explorer should have no trouble consuming and digesting them (choice C can be eliminated). Item II Is false: cellulose contains β-glycosidic linkages. If the natives can digest cellulose, but not glycogen, then they cannot digest α-glycosidic linkages (choice D can be eliminated). Item III is false: starch also contains a α-glycosidic linkages. If the natives cannot digest glycogen, then they likely cannot digest starch either (choice B can be eliminated, and choice A is true).

SOLUTIONS TO CHAPTER 3 PRACTICE PASSAGE

1. **B** The passage states that the ion is attracted to Photosystem 1 by the attraction of opposite charges (positively charged photosystem and negatively charged hexachloroplatinate ion).

2. **A** The main result of the light phase, as depicted in Figure 1, is the reduction of $NADP^+$ to make NADPH (choice A is correct). Choice B is wrong since $NADP^+$ is converted into NADPH, not vice versa. Choice C is incorrect since in any system, mass and charge are conserved. Electrons move from one molecule to another, but they are not created or destroyed in a chemical reaction. Choice D can be eliminated since Figure 1 depicts electrons moving from Photosystem 2 to Photosystem 1.

3. **C** NADPH contains ribose, a pentose. Choice C is correct.

4. **B** The light phase makes NADPH, and the dark phase consumes it. In the absence of the dark phase, NADPH will continue to be produced, but none will be consumed, making NADPH levels rise (choice B is correct). Choice C is wrong since the dark phase is responsible for biosynthesis, such as carbohydrate production, so this will decrease, not increase. Choice D can be eliminated since the amount of light and photoactivation should remain the same.

5. **B** Proteins are composed of amino acid residues which are joined together by peptide bonds during the translation process. To split the protein into smaller pieces, proteases and chemical reagents act to hydrolyze the peptide bond, reversing the biosynthetic process.

6. **C** A racemic mixture is one which contains equal quantities of two stereoisomers that rotate plane-polarized light in opposite directions. Since there are equal quantities of both, racemic mixtures are optically inactive. Thus, choice C, which states that the sample rotates light, is inconsistent with the conclusion that the sample is racemic and is the correct answer choice. All other choices are consistent with the conclusion that the sample is a racemic mixture of glucose. Carbohydrates, of which glucose is one, are made of only carbon, hydrogen, and oxygen (choice A is consistent and can be eliminated). Glucose, with six carbons and a carbonyl group on the 6th carbon, is an aldohexose (choice B is consistent and can be eliminated), and racemic mixtures do not rotate light (choice D is consistent and can be eliminated).

Chapter 4
Molecular Biology

It was once thought that simple living organisms were generated spontaneously from nonliving matter. When a steak went bad and became infested with larvae, it was because the decomposing meat actually became squirming worms. Most religions have traditional explanations for the origin of human life, too. Children are derived from adults due to the will of a deity; the original adults were placed on the Earth by that deity. But as empiricism developed during the Enlightenment, rigorous experiments were used to explain life, resulting in "scientific" models that gradually replaced more traditional explanations.

One early conclusion was that simple organisms were derived not from decomposing matter but from parental organisms. Subsequently, it was found that some organisms are too small to be seen with the naked eye. These "germs" were eventually implicated as the cause of most major diseases. Gradually, the scientific community came to the conclusion that all life was derived from other life. The patterns of inheritance and evolution were elucidated by a chain of scientists, from Mendel through Darwin. But the mechanism remained a mystery. Finally, cellular biology advanced to the point that scientists were aware of two substances found in cells that seemed appropriate vehicles for the transmission of inherited information: DNA and protein. The extreme length and orderly arrangement of repeating units in DNA and protein made it seem very likely that they could contain information. Researchers had waded through a chemical ocean of alphabet soup and suddenly come upon long strings of what looked like letters.

This is where biology stood in the early 1940s. In the '40s and '50s, two monumental achievements in microbiology finally clarified the gears in the clock of evolution and how they turn. One was the elucidation of the structure of DNA by Watson and Crick. The other was the proof by Avery, Herriott, Hershey, Chase, and their coworkers that DNA was the fundamental unit of genetic inheritance in microorganisms. In the following discussion, we will summarize the wealth of information that has been built upon these two prescient cornerstones.

4.1 DNA STRUCTURE

General Overview

Significant detail about the structure of DNA and RNA is provided in *MCAT Biochemistry Review;* here we will give a brief overview of this topic. DNA is short for **d**eoxyribo**n**ucleic **a**cid. DNA and RNA (**ribon**ucleic **a**cid) are called **nucleic acids** because they are found in the nucleus and possess many acidic phosphate groups.

The building block of DNA is the **d**eoxyribo**n**ucleoside 5' **tri**phosphate (dNTP, where N represents one of the four basic nucleosides). Deoxyadenosine 5' triphosphate (dATP) is shown in Figure 1; the other bases are shown in Figure 2. Nucleotides are built from three components: a sugar (deoxyribose for DNA, ribose for RNA), an aromatic, nitrogenous base, and 1-3 phosphate groups. The bases G and A are derived from a precursor called purine, so they are referred to as **the purines**. C, T, and U are **the pyrimidines**.[1]

A nucleo*side* is ribose or deoxyribose with a purine or pyrimidine linked to the 1' carbon; nucleo*tides* are phosphate esters of nucleosides, with one, two, or three phosphate groups joined to the ribose ring by the 5' hydroxy group. When nucleotides contain three phosphate residues, they are also referred to as **nucleoside triphosphates**, abbreviated **NTP** (if the sugar is deoxyribose, they are abbreviated **dNTP**). In individual nucleotides, N is replaced by A, G, C, T, or U.

Figure 1 Deoxyadenosine Triphosphate (dATP)

---

[1] A mnemonic for this is Pyramids (pyrimidines) have sharp edges, so they CUT. Another mnemonic is CUT the Py.

The sugar + phosphate portion of the nucleotide is referred to as the **backbone** of DNA, because it is invariant. The base is the variable portion of the building block.

PYRIMIDINE BASES

cytosine   thymine   uracil
                  (DNA only)   (RNA only)

PURINE BASES

adenine   guanine

Figure 2   Aromatic Bases of DNA and RNA

Polynucleotides

Nucleotides in the DNA chain are covalently linked by **phosphodiester bonds** between the 3' hydroxy group of one deoxyribose and the 5' phosphate group of the next deoxyribose (Figure 3). A polymer of several nucleotides linked together is termed an *oligo*nucleotide, and a polymer of many nucleotides is a *poly*nucleotide. Since the only unique part of the nucleotide is the base, the sequence of a polynucleotide can be abbreviated by simply listing the bases attached to each nucleotide in the chain. The end of the chain with a free 5' phosphate group is written first in a polynucleotide, with other nucleotides in the chain indicated in the 5' to 3' direction.

Figure 3 The Polymerization of Nucleotides

The Watson-Crick Model of DNA Structure

James Watson and Francis Crick (with the help of Maurice Wilkins and Rosalind Franklin) developed a model of the structure of DNA in the cell. According to the **Watson-Crick model**, cellular DNA is a right-handed double helix held together by hydrogen bonds between bases. It is important to understand each facet of this model.

In the cell, DNA does not exist in the form of a single long polynucleotide. Instead, the DNA found in the nucleus is double-stranded (**ds**). In ds-DNA, two very long polynucleotide chains are hydrogen-bonded together in an **antiparallel** orientation. Antiparallel means the 5' end of one chain is paired with the 3' end of the other. The H-bonds in ds-DNA are between the bases on adjacent chains. This H-bonding is very specific: A is always H-bonded to T, and G is always H-bonded to C (Figure 4). Note that this means an H-bonded pair always consists of a *purine plus a pyrimidine.*[2] Thus, both types of base pairs (AT or GC) take up the same amount of room in the DNA double helix. The GC pair is held together by three hydrogen bonds, the AT pair by two. Two chains of DNA are said to be complementary if the bases in each strand can hydrogen bond when the strands are oriented in an antiparallel fashion. If we are talking about ds-DNA 100 nucleotides long, we would say it is 100 base pairs (bp) long. A kbp (kilobase pair) is ds-DNA 1000 nucleotides long.

Figure 4   Base Pairing

The binding of two complementary strands of DNA into a double-stranded structure is termed **annealing**, or **hybridization**. The separation of strands is termed **melting**, or **denaturation**.

- Which of the following is/are true about ds-DNA?[3]
    - I.   If the amount of G in a double helix is known, the amount of C can be calculated.
    - II. If the fraction of purine nucleotides and the total molecular weight of a double helix are known, the amount of cytosine can be calculated.
    - III. The two chains in a piece of ds-DNA containing mostly purines will be bonded together more tightly than the two chains in a piece of ds-DNA containing mostly pyrimidines.
    - IV. The oligonucleotide ATGTAT is complementary to the oligonucleotide ATACAT.

---

[2]   This fact has a fringe benefit: we can calculate the number of purines if we know the number of pyrimidines. We can actually calculate several variables. Chargaff's Rule rule states that [A] = [T] and [G] = [C]; and [A] + [G] = [T] + [C].

[3]   **Item I: True.** For every G, there is a C; and for every A there is a T. Item II: False. The ratio of purines to pyrimidines is always the same (50:50) since each purine is paired with a pyrimidine. In order to calculate the amount of any one base, you have to know the ratio of AT to GC pairs. Item III: False. Again, the ratio of purines to pyrimidines is always the same; 50:50. However, two chains containing mostly GC pairs will bond more tightly than two chains containing mostly AT pairs, since GC pairs are held together by 3 H-bonds while AT pairs have only 2. **Item IV: True.** Remember: the strands are antiparallel, A and T pair, G and C pair, and the 5' end is always written first.

There is another important detail about DNA structure: not only is it double-stranded, it is also *coiled*. In ds-DNA, the two hydrogen-bonded antiparallel DNA strands form a **right-handed double helix** (meaning it corkscrews in a clockwise motion) with the bases on the interior and the ribose/phosphate backbone on the exterior. The double helix is stabilized by van der Waals interactions between the bases, which are stacked upon each other.

Figure 5   A Small Section of a DNA Double Helix

Chromosome Structure and Packing

The sum total of an organism's genetic information is called its **genome**. Eukaryotic genomes are composed of several large pieces of linear ds-DNA; each piece of ds-DNA is called a **chromosome**. Humans have 46 chromosomes, 23 of which are inherited from each parent. Prokaryotic (bacterial) genomes are composed of a **single circular chromosome**. Viral genomes may be linear or circular DNA or RNA. The human genome consists of over 10^9 base pairs, while bacterial genomes contain only 10^6 base pairs. But there is no direct correlation between genome size and evolutionary sophistication, since the organisms with the largest known genomes are amphibians. Much of the size difference in higher eukaryotic genomes is the result of repetitive DNA that has no known function.

If the DNA remained as a simple double helix floating free in the cell, it would be very bulky and fragile. Prokaryotes have a distinctive mechanism for making their single circular chromosome more compact and sturdy. An enzyme called **DNA gyrase** uses the energy of ATP to twist the gigantic circular molecule. Gyrase functions by breaking the DNA and twisting the two sides of the circle around each other. The resulting structure is a twisted circle that is composed of ds-DNA. As discussed earlier, the two strands are already coiled, forming a helix. The twists created by DNA gyrase are called **supercoils**, since they are coils of a structure that is already coiled.

Since eukaryotes have even more DNA in their genome than prokaryotes, the eukaryotic genome requires denser packaging to fit within the cell (Figure 6). To accomplish this, eukaryotic DNA is wrapped around globular proteins called **histones**. After being wrapped around histones, but before being completely packed away, DNA has the microscopic appearance of beads on a string. The beads are called **nucleosomes**; they are composed of DNA wrapped around an octamer of histones (a group of eight). The string between the beads is a length of double-helical DNA called linker DNA and is bound by a single linker histone. Fully packed DNA is called **chromatin**; it is composed of closely stacked nucleosomes.

Figure 6   DNA Packaging

To look for patterns and morphology, chromosomes can be stained with chemicals. Usually, condensed metaphase chromosomes are used, as they are compact and easier to see. When chromosomes are treated, distinct light and dark regions become visible. The darker regions are denser and are called **heterochromatin**. Heterochromatin is rich in repeats; the lighter regions are less dense and are called **euchromatin**. Density gives a sense of DNA coiling or compactness, and these patterns are constant and heritable. It's now known that the lighter regions have higher transcription rates and therefore higher gene activity. The looser packing makes DNA accessible to enzymes and proteins.

Centromeres

A centromere is the region of the chromosome to which spindle fibers attach during cell division. The fibers attach via **kinetochores**, multiprotein complexes that act as anchor attachment sites for spindle fibers. Other protein complexes also bind the centromere after DNA replication to keep sister chromatids attached to each other. Centromeres are made of heterochromatin and repetitive DNA sequences. Chromosomes have p (short) and q (long) arms, and centromere position defines the ratio between the two (Figure 7).

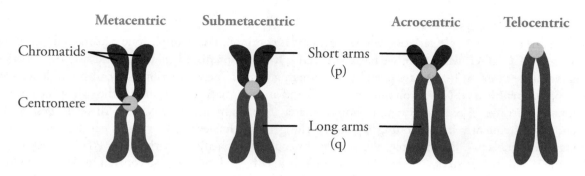

Figure 7   Centromere Positions

Telomeres

The ends of linear chromosomes are called **telomeres**. At the DNA level, these regions are distinguished by the presence of distinct nucleotide sequences repeated 50 to several hundred times. The repeated unit is usually 6–8 base pairs long and guanine-rich. Many vertebrates (including humans and mice) have the same repeat: 5'-TTAGGG-3'. Telomeres are composed of both single- and double-stranded DNA. Single stranded DNA is found at the very end of the chromosome and is about 300 base pairs in length. It loops around to form a knot, held together by many telomere-associated proteins. This stabilizes the end of the chromosome; specialized telomere cap proteins distinguish telomeres from double-stranded breaks (Section 4.4), and this prevents activation of repair pathways.

Telomeres function to prevent chromosome deterioration and also prevent fusion with neighboring chromosomes. They function as disposable buffers, blocking the ends of chromosomes. DNA replication of telomeres represents a special challenge to cellular machinery (see Section 4.4). Since most prokaryotes have circular genomes, their DNA does not contain telomeres.

4.2   GENOME STRUCTURE AND GENOMIC VARIATIONS

The human genome contains 24 different chromosomes (22 autosomes, plus two different sex chromosomes), 3.2 billion base pairs, and codes for about 21,000 genes. The sequence of the human genome was reported by two independent groups in 2001 (the publicly funded Human Genome Project lead by Dr. Francis Collins, and Dr. J. Craig Venter and his firm Celera Genomics).

The human genome has numerous regions with high transcription rates, separated by long stretches of intergenic space. **Intergenic regions** are composed of noncoding DNA; they may direct the assembly of specific chromatin structures and can contribute to the regulation of nearby genes, but many have no known function. Tandem repeats and transposons are major components of intergenic regions.

Genomic regions with high transcription rates are rich in genes. A gene is a DNA sequence that encodes a gene product. It includes both regulatory regions (such as promoters and transcription stop sites), and a region that codes for either a protein or a non-coding RNA.

Nucleotide Variation

Small-scale and large-scale variation across a genome is common. For example, one person could have the sequence CCCGGG, while another has CCTGGG. It's been predicted that there are single nucleotide changes once in every 1,000 base pairs in the human genome. These variations are called **single nucleotide polymorphisms** (SNPs, pronounced "snips") and are essentially mutations. [If the size of the human genome is just over 3 billion base pairs, approximately how many human SNPs are there?[4]] These SNPs occur most frequently in noncoding regions of the genome; however, some SNPs can lead to specific traits and phenotypes. For example, about 70% of people taste phenylthiocarbamide (PTC) as very bitter, and the remaining 30% don't taste PTC at all. You may have done this test yourself, as PTC response is commonly used as an example in genetics classes. This ability is a dominant genetic trait and is determined by a gene on chromosome 7. Three SNPs in this gene determine PTC taste sensitivity.

Copy-Number Variation

Copy-number variations (CNVs) are structural variations in the genome that lead to different copies of DNA sections. Large regions of the genome (10^3 to 10^6 base pairs) can be duplicated (increasing copy number) or deleted (decreasing copy number). The specific mechanism by which this occurs is not clear, but it may be due to misalignment of repetitive DNA sequences during synapsis of homologous chromosomes in meiosis. These changes therefore apply to much larger regions of the genome compared to SNPs. They are a normal part of our genome (0.4% of the genome can have CNV), but have also been associated with cancer and other diseases. Genes involved in immune system function, as well as brain development and activity, are often enriched in CNVs.

Repeated Sequences: Tandem Repeats

Much of our genome is single copy, meaning there is one copy of the gene in a haploid set of the genome. This is true for most eukaryotic genes that code for proteins. However, genomes also have regions of **tandem repeats**, where short sequences of nucleotides are repeated one right after the other, from as little as three to over 100 times. The human genome has over a thousand regions of tandem repeats. Repeats can be unstable, when the repeating unit is short (such as di- or trinucleotides) or when the repeat itself is very long. Unstable tandem repeats can lead to chromosome breaks and some have been implicated in disease. Tandem repeats often show variations in length between individuals, which can be useful in DNA fingerprinting. Heterochromatin, centromeres, and telomeres are all rich in repeats.

4.3   THE ROLE OF DNA

DNA encodes and transmits the genetic information passed down from parents to offspring. Before 1944 it was generally believed that protein, rather than DNA, carried genetic information, since proteins have an "alphabet" of 20 letters (the amino acids), while DNA's "alphabet" has only 4 letters (the four nucleotides). But in that year, Oswald Avery showed that DNA was the active agent in bacterial transformation. In short, this means he proved that pure DNA from one type of *E. coli* bacteria could transform *E. coli* of another type, causing it to acquire the genetic nature of the first type. Later Hershey and Chase proved that DNA was the active chemical in the infection of *E. coli* bacteria by bacteriophage T2.[5] These experiments will be discussed in more detail in Chapter 7.

---

[4] 3×10^9 base pairs × 1 SNP/1000 base pairs = 3×10^6 SNPs, or approximately 3 million human SNPs.

[5]   Transformation and bacteriophage will be discussed in Chapter 5.

The Genetic Code

DNA does not directly exert its influence on cells, but merely contains sequences of nucleotides known as **genes** that serve as **templates** for the production of another nucleic acid known as RNA. The process of reading DNA and writing the information as RNA is termed **transcription**. This can generate either a final gene product (as in the case of all non-coding RNAs, discussed below), or a messenger molecule. The messenger RNA (mRNA) is then read, and the information is used to construct protein. The synthesis of proteins using RNA as a template is termed **translation** and is accomplished by the **ribosome**, which is a massive enzyme composed of many proteins and pieces of RNA (known as ribosomal RNA or rRNA).[6]

The overall process looks like this: DNA → RNA → protein. This unidirectional flow equation represents the **Central Dogma** (fundamental law) of molecular biology. This is the mechanism whereby inherited *information* is used to create actual *objects*, namely enzymes and structural proteins.

This language used by DNA and mRNA to specify the building blocks of proteins is known as the **Genetic Code**. The alphabet of the genetic code contains only four letters (A, T, G, C). How can four letters specify the ingredients of the multitude of proteins in every cell? [What is the smallest "word" size that would allow this four-letter alphabet to encode twenty different amino acids?[7]] A number of experiments confirmed that the genetic code is written in three-letter words, each of which codes for a particular amino acid. A nucleic acid word (3 nucleotide letters) is referred to as a **codon**.

The genetic code is represented in Figure 8, on the next page. The first nucleotide in a codon is given at the left, the second on top, and the third on the right. At the intersection of these three nucleotides is the amino acid called for by that codon. [Why is uracil (U) shown in the chart, and why is thymine (T) absent?[8] The codon GTG in DNA is transcribed in RNA as __, which the ribosome translates into what amino acid?[9]]

---

[6] To *transcribe* a letter is to listen to spoken words and write them down as printed text. The message doesn't change, and the language doesn't change. To *translate* a letter is to change it from one language to another. Cellular transcription is the process whereby a code is read from a nucleic acid (DNA) and written in the language of another nucleic acid (RNA), so the language is the same. In cellular translation, nucleic acids are read and polypeptides are written, so here the language does change.

[7] With four nucleotides, if a "word" (codon) is two nucleotides long, there are $4^2 = 16$ possible codons; too few to specify 20 unique amino acids. However, there are $4^3 = 64$ possible 3-letter "words," and 64 is more than enough different codons to specify 20 unique amino acids. Thus, three nucleotides is the minimum codon size.

[8] RNA is the nucleic acid that actually encodes protein during translation. RNA has U instead of T.

[9] The RNA codon transcribed from the DNA will be CAC, coding for histidine.

4.3

1st Position (5' End)	2nd Position				3rd Position (3' End)
	U	C	A	G	
U	Phe	Ser	Tyr	Cys	U
	Phe	Ser	Tyr	Cys	C
	Leu	Ser	**Stop**	**Stop**	A
	Leu	Ser	**Stop**	Trp	G
C	Leu	Pro	His	Arg	U
	Leu	Pro	His	Arg	C
	Leu	Pro	Gln	Arg	A
	Leu	Pro	Gln	Arg	G
A	Ile	Thr	Asn	Ser	U
	Ile	Thr	Asn	Ser	C
	Ile	Thr	Lys	Arg	A
	Met	Thr	Lys	Arg	G
G	Val	Ala	Asp	Gly	U
	Val	Ala	Asp	Gly	C
	Val	Ala	Glu	Gly	A
	Val	Ala	Glu	Gly	G

Figure 8 The Genetic Code

- The genetic code was studied by experimenters using a cell-free protein synthesis system. All of the materials necessary for protein synthesis (ribosomes, amino acids, tRNA, GTP, ATP) were purified and placed in a beaker. Then synthetic RNA was added, and protein was translated from this template. For example, when synthetic RNA containing only cytosine (CCCCC…) was added, polypeptides containing only proline (polyproline) resulted. What kind of synthetic RNA would give rise to a mixture of polyproline, polyhistidine, and polythreonine?[10]

There are 64 codons. Sixty-one of them specify amino acids; the remaining three are called **stop codons**. Their function is to notify the ribosome that the protein is complete and cause it to stop reading the mRNA (see Section 4.5). Stop codons are also called **nonsense codons**, since they don't code for any amino acid. Note that most of the twenty amino acids can be coded for by more than one codon. Often, all four of the codons with the same first two nucleotides (e.g., CU_) encode the same amino acid. [If the last nucleotide in the codon CUU is changed in a gene that codes for a protein, will the protein be affected?[11]] Two or more codons coding for the same amino acid are known as **synonyms**. Because it has such synonyms, the genetic code is said to be **degenerate**. However, it is very important to realize that though an amino acid may be specified by several codons, *each codon specifies only a single amino acid*. This means that each piece of DNA can be interpreted only one way: the code has no **ambiguity**.

---

[10] The RNA would have to be CCACCACCACCACCACCAC…. This would yield polyproline if read as CCA, CCA, CCA. But if it were read as CAC, CAC, CAC, it would give rise to polyhistidine. If it were read ACC, ACC, ACC, it would encode polythreonine.

[11] No, since CUN codes for leucine, regardless of what N is. Notice that switching the third nucleotide in the majority of codons will have no effect.

The code in Figure 8 is the standard genetic code and is used by most organisms. However, some protists use an alternate genetic code, and the mitochondrial genome of many organisms (including humans and many other vertebrates) uses a slightly different code.

Beyond the Central Dogma

There are several aspects of molecular biology that aren't explicitly stated in the Central Dogma.

- Some viruses (retroviruses) make DNA from RNA using the enzyme reverse transcriptase.
- Information can also be transferred in other ways. For example, DNA methylation and post-translational modification of proteins can alter gene expression and convey information, despite the fact that neither is directly included in the Central Dogma.
- Many final gene products are not proteins but are RNAs instead.

4.4   DNA REPLICATION

The DNA genome is the control center of the cell. When mitosis produces two identical daughter cells from one parental cell, each daughter must have the same genome as the parent. Therefore, cell division requires duplication of the DNA, known as **replication**. This is an enzymatic process, just as the Krebs cycle and glycolysis are enzymatic processes. It occurs during **S** (synthesis) **phase** in interphase of the cell cycle (Chapter 6). Let's go through the process of replication, stopping to add essential facts to a list of things to memorize. But before we get bogged down with details, we should have a look at the big picture.

There is only one logical way to make a new piece of DNA that is identical to the old one: copy it. The old DNA is called **parental** DNA, and the new is called **daughter** DNA. What is the relationship between parental and daughter DNA after replication? There are several possibilities (Figure 9 on the next page). In other words, where do the atoms from the parent go when the daughters are made?

Experiments done by Meselson and Stahl in 1958 aimed to determine if DNA replication is semiconservative, conservative, or dispersive (Figure 9 on the next page). In *conservative* replication, the parental ds-DNA would remain as-is while an entirely new double-stranded genome was created. The *dispersive* theory said that both copies of the genomes were composed of scattered pieces of new and old DNA. Meselson and Stahl showed that replication is semiconservative; after replication, one strand of the new double helix is parental (old) and one strand is newly synthesized daughter DNA.

4.4

Semiconservative Replication

Parental DNA

Conservative Replication

Parental DNA

Dispersive Replication

Parental DNA

Figure 9   Meselson-Stahl Experiments

Let's begin the list of things to memorize here:

1) **DNA replication is semiconservative.**

Individual strands of the double-stranded parent are pulled apart, and then a new daughter strand is synthesized using the parental DNA as a template to copy from.[12] Each new daughter chain is perfectly __[13] to its template or parent.

Now we'll look at replication at the molecular level. When it is not being replicated, DNA is tightly coiled. The replication process cannot begin unless the double helix is uncoiled and separated into two single strands. The enzyme that unwinds the double helix and separates the strands is called helicase. [Would you expect helicase to use the energy of ATP hydrolysis to do its job?[14]] The place where the helicase begins to unwind is not random. It is a specific location (sequence of nucleotides) on the chromosome called the **origin of replication** (abbreviated ORI). This sequence is found by proteins with tertiary structures to specifically recognize a particular pattern of nucleotides. They scan along the chromosome (like a train on a track) until they find the right spot; then they call in helicase and other enzymes to initiate DNA replication. In prokaryotes, a protein called DnaA finds the ORI to initiate DNA replication. In eukaryotes, three proteins cooperate to find the ORI, two of which are synthesized during M and G_1 phases of the cell cycle (see Chapter 6) but rapidly destroyed once the S phase begins. This means these two proteins link DNA replication to the cell cycle, ensuring DNA replication doesn't initiate during other phases of the cell cycle.

---

[12] A template is something that is copied. The metal plates used in printing presses are an example.

[13] complementary

[14] Yes. Separating the strands requires the breaking of many H-bonds.

When helicase unwinds the helix at the origin of replication, the helix gets wound more tightly upstream and downstream from this point.[15] The chromosome would get tangled and eventually break, except that enzymes called **topoisomerases** cut one or both of the strands and unwrap the helix, releasing the excess tension created by the helicases. Another potential problem is that single-stranded DNA is much less stable than ds-DNA. **Single-strand binding proteins (SSBPs)** protect DNA that has been unpackaged in preparation for replication and help keep the strands separated. The separated strands are referred to as an **open complex**. Replication may now begin.

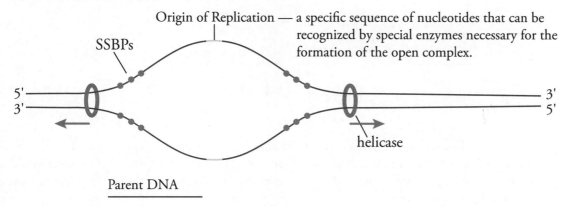

Figure 10   Initiation—The Open Complex

An RNA primer must be synthesized for each template strand. This is accomplished by a set of proteins called the primosome, of which the central component is an RNA polymerase called **primase**. Primer synthesis is important because the next enzyme, DNA polymerase, cannot start a new DNA chain from scratch. It can only add nucleotides to an existing nucleotide chain. The RNA primer is usually 8–12 nucleotides long, and is later replaced by DNA.

Daughter DNA is created as a growing polymer. **DNA polymerase** (DNA pol) catalyzes the elongation of the daughter strand using the parental template, and elongates the primer by adding dNTPs to its 3' end. In fact, the 3' hydroxyl group acts as a nucleophile in the polymerization reaction to displace 5' pyrophosphate from the dNTP to be added. [The template strand is read in what direction?[16]] DNA pol is part of a large complex of proteins called the replisome. Other accessory proteins in this complex help DNA polymerase and allow it to polymerize DNA quickly. The prokaryotic replisome contains 13 components, and the eukaryotic replisome contains 27 proteins; additional complexity in the eukaryotic system is required because replication machinery must also unwind DNA from histone proteins.

Rapid elongation of the daughter strands follows. Since the two template strands are antiparallel, the two primers will elongate toward opposite ends of the chromosome. After a while it looks like this:

---

[15] Imagine two long ropes wound around each other. What happens if you pull them apart in the middle?

[16] If the daughter is made 5' to 3', and the two strands have to end up antiparallel, the template must be read 3' to 5'.

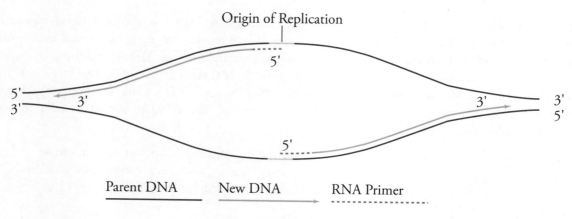

Figure 11 Elongation

DNA polymerase checks each new nucleotide to make sure it forms a correct base-pair before it is incorporated in the growing polymer. The thermodynamic driving force for the polymerization reaction is the removal and hydrolysis of pyrophosphate ($P_2O_7^{4-}$) from each dNTP added to the chain. Here are some more replication rules to memorize:

2) **Polymerization occurs in the 5' to 3' direction, without exception.** This means the existing chain is always lengthened by the addition of a nucleotide to the 3' end of the chain. There is never 3' to 5' polymerase activity.

3) **DNA pol requires a *template*.** It cannot make a DNA chain from scratch but must copy an old chain. This makes sense because it would be pretty useless if DNA pol just made a strand of DNA randomly, without copying a template.

4) **DNA pol requires a *primer*.** It cannot start a new nucleotide chain.

• Can DNA polymerase make the following partially double-stranded structure completely double stranded in the presence of excess nucleotides, using the top strand as a primer?[17]

---

[17] No. The DNA strands are antiparallel, meaning that the upper strand would have to be extended in a 3' to 5' direction, which is impossible. Note that the phrase "in the presence of excess nucleotides" is extraneous. It just means there are plenty of building blocks around. Typical MCAT smokescreen.

Replication proceeds along in both directions away from the origin of replication. Both template strands are read 3' to 5' while daughter strands are elongated 5' to 3'. The areas where the parental double helix continues to unwind are called the **replication forks.** Let's split Figure 11 and look at an enlargement of the right side:

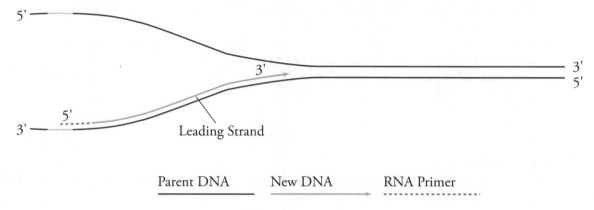

Figure 12 Leading Strand

See how it looks like a big fork? In examining these pictures, you have probably become aware of a problem. It seems like only half of each template strand will be replicated (in Figure 12, the right half of the bottom strand and the left half of the top strand). The problem is that chain elongation can only proceed in one direction, 5' to 3', but in order to replicate the right half of the top chain and the left half of the bottom one continuously, we would have to go in the opposite direction. Here's the solution:

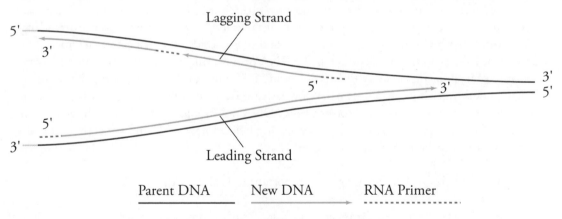

Figure 13 Leading and Lagging Strands

The solution to this problem involves building strands of DNA on opposite sides of the ORI using different methods. As the bottom chain on the right is elongated continuously, the replication fork widens. After a good bit of the top template chain becomes exposed, primase comes in and lays down a primer, which DNA pol can elongate. Then, when the replication fork widens again and more of the top template becomes exposed, these events are repeated. The bottom daughter on the right side, and the top daughter on the left side are called the **leading strands** because they elongate continuously right into the widening replication fork. The top daughter on the right, and the bottom daughter on the left are called the **lagging strands** because they must wait until the replication fork widens before beginning to polymerize.

The small chunks of DNA comprising the lagging strand are called **Okazaki fragments**, after their discoverer. [As the replication forks grow, does helicase have to continue to unwind the double helix and separate the strands?[18]] Let's continue our memorization list:

5) **Replication forks grow away from the origin in both directions.** Each replication fork contains a **leading strand** and a **lagging strand**.

6) Replication of the leading strand is **continuous** and leads into the replication fork, while replication of the lagging strand is **discontinuous**, resulting in Okazaki fragments.

7) Eventually **all RNA primers are replaced by DNA**, and the **fragments are joined by an enzyme called DNA ligase**.

DNA Polymerase

DNA polymerase can rapidly build DNA and is able to add tens of thousands of nucleotides before falling off the template. It is therefore said to be *processive*.

Eukaryotes have several different DNA polymerase enzymes, and their mechanisms of action are complex. You do not need to worry about this complexity.

Prokaryotes, on the other hand, have five types of DNA polymerases, called DNA polymerase I, II, III, IV, and V. You should definitely know the functions of DNA pol III and DNA pol I:

1) **DNA pol III** is responsible for the super-fast, super-accurate elongation of the leading strand. In other words, it has high processivity. It has 5' to 3' polymerase activity as well as 3' to 5' exonuclease[19] activity. This is when the enzyme moves backward to chop off the nucleotide it just added if it was incorrect; the ability to correct mistakes in this way is known as **proofreading function**. It has no known function in repair, and so is considered a replicative enzyme.

2) **DNA pol I** starts adding nucleotides at the RNA primer; this is 5' to 3' polymerase activity. Because of its poor processivity (it can only add 15-20 nucleotides per second), DNA pol III usually takes over about 400 base pairs downstream from the ORI. DNA pol I is also capable of 3' to 5' exonuclease activity (proofreading). DNA pol I removes the RNA primer via 5' to 3' exonuclease activity, while simultaneously leaving behind new DNA in __[20] activity. Finally, DNA pol I is important for excision repair.

The functions of DNA pol II, IV, and V are less important to know for the MCAT:

3) DNA pol II has 5' to 3' polymerase activity, and 3' to 5' exonuclease proofreading function. It participates in DNA repair pathways and is used as a backup for DNA pol III.

4) DNA pol IV and DNA pol V have similar characteristics. They are error prone in 5' to 3' polymerase activity, but function to stall other polymerase enzymes at replication forks when DNA repair pathways have been activated. This is an important part of the prokaryotic checkpoint pathway.

---

[18] Yes.

[19] **Exonuclease** means "cutting a nucleic acid chain at the end." An **endonuclease** will cut a polynucleotide acid chain in the middle of the chain, usually at a particular sequence. Two important types of endonucleases are: **repair enzymes** that remove chemically damaged DNA from the chain, and **restriction enzymes**, which are endonucleases found in bacteria. Their role is to destroy the DNA of infecting viruses, thus restricting the host range of the virus.

[20] 5' to 3' polymerase; remember, all polymerization is 5' to 3'.

If a bacterium possesses a mutation in the gene for DNA polymerase III, resulting in an enzyme without the 3' to 5' exonuclease activity, will mutations occur more often than in bacteria with a normal DNA polymerase gene?[21]

Prokaryotic vs. Eukaryotic Replication

Prokaryotes have only one chromosome, and this one chromosome has only one origin. Because the chromosome is circular, as replication proceeds the partially duplicated genome begins to look like the Greek letter θ (theta). Hence the replication of prokaryotes is said to proceed by the **theta mechanism** and is referred to as **theta replication** (see Figure 14).

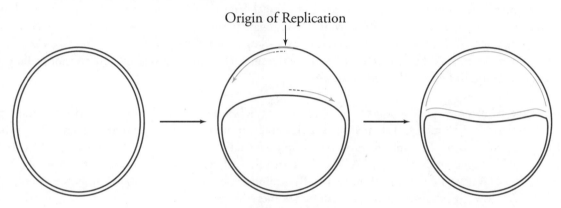

Figure 14 Theta (θ) Replication

In eukaryotic replication, each chromosome has several origins. This is necessary because eukaryotic chromosomes are so huge that replicating them from a single origin would be too slow. As the many replication forks continue to widen, they create an appearance of bubbles along the DNA strand, so they are referred to as "replication bubbles." Eventually the replication forks meet, and the many daughter strands are ligated together.

Figure 15 Eukaryotic Replication

---

[21] Yes. The 3' to 5' exonuclease activity is the polymerase's way of editing its work. Without this editing function, many more point mutations would occur due to the incorporation of wrong nucleotides. The normal polymerase is remarkably adept at sensing correct base pairing and removing bases that don't belong.

Replicating Telomeres in Eukaryotes

DNA polymerase can only build DNA in one direction (5' to 3'), and it requires both a template and a primer. These requirements lead to a roadblock at chromosome ends. Eventually there will be no place on the lagging strand to lay down a primer, and primers close to the end of DNA cannot be replaced with DNA because there is nothing on the other side (DNA polymerase usually uses a previous length of upstream DNA to replace the primer, but this isn't available at the end of a chromosome). This means that DNA replication machinery is unable to replicate sequences at the very ends of chromosomes, and after each round of the cell cycle and DNA replication, the ends of chromosomes shorten. **Telomeres** are disposable repeats at the end of chromosomes. They are consumed and shorten during cell division, becoming between 50 and 200 base pairs shorter.

When telomeres become *too* short, they reach a critical length where the chromosome can no longer replicate. As a consequence, cells can activate DNA repair pathways, enter a senescent state (where they are alive but not dividing), or activate apoptosis (pre-programmed cell death). The *Hayflick limit* is the number of times a normal human cell type can divide until telomere length stops cell division. Many age-related diseases are linked to telomere shortening.

Telomerase is an enzyme that adds repetitive nucleotide sequences to the ends of chromosomes and therefore lengthens telomeres. Telomerase is a ribonucleoprotein complex, containing an RNA primer and reverse transcriptase enzyme. Reverse transcriptases read RNA templates and generate DNA. In humans, the RNA template is 3' CCCAAUCCC 5', and this allows for chromosome extension, one DNA repeat (5'-TTAGGG-3') at a time (Figure 16). The telomerase complex continuously polymerizes, then translocates, allowing extension of six-nucleotide telomere repeats.

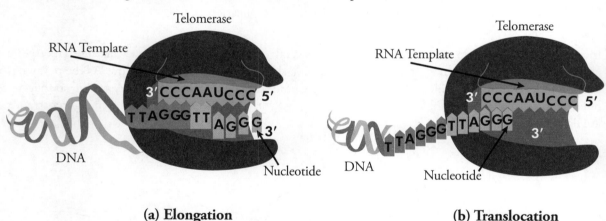

Figure 16 Telomerase and Telomere Lengthening

In most organisms, telomerase is only expressed in the germ line, embryonic stem cells, and some white blood cells. However, cancer cells can also express telomerase, which can help the cells immortalize. Telomere extension allows the cells to bypass senescence and apoptosis, and can therefore contribute to their transformation to a pre-cancerous state.

4.5 GENETIC MUTATION

Genetic mutation refers to any alteration of the DNA sequence of an organism's genome. These can be inherited or acquired throughout life. Mutations that can be passed onto offspring are called germline mutations, since they occur in the germ cells (which give rise to gametes). Somatic mutations occur in somatic (non-gametic) cells and are not passed onto offspring. In other words, somatic mutations can have a major effect on an individual, but will not be passed on to future individuals in that population. Our cells have evolved elaborate repair pathways to help deal with mutations, and these will be discussed in the next section.

4.5

Causes of Mutation

There are many causes of mutation. Most are induced by an environmental or chemical factor; however, they can also occur spontaneously.

Physical Mutagens

Ionizing radiation (such as X-rays, alpha particles, and gamma rays) can cause DNA breaks. If these only occur on one strand (Figure 17, left), they can be easily patched up because the DNA helix is still held together in one piece. However, if both backbones are broken close to each other on a segment of DNA, a double-strand break (DSB) occurs (Figure 17, right). Here, the chromosome has been split into two pieces and it's much more difficult to piece them back together.

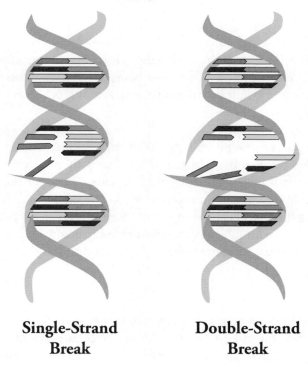

Single-Strand Break

Double-Strand Break

Figure 17   Single- and Double-Strand Breaks in DNA

UV light causes photochemical damage to DNA. For example, if two pyrimidines (two Cs or two Ts) are beside each other on a DNA backbone, UV light can cause them to become covalently linked. These pyrimidine dimers distort the DNA backbone (Figure 18) and can cause mutations during DNA replication if they are not repaired.

Figure 18   Pyrimidine Dimers in the DNA Helix

Reactive Chemicals

Many chemicals interact directly with DNA, and many others turn into damaging agents as they're being processed by a cell. Chemicals can covalently alter bases or can cause cross-linking or strand breaks. Cross-links are abnormal covalent bonds between different parts of DNA. Any compound that can cause mutations is called a **mutagen**.

Compounds that look like purines and pyrimidines (with large flat aromatic ring structures) cause mutations by inserting themselves between base pairs, or *intercalating*, thereby causing errors in DNA replication. Ethidium bromide is often used to visualize nucleic acids during gel electrophoresis in molecular biology labs. This chemical is used because it is planar (and therefore intercalates with the DNA ladder), and glows orange when exposed to UV light (meaning nucleic acids in a gel can be easily visualized). However, because it intercalates with DNA, is also distorts the structure and can therefore disrupt DNA replication and transcription. Thus, ethidium bromide is a mutagen.

Biological Agents

Biological agents can also cause mutations. For example, although DNA polymerase has proofreading and correction abilities, it can still make a mistake. An incorrect base pair may be repaired (see Section 4.6), but if not, it will be passed on to all daughter cells. In this case, there is no mutagen. The mistake is spontaneous. Viruses can also affect DNA. Lysogenic viruses insert into the genome of the host cell (see Chapter 5), and this can cause mutations and disrupt genetic function. Some viruses can cause cancer because of this function. And finally, transposons can induce mutations. This will be described in the next section.

Types of Mutations

Based on structure, there are seven kinds of mutations:

1) Point mutations
2) Insertions
3) Deletions
4) Inversions
5) Amplifications
6) Translocations and rearrangements
7) Loss of heterozygosity

Point mutations are single base pair substitutions (A in place of G, for example). Point mutations can be *transitions* (substitution of a pyrimidine for another pyrimidine or substitution of a purine for another purine) or *transversions* (substitution of a purine for a pyrimidine or vice versa). There are three types of point mutations:

1) **Missense mutation**: This causes one amino acid to be replaced with a different amino acid. This may not be serious if the amino acids are similar. [How can this occur?[22]]
2) **Nonsense mutation**: A stop codon replaces a regular codon and prematurely shortens the protein.
3) **Silent mutation**: A codon is changed into a new codon for the same amino acid, so there is no change in the protein's amino acid sequence.

Insertion refers to the addition of one or more extra nucleotides into the DNA sequence, and deletion is the removal of nucleotides from the sequence. Both of these mutations can cause a shift in the reading frame. For example, AAACCCACC is read as AAA, CCC, ACC. It would code for Lys-Pro-Thr. Inserting an extra G into the first codon could produce this: AGAACCCACC. This would be read AGA, ACC, CAC, C. It now codes for Arg-Thr-His (plus there's an extra C). Not only has the first codon and amino acid changed, the whole gene will be read differently and all amino acids in the protein from that point on will change. Mutations that cause a change in the reading frame are called **frameshift mutations**. Generally speaking, frameshift mutations are very serious. Note that a frameshift can lead to premature termination of translation (yielding an incomplete polypeptide) if it results in the presence of an abnormal stop codon. [Are all insertions and deletions frameshift mutations?[23] If the following oligonucleotide is mutated by inserting a G between the fifth and sixth codons, what effect will this have on the oligopeptide it encodes: AUG AAG GGG CCC UUU AAA UGA CCC?[24] For each type of mutation, does it involve a change in the genotype, the phenotype, or both?[25]]

---

[22] For example, substituting a small hydrophobe such as valine for another small hydrophobe like leucine will probably cause little disruption of protein structure. Another way of defining conservative mutations is that they cause changes in primary structure but do not affect secondary, tertiary, or quaternary structure.

[23] No. If you insert or delete one whole codon or several whole codons, you add or remove amino acids to the polypeptide without changing the reading frame.

[24] The original RNA codes for Met-Lys-Gly-Pro-Phe-Lys. After the insertion, the oligonucleotide will code for Met-Lys-Gly-Pro-Phe-Glu-Met-Thr. Note that this contains different amino acids and it's longer. The extra length is due to the fact that a stop codon, UGA, changed by the frameshift.

[25] By definition, all mutations involve a change in the genotype. Most mutations also cause a change in the phenotype, but in the case of conservative mutations, it is a very subtle change that would be hard to detect.

In addition to mutations at individual nucleotides, larger-scale mutations are also common. Insertions and deletions can involve thousands of bases. An **inversion** is when a segment of a chromosome is reversed end-to-end. The chromosome undergoes breakage and rearrangement within itself (Figure 19). Insertions, deletions, and inversions can be caused by transposons (see below).

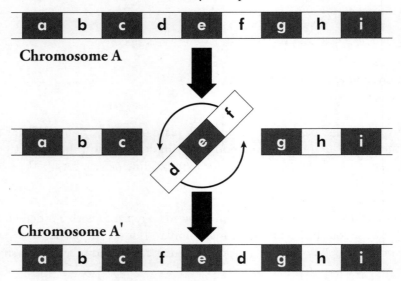

Figure 19   Chromosome Inversion

Chromosome amplification is when a segment of a chromosome is duplicated. **Translocations** result when recombination occurs between nonhomologous chromosomes (Figure 20). This can create a gene fusion, where a new gene product is made from parts of two genes that were not previously connected. This is a common occurrence in many types of cancer. Translocations can be balanced (where no genetic information is lost), or unbalanced (where genetic information is lost or gained).

Figure 20   Chromosome Translocation

Transposons

Both prokaryotes and eukaryotes have mobile genetic elements in their genomes, called transposable elements or **transposons**. It is thought that many eukaryotic transposons are degenerate (old and defective) retroviruses. "Genetic mobility" means that these short segments can jump around the genome. Transposons can cause mutations and chromosome changes such as inversions, deletions, and rearrangements.

There are three common types of transposons, each with a different structure. The first type is the simplest and is called an IS element (Figure 21, top). It is composed of a transposase gene (discussed below), flanked by inverted repeat sequences. The structure of an example inverted repeat is shown in Figure 22. Some transposons are more complex, in that they also contain additional genes (Figure 21, middle). For example, some transposons contain genes for antibiotic resistance. Finally, composite transposons have two similar or identical IS elements with a central region in between (Figure 21, bottom).

Figure 21   Transposon Structure

Figure 22   Inverted Repeats

All transposons contain a gene that codes for a protein called **transposase**. This enzyme has "cut and paste" activity, where it catalyzes mobilization of the transposon (excision from the donor site) and integration into a new genetic location (the acceptor site). Sometimes the transposon sequence is completely excised and moved, and sometimes it is duplicated and moved while still maintained at the original location (Figure 23, next page). The inverted repeats are important for this mobilization.

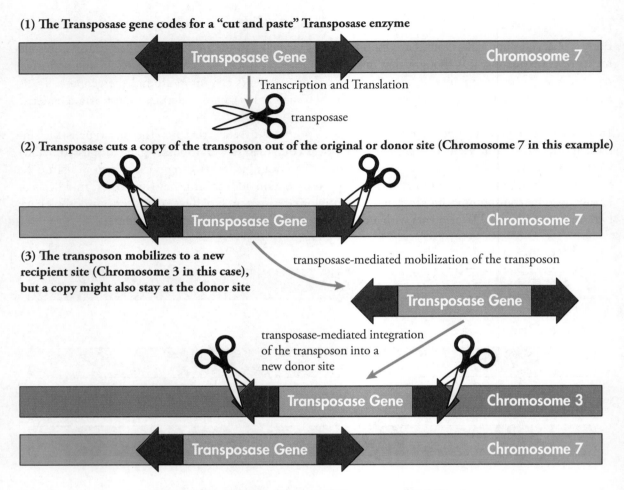

(1) The Transposase gene codes for a "cut and paste" Transposase enzyme

Transcription and Translation

transposase

(2) Transposase cuts a copy of the transposon out of the original or donor site (Chromosome 7 in this example)

(3) The transposon mobilizes to a new recipient site (Chromosome 3 in this case), but a copy might also stay at the donor site

transposase-mediated mobilization of the transposon

transposase-mediated integration of the transposon into a new donor site

Figure 23 The Mechanism of Transposon Mobilization

Many mobilizations have no effect because the transposon inserts into a relatively unimportant part of the genome. However, transposons can cause mutations if they jump into an important part of the genome.

When transposons are mobilized, they can insert in any part of the genome, and this can affect gene expression or cause mutations. They can jump into a promoter and turn gene expression off. They can jump into a protein-coding region and disrupt (or mutate) the sequence. They can also jump into regulatory parts of the genome and ramp up gene expression at a nearby site.

In addition to jumping around the genome, transposons can cause structural changes to chromosomes when they work in pairs. Directionality of the transposon is important here, as it determines what happens to the chromosome. If a chromosome has two transposons with the same direction (Figure 24), the transposons can line up beside each other, so they are parallel. This causes the chromosomal segment between them to loop around. Recombination occurs between the transposons, and this causes deletion of the DNA between the two transposons. The original chromosome therefore completely loses the DNA segment between the transposons (a deletion). The segment of DNA that is lost takes one transposon with it, meaning it can actually jump back into the genome somewhere else, causing chromosome rearrangement: one chunk of a chromosome has moved to a new location in the genome.

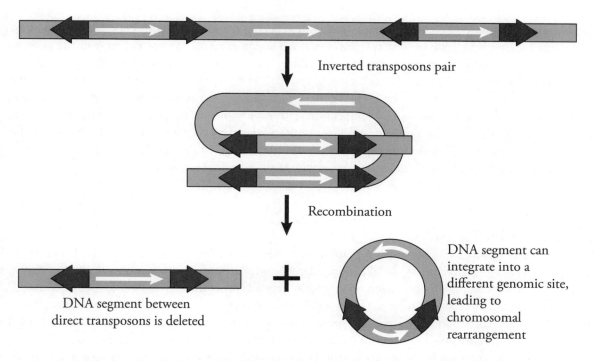

Figure 24 Deletion and Chromosomal Rearrangements via Transposons

If a chromosome has two transposons with inverted orientations (Figure 25), they can again pair and align with each other. After recombination, the sequence of DNA between the two transposons ends up inverted.

DNA segment between inverted transposons is inverted

Figure 25 Chromosome Inversion via Transposons

Diploid organisms have two copies of each gene, and generally a mutation in one copy is tolerated as long as the other copy of the gene is normal. However, if a deletion removes the normal copy of the gene, the only remaining copy is the mutated version. This is referred to as **loss of heterozygosity**. This makes the locus **hemizygous**: there is only one gene copy in the diploid organism. If the remaining allele is mutant or defective, all gene expression of the normal gene product is lost. For example, hereditary retinoblastoma is a type of retinal cancer common in young children. It occurs when a child receives a flawed copy of the tumor suppressor Rb1 from one parent, and a loss of heterozygosity event leads to loss of the normal allele (from the other parent). With no functional Rb protein (due to having only one copy of Rb1, and it being a flawed or mutant copy), the child almost invariably develops retinoblastoma.

Effects of Mutations

There are many mechanisms by which mutations can exert their effects on the cell. A single amino acid change can affect protein activity, localization, degradation, half-life, or interactions, or, it may have no effect at all. The outcome of a mutation on a protein depends on where the mutation occurs. Mutations on sex chromosomes typically have a greater effect than mutations on autosomes since autosomes are present in double copies. Males have only one X chromosome and one Y chromosome, with no back-up copy of either. Similarly, most females only express one of their X chromosomes (see Section 4.9), and so they, too, often don't have a back-up copy. Haploid expression in a diploid organism is **hemizygosity**, and this can lead to an increased effect of mutations on these chromosomes.

Gain-of-function mutations increase the activity of a certain gene product, or change it such that it gains a new and abnormal function. Loss-of-function mutations are the opposite; they result in the gene product having less or no function. In **haploinsufficiency**, a diploid organism has only a single functional copy of a gene, and this single copy is not enough to support a normal state. Haploinsufficiency highlights the importance of gene dose: many times, just expressing a gene is not enough. You must express *enough* of the gene to maintain good health.

Good and Bad Mutations

Despite the bad reputation they have, not all mutations are bad. Many mutations are neutral, and have no effect. Evolution is based on mutations and selection, and some mutations are beneficial. Those that confer a survival advantage will be selected for in a population.

There are examples of beneficial mutations in humans:

- Sickle-cell anemia is caused by mutations in the gene for hemoglobin (Hb). One of the most common mutations allows deoxygenated Hb to dimerize and form long chains, which distorts the red blood cell shape, causing it to sickle. These deformed cells cannot function properly and are prematurely destroyed, leading to anemia. However, people who carry this gene also have an advantage in that they are more resistant to malaria. In areas where malaria is common, this is an important benefit.

- Some humans are missing 32 base pairs in a gene called CCR5. This deletion confers HIV resistance to homozygotes and delays AIDS onset in heterozygotes. This mutation may have also conferred resistance to diseases in the past (such as the bubonic plague or smallpox), explaining its prevalence in populations of European descent, where these diseases were prevalent.

Mutations can also be disease *causing*. In some cases, one mutation is sufficient to induce a diseased state. In other cases, many mutations have to cooperate and occur together to cause a disease.

Inborn errors of metabolism are a huge group of genetic diseases that involve disorders of metabolism. Most of these are due to a single mutation in a single gene that codes for some sort of metabolic enzyme. Symptoms are caused by either the build-up of a toxic compound that can't be broken down or by the deficiency of an essential molecule that cannot be synthesized. Because cellular metabolism is crucial, many symptoms are possible and a wide range of systems can be affected. Inborn errors of metabolism are typically organized into groups of disorders, depending on what type of metabolic pathways they affect: carbohydrate, amino acid, urea cycle, organic acids, fatty acid oxidation, mitochondrial, porphyrin, purine or pyrimidine, steroid, peroxisomal function, or lysosomal storage.

Cancer is driven by mutation accumulation. These mutations can either be inherited or can be caused by carcinogen exposure. A carcinogen is a mutagen that is directly involved in causing cancer. Tumors typically have hundreds of mutations, ranging from point mutations to massive chromosomal changes. These mutations are often in oncogenes and tumor suppressors. An oncogene is a gene that can cause cancer when it is mutated or expressed at high levels. Tumor suppressors are the opposite in that their deletion (or expression at decreased levels) can cause cancer. Some mutations will drive tumor growth and are highly selected for. These mutations are the most promising targets for developing cancer treatments, as the cancer cells rely on these mutations for growth.

4.6   DNA REPAIR

Cells have developed several mechanisms to deal with DNA damage. First, cell cycle checkpoints are activated, and arrest cell cycle progression. In eukaryotes, checkpoint pathways function at phase boundaries (such as the G_1/S transition, and the G_2/M transition), and can also be activated within some phases. Extensive DNA damage can induce apoptosis in eukaryotes, but before this happens, cells try to repair the DNA damage. This is important so that defective DNA isn't passed on to daughter cells. There are several types of DNA repair.

Direct Reversal

Many types of DNA damage are irreversible and require repair pathways to fix the damage. However, a few can be directly reversed. For example, some enzymes can repair UV-induced pyrimidine photodimers using visible light. This process is called photoreactivation, and directly repairs the UV damage to DNA. This is commonly performed by bacteria and many plants. If pyrimidine dimers are not directly reversed, nucleotide excision repair can be used instead. Nucleotide excision repair is the main mechanism of repair in humans, but it can introduce a mutation when trying to complete the repair. If left unrepaired, pyrimidine dimers in humans may lead to melanoma, a type of very dangerous and malignant skin tumor.

Homology-Dependent Repair

One of the benefits of DNA structure is the presence of a back-up copy; because DNA is double stranded, mutations on one strand of DNA can be repaired using the undamaged, complementary information on the other strand. Repair pathways that rely on this characteristic of DNA are called **homology-dependent repair pathways**. These can be divided into repair that happens before DNA replication (**excision repair**), or repair that happens during and after DNA replication (**post-replication repair**).

Excision Repair

Excision repair involves removing defective bases or nucleotides and replacing them. If these bases are not repaired, they can induce mutations during DNA replication, since replication machinery cannot pair them properly.

Post-Replication Repair

The **mismatch repair pathway** (MMR) targets mismatched Watson-Crick base pairs that were not repaired by DNA polymerase proofreading during replication. To do this, mispaired bases must be identified and fixed, but the crucial question is: which base is the correct one and which is the mistake? For example, if DNA contains an AC base pair, is the adenine correct and C should be removed and replaced with T? Or is the cytosine correct and A should be removed and replaced with G?

Some bacteria use genome methylation to help differentiate between the older DNA template strand and the newly synthesized daughter strand. Methylation takes a while to complete, which means that shortly after DNA synthesis, the parental template strand will be labeled with methylated bases and the new daughter strand will not. Bacterial machinery can read these methyl tags and know which base is the correct one (the one on the older strand) and which needs to be replaced (the newer one).

Other prokaryotes and most eukaryotes use a different system, where the newly synthesized strand is recognized by the free 3'-terminus on the leading strand, or by the presence of gaps between Okazaki fragments on the lagging strand.

Double-Strand Break Repair

DNA double-strand breaks (DSBs) can be caused by reactive oxygen species, ionizing radiation, UV light or chemical agents. Cells have two pathways to help in DSB repair: homologous recombination and nonhomologous end-joining. The goal of both is to reattach and fuse chromosomes that have come apart because of DSB. If done incorrectly, this can lead to deletions (where genetic information is lost) or translocations (where chromosome segments move to other chromosomes).

Homologous Recombination

After DNA replication, the genome contains identical sister chromatids. Homologous recombination is a process where one sister chromatid can help repair a DSB in the other. First, the DSB is identified and trimmed at 5' ends to generate single-stranded DNA (Figure 26). This is done by nucleases (which break phosphodiester bonds) and helicase (to unwind the DNA). Many proteins bind these ends and start a search of the genome to find a sister chromatid region that is complementary to the single-stranded DNA. Once found, the complementary sequences are used as a template to repair and connect the broken chromatid. This requires a "joint molecule," where damaged and undamaged sister chromatids cross over. DNA polymerase and ligase build a corrected DNA strand.

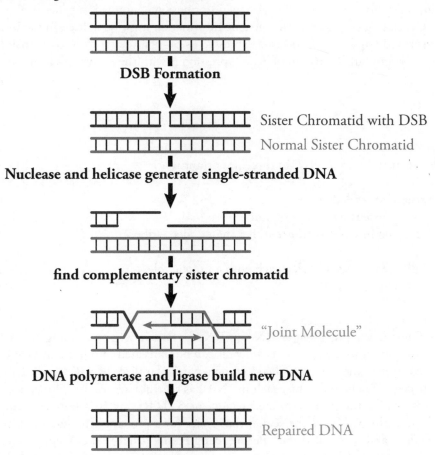

DSB Formation

Sister Chromatid with DSB
Normal Sister Chromatid

Nuclease and helicase generate single-stranded DNA

find complementary sister chromatid

"Joint Molecule"

DNA polymerase and ligase build new DNA

Repaired DNA

Figure 26   Homologous Recombination to Repair Double-Strand Breaks

Nonhomologous End Joining

Cells that aren't actively growing or cycling through the cell cycle don't have the option of using sister chromatids to repair DSBs in an error-free way. Since DNA replication isn't happening, there is no chromosome backup to use. In this case, even a poorly repaired chromosome is better than one with a DSB, since chromosome breaks can lead to rearrangements.

Nonhomologous end joining is used to accomplish repair in this case. This process is common in eukaryotes but relatively uncommon in prokaryotes. First, broken ends are stabilized and processed, then DNA ligase connects the fragments. Nothing about this process requires specificity; the goal is just to reconnect broken chromosomes. Often this can result in base pairs being lost or chromosomes being connected in an abnormal way.

4.6

4.7 GENE EXPRESSION: TRANSCRIPTION

Gene expression refers to the process whereby the information contained in genes begins to have effects in the cell. The Central Dogma tells us that genetic information must be written in the form of RNA (i.e., it must be **transcribed**); and then it must be expressed as protein (i.e., it must be **translated**). Therefore, the logical place to begin our discussion of gene expression is with the nature of RNA and transcription.

Characteristics of RNA

RNA is chemically distinct from DNA in three important ways:

1) RNA is **single-stranded**, except in some viruses.
2) RNA contains **uracil** instead of thymine.
3) The pentose ring in RNA is **ribose** rather than 2' deoxyribose.

There are several different types of RNA, each with a unique role.

Coding RNA

You are already familiar with **messenger RNA** (mRNA), the only type of coding RNA. This molecule carries genetic information to the ribosome, where it can be translated into protein; each unique polypeptide is created according to the sequence of codons on a particular piece of mRNA, which was transcribed from a particular gene. To allow for this, each mRNA has several regions. The 5' region is not translated into protein (so it's called the 5' untranslated region, or **5'UTR**), but it is important in initiation and regulation. Following the 5'UTR is the region that codes for a protein. This starts at a start codon and ends at a stop codon, and it is called the **open reading frame** (ORF). The 3' end of the mRNA (after the stop codon) isn't translated into protein, but it often contains regulatory regions that influence post-transcriptional gene expression (see Section 4.9).

Eukaryotic mRNA is usually **monocistronic** and obeys the "one gene, one protein" principle. This means that each piece of mRNA encodes only one polypeptide (and so contains one ORF). Hence, there are as many different mRNAs as there are proteins. Because each mRNA can be read many times, each transcript can be used to make many copies of its polypeptide. There are a few exceptions to the "one gene, one protein" principle; recently, some polycistronic eukaryotic mRNAs have been discovered, and these will be discussed below.

In contrast, prokaryotic mRNA often codes for more than one polypeptide and is termed **polycistronic**. Different open reading frames on the same polycistronic mRNA are generally related in function.[26] Translation termination and initiation sequences are found between the ORFs. The termination information helps finish the previous peptide chain, and initiation information helps start translation of the next open reading frame on the transcript.

---

[26] For instance, if five enzymes are necessary for the synthesis of a particular molecule, then all five enzymes might be encoded on a single piece of mRNA.

Messenger RNA is constantly produced and degraded, according to the cell's need for the protein encoded by each piece of mRNA. In fact, this is the principal means whereby cells regulate the amount of each particular protein they synthesize. This is an important point that will be emphasized later. Note that in eukaryotes, the first RNA transcribed from DNA is an immature or precursor to mRNA called **heterogeneous nuclear RNA** (hnRNA). Processing events (such as addition of a cap and tail, and splicing) are required for hnRNA to become mature mRNA. Since prokaryotes do not process their primary transcripts, hnRNA is only found in eukaryotes.

Non-Coding RNA

Non-coding RNA (ncRNA) is a functional RNA that is not translated into a protein. The human genome codes for thousands of ncRNAs, and there are several types. The two major types to know for the MCAT are transfer RNA (tRNA) and ribosomal RNA (rRNA).

Transfer RNA (tRNA) is responsible for translating the genetic code. Transfer RNA carries amino acids from the cytoplasm to the ribosome to be added to a growing protein. The structure of tRNA and how it does its job will be discussed in Section 4.8. [Estimate how many different tRNAs there are.[27]]

Ribosomal RNA (rRNA) is the major component of the ribosome. Humans have only four different types of rRNA molecules (18S, 5.8S, 28S and 5S), although almost all the RNA made in a given cell is rRNA. All rRNAs serve as components of the ribosome, along with many polypeptide chains. One rRNA provides the catalytic function of the ribosome, which is a little odd. In most other cases, enzymes are made from polypeptides. Catalytic RNAs are also called **ribozymes** (or ribonucleic acid enzymes), since they are capable of performing specific biochemical reactions, similar to protein enzymes. There are additional examples of ribozymes, including snRNA (discussed below) and some introns that are self-splicing.

Some other interesting non-coding RNAs are:

- **Small nuclear RNA** (snRNA) molecules (150 nucleotides) associate with proteins to form snRNP (small nuclear ribonucleic particles) complexes in the spliceosome.
- **MicroRNA** (miRNA) and **small interfering RNA** (siRNA) function in RNA interference (RNAi), a form of post-transcriptional regulation of gene expression. Both can bind specific mRNA molecules to either increase or decrease translation. This will be discussed more in Section 4.9.
- **Long ncRNAs** are longer than 200 nucleotides. They help control the basal transcription level in a cell by regulating initiation complex assembly on promoters. They also contribute to many types of post-transcriptional regulation by controlling splicing and translation, and they function in imprinting and X-chromosome inactivation (see Section 4.9).

4.7

---

[27] Each tRNA must recognize a codon on mRNA and respond by delivering the appropriate amino acid to the ribosome. There are 20 different amino acids, so there at least 20 different tRNAs. However, there are 61 possible codons, so there could be as many as 61 different tRNAs. The actual number is between 20 and 61, because the third nucleotide of the codon is often not needed for specificity of the amino acid.

Replication vs. Transcription

Transcription is the synthesis of RNA (usually mRNA, tRNA, or rRNA) using DNA as the template. The word *transcription* indicates that in the process of reading and writing information, the language does not change. Information is transferred from one polynucleotide to another. This should lead you to expect transcription to be fairly similar to replication. And it is.

Both replication and transcription involve **template-driven polymerization**. [Because of this, the RNA transcript produced in transcription is ___[28] to the DNA template, just as the daughter strand produced in replication was.] The *driving force* for both processes is the removal and subsequent hydrolysis of pyrophosphate from each nucleotide added to the chain, with the existing chain acting as nucleophile. [Transcription, like replication, can occur only in the ___[29] direction. Do the polymerase enzymes in both replication and transcription require a primer?[30]] Another important difference between transcription and DNA replication is that RNA polymerase has not been shown to possess the ability to remove mismatched nucleotides (it lacks exonuclease activity); in other words, it cannot correct its errors. Thus, transcription is a lower fidelity process than replication. [A virus possessing an RNA genome relies on RNA polymerase rather than DNA polymerase to replicate its genome. Will this virus have a higher or a lower rate of spontaneous mutation than organisms with ds-DNA genomes?[31]]

Another similarity is that transcription, like replication, begins at a specific spot on the chromosome. The name of the site where transcription starts (the **start site**) is different from the name of the place where replication begins, ___.[32] The sequence of nucleotides on a chromosome that activates RNA polymerase to begin the process of transcription is called the **promoter**, and the point where RNA polymerization actually *starts* is called the start site. In fact, from this point forward, just about every event in transcription is given a different name from the events in replication.

Reference Points in Transcription

Before we discuss the mechanics of transcription, we need to clarify a few reference points (see Figure 27). We noted previously that the chromosome is referred to as the *template*, not *parent*. What about the individual strands of the chromosome? Are they both templates for the same mRNA? Let's answer with a thought experiment. Say there is a strand of DNA which has the sequence AAAAAAAAA. If we transcribe this strand, the resulting mRNA will look like: UUUUUUUUU. When it is translated, this mRNA will result in an oligopeptide with this primary structure: Phe-Phe-Phe. (Refer to the genetic code table in Section 4.3.) Now, what if we transcribe the other strand of the chromosome? What is its DNA sequence? What will the transcript look like? And the oligopeptide?[33] Our conclusion is that only one of the strands of the DNA template encodes a particular mRNA molecule. But it makes sense: paired DNA

---

[28] complementary

[29] 5' to 3'

[30] No, RNA pol does not require a primer. Remember, the primer in replication is a piece of RNA, made by an RNA polymerase.

[31] The virus will have a very high rate of mutation. It is a general law that most mutations are harmful. Hence, individual viruses will be far less likely to survive than organisms with DNA genomes. However, the high mutation rate will allow the entire species of virus to evolve very rapidly, making it very successful as a parasite (since it will evade host defense systems).

[32] the origin

[33] The DNA strand must be complementary to the first strand we discussed. So the sequence must be TTTTTTTTT. Thus, the transcript will have to be AAAAAAAAA. Because AAA codes for lysine, the oligopeptide would be Lys-Lys-Lys.

4.7

strands are *complementary*, not *identical*. The strand which is actually transcribed is called the **template**, **non-coding**, **transcribed**, or **antisense strand**; it is complementary to the transcript. The other DNA strand is called the **coding** or **sense strand**; it has the same sequence as the transcript (except it has T in place of U). It is customary to say that transcription starts at a point and proceeds **downstream**, which means toward the 3' end of the coding strand and transcript. **Upstream** means toward the 5' end of the coding strand, beyond the 5' end of the transcript. Upstream nucleotide sequences are referred to using negative numbers, and downstream sequences are referred to using positive numbers. The first nucleotide on the template strand which is actually transcribed is called the start site. The corresponding nucleotide on the coding strand is given the number +1. As we'll see below, regulatory sequences on the chromosome are referred to by where they occur on the coding strand.

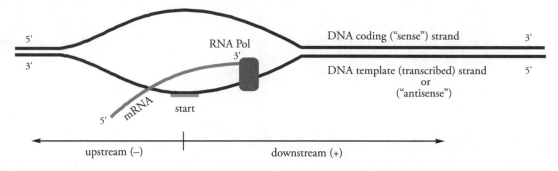

Figure 27 Reference Points in Transcription

- The figure above labels the transcript "mRNA." Is this accurate in all life forms? (Hint: in eukaryotes, is the initial transcript mature mRNA ready to be translated?)[34]

Prokaryotic Transcription

It is important to understand all the vocabulary and general principles presented above. In this section and the next, we will present some more detailed information.

In bacteria (prokaryotes), all types of RNA are made by the same RNA polymerase. Prokaryotic RNA polymerase is a large enzyme complex consisting of five subunits: two alpha subunits, a beta subunit, a beta' subunit, and an omega subunit ($\alpha_2\beta\beta'\omega$). This is the **core enzyme** responsible for rapid elongation of the transcript. However, the core enzyme alone cannot initiate transcription. An additional subunit termed the **sigma factor** (σ) is required to form what is sometimes referred to as the **holoenzyme** (*holo* = complete), which is responsible for initiation.

Transcription occurs in three stages: **initiation**, **elongation**, and **termination**. Initiation occurs when RNA polymerase holoenzyme binds to a promoter. The typical bacterial promoter contains two primary sequences: the **Pribnow box** at −10 and the **−35 sequence**. Holoenzyme scans along the chromosome like a train on a railroad track until it recognizes a promoter and then stops, forming a **closed complex**. The RNA polymerase must unwind a portion of the DNA double helix before it can begin to synthesize

---

[34] No, it is accurate for prokaryotes only. In eukaryotes, the RNA transcript must be processed (spliced) and transported out of the nucleus before it can be translated. We will discuss this in-depth later in the chapter.

RNA. The RNA polymerase bound at the promoter with a region of single-stranded DNA is termed the **open complex**. Once the open complex has formed, transcription can begin.

The sigma factor plays two roles in helping the polymerase find promoters. The first is to greatly increase the ability of RNA polymerase to recognize promoters. The second is to decrease the nonspecific affinity of holoenzyme for DNA. Once the open complex and several phosphodiester bonds have been formed, the sigma factor is no longer necessary and leaves the RNA polymerase complex.

The core enzyme elongates the RNA chain *processively*, with one polymerase complex synthesizing an entire RNA molecule. As the core enzyme elongates the RNA, it moves along the DNA downstream in a **transcription bubble** in which a region of the DNA double helix is unwound to allow the polymerase to access the complementary DNA template. When a termination signal is detected, in some cases with the help of a protein called rho, the polymerase falls off of the DNA, releases the RNA, and the transcription bubble closes.

Comparing Prokaryotic and Eukaryotic Transcription

Eukaryotic and prokaryotic transcription are similar, but you need to be aware of four major differences. Differences in location, RNA polymerases, and primary transcripts are discussed here. Regulation of transcription is another major difference and is discussed in Section 4.9.

Location

Eukaryotic means "true-kernelled." Prokaryotic means "before-the-kernel." The **karyon** (kernel) is, of course, the nucleus. The fact that prokaryotes have no nucleus means transcription occurs free in the cytoplasm, in the same compartment where translation occurs, and transcription and translation can occur *simultaneously*. Eukaryotes must transcribe their mRNA in the nucleus, modify it (see below), and then transport it across the nuclear membrane to the cytoplasm where it can be translated. Transcription and translation in eukaryotes *do not* occur simultaneously.

Another important difference between prokaryotic and eukaryotic gene expression is that the primary transcript in prokaryotes is mRNA. In other words, the product of transcription by prokaryotic RNA polymerase is ready to be translated. In fact, translation of prokaryotic mRNA begins before transcription is completed!

In contrast, the eukaryotic primary transcript (hnRNA made by RNA pol II, see below for info on eukaryotic RNA polymerases) is modified extensively before translation (Figure 30). The most important example is **splicing**. Eukaryotic DNA has non-coding sequences intervening between the segments that actually code for proteins. Sometimes these intervening sequences contain enhancers or other regulatory sequences and they can be quite long. The average size of a mammalian intron, for example, is about 2,000 nucleotides. *Int*ervening sequences in the RNA are called **introns**. Note that introns are intragenic regions (and not intergenic space, discussed in Section 4.2). Protein-coding regions of the RNA are termed **ex**ons because they actually get **ex**pressed. Before the RNA can be translated, introns must be removed and exons joined together; this is accomplished via splicing.

Splicing is mediated by the **spliceosome**, a complex that contains over 100 proteins and 5 small nuclear RNA (snRNA) molecules. About half the proteins stably bind snRNAs, and these form three small nuclear ribonucleic particles (snRNPs). Each snRNP is therefore made of proteins and snRNAs. The spliceosome assembles around each intron that needs to be removed. This happens in a series of steps, where different snRNP components are recruited and released as the reaction proceeds.

To catalyze the splicing reaction, snRNPs recognize and hydrogen bond to conserved nucleotides in the intron: typically GU at the 5' end, AG at the 3' end, and an adenine 15–45 bases upstream of the 3' splice site. This aligns the hnRNA such that the splicing mechanism can take place (Figure 28). Two splicing reactions are catalyzed by the spliceosome. The first reaction attaches one end of the intron to the conserved adenine. This causes the intron to form a looped structure, then the second reaction joins the two exons (Figure 28) and releases the loop. The five conserved nucleotides necessary for this reaction (GU, A and AG) are found in all genes and across all eukaryotic species.

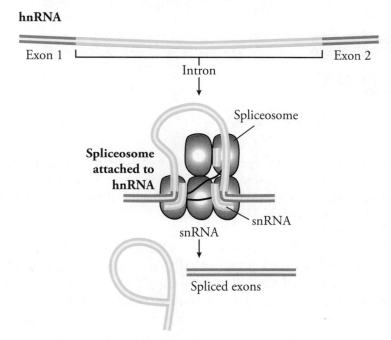

Figure 28   Mechanism of Splicing

For a given gene, there are often different options or patterns of splicing, a phenomenon called **alternative splicing**. One gene could have different promoters in the 5' region, which can change where/how the RNA begins. There can be alternative 5' exons or 3' exons, which can affect either end of the RNA. In the middle, too, some exons can be included or skipped. Finally, there could be mutually exclusive exons, where sometimes one is included and sometimes the other is kept. This leads to different mRNAs being made from one DNA gene sequence; the mRNAs can be different in length and sequence. Shuffling exons in this way is one way to increase the complexity of gene expression (Figure 29 on the following page).

Figure 29   An Example of Alternative Splicing

Alternative splicing is mediated by introns and exons, as well as by the proteins that can bind to these sequences. There are almost 200,000 introns in the human genome, with an average of about seven per gene. It was initially thought that introns were unimportant and had no function, but the current picture of introns is a little more complicated than first believed.

Eukaryotic hnRNA must be modified in two other ways before translation can occur. A tag is added to each end of the molecule: a **5' cap** and a **3' poly-A tail**. The 5' cap is a methylated guanine nucleotide stuck on the 5' end [which is the end made __ (first or last?)[35]]. The poly-A tail is a string of several hundred adenine nucleotides. The cap is essential for translation, while both the cap and the poly-A tail are important in preventing digestion of the mRNA by exonucleases that are free in the cell.

---

[35] It is made first, since transcription proceeds from 5' to 3'.

- Why would active exonucleases be floating free in the cell?[36]

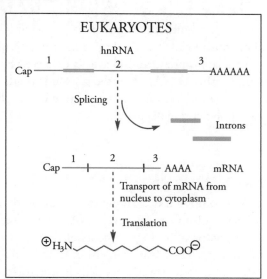

Figure 30 Comparison of Prokaryotic and Eukaryotic Gene Expression

- One piece of RNA isolated from a human cell is found to produce two different polypeptides when added to a cell-free protein synthesis system containing all the enzymes necessary for eukaryotic gene expression. When the two polypeptides are separated and digested with trypsin, they produce fragments of the following molecular weights:
  Polypeptide 1: 5 kD, 8 kD, 12 kD, and 14 kD
  Polypeptide 2: 3 kD, 5 kD, 8 kD, 10 kD, 12 kD, and 14 kD
  How can we explain the synthesis of two different polypeptides from one piece of RNA?[37]

RNA Polymerase

In prokaryotes, all RNA is made by the $\alpha_2\beta\beta'\omega\sigma$ RNA polymerase complex. In eukaryotes, there are many different RNA polymerases:

- **RNA polymerase I transcribes most rRNA**
- **RNA polymerase II transcribes hnRNA** (so ultimately mRNA), most snRNA, and some miRNA
- **RNA polymerase III transcribes tRNA**, long ncRNA, siRNA, some miRNA, and a subset of rRNA

Please note: In our discussion of replication, you learned about many *prokaryotic DNA* polymerases. In contrast, here you learned about many eukaryotic RNA polymerases. Don't get mixed up!

---

[36] Two conceivable reasons: 1) *mRNA has a very short lifespan;* it is degraded rapidly, and more must be made if the protein is still needed. Note that this is consistent with the idea that regulation of gene expression occurs primarily at the transcriptional level since this is more efficient. 2) Viruses may inject RNA into the cell. If it does not have the correct cap and tail modifications, exonucleases will destroy it.

[37] Here is an example of the use of splicing for the regulation of gene expression. The piece of RNA must have been hnRNA. In the cell-free system it underwent **differential splicing** to produce one of two different mRNA molecules. Apparently, Polypeptide 1 came from an mRNA which had more material spliced out than the mRNA coding for Polypeptide 2.

4.8 GENE EXPRESSION: TRANSLATION

Translation is the synthesis of polypeptides according to the amino acid sequence dictated by the sequence of codons in mRNA. During translation, an mRNA molecule attaches to a ribosome at a specific codon, and the appropriate amino acid is delivered by a tRNA molecule. Then the second amino acid is delivered by another tRNA. Then the ribosome binds the two amino acids together, creating a dipeptide. This process is repeated until the polypeptide is complete, at which point the ribosome drops the mRNA and the new polypeptide departs.

Transfer RNA (tRNA)

Each tRNA is composed of a single transcript produced by RNA polymerase III. The tertiary structure of every tRNA molecule is similar. tRNAs have a stem-and-loop structure stabilized by hydrogen bonds between bases on neighboring segments of the RNA chain (Figures 31 and 32). Several modified nucleotides are found in tRNA (e.g., dihydrouridine). One end of the structure is responsible for recognizing the mRNA codon to be translated. This is the **anticodon**, a sequence of three ribonucleotides which is complementary to the mRNA codon the tRNA translates. A key step in translation is *specific base pairing between the tRNA anticodon and the mRNA codon*. It is this specificity that dictates which amino acid of the twenty will be added to a growing polypeptide chain by the ribosome. [Is it likely that the three nucleotides of the anticodon contribute to the tertiary structure of tRNA by base-pairing with other nucleotides in the chain?[38]] The other end of the tRNA molecule has the **amino acid acceptor site**, which is where the amino acid is attached to the tRNA. [If you analyzed a thousand tRNA molecules, which region would you expect to vary the most?[39]] Since there is a tRNA for each codon, each tRNA is specific for one amino acid, while each amino acid may have several tRNAs. Each tRNA can be named according to the amino acid it's specific for. For example, a tRNA for valine would be written $tRNA_{Val}$. When the amino acid is attached, the tRNA is written this way: $Val\text{-}tRNA_{Val}$.

Figure 31 Cloverleaf (Two-Dimensional) Structure of tRNA

Figure 32 Three-Dimensional Structure of tRNA

---

[38] No. They must be available for base pairing with the codon.

[39] The anticodon is different for each of the different tRNA molecules. Part of the rest of the molecule varies from one tRNA to the next, but about 60 percent is constant. The amino acid binding site is always the same: CCA (at the 3' end of the tRNA molecule).

tRNA molecules often contain nitrogenous bases in many positions that have been covalently modified. Base methylation is particularly common. Some specific examples are inosine (derived from adenine), pseudouridine (derived from uracil), or lysidine (derived from cytosine). Inosine in particular plays an important role in wobble base pairing.

The Wobble Hypothesis

Using the standard genetic code, you would guess that organisms have 61 distinct tRNA molecules to recognize the 61 amino acid-coding codons possible in mRNA. In actual fact, most organisms have fewer than 45 different types of tRNAs, meaning some anticodons must pair with more than one codon. Francis Crick's **Wobble Hypothesis** explains this and states that the first two codon-anticodon pairs obey normal base pairing rules, but the third position is more flexible (Figure 33). This allows for non-traditional pairing and explains why a smaller number of tRNAs are possible.

Figure 33   Wobble Base Pairing Between a tRNA Anticodon and an mRNA Codon

A modified inosine base (I) at the 5' end of the anticodon is particularly wobbly, as it can bond to three different codon bases (A, U, or C). Some common wobble pairing combinations are:

5' Base in Anticodon (tRNA)	3' Base in Codon (mRNA)
G	C (Watson-Crick base) or U (wobble base)
C	G
A	U
U	A (Watson-Crick base) or G (wobble base)
I	A, U, or C (all wobble bases)

In other words, the most common wobble base pairs are guanine-uracil, inosine-uracil, inosine-adenine, and inosine-cytosine (G-U, I-U, I-A, and I-C). Both the wobble base pair and the normal Watson-Crick base pair have similar thermodynamic stabilities.

Amino Acid Activation

Peptide bond formation during protein synthesis is a process that requires a lot of energy because the peptide bond has unfavorable thermodynamics ($\Delta G > 0$) and slow kinetics (high activation energy). Reaction coupling is used to power the process: two high-energy phosphate bonds are hydrolyzed to provide the energy to attach an amino acid to its tRNA molecule. This process is called **tRNA loading** or **amino acid activation**, and it is useful because breaking the aminoacyl-tRNA bond will drive peptide bond formation forward. Amino acid activation occurs in several steps:

1) An amino acid is attached to AMP to form *aminoacyl* AMP. In this reaction, the nucleophile is the acidic oxygen of the amino acid, and the leaving group is PP_i.

2) The pyrophosphate leaving group is hydrolyzed to 2 orthophosphates. This reaction is highly favorable ($\Delta G \ll 0$).

3) tRNA loading, an unfavorable reaction, is driven forward by the destruction of the high-energy aminoacyl—AMP bond created in Step 1.

Figure 34 Amino Acid Activation as an Example of Reaction Coupling
Note: water as a reactant has been left out of all reactions in this figure.

Overall, amino acid activation requires 2 ATP equivalents because it uses two high-energy bonds. An ATP equivalent is a single high-energy phosphate bond. You can get 2 ATP equivalents by hydrolyzing 2 ATP to 2 ADP + 2 P_i or by hydrolyzing 1 ATP to AMP + 2 P_i.

Eventually, the bond between the amino acid and the tRNA molecule will be broken. This hydrolysis will power peptide bond formation: the nitrogen of another amino acid will nucleophilically attack the carbonyl carbon of this amino acid, and tRNA will be the leaving group.

Aminoacyl-tRNA Synthetases

We have stated that incorporation of the appropriate amino acid in a growing polypeptide depends on the delivery of the correct amino acid by a specific tRNA. But we also noted that the amino acid acceptor sites of all tRNA molecules are the same. How is the attachment of the appropriate amino acid to each tRNA molecule accomplished? **Aminoacyl-tRNA synthetase enzymes** are specific to each amino acid, and there is at least one aminoacyl-tRNA synthetase for every amino acid. This family of enzymes recognizes both the tRNA and the amino acid based on their three-dimensional structures. They are highly specific, which is important because joining the wrong amino acid to a tRNA would result in the wrong amino acid being incorporated into a polypeptide. Given that some amino acids differ only by a single methyl group, this specificity is quite amazing. Aminoacyl-tRNA synthetases also function with a very low error rate. [If there is a 1/1000 error rate in amino acid incorporation, what percentage of polypeptides that are 500 amino acid residues long will not contain any errors?[40]]

Overall then, **amino acid activation** serves two functions. One is specific and accurate amino acid delivery, and the other is thermodynamic activation of the amino acid.

- A bacterial strain with a point mutation in the gene for hexokinase is not able to metabolize glucose. The mutation causes a substitution of arginine for serine. These bacteria are used to test whether chemicals are mutagenic. The chemical is added to a culture of bacteria with glucose as the only carbon source. Any bacteria that grow must have undergone a mutation which remedied the problem (this is called *suppression* of the original mutation). When a particular hair spray ingredient is tested, several colonies grow on the glucose-only medium. Which one of the following might act as a suppressor of the first mutation?[41]
    A) A point mutation during replication of a tRNA gene
    B) A mutation in RNA polymerase that increases the rate of promoter recognition
    C) A base pair deletion in the hexokinase gene
    D) A point mutation during transcription of a tRNA molecule

The Ribosome

The ribosome is composed of many polypeptides and rRNA chains held together in a massive quaternary structure. Ribosomes float around in the cytoplasm, and each has a small subunit and a large subunit. The unit of measurement is the Svedberg, or S, unit. Svedbergs are a measure of sedimentation rate, that is, how quickly something will sink in a gradient during centrifugation, thus the sum of the small and large subunits' S values is not the same as the S value of the whole ribosome.

---

[40] The easiest way to calculate this is to figure out the probability of getting *all* amino acids in the protein correct, in other words, we must use the *non*-error rate for our calculation, not the error rate. If the error rate is 1/1000, then the non-error rate is 999/1000. The probability of having no errors is $.999^n$, where n = the number of amino acid residues. In other words, a single amino acid has .999 probability, or 99.9% probability of being correct. Two amino acids correct in a row have a $.999 \times .999$ probability ($.999^2$), or .998, or 99.8% probability of happening. Continuing in this manner, a 500-amino acid protein has a $.999^{500}$ probability of being entirely correct, or .606, approximately a 60% probability. Longer proteins have a higher chance of containing errors.

[41] A single base change in the anticodon of the tRNA for arginine could cause it to recognize the codon for serine. If that happened in the mutant bacteria, problems might ensue, but one good result would be that the correct amino acid would be incorporated at the mutated site in hexokinase (choice **A** is correct; note that point mutations in tRNA genes are actually a common means of suppression in bacteria). Increasing the rate at which RNA polymerase recognizes the promoter might increase the rate of transcription, but it would not fix a mutant enzyme (choice B is wrong), and a base pair deletion in the hexokinase gene would cause a frameshift mutation and a serious significant change in protein structure and function (choice C is wrong). A point mutation during transcription of a tRNA molecule might have a temporary effect on a single bacterium, but it would not be passed on to its progeny; remember than only DNA mutations have lasting effects and errors made during transcription are generally insignificant (choice D is wrong).

The prokaryotic ribosome sediments in a gradient at a rate of 70S, so it is referred to as the **70S ribosome**. It is composed of a 30S small subunit and a 50S large subunit. Eukaryotes have an **80S ribosome**. It also has a small and large subunit. The large subunit sediments in a gradient at a rate of 60S. The small subunit sediments in a gradient at a rate of 40S. The large and small subunits of both prokaryotic and eukaryotic ribosomes are made up of many smaller peptides and several rRNA molecules (see Figure 35). The ribozymic activity of both prokaryotic and eukaryotic ribosomes is found in the large subunit and is associated with the rRNAs.

Figure 35   Ribosome Components

In both prokaryotes and eukaryotes, the complete ribosome (both subunits together) has three special binding sites. The **A site** (*a*minoacyl-tRNA site) is where each new tRNA delivers its amino acid. The **P site** (*p*eptidyl-tRNA site) is where the growing polypeptide chain, still attached to a tRNA, is located during translation. The **E site** (*e*xit-tRNA site) is where a now-empty tRNA sits prior to its release from the ribosome. [During translation, the next codon to be translated is exposed in the __[42].] tRNAs move through the sites from **A → P → E**.

---

[42] A site, since this is where the next amino acid to be added must bind.

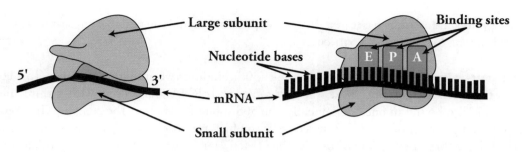

Figure 36 The Ribosome

Prokaryotic Translation

In prokaryotes, translation occurs in the same compartment and at the same time as transcription. In other words, *while the mRNA is being made*, ribosomes attach and begin translating it. [Does this mean that the first end of the mRNA to be translated is 5' or 3'?[43]] Note that it says ribosome**s** above. Several ribosomes attach to the mRNA and translate it simultaneously (see Figure 37; you may hear the term *polyribosome* used to describe this arrangement; polyribosomes are seen in both prokaryotes and eukaryotes). [You figured out the direction of translation on the mRNA from what you already know. Do you have any previous knowledge that would help you answer this: Does translation always begin at the 5' end of the mRNA, or somewhere up the chain?[44]]

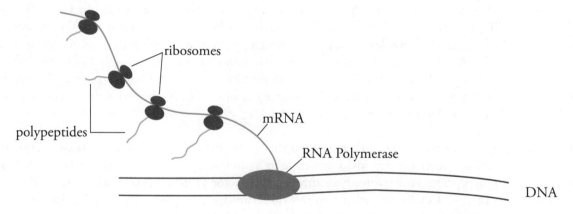

Figure 37 A Prokaryotic Polyribosome

Because prokaryotes often have polycistronic mRNAs, their ribosomes can also start translation in the middle of the chain. This means termination and initiation sequences are found between each ORF. Even for the first open reading frame on a transcript, translation doesn't begin right at the 5' end. An upstream regulatory sequence is essential for initiation, just as in transcription. Here, instead of a promoter, we have a **ribosome binding site**, also known as the **Shine-Dalgarno sequence**, located at −10 (ten ribonucleotides upstream, or on the 5' side of the start codon). The Shine-Dalgarno sequence is complementary to a pyrimidine-rich region on the small subunit, and thus helps position the initiation machinery on the transcript.

---

[43] 5' first, since the mRNA is made 5' end first. Transcription and translation go in the same direction on mRNA.

[44] It does not always occur at the very end. You can deduce this from the fact that mRNA is polycistronic. If there are more than one translation start sites on the mRNA, they can't all be at the 5' end.

Like transcription, translation has three distinct stages: initiation, elongation, and termination. Many antibiotics function by inhibiting a particular stage.[45]

Initiation starts with the small ribosomal subunit (30S) binding two initiation proteins. This complex then binds the mRNA transcript. Next, the first aminoacyl-tRNA joins, along with a third initiation factor, which is also bound to one GTP. Finally, the 50S subunit completes the complex. This process is powered by the hydrolysis of one GTP molecule.[46] The first aminoacyl-tRNA is special; it is called the **initiator tRNA**, abbreviated **fMet-tRNA$_{fMet}$**. The "fMet" stands for *formylmethionine*, which is a modified methionine used as the first amino acid in all prokaryotic proteins.[47] The initiator tRNA sits in the P site of the 70S ribosome, hydrogen-bonded with the **start codon**. [What is the start codon? Does this codon initiate translation wherever it appears?[48]] Before elongation, all initiation factors dissociate from the complex.

Elongation, a three-step cycle, may now begin. In the first step, the second aminoacyl-tRNA enters the A site and hydrogen bonds with the second codon. This process requires the hydrolysis of one phosphate from GTP. This is done by an elongation factor protein, which is a GTPase. In the second step, the **peptidyl transferase** activity of the large ribosomal subunit catalyzes the formation of a peptide bond between fMet and the second amino acid. The amino group of amino acid #2 acts as nucleophile, and tRNA$_{fMet}$ is the leaving group; it dissociates from the ribosome. A new dipeptide is now attached to tRNA #2. Now you can figure out the direction of translation from the point of view of the polypeptide; you won't have to memorize it.[49] The third step is **translocation**, in which tRNA #1 (now empty) moves into the E site, tRNA #2 (holding the growing peptide) moves into the P site, and the next codon to be translated moves into the A site. An elongation factor helps with translocation, and this process costs one GTP. The new dipeptide is still attached to tRNA #2, and tRNA #2 is still H-bonded to codon #2. The presence of tRNA #1 in the E site (still H-bonded to codon #1), is thought to help maintain the reading frame of the mRNA (disruption of tRNA binding to the E site results in an increase in the number of frameshift mutations in the resulting protein). [Does the ribosome move relative to the mRNA during translocation?[50]] These three steps repeat over and over again, connecting amino acids in the order their codons appear along the mRNA strand (and thus appear in the A site).

Termination occurs when a stop codon appears in the A site. Instead of a tRNA, a **release factor** now enters the A site. This causes the peptidyl transferase to hydrolyze the bond between the last tRNA and the completed polypeptide. Prokaryotes have three release factor proteins, two of which recognize stop codons and one that works with the other two to help terminate translation. Finally, the ribosome separates into its subunits and releases both mRNA and polypeptide.

---

[45] For example, streptomycin and tetracycline bind to the 30S subunit of the prokaryotic ribosome. Chloramphenicol and erythromycin bind to the 50S subunit.

[46] This may seem odd, as ATP is normally the energy molecule. But a high-energy phosphate is a high-energy phosphate. Another example is the GTP produced in the Krebs cycle.

[47] In fact, cells of our immune system release cytotoxins when they sniff out fMet, because this chemical is a sure sign that bacteria are busily translating.

[48] Refer to the genetic code table. The codon for methionine is AUG; that's the start codon. It only initiates translation when it is preceded by a Shine-Dalgarno sequence (prokaryotes).

[49] The direction of synthesis is N → C, since the N of amino acid #2 binds to the C of #1. As the polypeptide elongates, its N terminus will come snaking out of the ribosome.

[50] It must, if the tRNA remains H-bonded to the mRNA while moving to another spot in the ribosome.

4.8

Figure 38 Translation Elongation

Let's focus for a moment on the energetics of translation. Why doesn't peptide bond formation require GTP hydrolysis, like the other steps in translation?[51] You should be able to answer questions like this: How many high-energy phosphate bonds are required to make a 50 amino acid polypeptide chain, including the energy used to activate amino acids to aminoacyl-tRNAs?[52]

4.8

Eukaryotic Translation

There are several differences between eukaryotic and prokaryotic translation. Many of these have already been mentioned: the ribosome is larger (80S) and has different components than the prokaryotic ribosome, the mRNA must be processed before it can be translated (spliced, with cap and tail added), and the N-terminal amino acid is different (Met instead of fMet). Also remember that eukaryotic mRNA must not only be spliced, capped, and tailed, but it also requires transport from nucleus to cytoplasm, thus transcription and translation *cannot* proceed simultaneously.

Eukaryotes do not use the Shine-Dalgarno sequence to initiate translation. There are 5' UTR sequences in eukaryotes that function in starting translation; a common one is the *Kozak sequence*, which is a consensus sequence typically located a few nucleotides before the start codon.

Eukaryotic translation begins with formation of the initiation complex. The assembled complex is recruited to the 5' capped end of the transcript, by an initiation complex of proteins. Additional proteins are recruited (such as a poly-A tail binding protein) and the initiation complex starts scanning the mRNA from the 5' end, looking for a start codon. Once the start codon has been found, the large ribosomal subunit (60S) is recruited and translation can begin.

---

[51] Because the bond between each amino acid and its tRNA is a high-energy bond whose hydrolysis drives peptide bond formation. Remember that the aminoacyl-tRNA bond was formed using the energy of two phosphate bonds from ATP.

[52] There are two phosphate bonds hydrolyzed per amino acid to make the aminoacyl-tRNAs, or 100 for the 50 amino acid polypeptide. Two phosphate bonds are required for each elongation step, one for the entrance of each new aminoacyl-tRNA into the ribosomal A site and the other for translocation. Since there are 49 elongation steps for a 50-amino acid protein, 98 high-energy bonds are hydrolyzed during elongation. Finally, one GTP is hydrolyzed during initiation to position the first tRNA and mRNA on the ribosome, and one GTP is hydrolyzed in termination. Thus, a total of 200 high-energy bonds are required for the translation of a 50-amino acid protein. In other words, it costs $4n$ high-energy bonds to make a peptide chain, where n is the number of amino acids in the chain.

The order in which the initiation complex is formed is different in eukaryotes. [Are the nascent (newly formed) polypeptide chains emerging from a polyribosome in a eukaryote all the same?[53]] Eukaryotic translation termination involves two release factors, that, like their prokaryotic counterparts, recognize stop codons and work together to end translation and release the completed polypeptide.

- Which one of the following pairs of processes may occur simultaneously on the same RNA molecule in a eukaryotic cell?[54]
    A) Translation and transcription
    B) Transcription and splicing
    C) Splicing and translation
    D) Messenger RNA degradation and transcription

Cap-Independent Translation

It was long thought that all eukaryotic translation started at the 5' end of an mRNA. In other words, all eukaryotic transcripts were assumed to be monocistronic, and coded for only one polypeptide chain. It is true that this mechanism is by far the major one in eukaryotic cells. Because of the important role of 5' mRNA cap recognition, it's called **cap-dependent translation**.

However, it's recently been discovered that eukaryotes are sometimes capable of starting translation in the middle of an mRNA molecule, a process called **cap-independent translation** (because the beginning of translation doesn't require the 5' cap of the mRNA). To do this, the transcript must have an internal ribosome entry site, or IRES. This is a specialized nucleotide sequence, and was first discovered in viruses. Since then, IRESs have been found in a number of eukaryotic transcripts. Most code for proteins that help the cell deal with stress, or help activate apoptosis. In other words, the IRESs found so far make sure the cell can make essential proteins when under sub-optimal growth conditions. Cells under stress generally inhibit translation (via inhibiting translation initiation), and cap-independent translation allows the cell to make proteins when doing so is crucial for survival or programmed cell death. Activation of translation using an IRES requires different proteins than normal initiation.

Additional nucleotide sequences have been identified, which allow cap-independent translation in eukaryotes. While some of these are used in molecular biology labs, it's unclear how or if they function in normal eukaryotic cells.

---

[53] In eukaryotes, the answer is: yes, always, because eukaryotic mRNA is monocistronic. In prokaryotes, however, different polypeptides may be translated from a single piece of mRNA, since prokaryotic mRNA is polycistronic.

[54] In order for processes in eukaryotes to occur simultaneously, they must occur in the same compartment. Transcription and splicing both occur in the nucleus and could therefore occur simultaneously (choice **B** is correct). Translation occurs in the cytoplasm, while transcription and splicing occur in the nucleus, thus translation cannot occur at the same time as either of these processes (choices A and C are wrong). mRNA degradation and transcription cannot occur at the same time; if this were true, no mRNA molecules would survive to be translated (choice D is wrong).

4.9 CONTROLLING GENE EXPRESSION

Adult humans have over 220 different types of cells, all with the same genome, but with different attributes such as morphology, lifespan, function, ability to secrete, response to signaling molecules, mobility, etc. These changes are due to differences in gene expression and protein function. In each cell type, some genes are expressed and others are silenced; further, genes that are expressed can have different levels of expression, where in one cell type the gene is expressed at a high level (to produce lots of ncRNA or protein), and in a different cell type the same gene is expressed at a low level. They can also have varying activity, stability, and half-life. These variations in gene expression can be altered using many different mechanisms:

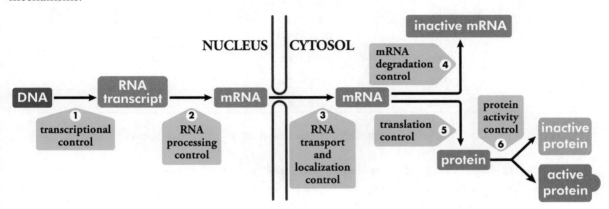

Figure 39 Mechanisms of Controlling Gene Expression in Eukaryotes

Transcription is the principle site of the regulation of gene expression in both eukaryotes and prokaryotes. This means that the amount of each protein made in every cell is affected by the amount of mRNA that gets transcribed. Gene expression can also be controlled epigenetically. Broadly speaking, **epigenetics** focuses on changes in gene expression that are not due to changes in DNA sequences, but are either heritable or have a long-term effect. The three most commonly studied areas in this field are DNA methylation, chromatin remodeling, and RNA interference. Let's look at the regulation of gene expression, starting with DNA and working down toward proteins.

Controlling Gene Expression at the DNA Level

DNA Methylation and Chromatin Remodeling

Both prokaryotic and eukaryotic DNA can be covalently modified by adding a methyl group. Bacteria methylate new DNA shortly after synthesis, and the brief delay is useful in mismatch repair pathways (see above). Methylation can also control gene expression in prokaryotes, either by promoting or inhibiting transcription.

Eukaryotic DNA methylation has been found in every vertebrate genome studied so far. Broadly speaking, it plays an important role in controlling gene expression (especially during embryonic development), and has also been implicated in several diseases.

DNA methylation turns off eukaryotic gene expression two ways:

1) Methylation physically blocks the gene from transcriptional proteins.
2) Certain proteins bind methylated CpG groups and recruit chromatin remodeling proteins that change the winding of DNA around histones.

- Regulation of a gene is examined *in vitro* in the presence and absence of chromatin assembly, and in the presence and absence of a sequence-specific regulator of transcription. Transcription is quantitated after the experiment and the following results are obtained:

	Sequence-Specific Factor	DNA	Relative Amount of Transcription
1.	None	unpackaged	0.74
2.	None	packaged	0.07
3.	Present	unpackaged	1.0
4.	Present	packaged	0.59

Which one of the following conclusions can be drawn from this experiment?[55]

A) The degree of activation by the sequence-specific factor is greater in the presence of chromatin assembly than in its absence.
B) The sequence-specific factor acts to repress transcription.
C) The histones increase the rate of transcription.
D) The sequence-specific factor increases the rate of transition from a closed complex to an open complex.

Gene Dose

One way to increase gene expression is to increase the copy number of a gene by amplification. Increasing gene dose will allow a cell to make large quantities of the corresponding protein. Similarly, gene deletion causes a decrease in gene expression. Both are examples of copy number variation, discussed earlier in Section 4.2.

Imprinting

Genomic imprinting is when only one allele of a gene is expressed. In some situations, the maternal allele is expressed, and in others, the paternal allele is expressed. Imprinted genes tend to be clustered together on chromosomes. Imprinting is a dynamic process and can change from generation to generation. In other words, a gene that is imprinted in an adult may be "unimprinted" and expressed in that adult's offspring. This observation led to the notion that imprinting is an epigenetic process. Silencing of a certain gene involves DNA methylation, histone modification, and binding of long ncRNAs. These epigenetic marks are established in the germline and are maintained throughout life and mitotic divisions.

---

[55] A quick glance at the data indicates that transcription is increased in the presence of the sequence-specific factor (compare lines 1 and 2 with lines 3 and 4; choice B is wrong), and that histones decrease the rate of transcription (packaged DNA has a lower rate of transcription than unpackaged; choice C is wrong). Looking closer, it appears that the sequence specific factor causes an approximate 8-fold increase in the transcription rate of packaged DNA (compare lines 2 and 4), but it doesn't even double the rate of transcription of unpackaged DNA (compare lines 1 and 3). It might be that this occurs because the factor increases the rate of transition to an open complex, but there is no data to support this (choice **A** is a better answer than choice D). Don't confuse "open complex" (which means separated DNA strands) with "unpackaged" (which means not wrapped around histones).

X Chromosome Inactivation

Female mammals have two X chromosomes, one of which is active (called Xa) and one of which is silenced, or inactive (and is called Xi). In humans, X-inactivation occurs early in development, at the blastocyst stage (Chapter 13). Each cell in the inner cell mass randomly inactivates an X chromosome, and this decision is irreversible. This means every cell derived from each cell in the inner cell mass will have the same X chromosome inactivated, however, because each cell makes its own decision, an adult can have different X chromosomes inactivated in different tissues and cells. Because of X-inactivation, all humans have the same number of gene products for the X chromosome; males have only one X chromosome, and females have only one *active* X chromosome. Not all animals behave the same when it comes to X-inactivation. Some animals (such as marsupials) consistently silence one X chromosome; in the case of marsupials, the paternally derived X chromosome is inactivated and the maternal X chromosome is active. Xi is very condensed, and packaged in heterochromatin. It has high levels of DNA methylation.

Controlling Gene Expression at the RNA Level: Regulation of Transcription in Prokaryotes

Regulation of transcription is the primary method of regulation of gene expression in prokaryotes. One simple mechanism of transcriptional regulation in bacteria is that some promoters are simply stronger than others. The problem with this mechanism of regulation is that it is "pre-set" and cannot respond to changing conditions within the cell. Bacteria also possess far more complex regulatory mechanisms, which activate or suppress transcription depending on current needs for specific gene products. For example, bacteria only produce the enzyme β-galactosidase and other proteins required for lactose catabolism when lactose is present. [Assuming these protein products do not have a harmful effect on the cell, what advantage might there be in turning off the genes when the protein products are not required?[56]]

- Are the terms *polypeptide enzyme* and *gene product* synonymous? Or are there gene products that are not polypeptide enzymes? Are there polypeptides which are not enzymes?[57]

Enzymes involved in anabolism (biosynthesis) should be produced when the item they help make (their product) is scarce. Enzymes involved in catabolism (degradative metabolism) should be produced when the item they help break down (their substrate) is abundant, such as food. Thus, there are two basic ways we can imagine how transcription is regulated. The transcription of enzymes involved in biosynthetic pathways should be inhibited by their product. The transcription of enzymes involved in catabolic pathways should be automatically inhibited whenever the substrate is not around, and activated when it is. That is in fact exactly what happens. Anabolic enzymes whose transcription is inhibited in the presence of excess amounts of product are **repressible**. Catabolic enzymes whose transcription can be stimulated by the abundance of a substrate are called **inducible enzymes**.[58]

---

[56] It takes a great deal of ATP to synthesize RNA and protein, so it's more energy-efficient to transcribe and translate only the proteins that are needed.

[57] They are not synonymous. All polypeptides are gene products, but some gene products are not polypeptides and some polypeptides are not enzymes. Transfer RNA and rRNA are gene products, but not polypeptides. Microfilaments and other elements of the cytoskeleton, as well as collagen and many other polypeptides, are not enzymes.

[58] So note: the default for repressible systems is "ON"; for inducible systems the default is "OFF."

There are two common examples of this. The **lac operon** is inducible, since the enzymes it codes for are part of lactose catabolism, and the **trp operon** is repressible, since the enzymes it codes for mediate tryptophan biosynthesis or anabolism. An operon has two components, a coding sequence for enzymes, and upstream regulatory sequences or control sites. Operons may also include genes for regulatory proteins, such as repressors or activators, but they don't have to. These genes can be located elsewhere in the genome and typically have their own promoters.

The Lac Operon

The lac operon contains several components:

1) P region: the promoter site on DNA to which RNA polymerase binds to initiate transcription of *Y*, *Z*, and *A* genes
2) O region: the operator site to which the Lac repressor binds
3) *Z* gene: codes for the enzyme β-galactosidase, which cleaves lactose into glucose and galactose
4) *Y* gene: codes for permease, a protein which transports lactose into the cell
5) *A* gene: codes for transacetylase, an enzyme which transfers an acetyl group from acetyl-CoA to β-galactosides (note that this function is not required for lactose metabolism)

Additionally, there are two genes, each with their own promoter, that code for proteins important in the regulation of the lac operon:

1) *crp* gene: located at a distant site, this gene codes for a catabolite activator protein (CAP) and helps couple the lac operon to glucose levels in the cell
2) *I* gene: located at a distant site, this gene codes for the Lac repressor protein

So overall, there are five protein coding genes and two regulatory sequences. Both *crp* and *I* have their own promoters. The protein products of these two genes control gene expression of *Z*, *Y*, and *A*.

Bacterial cells preferentially use glucose as an energy source. This means that in the presence of glucose, the lac operon will be off, or expressed at low amounts (see Figures 40 and 41). This is mediated by the CAP and repressor proteins. Glucose levels control adenylyl cyclase, which converts ATP to cAMP. In high glucose conditions, adenylyl cyclase is inactivated and cAMP levels are very low. In low glucose conditions, the opposite is true: adenylyl cyclase is activated and cAMP levels are high. CAP binds cAMP and this complex binds the promoter of the lac operon (Figure 42). This helps activate RNA polymerase at the lac operon and contributes to the operon being turned on when glucose levels are low.

The *I* gene codes for a repressor protein, which binds the operator of the lac operon. This prevents RNA pol from binding the promoter and transcribing *Z*, *Y*, and *A* genes, thereby blocking transcription of the operon when lactose is absent (Figure 40). The repressor protein can also bind lactose, and this blocks its activity on the operator. This binding is allosteric, and it causes a conformational change in the tertiary structure of the repressor protein, such that it is no longer capable of binding to the operator. As a consequence, it falls off the DNA (Figures 41 and 42).

High transcription of *Z*, *Y*, and *A* genes occurs when glucose is absent and lactose is present (Figure 42, page 116). Low glucose results in an increased amount of cAMP, which binds to CAP and helps activate RNA polymerase activity at the lac operon. Lactose presence means the Lac repressor protein is unable to bind the lac operator and negatively regulate transcription; thus, the polycistronic mRNA is transcribed at high levels. When the supply of lactose becomes very scarce, there isn't enough to bind to the repressors, and most of the repressor proteins return to their original structure. They now rebind to the operator, decreasing transcription of *Z*, *Y*, and *A* genes.

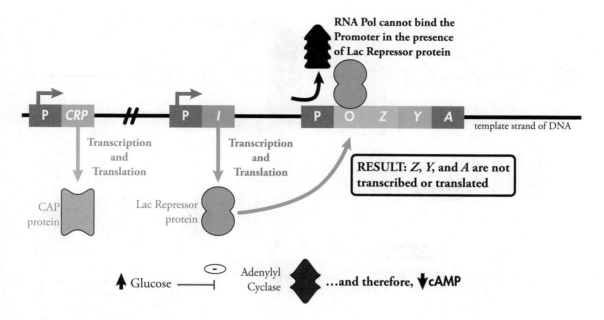

RNA Pol cannot bind the Promoter in the presence of Lac Repressor protein

RESULT: *Z, Y,* and *A* are not transcribed or translated

↑ Glucose ⊖ Adenylyl Cyclase ...and therefore, ↓cAMP

Figure 40 The Lac Operon in the Presence of Glucose and Absence of Lactose

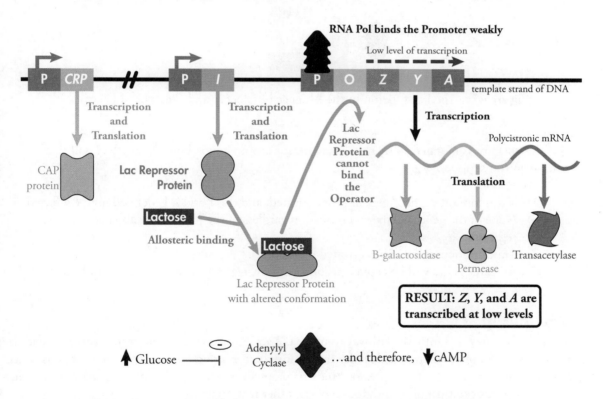

RNA Pol binds the Promoter weakly

Low level of transcription

Transcription

Polycistronic mRNA

Translation

Lac Repressor Protein cannot bind the Operator

B-galactosidase   Permease   Transacetylase

RESULT: *Z, Y,* and *A* are transcribed at low levels

Allosteric binding

↑ Glucose ⊖ Adenylyl Cyclase ...and therefore, ↓cAMP

Figure 41 The Lac Operon in the Presence of both Glucose and Lactose

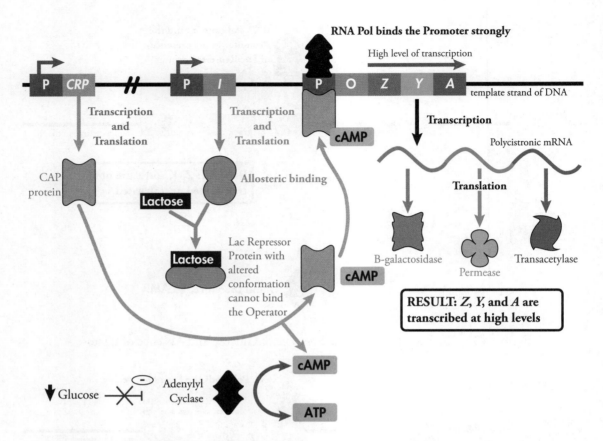

Figure 42 The Lac Operon in the Absence of Glucose and Presence of Lactose

- If the operator is mutated so that the lac repressor can no longer bind, what effect will this have on transcription?[59]

  A) Transcription of the *Z* gene will be activated, and the *Y* and *A* genes will not be affected.
  B) None of the genes will be transcribed, regardless of the presence or absence of lac repressor.
  C) Transcription will still be activated by lactose.
  D) All three genes will be expressed constitutively, regardless of the presence of lactose.

The Trp Operon

Bacteria use a five enzyme synthetic pathway to make the amino acid tryptophan from chorismic acid. In the presence of tryptophan, there is little point in making these enzymes, so the repressor protein is coded by the *trpR* gene (Figure 43). The repressor binds tryptophan when it is present, and the two together then bind the operator to turn off transcription of the other five trp genes.

---

[59] If the repressor cannot bind to the operator, nothing will prevent RNA polymerase from transcribing all the genes on the operon in an unregulated, constitutive (or continuous) fashion (choice **D** is true and choice B is false). All genes on the operon are expressed or repressed together (choice A is false), and lactose will no longer have any effect (the expression of the genes is unregulated, so choice C is false).

With no tryptophan present, the repressor protein cannot bind the operator. Without this block, RNA polymerase transcribes the five genes in the trp operon, and the five gene products allow the cell to make tryptophan. This is an example of anabolic repressible transcription.

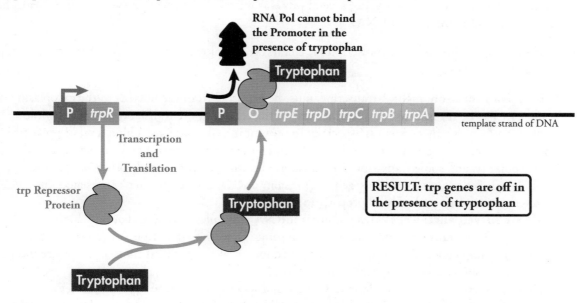

Figure 43 The Trp Operon in the Presence of Tryptophan

Control of Gene Expression at the RNA Level: Regulation of Transcription in Eukaryotes

Given the complexity of eukaryotes compared to prokaryotes, it is not surprising that the regulation of eukaryotic transcription is also more complex. Most of this regulation happens at initiation.

For protein-coding genes, there are upstream control elements (UCEs), usually about 200 bases upstream of the initiation site, a core promoter containing binding sites for the basal transcription complex and RNA polymerase II (about 50 bases upstream of the transcription start site), and a TATA box at –25. The TATA box is a highly conserved DNA recognition sequence for the TATA box binding protein (TBP). Binding of TBP to the TATA box initiates transcription complex assembly at the promoter.

Enhancer sequences in DNA are bound by **activator proteins**, and this is another kind of transcriptional regulation. The enhancer may be located many thousands of base pairs away from a promoter (either upstream or downstream) and still regulate transcription. This is likely done by DNA looping so enhancers and their activator proteins can get close to transcriptional machinery.

Eukaryotes also have **gene repressor proteins**, which inhibit transcription; this can also be done by modifying chromatin structure. *Transcription factors* have DNA-binding domains and are crucial in transcription regulation. They can bind promoters or other regulatory sequences. In fact, in many cases, transcription levels in eukaryotes are controlled by huge committees of proteins. This produces a combinatorial effect, where each protein contributes to regulation, and can itself be regulated. These complex networks help link transcription to cell signaling and status. The binding of transcriptional machinery to DNA is often regulated by extracellular signals. For example, steroid hormones bind to receptors in the cell, and this sends the receptor to the nucleus. The complex binds DNA to regulate transcription. [If a mutation in a eukaryotic fat cell reduces the level of several proteins related to fat metabolism, does this mean the proteins are encoded by the same mRNA?[60]]

Beyond regulating the initiation of transcription, eukaryotes employ several other methods of transcriptional regulation, including:

- **RNA Translocation**: mRNA transcripts must be exported from the nucleus to the cytoplasm and can also be transported to different areas of the cell. They are translationally silent while this is happening. This system is especially important in cells that have a high level of polarity, where one area or end of the cell is distinctly different from the other. For example, neurons have polarity, and some transcripts are transported to the dendrites, while others stay in the soma. This is a way of controlling gene expression: mRNA transcripts aren't translated into proteins until they are localized properly in the cell.
- **mRNA Surveillance**: Cells closely monitor mRNA molecules to ensure that only high-quality mRNA transcripts are read by the ribosome. Defective transcripts (such as those with premature stop codons, or those without stop codons at all) and stalled transcripts (where the ribosome is stalled in translation) are degraded.
- **RNA Interference**: RNA interference (RNAi) is a way to silence gene expression after a transcript has been made. It is mediated by miRNA and siRNA (Section 4.7). Molecular biology labs often use the RNAi system experimentally, as a way to decrease protein expression (see Appendix). Generally speaking, the siRNAs bind complementary sequences on mRNAs, and this ds-RNA is then degraded. The amount of transcript in the cell decreases, and gene expression is thus negatively regulated.

Control of Gene Expression at the Protein Level: Translation Initiation

We've already discussed the complex process of assembling translational machinery. In both prokaryotes and eukaryotes, this is a highly regulated process that links protein synthesis with upstream signaling pathways. Otherwise there is little control at the level of translation.

Post-Translational Modification

Newly synthesized proteins released from the ribosome are rarely able to function. They need to be correctly folded, modified, or processed, and transported to where they function in the cell. These modifications are called post-translational events, since they occur after protein synthesis.

---

[60] No, it does not. *Eukaryotic mRNA is monocistronic.* A more likely explanation is that a number of different genes located throughout the genome have related regulatory sequences that bind the same sequence-specific transcription factors. This is the means used by eukaryotes to achieve coordinated expression of genes. Related proteins are clumped together on the same piece of mRNA in prokaryotes only.

Protein Folding

First, the newly synthesized nascent protein is folded into its correct three-dimensional shape. This is accomplished by a family of proteins called **chaperones**. If folded correctly, the protein is said to be in its native conformation. If the protein is unfolded or misfolded, it's said to be in its non-native state. Chaperone proteins are found across all types of organisms (from bacteria to plants to mammals), and also function in assembly or folding of other macromolecular structures. For example, chaperone proteins assist in nucleosome assembly from folded histones and DNA. In eukaryotic cells, chaperones are found in many subcellular compartments.

Covalent Modification

Many proteins are covalently modified. Some have hydrophobic groups added to facilitate membrane localization. For example, the addition of a fatty acid can target a protein to a membrane (either the plasma membrane or an organelle membrane).

Smaller chemical groups can also be added. For example, proteins can be:

- Acetylated: addition of an acetyl group ($-C(O)CH_3$), usually at the N-terminus of a protein, or at a lysine amino acid
- Formylated: addition of a formyl group ($-C(O)H$)
- Alkylated: addition of an alkyl group (such as methyl, ethyl, etc.). Methylation is a common post-translational modification, and is usually done to lysine or arginine amino acids.
- Glycosylated: addition of a glycosyl group to arginine, asparagine, cysteine, serine, threonine, tyrosine, or tryptophan amino acids. A glycosyl group is the substituent form of a cyclic mono- , di-, or oligosaccharide. This results in a glycoprotein.
- Phosphorylated: addition of a phosphate group (PO_4^{3-}) to a serine, threonine, tyrosine, or histidine amino acid
- Sulphated: addition of a sulphate group (SO_4^{2-}) to a tyrosine amino acid

Proteins can also be linked to other proteins. For example, in ubiquitination, proteins are covalently linked to ubiquitin.

There are many other examples of protein covalent modification. Overall, these modifications can have many effects on a protein and its function. They can change protein subcellular localization, target a protein for degradation, change interactions between proteins and other molecules, activate or inhibit enzyme activity, or change enzyme affinity for substrates. These modifications are typically studied in the lab using mass spectrometry (see *MCAT Organic Chemistry Review*), western blotting, or eastern blotting (see Appendix).

Processing

Many proteins require cleavage of some sort to become mature or functional. Cleavage can occur at either end of a peptide chain, or in the middle. Protein precursors are often used when the mature protein may be dangerous to the organism. Because the precursor is already made, it allows large quantities of mature protein to be available on short notice. Enzyme precursors are called **zymogens** or **proenzymes**.

A well-known example of post-translational processing is insulin. Insulin is made from a prohormone (Figure 44, next page); preproinsulin is the primary translational product of the human *INS* gene. This peptide is 110 amino acids in length. To form proinsulin, an N-terminus signal peptide is removed and

4.9

disulphide bonds form in the endoplasmic reticulum. Three cleavage events are necessary to process pro-insulin: the C peptide is removed by a family of enzymes called proprotein convertases, and a dipeptide fragment is removed from the C-terminus of the B chain peptide by a carboxypeptidase. These cleavage events occur in a secretory vesicle. The biological effects of insulin are well known, but it's recently been shown that peptide C also has signaling properties.

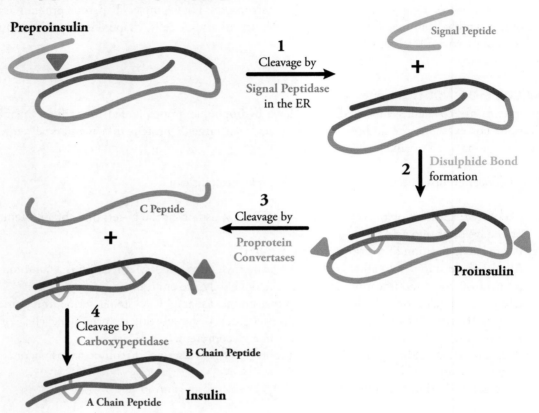

Figure 44   Insulin Processing: An Example of Post-Translational Modification

4.10   RETURN TO GENE STRUCTURE: A SUMMARY

Now that we have been through all the processes that a cell uses to turn a gene into a protein, and control this process, let's review the components once again (Figure 45). Transcription begins at a start site but needs a promoter upstream of this. It ends at a termination signal. The RNA transcript contains the open reading frame (which goes from start codon to stop codon), as well as both 5' and 3' regulatory regions.

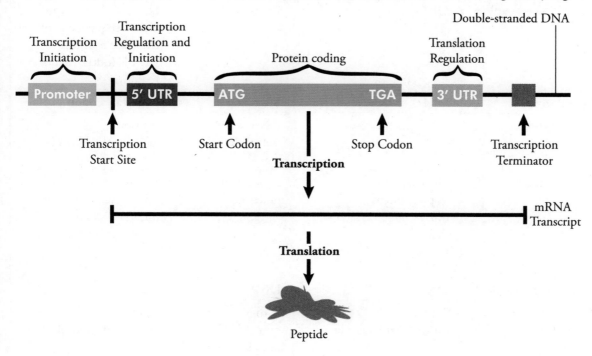

Figure 45   Gene Structure and Protein Expression

DNA replication, transcription, and translation have many similarities and some differences, and these are summarized in Table 1.

Table 1 A Review of Molecular Biology Processes

	DNA Replication	Transcription	Translation
Signal to get ready	ORI	Promoter	• Shine-Dalgarno (prok) • Kozak sequence (euk) • these are found in 5'UTR (untranslated region)
Signal to start	ORI	Start site	AUG start codon
Key synthesis enzyme	DNA polymerase	RNA polymerase	Ribosome (made of rRNA and peptides)
Other important enzymes	Helicase Topoisomerase SSBPs Primase Ligase Telomerase	Spliceosome machinery	Aminoacyl tRNA synthetases Initiation factors Elongation factors Release factors
Template molecule	DNA	DNA	mRNA
Read direction	3' to 5' on the DNA template	3' to 5' on the DNA template	5' to 3' on the RNA template
Molecule synthesized	DNA	RNA (mRNA in prok, hnRNA in euk)	Peptides
Build direction	5' to 3'	5' to 3'	N-terminus to C-terminus
Prokaryotic location	Cytoplasm	Cytoplasm	Cytoplasm
Eukaryotic location	Nucleus	Nucleus	Cytoplasm
Signal to stop	When the replication bubbles or newly synthesized strands meet and are ligated together	Transcription stop sequence or poly-A sequence	Stop codon (UAG, UGA, UAA)

4.10

Chapter 4 Summary

- DNA is the fundamental unit of inheritance in cells.

- DNA and RNA are polymers, made of nucleotide monomers. A nucleotide contains phosphate group(s), a sugar (either deoxyribose for DNA or ribose for RNA), and a nitrogenous base, either a purine (adenine or guanine) or a pyrimidine (thymine, cytosine, or uracil).

- In DNA, adenine always pairs with thymine via two hydrogen bonds, and cytosine always pairs with guanine via three hydrogen bonds.

- Uracil replaces thymine in RNA, and the ribose in RNA has an OH group on carbon 2.

- DNA is supercoiled in prokaryotes and packaged around histone proteins in eukaryotes.

- Eukaryotic DNA is divided into several linear chromosomes which have unique structures, including the long (q) and short (p) arms, centromere and telomeres on the ends.

- Genomes have extensive variation, including single nucleotide polymorphisms and copy number variation; transposons are mobile genetic elements which also contribute to genomic variation.

- Mutations can occur spontaneously, or can be caused by environmental factors (such as ionizing radiation), chemicals, or biological agents.

- Point mutations are classified based on their effect on the DNA (transition/transversion) or their effect on the amino acid sequence (missense, nonsense, or silent).

- Frameshift mutations are caused by insertions or deletions in the DNA base sequence that affect the reading frame of a gene. These are generally very serious mutations because they affect every amino acid codon from the point of the mutation on.

- Other types of mutations include inversions, translocations, and rearrangements.

- Transposons are mobile genetic elements that can "jump" from chromosome to chromosome. This can lead to deletions, insertions, and mutations. They consist of two inverted repeats flanking the gene for transposase and may include other genes as well.

- DNA replication occurs in the S-phase of the cell cycle and is semiconservative in nature.

- Several enzymes are involved in DNA replication. Helicases unwind the parental DNA at the origin of replication. Primases synthesize an RNA primer. DNA polymerase synthesizes new DNA, proofreads, and replaces the RNA primer. DNA ligase attaches the Okazaki fragments in the lagging strand.

- Cells have developed several ways to fix mutations, including: direct reversal, homology-dependent repair pathways (such as excision repair and post-replication repair), double-strand break repair (such as homologous recombination and nonhomologous end joining), and SOS repair.

- Transcription is the first part of protein synthesis; it is the creation of an RNA transcript by an RNA polymerase that reads the DNA template. Translation is the second part of protein synthesis; it is the creation of a polypeptide chain by ribosomes that read the mRNA transcript.

- There are several types of RNA that do not encode proteins. Some are directly involved in translation (rRNA and tRNA), while others play a role in gene expression (snRNA, miRNA, siRNA).

- Key info about prokaryotes: theta replication, genome is a single circular piece of DNA, three different DNA polymerases, one RNA polymerase, no mRNA processing, polycistronic mRNA, simultaneous transcription/translation, smaller ribosomes.

- Key info about eukaryotes: replication bubbles, genome is several linear pieces of DNA, one DNA polymerase, three RNA polymerases, capping, tailing, and splicing of mRNA prior to translation, monocistronic mRNA, transcription in nucleus, translation in cytosol, larger ribosomes.

CHAPTER 4 FREESTANDING PRACTICE QUESTIONS

1. A competitive inhibitor of eukaryotic RNA polymerase III would have the greatest effect on:

A) replication.
B) reverse transcription.
C) translation.
D) mutation.

2. In the lac operon, transcription is regulated by a repressor protein and only takes place in the presence of lactose. Which of the following statements is correct?

A) The repressor protein binds to the promoter site to inhibit transcription.
B) Lactose binds to the promoter site to initiate transcription.
C) Lactose binds to the repressor protein to inhibit transcription.
D) The repressor protein binds the operator site to inhibit transcription.

3. Which of the following could not be caused by a single point mutation in the DNA?

A) Ala-Gln-Cys-Asp-Leu → Ala-Gln
B) Ala-Gln-Cys-Asp-Leu → Ala-Gln-Cys-Asp-Leu
C) Ala-Gln-Cys-Asp-Leu → Ala-Gln-Cys-His-Lys
D) Ala-Gln-Cys-Asp-Leu → Ala-Gln-Cys-His-Leu

4. Which of the following is/are true with respect to eukaryotic mRNA?

   I. Monocistronic
   II. Transcription stops at the stop codon
   III. Has the same sequence as the template DNA that it was transcribed from

A) I only
B) I and II
C) II and III
D) I, II, and III

5. Which of the following is NOT a similarity between replication and transcription?

A) Both processes occur with the same fidelity.
B) Polymerization in both processes is based on reading a template.
C) A pyrophosphate is removed from every nucleotide as polymerization occurs.
D) Both processes occur in the 5' to 3' direction.

6. Which of the following functions is NOT typically attributed to small nuclear RNA (snRNA)?

A) Processing of pre-mRNA
B) Regulation of transcription factors
C) Coordinating amino acid addition in translation
D) Maintaining telomeres

7. Organisms with a higher degree of complexity do not necessarily have more diverse genomes than less complex organisms, in spite of the need for a greater diversity of proteins. Post-translational modification is one method used by more complex organisms to produce proteins that serve a wider variety of distinct functions. Which of the following explains this phenomenon?

A) The genome itself is manipulated by the agents responsible for post-translational modification in order to yield an increase in the number of transcriptional products.
B) Post-translational modification alters the structures and functions of proteins produced from a relatively smaller number of genes.
C) hnRNA is modified by the actions of post-transcriptional agents to provide increased variety in the mRNA used for translation.
D) Post-translational modifications enhance the ability of the ribosome to produce distinct protein products.

CHAPTER 4 PRACTICE PASSAGE

Protein synthesis involves a number of complex steps, from transcription of the gene through to translation and post-translational modification. After mRNA is transcribed in eukaryotes, it must be processed (capped, poly-A tailed, and spliced) before it can be translated. Prokaryotes do not need to process their mRNA.

Due to the exonuclease activity of DNA polymerase, DNA replication is generally a high-fidelity process. Random errors occasionally occur and these mutations are classified as *frameshift mutations* (insertions or deletions in the base sequence) or *point mutations* (a single base pair change). Any mutation is subject to natural selection, with advantageous mutations preserved and the most deleterious mutations eliminated quickly. Thus, areas of the genome that appear to evolve very slowly (i.e., have a slower rate of mutation than other areas) do not actually have a slower rate; rather, that area is highly critical to normal functioning of the organism involved.

Point mutations can be further classified by their final effect on the mature protein. Because of the redundancy of the genetic code, some mutations do not alter the final amino acid sequence of the protein and are referred to as *silent mutations*. However, it was discovered that all redundant codons are not equal; some are used preferentially to enhance the speed or accuracy of protein translation. tRNAs corresponding to redundant codons are not found equally in the cell; some tRNAs are more common than others. Silent mutations can cause phenotypic changes by altering mRNA stem-and-loop folding, half-life, and splicing sites. Thus, mutations formerly considered "silent" have now been implicated in a number of different disorders, such as Marfan syndrome, phenylketonuria, Seckel syndrome, and increased pain sensitivity.

1st Position (5' End)	2nd Position				3rd Position (3' End)
	U	C	A	G	
U	Phe	Ser	Tyr	Cys	U
	Phe	Ser	Tyr	Cys	C
	Leu	Ser	**Stop**	**Stop**	A
	Leu	Ser	**Stop**	Trp	G
C	Leu	Pro	His	Arg	U
	Leu	Pro	His	Arg	C
	Leu	Pro	Gln	Arg	A
	Leu	Pro	Gln	Arg	G
A	Ile	Thr	Asn	Ser	U
	Ile	Thr	Asn	Ser	C
	Ile	Thr	Lys	Arg	A
	Met	Thr	Lys	Arg	G
G	Val	Ala	Asp	Gly	U
	Val	Ala	Asp	Gly	C
	Val	Ala	Glu	Gly	A
	Val	Ala	Glu	Gly	G

Figure 1 The Genetic Code

1. Based on information in the passage, genes coding for particularly abundant proteins in a cell would have all of the following EXCEPT:

A) codons corresponding to abundant tRNAs.
B) equal use of redundant codons.
C) greater use of preferential codons.
D) high-fidelity replication.

2. Which of following could account for the changes brought on by silent mutations in both eukaryotes and prokaryotes?

   I.   Decrease in mRNA half-life
  II. Disruption of splicing sites
 III. Changes in mRNA folding

A) I and II only
B) II and III only
C) I and III only
D) I, II, and III

3. Researchers studying a gene associated with breast cancer found that regions where silent mutations occur ("silent sites") in this gene evolve very slowly compared to other regions within this gene. Comparisons were made between mice and humans. Which of the following is most likely true about this gene?

A) Mutations at other sites are more detrimental to the health of the organism than mutations at the silent sites.
B) Mutations at the silent sites increase the accuracy of mRNA splicing.
C) Mutations within the silent sites often lead to the death of the organism.
D) The silent sites are less critical to overall function than the other sites.

4. Researchers studying the DNA polymerase activity in several different organisms discovered a mutant *E. coli* polymerase that retained almost 100% of wild-type activity. Which of the following active-site missense mutations is LEAST likely to affect enzyme activity?

A) A → D
B) V → L
C) R → G
D) L → W

5. Point mutations are found in three subclasses: nonsense mutations, missense mutations, and silent mutations. Which of the following represents a silent mutation?

A) UGC to UGA
B) UUA to CUA
C) CAC to CAA
D) CAU to CUU

6. How could changing the half-life of an mRNA lead to phenotypic changes?

A) A shorter mRNA half-life would lead to a truncated protein.
B) A longer mRNA half-life would increase the amount of time the mRNA stays bound to the template strand of DNA, and reduce the amount of protein translated.
C) Differences in mRNA folding could alter the rates of translation.
D) More or less of the protein encoded by that mRNA would be translated.

SOLUTIONS TO CHAPTER 4 FREESTANDING PRACTICE QUESTIONS

1. **C**   RNA polymerase III transcribes transfer RNA (tRNA), which then carries amino acids to ribosomes for use in translation. This polymerase plays no role in replication (choice A is wrong), and reverse transcription uses a DNA polymerase (in any case, it is not carried out by eukaryotes; choice B is wrong). Blocking the action of this enzyme would not alter the base sequence, so mutation would not be affected (choice D is wrong).

2. **D**   The lac operon includes an operator site to which a repressor protein binds (choice A is wrong). The operator site is located between the promoter region and the start transcription site. When the repressor is bound, RNA polymerase (which binds to the promoter site; choice B is wrong) cannot move forward to the start site; thus, transcription is inhibited (choice D is correct). Lactose binds to the repressor protein at an allosteric site, causing a conformational change so that the repressor protein can no longer bind to the operator. When this happens, RNA polymerase can move forward to the start site and transcription will occur (choice C is wrong).

3. **C**   A point mutation is a single base pair substitution. There are few possibilities that can result if a single base is substituted. If the new codon is now a stop codon, then the polypeptide will be truncated (choice A could result from a point mutation and can be eliminated). If the new codon codes for the same amino acid as before the mutation, then a silent point mutation has occurred and no change will be seen in the amino acid sequence (choice B could result from a point mutation and can be eliminated). If the mutation leads to a single new amino acid, then a missense point mutation has occurred (choice D could result from a point mutation and can be eliminated). However, if more than one base was changed, or bases were added/deleted (a frameshift mutation), this would lead to multiple new amino acids (choice C could not result from a point mutation and is the correct answer choice).

4. **A**   Item I is true: Eukaryotic mRNA is monocistronic, meaning that only one protein is transcribed from each mRNA (choice C can be eliminated). Item II is false: transcription does not stop at a stop codon; *translation* stops at a stop codon (choices B and D can be eliminated, and choice A is the correct answer). Transcription stops when a termination signal is reached. Item III is also false: when mRNA is transcribed, it is complementary to the template strand, not identical to it.

5. **A**   Fidelity refers to accuracy. Because RNA polymerases do not proofread, transcription is less accurate (i.e., a lower-fidelity process; choice A is not a similarity and is the correct answer choice). Both replication and transcription use DNA as a template (choice B is a similarity and can be eliminated). In both cases, the removal of pyrophosphate provides the energy for polymerization to occur (choice C is a similarity and can be eliminated). Lastly, although RNA polymerase (in transcription) and DNA polymerase (in replication) move along the parent chain in the 3' → 5' direction, the new chain is made in the 5' → 3' direction.

6. **C**   Transfer RNA (tRNA), not snRNA, is typically involved in the process of coordinating the amino acids that are added to a growing protein during translation (choice C is not a function of snRNA and is the correct answer choice). It should also be noted that translation is NOT taking place in the nucleus, which is the location of snRNA. Processing of

pre-mRNA, regulation of transcription factors, and maintenance of telomeres are all functions typically attributed to snRNA and take place in the nucleus (choices A, B, and D are all functions that include snRNAs and can be eliminated).

7. **B** Post-translational modification is, by definition, the manipulation of protein products after translation; the primary purpose of these modifications is to allow for a large increase in the number of possible protein products from a relatively small genome (choice B is correct). The genome itself is not changed during post-translational modification (choice A is wrong). hnRNA is processed in the nucleus after transcription to yield a variety of mRNA transcripts (and this is the other primary way that protein diversity can be achieved), but the question specifically asks about post-translational modification, not post-transcriptional effects (choice C is wrong). The ribosome is essentially a factory that reads the code on an mRNA and links amino acids together, and that's it. Ribosomes create the primary protein structure; this IS translation. Post-translational modification happens after this step (choice D is wrong).

SOLUTIONS TO CHAPTER 4 PRACTICE PASSAGE

1. **B** Proteins that are abundant require speed and accuracy during translation, and the passage states that this can be accomplished by using preferential codons (choice C is true and can be eliminated; choice B is false and the correct answer choice). Likewise, codons corresponding to abundant tRNAs would be used instead of those corresponding to the more rare tRNAs (choice A is true and can be eliminated). Choice D is true of all genes, abundant proteins or not (choice D can be eliminated).

2. **C** The passage states that silent mutations can lead to all three of the Roman numeral items listed; however, prokaryotes do not undergo mRNA splicing. Thus, Item I is true for both eukaryotes and prokaryotes (choice B can be eliminated), Item II is only true for eukaryotes (choices A and D can be eliminated), and Item III is true for both.

3. **C** According to the passage, areas of the genome that appear to evolve very slowly are highly critical to normal functioning of the organism. Thus, mutations in these areas most likely disrupt function in a major way, leading to the death of the organism and thus the loss of the mutation (hence the reason it appears to evolve very slowly; choice C is correct, and choice D is wrong). If other sites appear to evolve more quickly, mutations at those sites must be less detrimental (choice A is wrong). If mutations at the silent sites increase the accuracy of mRNA splicing, this would be beneficial and thus preserved (choice B is wrong). Note that the information on breast cancer and humans versus mice is not necessary to answer the question and is there solely to distract you. Focus on what the question is asking you.

4. **B** In order for a mutation to have a minimal effect on enzyme activity, it must be a relatively conservative mutation. Both valine (V) and leucine (L) are nonpolar amino acids; the substitution of L for V is not likely to have a significant effect on enzyme activity (choice B is correct). Alanine (A) is nonpolar, and aspartic acid (D) is acidic (and polar). The substitution of D for A would likely be disruptive (choice A is wrong). Arginine (R) is basic (polar)

and glycine (G) is nonpolar; the substitution of G for R would likely be disruptive (choice C is wrong). Leucine (L) is nonpolar, as is tryptophan (W); however, the structure of tryptophan is significantly different than leucine. Tryptophan has a large double-ring side chain, while the side chain of leucine is a short hydrocarbon, $-CH_2CH(CH_3)_2$, very similar to valine, $-CH(CH_3)_2$. The substitution of leucine for valine is likely to be much better tolerated than the substitution of tryptophan for leucine (choice B is better than choice D).

5. **B** Nonsense mutations convert a codon for an amino acid into a stop codon, missense mutations lead to amino acid substitutions, and silent mutations do not affect the amino acid sequence of a protein. To answer this question, you must use the genetic code in Figure 1. UGC codes for cysteine and UGA is a STOP codon, making this a nonsense mutation (choice A is wrong). The codons UUA and CUA both code for leucine, making this a silent mutation (choice B is correct). CAC codes for histidine and CAA codes for glutamine; this is a missense mutation (choice C is wrong). CAU codes for histidine and CUU codes for leucine; this is also a missense mutation (choice D is wrong).

6. **D** If the half-life of an mRNA is increased, it will stay in the cell longer and more of the protein would be translated. Likewise, if the mRNA's half-life is decreased, it will be eliminated from the cell more quickly, and less of the protein would be translated. The mRNA half-life has nothing to do with the length of the protein; protein size is dictated by the length of the open reading frame on the mRNA molecule and the number of codons in the translated region (choice A is wrong). mRNA does not stay bound to the DNA template strand for any length of time, regardless of half-life. As mRNA is transcribed, the DNA helix reforms immediately behind it, releasing the mRNA from the transcription bubble as it is synthesized (choice B is wrong). Choice C is a true statement but does not address the question of half-life (choice C is wrong).

Chapter 5
Microbiology

A milestone in microbiology was the demonstration by Louis Pasteur in 1861 that microbes do not spontaneously arise in boiled broth; they must arrive there by contamination. This put the last nail in the coffin of the idea of spontaneous generation of life. Another major contribution to the golden age of microbiology was the isolation of the bacteria responsible for anthrax in 1876 by a physician named Robert Koch. This and other experiments led to the germ theory of disease, the idea that disease was not caused by bad air ("malaria"), but by microorganisms. In this chapter, we will examine three major groups of disease-causing organisms, beginning with the smallest (viruses) and ending with the largest (fungi—which are often not microscopic at all but visible with the naked eye).

5.1 VIRUSES

With the identification of bacteria as the cause of anthrax and other diseases, medical science appeared in the late 1800s to be headed toward explanation of all infectious disease. Researchers soon found, however, that some infectious agents could not be trapped by passage through filters in the same manner as bacteria. These agents also proved invisible to the light microscope, unlike bacteria. With the advent of electron microscopy, the tiny infectious agents known as **viruses** were finally visualized. Today, molecular biology has shed great light onto viruses, down to the nucleotide sequence of entire viral genomes. However, viruses such as HIV still remain one of the most serious threats to health, indicating there is still much to learn.

Viruses infect all life forms on Earth, including plants, animals, protists, and bacteria. A virus is an **obligate intracellular parasite**. As such, they are only able (*obligated*) to reproduce within (*intra*) cells. While within cells, viruses have some of the attributes of living organisms, such as the ability to reproduce; but outside cells, viruses are without activity. Viruses on their own are unable to perform any of the chemical reactions characteristic of life, such as synthesis of ATP and macromolecules.[1] *Viruses are not cells or even living organisms.* To reproduce, they commandeer the cellular machinery of the host they infect and use it to manufacture copies of themselves. In the final analysis, a virus is nothing more than a package of nucleic acid that says: "Pick me up and reproduce me." Remember this crucial definition: a virus is an obligate intracellular parasite that relies on host machinery whenever possible. In the following sections, we will look at some of the variations on this basic theme.

- Cyanide (an inhibitor of the electron transport chain) is added to a culture of virus-infected mammalian cells. The virus has none of the components of electron transport or any other proteins that are inhibited by cyanide. Which one of the following best describes the effect of cyanide?[2]
    - A) The mammalian cells will die, and all viruses will be destroyed as well, regardless of their stage of development.
    - B) Mammalian cells are killed, and viral replication halted, but the culture remains infectious.
    - C) Mammalian cells stop growing, and viral replication is unaffected.
    - D) Mammalian cells continue to grow, but viral replication is halted.

Viral Structure and Function

The structure of viruses reflects their life cycle. In general, all viruses possess a nucleic acid genome packaged in a protein shell. The exterior protein packaging helps to convey the genome from one cell to infect other cells. Once in a cell, the viral genome directs the production of new copies of the genome and of the

---

[1] Note, however, that some viruses store some ATP in their capsids. They acquired this ATP from the previous host and typically use it to power penetration (see below).

[2] The mammalian cells are directly dependent on the ATP generated by the electron transport chain, so if cyanide inhibits the electron transport chain, the mammalian cells will die (choice D is wrong). The viruses are dependent on the mammalian cells for the ATP and enzymes needed for replication, so if the mammalian cells die, viral replication will stop (choice C is wrong). However, any viruses that had already completed the replication process when the cyanide was added will not be affected, and will remain infectious (choice **B** is correct, and choice A is wrong).

protein packaging needed to produce more virus. However, the nature of the genome, the protein packaging, and the viral life cycle vary tremendously between different viruses.

A viral genome may consist of either DNA *or* RNA that is either single- *or* double-stranded and is either linear *or* circular. Viruses utilize virtually every conceivable form of nucleic acid as their genome. However, a given type of virus can have only one type of nucleic acid as its genome, and a mature virus does not contain nucleic acid other than its genome.[3] [If the ratio of adenine to thymine in a DNA virus is not one to one, what can be said about the genome of this virus?[4] A disease agent that is isolated from a human cannot reproduce on its own in cell-free broth but can reproduce in a culture of human cells. In its pure form, it possesses both RNA and DNA. Is it possible that the disease agent is a virus?[5]]

A factor that influences all viral genomes, regardless of the form of the nucleic acid used as genome, is size as a limiting factor. Viruses are much smaller than the hosts they infect, both prokaryotic and eukaryotic. Figure 1 depicts the relative size of a **bacteriophage** (a virus that infects bacteria) and its host.

E. coli bacterium
(avg. 1–2 microns)

a small eukaryotic cell
(avg. 10–20 microns)

a complex
bacteriophage
(avg. 100–200 nanometers)

Figure 1   The Relative Size of a Virus

Not only are viruses small, but the exterior protein shell of a virus is typically a rigid structure of fixed size that cannot expand to accommodate a larger genome. [What is the likely result if a viral genome is tripled in size?[6]] To adapt to this size constraint, viral genomes have evolved to be extremely economical. One adaptation is for the viral genome to carry very few genes and for the virus to rely on host-encoded proteins for transcription, translation, and replication. [How do ribosomes used to translate viral proteins compare to host ribosomes?[7]] Another adaptation found in viral genomes is the ability to encode more than one protein in a given length of genome. A virus can accomplish this feat by utilizing more than one reading frame within a piece of DNA so that genes may overlap with each other.

---

[3] There are exceptions. For example, it has recently been discovered that the Hepatitis B virus has a circular DNA genome which is part single-stranded and part double-stranded. The take-home point here is that when a virus is not inside a host cell, it contains only its genome, which is always the same (except in special situations such as when a piece of host genome accidentally becomes incorporated in the viral genome). In contrast, a true cell contains not only its genome, but also mRNA, rRNA, and tRNA.

[4] Adenine base pairs with thymine in double-stranded DNA. Thus, for every A, there should be one T, for a one to one ratio of A to T. If the ratio differs from this, the genome must be single-stranded DNA, or RNA, which has no T.

[5] No, it cannot be a virus. Viruses possess only one kind of nucleic acid. The disease agent is another kind of obligate intracellular parasite (certain bacteria can only reproduce inside host cells, e.g., *Chlamydia*).

[6] The viral genome will probably no longer fit within the normal viral structure, and the genome will therefore not be packaged into infectious viral particles.

[7] Viruses use host ribosomes. Viral and host proteins are translated by the same ribosomes.

- A 1000 base pair region of viral genome is found to encode two polypeptides unrelated in amino acid sequence during infection of eukaryotic cells. If one of these polypeptides is 250 amino acids in length and the other is 300, what is the best explanation for this?[8]
  - A) A missense mutation
  - B) Viruses use a different genetic code than eukaryotes do
  - C) Overlapping multiple reading frames
  - D) The polypeptides are splicing variants

Surrounding the viral nucleic acid genome is a protein coat called the **capsid**. The capsid provides the external morphology that is used to classify viruses. It is made from a repeating pattern of only a few protein building blocks. *Helical* capsids are rod-shaped, while *polyhedral* capsids are multiple-sided geometric figures with regular surfaces. Complex viruses may contain a mixture of shapes. For example, the T4 bacteriophage has a helical sheath and a polyhedral head (Figure 2). This virus is commonly used in research; its host is the bacterium *E. coli*. The genome is located within the capsid **head**. Other parts of the capsid are used during infection of the host. The **tail fibers** attach to the surface of the host cell, as does the **base plate**. The **sheath** contracts using the energy of stored ATP, injecting the genome into the host. [Why might a bacteriophage inject its DNA, while animal viruses do not?[9]]

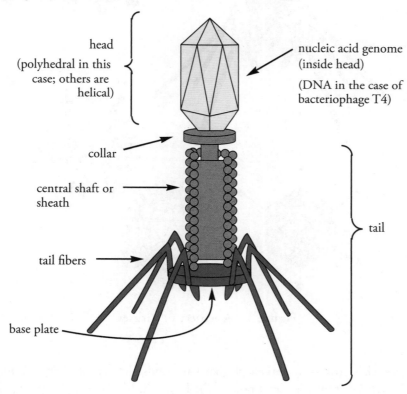

head
(polyhedral in this case; others are helical)

nucleic acid genome
(inside head)

(DNA in the case of bacteriophage T4)

collar

central shaft or sheath

tail fibers

base plate

tail

Figure 2 Bacteriophage T4

---

[8] The problem is that the virus must contain at least 750 bp (250 amino acids) and 900 bp (300 amino acids) of genetic information for unrelated polypeptides in 1000 bp of DNA. The only way to do this is overlapping multiple reading frames (choice **C**).

[9] Phage must puncture the bacterial cell wall, while animal viruses can be internalized whole into animal cells (since they do not have a cell wall).

The most important thing to understand is that the entire viral capsid is composed of protein, while the viral genome is composed of nucleic acid (DNA or RNA). Most viruses are not as structurally complex as the bacteriophage shown in Figure 2. See Figure 3 for more examples.

Figure 3   A Variety of Viruses

Many animal viruses also possess an **envelope** that surrounds the capsid. This is a membrane on the exterior of the virus derived from the membrane of the host cell. It contains phospholipids, proteins, and carbohydrates from the host membrane, in addition to proteins encoded by the viral genome. Enveloped viruses acquire this covering by **budding** through the host cell membrane. To infect a new host, some enveloped viruses fuse their envelope with the host's plasma membrane, which leaves the de-enveloped capsid inside the host cell. Viruses which do not have envelopes are called **naked viruses**. All phages and plant viruses are naked. [Can you imagine why this might be true?[10]]

---

[10]   Remember: viruses acquire envelopes by budding through host membranes. Phages and plant viruses infect hosts that possess cell walls. When viruses begin to exit the cell, the cell wall is destroyed, and host membranes rupture. Thus, there is no membrane through which the remaining viruses must bud; they simply escape in a lytic explosion.

Whether enveloped or naked, the surface of a virus determines what host cells it can infect. Viral infection is not a random process, but highly specific. A virus binds to a specific receptor on the cell surface as the first step in infection. After binding, the virus will be internalized, either by fusion with the plasma membrane or by receptor-mediated endocytosis. Only cells with a receptor that matches the virus will become infected, explaining why only specific species or specific cell types are susceptible to infection. The viral surface is also important for recognition by our immune system. [If antibodies to a viral capsid protein are ineffective in blocking infection, what might this indicate about the virus?[11]]

Bacteriophage Life Cycles

Since viruses lack the ability to produce energy and replicate on their own, they use the machinery of the cell they infect to carry out these processes. The viral genome contains genes that redirect the infected cell to produce viral products. The first step is binding to the exterior of a bacterial cell in a process termed **attachment** or **adsorption**. The next step is injection of the viral genome into the host cell in a process termed **penetration** or **eclipse**. It is called "eclipse" because the capsid remains on the outer surface of the bacterium while the genome disappears into the cell, removing infectious virus from the media. From this point forward, a phage follows one of two different paths: it enters either the **lytic cycle** or the **lysogenic cycle**.

The Lytic Cycle of Phages

As soon as the phage genome has entered the host cell, host polymerases and/or ribosomes begin to rapidly transcribe and translate it. One of the first viral gene products made is sometimes an enzyme called **hydrolase**, a hydrolytic enzyme that degrades the entire host genome. (Hydrolase is an example of an **early gene**; one of a group of genes that are expressed immediately after infection and which includes any special enzymes required to express viral genes.) Then multiple copies of the phage genome are produced (using the dNTPs resulting from degradation of the host genome), as well as an abundance of capsid proteins. Next, each new capsid automatically assembles itself around a new genome. Finally, an enzyme called **lysozyme** is produced. An example of a **late gene**, lysozyme is also present in human tears and saliva. It destroys the bacterial cell wall. Because osmotic pressure is no longer counteracted by the protection of the cell wall, the host bacterium bursts ("lyses," hence the name *lytic*), releasing about 100 progeny viruses, which can begin another round of the cycle (see Figure 4 on the next page). [If lysozyme were an early gene, would this be advantageous to the virus?[12]]

---

[11] It suggests that the virus is enveloped, so the antibody cannot reach its epitope on the capsid surface in infectious virus.

[12] No. The host cell would lyse before the phage had time to replicate and assemble.

1. Attachment of phage to *E. coli* and injection of phage chromosome

6. Release of progeny phage by lysis of bacterial wall

2. Breakdown of bacterial chromosome by phage-specific enzyme

Phage Chromosome

Bacterial (host) chromosome

Host *E. coli* cell

Phage Chromosome

Bacterial chromosome totally broken down

Phage heads being assembled

Phage sheath and base plate

5. Assembly of progeny phage particles

3. Replication of phage chromosome using bacterial materials and phage enzymes

4. Expression of phage genes to produce phage structural components

Figure 4   The Lytic Cycle

- When phage are first added to a bacterial culture, the number of infective viruses initially decreases before it later increases. Why does this occur?[13]
- Bacteria cultured in the presence of ^{35}S-labeled cysteine and ^{32}P-labeled phosphates are infected with phage T4. When phage from this culture are used to infect a new nonradiolabeled bacterial culture, which of the isotopes will be found in the interior of the newly infected bacteria?[14]
- A bacteriophage with an important capsid gene deleted infects the same cell as another virus with a normal copy of the same gene. At the time of host-cell lysis:[15]
  - A) all released viruses will be capable of infecting new hosts, but only some of these new infections will give rise to phage capable of infecting new hosts.
  - B) no infective viruses will be released.
  - C) each individual virus that is released will produce a mixture of infective and noninfective viruses in subsequent infections.
  - D) only normal viruses will be released.

---

[13] The initial decrease is due to the simple fact that many phage have injected their genomes into hosts and are no longer infectious.

[14] The ^{35}S cysteine will be incorporated into viral coat proteins and the ^{32}P phosphate will be incorporated into the viral nucleic acid genome in newly released viral particles. (Proteins contain no P and nucleic acids contain no S.) When these viruses infect bacteria, their nucleic acids are injected into the bacteria while the capsid proteins remain on the exterior, which means that only the ^{32}P will be found in the interior of the newly infected cells.

[15] When two viruses infect the same cell, it is called co-infection. Some normal viruses will result, and some genomes from defective viruses will get packaged into capsids made from proteins encoded by the normal virus. The latter will be capable of infecting new hosts, but when they do, their progeny will not survive due to the capsid abnormality. Choice **A** is correct, and choices B and D are wrong. Think about it: where did the phage with the deleted capsid gene come from?! The deficient virus must have come from a co-infection such as this. The deficient phage can only infect host cells and reproduce with the help of normal viruses. Note that because a single virus carries only a single genome, it can produce only one type of progeny (choice C is wrong).

The Lysogenic Cycle of Phages

The lytic cycle is an efficient way for a virus to rapidly increase its numbers. It presents a problem though: all host cells are destroyed. This is an evolutionary disadvantage. Some viruses are cleverer: they enter the **lysogenic cycle**. Upon infection, the phage genome is incorporated into the bacterial genome and is now referred to as a **prophage**; the host is now called a **lysogen** (Figure 5). The prophage is silent; its genes are not expressed, and viral progeny are not produced. This dormancy is due to the fact that transcription of phage genes is blocked by a phage-encoded repressor protein that binds to specific DNA elements in phage promoters (operators). The cleverness of the lysogenic cycle lies in the fact that every time the host cell reproduces itself, the prophage is reproduced too. Eventually, the prophage becomes activated. It now removes itself from the host genome (in a process called **excision**) and enters the lytic cycle.

One potential consequence of the lysogenic cycle is that when the viral genome activates, excising itself from the host genome, it may take part of the host genome along with it. When the virus replicates, the small piece of host genome will be replicated and packaged with the viral genome. In subsequent infections, the virus will integrate the "stolen" host DNA along with its own genome into the new host's genome. The presence of the new DNA will become evident if it codes for a trait that the newly infected host did not previously possess, such as the ability to metabolize galactose. This process is called **transduction**. [Why would a bacterial gene, carried with a virus and integrated with viral genes into a new bacterial genome, not be repressed along with the viral genes during lysogeny?[16]]

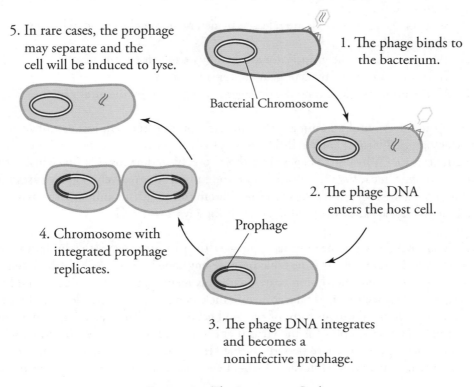

5. In rare cases, the prophage may separate and the cell will be induced to lyse.

Bacterial Chromosome

1. The phage binds to the bacterium.

2. The phage DNA enters the host cell.

4. Chromosome with integrated prophages replicates.

Prophage

3. The phage DNA integrates and becomes a noninfective prophage.

Figure 5   The Lysogenic Cycle

---

[16] Prophage latency results from a viral repressor protein binding to viral DNA in a sequence-specific manner. The specific DNA sequence to which the repressor binds is present in the viral genes but not in the bacterial genes, so the bacterial gene can be expressed while the viral genes are repressed.

Replication of Animal Viruses

There are a number of differences between phages and viruses which infect animal cells. (Animal viruses don't have a special name like "phage.") The general outline of the viral life cycle, however, remains the same. The virus must specifically bind to a proper host cell, release its genetic material into the host, take over host machinery, replicate its genome, synthesize capsid components, assemble itself, and finally escape to infect a new cell.

Animal cells have proteins on the surface of their plasma membranes that serve as specific receptors for viruses. These receptors play a role in normal cellular function; they do not exist simply for the benefit of the virus. Part of the tissue-specificity of animal viruses is due to the distribution of receptors necessary for adsorption. For example, the binding of the HIV virus protein gp120 to a T cell membrane protein termed CD4 is one of the first steps in HIV infection.

- Would treatment of an HIV-infected person with a soluble form of CD4 protein affect the infectivity of the virus?[17]
- Mutation of the cell-surface receptor that viruses attach to would be a means for an organism to become resistant to viral infection. Why is this mechanism not common?[18]
- Treatment of an enveloped animal virus with a mild detergent solubilizes several proteins from the virus, although the genome does not become accessible. Which one of the following is consistent with this scenario?[19]
    A) Some of the proteins that are released by detergent may be encoded by the genome of the infected cell.
    B) The infectivity of the virus is not affected by detergent treatment.
    C) The proteins released by detergent are capsid proteins.
    D) All the proteins released by the detergent are encoded by the viral genome.

The next step in the infection of an animal cell is penetration into the cell, just as in bacterial infection by a phage. Many animal viruses enter cells by **endocytosis** (a process whereby the host cell engulfs the virus and internalizes it). [Why don't phages enter their hosts by endocytosis?[20]] Once inside the host, the viral genome is *uncoated*, meaning it is released from the capsid. Alternatively, some viruses fuse with the plasma membrane to release virus into the cytoplasm. From this point, an animal virus may enter either a lytic cycle, a lytic-like cycle called the productive cycle, or a lysogenic cycle.

The lytic cycle in animal viruses is the same as in phages. The **productive cycle** is similar to the lytic cycle but does not destroy the host cell. It is possible because enveloped viruses exit the host cell by *budding through the host's cell membrane*, becoming coated with this membrane in the process. Budding does not necessarily destroy a cell since the lipid bilayer membrane can reseal as the virus leaves. Finally, in the animal virus lysogenic cycle the dormant form of the viral genome is called a **provirus** (analogous to a prophage). For example, Herpes simplex I is the virus that causes oral herpes. After infection, it may remain dormant as a provirus for an indefinite period of time. Then one day, usually when the host encounters stress (e.g., lack of sleep, upcoming professional school entrance exams), the virus reactivates.

---

[17] Yes, it would. The soluble CD4 protein would bind to the virus's CD4 receptor (gp120) and block attachment of the virus to the T cells.

[18] Two reasons: 1) The receptor has a specific role in the normal physiology of the host, which a mutation might compromise. 2) Viruses generally evolve so rapidly that they can keep up with any changes in the host, but this is not an absolute rule. Cells of our immune system keep us alive by keeping up with most microorganisms' tricks.

[19] The detergent solubilized the viral envelope (choice C is wrong). As stated in the text, some envelope proteins are encoded by the virus and some are derived from the host's membranes during budding (choice **A** is correct, and choice D is wrong). Removal of envelope proteins will impair viral adsorption and reduce infectivity (choice B is wrong).

[20] Bacteria do not perform endocytosis, in part because they have a rigid cell wall that does not permit them to.

Viral Genomes

Many factors determine the uniqueness of each virus. The type of genome, possession or lack of an envelope, nature of cell-surface proteins, and type of life cycle are examples. All of these parameters are used in the classification of viruses, and all are potential targets for therapeutic intervention. The nature of the genome is perhaps the most important of these and has important consequences for how infection by each virus proceeds. In the following discussion, we will look at a few viral genomes with an eye to *what proteins the virus must encode or actually carry in its capsid based on its genome type.* Our purpose is not to provide new information, but rather to demonstrate what conclusions can be drawn from what you already know (typical MCAT passage material). Do not memorize, but rather read for comprehension. We will not discuss ds-RNA or ss-DNA genomes, but by the end of this section, you should be able to imagine components they might require.

(+) RNA Viruses
—must *encode* RNA-dependent RNA pol (and do not have to carry it).

A (+) RNA virus, with a single-stranded RNA genome, is the simplest imaginable type of viral genome. (A piece of single-stranded viral RNA which serves as mRNA is called (+) RNA.) As soon as the (+) RNA genome is in the host cell, host ribosomes begin to translate it, creating viral proteins. The viral genome acts directly as mRNA. The technical way to describe this scenario is to say the genome is **infective**, meaning injecting an isolated genome into the host cell will result in virus production. In order for the virus to replicate itself, one of the proteins it encodes must be an **RNA-dependent RNA polymerase**, the role of which is __?[21] (+) RNA viruses cause the common cold, polio, and rubella. [Will an infectious virus be produced if the genome of an enveloped (+) strand RNA virus is added to an extract prepared from the cytoplasm of eukaryotic cells that retains translational activity but lacks DNA replication or transcription of host genes?[22] If a viral genome is (+) strand RNA, what is used as a template by the RNA-dependent RNA polymerase?[23]]

(−) RNA Viruses
—must *carry* RNA-dependent RNA pol (and, of course, encode it too).

The genome of a (−) RNA virus is *complementary* to the piece of RNA that encodes viral proteins. In other words, the genome of a (−) RNA virus is the template for viral mRNA production. If host ribosomes translate (−) RNA, useless polypeptides will be made. Hence, the virus must not only encode an RNA-dependent RNA polymerase, it must actually carry one with it in the capsid. When the virus enters the host cell, this enzyme will create a (+) strand from the (−) genome. Then the viral life cycle can proceed. (−) RNA viruses cause rabies, measles, mumps, and influenza. [Do (−) strand RNA viruses use host enzymes to catalyze RNA production in transcription or in replication of the genome?[24]]

---

[21] to copy the RNA genome for viral replication; the host never makes RNA from RNA.

[22] No. The (+) strand RNA virus will be able to produce viral genome and proteins, but progeny will not be able to acquire the envelope they need to be infectious.

[23] To make (+) strand copies of the genome, the virus needs the complementary strand as a template: the (−) strand RNA. Thus, the RNA-dependent RNA polymerase produces a (−) strand intermediate before generating new (+) strand genomes.

[24] Neither. Viral RNA-dependent RNA polymerase first makes (+) strand as mRNA and then uses the (+) strand as the template to replicate new (−) strand genomes.

Retroviruses
—must *encode* reverse transcriptase.

HIV, the virus that causes AIDS, and HTLV (Human T cell Leukemia Virus) are examples of retroviruses. These are (+) RNA viruses that undergo lysogeny. In other words, they integrate into the host genome as proviruses. In order to integrate into our double-stranded DNA genome, a viral genome must also be composed of double-stranded DNA. Since these viral genomes enter the cell in an RNA form, they must undergo **reverse transcription** to make DNA from an RNA template. This snubbing of the central dogma is accomplished by an **RNA-dependent DNA polymerase** (*reverse transcriptase*) encoded by the viral genome. Retroviruses are theoretically not required to carry this enzyme, only to encode it. [Why?[25]] The three main retroviral genes are *gag* (codes for viral capsid proteins), *pol* (polymerase codes for reverse transcriptase), and *env* (envelope codes for viral envelope proteins). [After integration of a retrovirus into the cellular genome, a reverse transcriptase inhibitor is added to the cell. Will the production of new viruses be blocked?[26]]

Double-Stranded DNA Viruses
—often *encode* enzymes required for dNTP synthesis and DNA replication.

These viruses often have large genomes that include genes for enzymes involved in deoxyribonucleotide synthesis (which we do whenever we make DNA) and DNA replication. [Given the limited information that viruses may contain in their genomes, why carry around genes for an enzyme possessed by the host?[27] Why don't RNA viruses do this?[28] What is a factor likely to limit the size of RNA genomes?[29] Some DNA viruses induce infected host cells to enter mitosis and may even override cellular inhibition of cell division so strongly that the cell becomes cancerous; what is the advantage to the virus of inducing host-cell division?[30]]

---

[25] Because the viral RNA genome can be translated by host ribosomes; thus, reverse transcriptase may be made after the viral genome enters the host. It just so happens that HIV does carry its reverse transcriptase within its capsid. You should understand why this is not a theoretical necessity.

[26] No, it will not. Reverse transcriptase is required for only one phase of the retrovirus life cycle: the copying of the viral RNA genome into DNA so that it can integrate into the host genome and be transcribed. Once the viral genome has integrated, transcription to produce viral mRNA and new viral RNA genomes does not involve reverse transcriptase. It can proceed with the normal host-cell enzymes.

[27] The host cell will only make dNTPs in preparation for replication. If the virus wants to reproduce without waiting for the host to do so, it must encode its own enzymes for the synthesis of DNA building blocks.

[28] Transcription is always occurring in all cells, so NTPs (not dNTPs) are always present.

[29] The error rate in RNA synthesis is much higher than in DNA synthesis, in part because there are mechanisms to proofread and correct errors in DNA synthesis (but not in RNA synthesis). If an RNA genome were too large, every copy of the viral genome synthesized would suffer from so many errors that no infectious virus would be produced.

[30] To replicate, the DNA virus must either provide all of the necessary components (such as dNTPs) itself, infect a cell that is already dividing, or induce the cell it infects to enter mitosis and produce the ingredients for DNA synthesis.

- Adenoviruses have a single linear ds-DNA genome which contains a number of different promoters that are regulated during infection. Although transcription is carried out by cellular RNA polymerase, the viral E1A gene product is required for transcription of most viral genes. If the E1A gene is deleted from the virus or if the gene product is inactivated, viral infection is unable to proceed. Adenoviruses also encode much of their own replication machinery, including DNA polymerase. If two different adenoviruses infect the same cell, one with a deleted E1A gene and another with a deleted DNA polymerase gene, will successful infection of the cell result?[31]

5.2 SUBVIRAL PARTICLES

Some infectious agents are even smaller and simpler than viruses and are termed **subviral particles**. These include prions and viroids.

Prions

As infectious agents, prions do not strictly follow the Central Dogma because they are self-replicating proteins [Why does this violate the Central Dogma?[32]]. The prion itself is a misfolded version of a protein that already exists (see Figure 6).

PrP^C
(normal protein)

PrP^{Sc}
(abnormal protein)

Figure 6   Comparison of the PrP^C structure to the PrP^{Sc} structure

---

[31] Yes, thanks to complementation. The mutant viruses will complement each other, one providing the E1A protein and the other providing DNA polymerase. Note that this had to have happened before; how else could defective viruses such as these exist? One virus which complements another is called a helper virus.

[32] The Central Dogma states that information flows in its nucleotide form from DNA to RNA (transcription), and then in its amino acid form from RNA to protein (translation). Prions take both transcription and translation out of the process and have proteins being shaped based on other proteins, hence the term "self-replicating."

When the normally folded protein (designated PrP^C) comes into contact with the prion (designated PrP^{Sc}), the prion acts as a template; the shape of the normal protein is altered and it too becomes infectious. Prions are responsible for a class of diseases in mammals referred to as the **transmissible spongiform encephalopathies** (TSEs). These diseases cause degeneration in the nervous system, especially the brain where characteristic holes develop, and are always fatal. The misfolded proteins are found in the nervous tissues and are very resistant to degradation by chemicals or heat, making them hard to destroy. Bovine spongiform encephalopathy (BSE, commonly called *mad cow disease*) is the prion disease found in cows; this was originally transmitted to cows from sheep because all types of tissue from sheep, including the brain and spinal cord, were used as a supplement in the feed for other farm animals. (Since this was discovered, strict rules have been put in place about which specific organs can be used to supplement animal feed, and those organs most likely to transmit prion disease are banned.) Though much less common, the disease *kuru* follows a similar transmission path in humans; it is only found in a limited number of tribes where consumption of the body, particularly of the brain, is part of honoring the dead (since identification of the transmission route, this practice has stopped and kuru has virtually disappeared).

However, prion diseases can also be genetically linked through mutations in the gene that codes for the prion protein. For example, fatal familial insomnia (FFI) is an autosomal dominant condition inherited on chromosome 20, and Creutzfeldt-Jakob disease (CJD) is also inherited. It is also possible for these diseases to arise spontaneously (through mutation) in someone with no prior family history. In general, however, prion diseases are very rare, striking only 1–2 people per million.

Whether transmitted, inherited, or spontaneously arising, prion diseases are characterized by their very long incubation periods, which can be several months to years in animals and several years to decades in humans. The misfolded proteins cause the destruction of neurons, particularly in the central nervous system, leading to loss of coordination, dementia, and death. Diagnosis is difficult, in part because of the long incubation periods and in part because the symptoms can be indicative of other conditions.

Viroids

Viroids consist of a short piece of circular, single-stranded RNA (200–400 bases long) with extensive self-complementarity (i.e., it can base-pair with itself to create some regions that are double-stranded; see Figure 7). Generally they do not code for proteins and they lack capsids. Some viroids are catalytic ribozymes, while others, when replicated, produce siRNAs that can silence normal gene expression.

Figure 7   Structure of a Viroid Showing Double-Stranded Regions

Replication of some viroids shares similarity to the replication of RNA viruses. A viroid RNA-dependent RNA polymerase synthesizes a (–) strand, which is circularized by an RNA ligase derived from the host;

this is then used as the round, rolling template to make more (+) copies that match the original RNA viroid sequence. An alternative to this mechanism leaves the (−) stand in a more linear state where it can still act as a template for (+) strand creation and then become circularized. In other cases, viroids somehow hijack the cell's DNA dependent RNA polymerase and direct it to read RNA templates. This mechanism is not well understood.

Most of the diseases caused by viroids are found in plants. The only human disease linked to viroids is Hepatitis D. The Hepatitis D viroid can only enter hepatocytes (liver cells) if it is contained in a capsid with a binding protein; since viroids do not have capsids, successful Hepatitis D infection required coinfection with Hepatitis B, from which it derives its capsid.

5.3   PROKARYOTES (DOMAIN BACTERIA)

Cell Theory

Advances in microbiology have been made possible by advancing technologies in magnification. Once humans were able to utilize basic, if crude, microscopy, the cell as the monomer of tissues and organs could be studied. In 1655, this led the English scientist, Robert Hooke, to define the Cell Theory based on his studies of cork. Its tenets are as follows:

1) All living organisms are composed of one or more cells and their products.
2) Cells are the monomer for any organism.
3) New cells arise from pre-existing, living cells.

Though these basic principles are still true, more modern extensions of Cell Theory also include the idea that no matter what the species, the chemical composition of cells is similar, that DNA is the source of hereditary programming information passed from cell to cell, that an organism's activity is determined by the total activity of its cells, and that biochemical energy flow occurs within cells. These additional principles have been explored and verified due to vast improvements both in microscopy as well as biochemical and genetic testing.

All living organisms (which does not include viruses) can be classified as either **prokaryotes** or **eukaryotes**. The classification of organisms into these groups is based on examination of their internal cellular structure. Representatives from both groups are able to carry out the basic biochemical processes of photosynthesis, the Krebs cycle, and oxidative phosphorylation to produce ATP. The primary feature of prokaryotes that distinguishes them from eukaryotes is that they do not contain **membrane-bound organelles** (nucleus, mitochondria, lysosomes, etc.). *Prokaryote* means "before the nucleus," and the lack of a nucleus indicates that prokaryotes are evolutionarily the oldest domains. Unlike viruses, however, prokaryotes possess all of the machinery required for life. They are true cells; true living organisms. The prokaryotes include **bacteria**, **archaea** (extremophiles), and **blue-green algae** (cyanobacteria).

The classification of living organisms, **taxonomy**, is an important part of biology because it is used to determine the evolutionary relationship of organisms to one another. The largest taxonomic division is the **domain**. There are three recognized domains: Bacteria, Archaea, and Eukarya. Domains Bacteria and Archaea include prokaryotic organisms, and Domain Eukarya includes eukaryotic organisms. Each domain can be further subdivided into **kingdoms**. Currently there are three well-recognized eukaryotic kingdoms (Animalia, Plantae, and Fungi), and great debate over the number of kingdoms that should be present in the other prokaryotic domains and in the single-celled eukaryotes (protists).

In this section, we will begin to study the most basic and ancient of organisms, the prokaryotes.

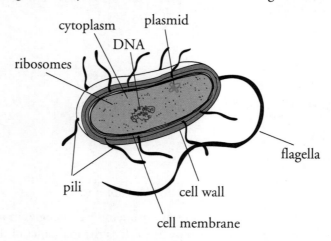

Figure 8   A Prokaryote

Bacterial Structure and Classification

Contents of the Cytoplasm

Unlike a eukaryotic cell, there are *no membrane-bound organelles* in prokaryotic cells (note that ribosomes, which are *not* membrane-bound, *are* found in bacteria). The prokaryotic genome is a single double-stranded circular DNA chromosome.[33] It is not located in a nucleus, and it is not associated with histone proteins as the eukaryotic genome is. In bacteria, transcription and translation occur in the same place at the same time. Ribosomes begin to translate mRNA before it is completely transcribed. Many ribosomes translating a single piece of mRNA form a structure known as a **polyribosome**.

[In Figure 9 on the next page, is the free end of the mRNA the 3' or the 5' end? Which end of the nascent polypeptides is the free end?[34]] Remember that the bacterial ribosome is structurally different from the eukaryotic ribosome, though both function the same way. The differences allow us to prescribe various antibiotics which interfere with bacterial translation without disrupting our own. (Examples are strepto-mycin and tetracycline, which bind only to bacterial ribosomes.)

---

[33] There are a few exceptions to this (e.g., bacteria with more than one chromosome and/or linear chromosomes), but you do not have to know them for the MCAT.

[34] The 5' end of the mRNA polymer is free, since elongation of mRNA proceeds 5' to 3'. Proteins are made N to C, so the free end of the polypeptides is the N terminus.

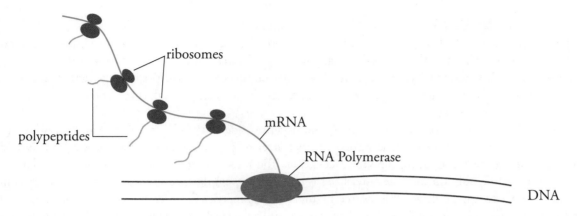

Figure 9 A Prokaryotic Polyribosome

One last genetic element that can be found in prokaryotic cells is the **plasmid**. This is a circular piece of double-stranded DNA which is much smaller than the genome. Plasmids are referred to as **extrachromosomal genetic elements**. They often encode gene products which may confer an advantage upon a bacterium carrying the plasmid. For example, plasmids frequently carry antibiotic-resistance genes (genes that encode proteins which can break down antibiotics). Many plasmids are capable of autonomous replication, which means that a single plasmid molecule within a bacterial cell may cause itself to be replicated into many copies. Plasmids are important not only because they may encode advantageous gene products, but also because they orchestrate bacterial exchange of genetic information, or **conjugation**, which is discussed below.

Bacterial Shape

Bacteria are often classified according to their shape. The three shapes and their proper names are organized in the following table:

Table 1 Bacterial Classification by Shape

Shape	Proper name (plural)	Proper name (singular)
round	cocci	coccus
rod-shaped	bacilli	bacillus
spiral-shaped	spirochetes or spirilla	spirochete, spirillum

The Cell Membrane and the Cell Wall

The bacterial cytoplasm is bounded by a lipid bilayer which is similar to our own plasma membrane. Outside the lipid bilayer is a rigid cell wall. It provides support for the cell, preventing lysis due to osmotic pressure. The bacterial cell wall is composed of **peptidoglycan**, a complex polymer unique to prokaryotes. It contains cross-linked chains made of sugars and amino acids, including D-alanine, which is not found in animal cells (our amino acids have the L configuration). The bacterial cell wall is the target of many antibiotics, such as penicillin. The enzyme *lysozyme*, which is found in tears and saliva and made by lytic viruses, destroys the peptidoglycan in the bacterial cell wall, resulting in an osmotically fragile structure called a **protoplast**. [Would a protoplast moved from salt water to fresh water shrivel or burst?[35]]

---

[35] It would burst, since water would flow into the cell by osmosis.

Gram Staining of the Cell Wall

As part of our tour of the bacterial cell, we will say a word about classification of bacteria according to two different types of cell wall. The method of classification is derived from the extent to which bacteria turn color in a procedure termed **Gram staining**. The two groupings are **Gram-positive**, which stain strongly (a dark purple color) and **Gram-negative** bacteria, which stain weakly (a light pink color).

Gram-positive bacteria have a thick peptidoglycan layer outside of the cell membrane and no other layer beyond this. Gram-negative bacteria have a thinner layer of peptidoglycan in the cell wall but have an additional outer layer containing lipopolysaccharide. The intermediate space in Gram-negative bacteria between the cell membrane and the outer layer is termed the **periplasmic space**, in which are sometimes found enzymes that degrade antibiotics (see Figure 10). The increased protection of Gram-negative bacteria from the environment is reflected in their weak staining, as well as in their increased resistance to antibiotics. [Which bacteria would be more susceptible to lysis when treated with lysozyme: Gram-positive or Gram-negative?[36]]

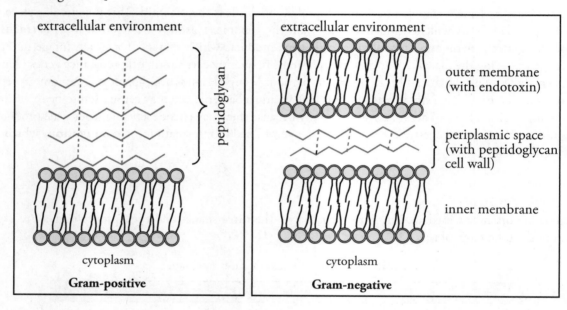

Figure 10   Gram-positive vs. Gram-negative Bacteria

---

[36] Lysozyme hydrolyzes linkages in peptidoglycan to weaken the cell wall. The peptidoglycan in Gram-positive cells is more accessible, since these cells do not possess an additional outer layer; therefore, Gram-positive cells will lyse more easily when treated with lysozyme.

Endotoxins vs. Exotoxins

Endotoxins are normal components of the outer membrane of Gram-negative bacteria that aren't inherently poisonous. However, they cause our immune system to have such an extreme reaction that we may die as a result. Endotoxins cause the most trouble when many bacteria die and their disintegrated outer membranes are released into the circulation. When this occurs, cells of the immune system release so many chemicals that the patient goes into what is called septic shock, in which much of the aqueous portion of the blood is leaked into the tissues, causing a drop in blood pressure, and other problems, which may be fatal. Endotoxins can have various chemical structures, including lipopolysaccharide, which contains sugars bound to lipids.

Exotoxins are very toxic substances secreted by both Gram-negative and Gram-positive bacteria into the surrounding medium. Exotoxins help the bacterium compete with other bacterial species, such as normal inhabitants of the mammalian gut. Some diseases that are caused by exotoxins are botulism, diptheria, tetanus, and toxic shock syndrome.

The Capsule

Another attribute which only some bacteria have is the **capsule** or **glycocalyx**. This is a sticky layer of polysaccharide "goo" surrounding the bacterial cell and often surrounding an entire colony of bacteria. It makes bacteria more difficult for immune system cells to eradicate. It also enables bacteria to adhere to smooth surfaces such as rocks in a stream or the lining of the human respiratory tract.

Flagella

Another item only some bacteria have are long, whip-like filaments known as **flagella**, which are involved in bacterial motility. [Can viruses move via flagellar propulsion to find host cells?[37]] A bacterium which possesses one or more flagella is said to be **motile**, because flagella are the only means of bacterial locomotion. Bacteria may be **monotrichous** (meaning they have a flagellum located at only one end), **amphitrichous** (meaning they have a flagellum located at both ends), or **peritrichous** (meaning that they have multiple flagella). The following is which?[38]

The structure of the flagellum is fairly complicated, with components encoded by over 35 genes, but it can be broken down into a few major components: the **filament**, the **hook**, and the **basal structure** (Figure 11 on the next page). The basal structure contains a number of rings that anchor the flagellum to the inner and outer membrane (for a Gram-negative bacterium) and serve to rotate the **rod** and the rest of the attached flagellum in either a clockwise or counterclockwise manner. The most important thing to remember about the prokaryotic flagellum is that its structure is different from the eukaryotic one (which contains a "9 + 2" arrangement of microtubules, discussed in Chapter 6).

---

[37] No. Viruses lack any means of energy production on their own and any means of active movement. They rely on diffusion to find host cells.

[38] Monotrichous

Figure 11   The Prokaryotic Flagellum

The rotation of the rod is powered by the diffusion of H^+ down the proton gradient generated across the inner membrane by electron transport. Bacterial motion can be directed toward attractants, such as food, or away from toxins, such as acid, in a process termed **chemotaxis**. The connection between chemotaxis and flagellar propulsion is dependent upon **chemoreceptors** on the cell surface that bind attractants or repellents and transmit a signal that influences the direction of flagellar rotation. The response of flagellar rotation to chemical attractants (or repellents) is not dependent on an *absolute* concentration, but to a *change* in the concentration over time. Thus, as the bacterium moves through the solution, it is able to detect whether it is moving toward or away from the highest concentration and respond accordingly.

Pili

Pili are long projections on the bacterial surface involved in attaching to different surfaces. The **sex pilus** is a special pilus attaching F^+ (male) and F^- (female) bacteria which facilitates the formation of **conjugation bridges** (discussed below). **Fimbriae** are smaller structures that are not involved in locomotion or conjugation but are involved in adhering to surfaces. [What other bacterial structure is involved in adhering to surfaces? Is it possible that the fimbriae play a role in infection by pathogenic organisms?[39]]

---

[39] The capsule, or glycocalyx is also involved in adherence. And yes, fimbriae do play a role in infection, by facilitating adhesion to cells so that the bacteria can colonize a tissue.

Bacterial Growth Requirements and Classification

Temperature

Another characteristic of bacteria used to categorize them is their ability to tolerate environmental variables, such as temperature. Though bacteria as a group can grow at a wide range of temperatures, each species has an optimal growth temperature. If the temperature is too high or too low, bacteria fail to grow and may be killed, hence the use of boiling to kill bacteria and refrigeration to slow bacterial growth and prevent food spoilage. Most bacteria favor mild temperatures similar to the ones that humans and other organisms favor (30°C); they are called **mesophiles** (moderate temperature lovers). **Thermophiles** (heat lovers) can survive at temperatures up to 100°C in boiling hot springs or near geothermal vents in the ocean floor. Bacteria that thrive at very low temperatures (near 0°C) are termed **psychrophiles** (cold lovers). [How might a decrease in temperature increase the bacterial growth rate?[40]]

Nutrition

Bacteria can be classified according to their *carbon source* and their *energy source.* **"Troph"** is a Latin root meaning "eat." **Autotrophs** utilize CO_2 as their carbon source. **Heterotrophs** rely on organic nutrients (glucose, for example) created by other organisms. **Chemotrophs** get their energy from chemicals. **Phototrophs** get their energy from light; not only plants but also some bacteria do this. Each bacterium is either a chemotroph or a phototroph and is either an autotroph or a heterotroph. There are thus four types of bacteria:

1) **Chemoautotrophs** build organic macromolecules from CO_2 using the energy of chemicals. They obtain energy by oxidizing inorganic molecules like H_2S.
2) **Chemoheterotrophs** require organic molecules such as glucose made by other organisms as their carbon source and for energy. (We are chemoheterotrophs.)
3) **Photoautotrophs** use only CO_2 as a carbon source and obtain their energy from the Sun. (Plants are photoautotrophs.)
4) **Photoheterotrophs** are odd in that the get their energy from the Sun, like plants, but require an organic molecule made by another organism as their carbon source.

- A bacterium that causes an infection in the bloodstream of humans is most likely to be classified as which one of the following?[41]
  - A) Chemoautotroph
  - B) Photoautotroph
  - C) Chemoheterotroph
  - D) Photoheterotroph

---

[40] Normally, you expect decreasing temperature to decrease the rate of all chemical, biochemical, and biological processes, since reactions accelerate when kinetic energy increases. However, bacteria that have evolved to live at low temperatures (psychrophiles) possess enzymes that may be optimally active at a low temperature, leading to better growth.

[41] Since there's no sunlight in the bloodstream, choices B and D are out. If it's a parasite, it most likely uses some of our chemicals, so it must be a heterotroph, which eliminates choice A. The answer is choice **C**.

- Which one of the following categories best describes an organism which uses sunlight to drive ATP production but cannot incorporate carbon dioxide into sugars?[42]
  - A) Chemoautotroph
  - B) Photoautotroph
  - C) Chemoheterotroph
  - D) Photoheterotroph

Growth Media

The environment in which bacteria grow is the **medium** (plural: **media**). In the lab, the most common solid medium is agar, a firm transparent gel made from seaweed. Bacteria live in the agar but do not metabolize it. The agar is usually kept in a clear plastic plate called a **Petri dish**, and the process of putting bacteria on such a plate is called **plating**. When one bacterium is plated onto a dish, if it grows, it will eventually give rise to many progeny in an isolated spot called a **colony**. **Minimal medium** contains nothing but glucose (in addition to the agar). More key terms: a **wild-type** bacterium (or a wild-type strain) is one which possesses all the characteristics normal to that particular species. The dense growth of bacteria seen in laboratory Petri dishes is known as a bacterial **lawn**. A **plaque** is a clear area in the lawn. Plaques result from death of bacteria and are caused by lytic viruses or toxins.

Bacteria can reproduce very rapidly, provided that the conditions of their environment are favorable and nutrients are abundant. The **doubling time** is the amount of time required for a population of bacteria to double its number. It ranges from a minimum of 20 minutes for *E. coli* to a day or more for slow growers, such as the bacteria responsible for tuberculosis and leprosy. The doubling time of a bacterial species will vary, depending upon the availability of nutrients and other environmental factors.

One other important term in bacterial nutrition is **auxotroph** (don't confuse this term with *auto*troph). This is a bacterium which cannot survive on minimal medium because it can't synthesize a molecule it needs to live. Therefore, it requires an *aux*iliary *troph*ic substance to live. For instance, a bacterium which is auxotrophic for arginine won't form a colony when plated onto minimal medium, but if the medium is supplemented with arginine, a colony will form. This arginine auxotrophy is denoted arg⁻. Auxotrophy results from a mutation in a gene coding for an enzyme in a synthetic pathway.

Bacteria can be differentiated not only by what substances they require, but also by what substances they are capable of metabolizing for energy. For instance, a strain of bacteria may be capable of surviving on minimal medium that has the disaccharide lactose as the only carbon source (no glucose). This would be denoted lac⁺. Mutation in a gene for the enzyme lactase would impair the bacterium's ability to survive on lactose-only medium. A bacterial strain incapable of growing with lactose as its only carbon source would be denoted lac⁻. Genetic exchange between bacteria by means of conjugation, transduction, or transformation (discussed below) can remedy these disabilities.

Oxygen Utilization and Tolerance

Oxygen metabolism is *aerobic* metabolism. Bacteria which require oxygen are called **obligate aerobes**. Bacteria which do not require oxygen are called **anaerobes**. There are three subcategories: **facultative anaerobes** will use oxygen when it's around, but they don't need it. [How much more ATP can they

---

[42] The ability to use sunlight indicates that the organism is a phototroph, and the inability to use carbon dioxide as a carbon source indicates that it is a heterotroph—it must use organic molecules as a carbon source. The answer is choice **D**.

make per glucose molecule when O_2 is present?[43]] **Tolerant anaerobes** can grow in the presence or absence of oxygen but do not use it in their metabolism. **Obligate anaerobes** are poisoned by oxygen. This is because they lack certain enzymes necessary for the detoxification of free radicals which form spontaneously whenever oxygen is around.[44] Obligate anaerobes commonly infect wounds.

- If a bacterium cannot use oxygen as an electron acceptor, is it an obligate anaerobe, a tolerant anaerobe, or a facultative anaerobe, or is it not possible to distinguish based on the information given?[45]

- A sample of bacteria is evenly mixed into a cool liquid agar nutrient mix in the absence of oxygen and then poured into a glass-walled tube that is open to the atmosphere on top. When the agar mix cools, it solidifies, and bacterial growth is observed as shown below. How would you classify the bacteria in terms of oxygen utilization and tolerance? (*Note*: Agar is practically impermeable to oxygen.)[46]

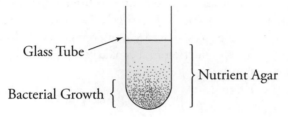

Glass Tube

Nutrient Agar

Bacterial Growth

Fermentation vs. Respiration

Respiration is glucose catabolism with use of an inorganic electron acceptor such as oxygen. In contrast, fermentation is glucose catabolism which does not use an electron acceptor such as O_2; instead, a reduced by-product of glucose catabolism such as lactate or ethanol is given off as waste. [Why is fermentation necessary whenever an external electron acceptor is not used?[47]]

Anaerobic Respiration

This is not a contradiction in terms! It refers to glucose metabolism with electron transport and oxidative phosphorylation relying on an external electron acceptor *other than* O_2. For example, instead of reducing O_2 to H_2O, some anaerobic bacteria reduce SO_4^{2-} to H_2S, or CO_2 to CH_4. Nitrate (NO_3^-) is another possible electron acceptor.

---

[43] Sixteen times as much. For more on this topic, see *MCAT Biochemistry Review*.

[44] The enzymes include superoxide dismutase (converts O_2^- to H_2O_2) and catalase (converts H_2O_2 to $H_2O + O_2$). An example of a harmful O_2 by-product is superoxide anion, O_2^-.

[45] The bacterium cannot be a facultative anaerobe, since the question states it cannot use O_2. It could be either an obligate or a tolerant anaerobe depending on its ability to neutralize harmful oxygen-free radicals.

[46] Since the bacteria grew only at the bottom of the tube, farthest away from any oxygen, this indicates that they could only grow in the absence of oxygen. Thus, they are obligate anaerobes.

[47] Because NAD^+ must be regenerated from NADH for glycolysis to continue. In fermentation, the electrons are passed from NADH to a molecule other than O_2, such as pyruvic acid.

- In an experiment, facultative anaerobic bacteria that are growing on glucose in air are shifted to anaerobic conditions. If they continue to grow at the same rate while producing lactic acid, then the rate of glucose consumption will:[48]
  - A) increase 16 fold.
  - B) decrease 16 fold.
  - C) decrease 2 fold.
  - D) not change.

Bacterial Life Cycle

Bacteria reproduce asexually. In asexual reproduction, there is no meiosis, no meiotic generation of haploid gametes, and no fusion of gametes to form a new individual organism. Instead, each bacterium grows in size until it has synthesized enough cellular components for two cells rather than one, replicates its genome, then divides in two. This process in bacteria is also known as **binary fission** (fission means "to split"). [In prokaryotes, does reproduction increase genetic diversity?[49] If a eukaryote reproduces strictly by asexual reproduction, how will this affect the genetic diversity of a population?[50] How is asexual reproduction in a eukaryote different from asexual reproduction in a prokaryote?[51]] Although bacteria do not reproduce sexually, they do possess a mechanism, termed **conjugation**, for exchanging genetic information (more on this later).

Growth of bacterial populations is described in stages (see Figure 12). Under ideal conditions, bacterial population growth is exponential, meaning that the number of bacterial cells increases exponentially with time. This also means the log of the population size grows linearly with time, hence the name **log phase.** [If 10 bacteria in log phase are placed in ideal growth conditions and the doubling time is 20 minutes, how many bacteria will there be after four hours?[52]]

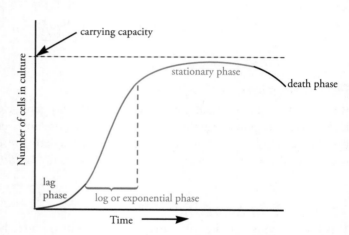

Figure 12   Bacterial Reproduction

---

[48] Aerobic respiration produces 32 ATP per glucose in prokaryotes compared to only 2 ATP per glucose in fermentation. If the rate of growth is to remain the same, the rate of ATP production must remain the same to drive biosynthetic pathways forward. Since fermentation produces 1/16 the amount of ATP per glucose, the rate of glucose consumption must increase sixteen fold to maintain the rate of growth at the same level. The answer is choice **A**. (In reality the growth rate would probably decrease.)

[49] No. Each daughter cell is identical to the parent cell (assuming no mutation took place).

[50] Many eukaryotes reproduce asexually. Sexual reproduction allows for generation of new allelic combinations through meiotic recombination and random union of gametes. Without this, diversity will decrease over time.

[51] In eukaryotes, asexual reproduction occurs through mitosis. Prokaryotes do not go through mitosis.

[52] Since four hours is equal to 240 minutes, the bacteria will divide twelve times. Therefore, one bacterium will produce $2^{12} = 4,096$ bacteria after 12 divisions. Since there are 10 bacteria initially, the total after four hours will be $10 \times 2^{12} = 40,960$.

Prior to achieving exponential growth, bacteria that were not previously growing undergo a **lag phase**, during which cell division does not occur even if the growth conditions are ideal.

- If growth conditions are ideal, why wouldn't cell division occur immediately?[53]
- Will bacteria that are transferred from a culture that is in log phase to a fresh new culture show a lag phase?[54]

As metabolites in the growth medium are depleted, and metabolic waste products accumulate, the bacterial population passes from log phase to **stationary phase**, in which cells cease to divide for lack of nutrients. The maximum population at the stationary phase is referred to as the **carrying capacity** for that environment. In the last stages of the stationary phase, cell death may occur as a result of the medium's inability to support growth. [If bacteria are grown in a medium with glucose as the main source of energy, when will the glycolytic pathway be more active: during the lag phase or during the stationary phase?[55]]

Endospore Formation

Some types of Gram-positive bacteria, such as the bacteria responsible for botulism, form **endospores** under unfavorable growth conditions. Endospores have tough, thick external shells comprised of peptidoglycan. Within the endospore are found the genome, ribosomes, and RNA which are required for the spore to become metabolically active when conditions become favorable. Endospores are able to survive temperatures above 100°C, which is why autoclaves or pressure cookers are required to completely sterilize liquids and substances that cannot be heated sufficiently in a dry oven. The metabolic reactivation of an endospore is termed **germination**. A single bacterium is able to form only one spore per cell. Thus, bacteria cannot increase their population through spore formation. [When are bacteria most likely to form endospores: during lag phase, log phase, or stationary phase? Is endospore formation a means for bacteria to reproduce?[56]]

Genetic Exchange Between Bacteria

Bacteria reproduce asexually, but genetic exchange is evolutionarily favorable because it fosters genetic diversity. Bacteria have three mechanisms of acquiring new genetic material: **transduction**, **transformation**, and **conjugation**. Note that none of these has anything to do with reproduction! Transduction was discussed in Section 5.1; it is the transfer of genomic DNA from one bacterium to another by a lysogenic phage. Transformation refers to a peculiar phenomenon: if pure DNA is added to a bacterial culture, the bacteria internalize the DNA in certain conditions and gain any genetic information in the DNA. Conjugation appears most likely to be related to normal bacterial function, however.

---

[53] Cells that are not growing are not actively producing components that are needed for cell division, such as dNTPs. The lag period is a time when biosynthetic pathways are very actively producing new cellular components so that cells can then begin to divide.

[54] No, since they will have all the gear necessary for population growth at the ready.

[55] The bacteria will use glucose during the lag phase to produce ATP and cellular machinery. During this period, glucose is abundant, and the cell is actively performing biosynthesis, so glycolysis is very active. During the stationary phase, however, the glucose will be depleted, and the rate of metabolism will have slowed dramatically, so the rate of glycolysis will decrease as well.

[56] Stationary. Forming an endospore is like hibernating, not reproducing. Bacteria do it in order to sleep through the bad times.

Conjugation

Although bacteria reproduce asexually, they have developed conjugation to exchange genetic information. In conjugation, bacteria make physical contact and form a bridge between the cells. One cell copies DNA, and this copy is transferred through the bridge to the other cell. A key to bacterial conjugation is an extrachromosomal element known as the **F (fertility) factor**. Bacteria that have the F factor are **male**, or F^+, and will transfer the F factor to female cells. Bacteria that do not contain the F factor are **female**, F^-, and will receive the F factor from male cells to become male. [If all cells in a population are F^+, will conjugation occur?[57]]

The F factor is a single circular DNA molecule. Although much smaller than the bacterial chromosome, the F factor contains several genes, many of which are involved in conjugation itself. [Which cell will produce sex pili: the male cell or the female cell?[58]] After the male cell produces sex pili and the pili contact a female cell, a **conjugation bridge** forms. The F factor is replicated and transferred from the F^+ to the F^- cell. DNA transfer between F^+ and F^- cells is unidirectional; it occurs in one direction only (see Figure 13).

Although the F factor is an extrachromosomal element, it does sometimes become integrated into the bacterial chromosomes through recombination. A cell with the F factor integrated into its genome is called an **Hfr (high frequency of recombination) cell**. [Will an Hfr cell undergo conjugation with an F^- cell?[59]] When an Hfr cell performs conjugation, replication of the F factor DNA occurs as in F^+ cells with the extra chromosomal F factor. Since the F factor DNA is integrated in the bacterial genome in Hfr cells, replication of F factor DNA continues into bacterial genes, and these too can be transferred into the F^- cell (see Figure 13).

- If bacteria contain only one copy of the bacterial genome, how can recombination occur?[60]
- If the F factor in an Hfr strain integrates near a gene required for lactose metabolism, is it likely that other genes involved in lactose metabolism will be transferred during conjugation at the same time?[61]

---

[57] No. Conjugation occurs only between F+ (male) and F^- (female).

[58] The male cell contains the F factor that encodes the genes for pili production and will produce pili.

[59] Yes. All of the genes of the F factor are still present and expressed normally in the Hfr cell.

[60] When an Hfr cell conjugates with an F^- cell and transfers a portion of the bacterial chromosomes, the F^- cell will have two copies of some genes, and recombination can occur between the two copies.

[61] Yes. Genes for proteins of related functions are often adjacent to each other in prokaryotes (in operons) and so will transfer to an F^- cell together.

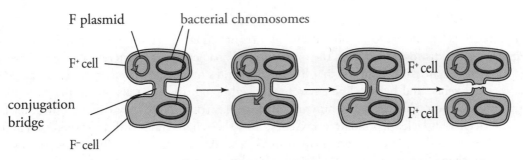

a) Conjugation and transfer of an F plasmid from an F⁺ donor to an F⁻ recipient

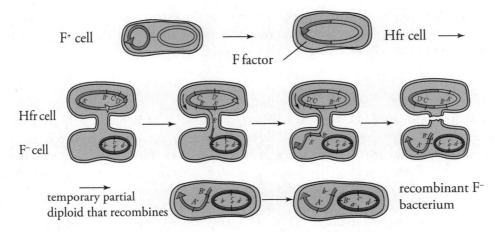

b) Conjugation and transfer of part of the bacterial chromosome from an Hfr donor to an F⁻ recipient, resulting in recombination

Figure 13 Conjugation

Conjugation Mapping

Hfr bacteria provide a mechanism of mapping the bacterial genome. By allowing Hfr cells to conjugate in the lab and stopping the conjugation process after different time intervals, researchers can figure out the order of the genes on the bacterial chromosome by analyzing recipient cells to see what genes were transferred.

For example, you have two strains of *E. coli*. One is a normal Hfr bacterium. The other is F⁻ and auxotrophic for arginine, leucine, and histidine (F⁻ Arg⁻ Leu⁻ His⁻). You allow conjugation to begin and stop it after 2 minutes. You find that all the recipients are now F⁻ Arg⁻ Leu⁻ His⁺. Then you take another bunch of bacteria and allow conjugation to proceed for 5 minutes. Now all the recipients are F⁻ Arg⁺ Leu⁻ His⁺. You do the experiment a third and final time, allowing 8 minutes of conjugation, and find the recipients to be F⁻ Arg⁺ Leu⁺ His⁺.

- What is the arrangement on the genome of the enzymes responsible for synthesis of each amino acid, relative to the site of F plasmid integration?[62]

---

[62] The experiments showed that the ability to make histidine was transferred in a short time. After a slightly longer time, the ability to make both histidine and arginine was transferred. Lastly, the ability to make leucine were transferred. So the arrangement on the genome (the map) must be: His-Arg-Leu-plasmid integration site.

Domain Archaea

Though all bacteria are prokaryotes, not all prokaryotes are equal. Certain prokaryotes belong to the domain *Archaea*, to be distinguished from the more "typical" bacteria (or eubacteria) which we have just discussed. The Archaea are the organisms that live in the world's most extreme environments, including hot springs, thermal vents, and hypersaline environments (although they can also be found in less extreme environments, such as soil, water, the human colon, etc.). Structurally, they differ from other bacteria because their cell wall lacks peptidoglycan. Genetically, they share traits with eukaryotes including the presence of introns and the use of many similar mRNA sequences. However, since they are single celled, they do reproduce via fission or budding. [What does this mean for their ability to increase their genetic diversity?[63]]

Since Archaea have to produce enzymes that can function in extreme environments, they are of great use in industrial applications, such as food processing and sewage treatment. The development of applications for products from these cells is an ongoing area of research.

Parasitic Bacteria

Parasitic bacteria can either be *obligate*, meaning that they must be inside a host cell to replicate, or *facultative*, meaning that they can live and replicate inside or outside of a host cell. In either case, the designation as a **parasite** means that damage is being done to the host cell. However, in order to ensure a continued supply of energy and cellular materials needed to survive and reproduce, parasitic bacteria need to modulate the course of that damage. [How is this model similar to viruses?[64]]

T cells (lymphocytes involved in immunity; see Chapter 9) are responsible for monitoring cellular contents; people who are T cell deficient have a hard time fighting off these types of bacterial infections, just as they would also struggle with viral infections. *Mycobacteria*, the genus of bacteria which encompasses the cause of tuberculosis as well as other diseases, has members which are obligate and others which are facultative, whereas the sexually transmitted disease chlamydia is caused solely by an obligate parasitic bacteria.

Symbiotic Bacteria

Symbiotic bacteria coexist with a host, where both the bacterial cell and the host cell derive a benefit. An example of this would be the *Rhizobia* genus, which is responsible for the fixing of nitrogen in the nodules that exist on the roots of legumes. Without these bacteria the legume plants would not be able to grow, as they would be unable to derive the necessary nitrogen from the soil on their own. Similarly, *Cyanobacteria* are responsible for nitrogen fixing in marine environments. Some of the bacterial flora in the human gut is also composed of symbionts which aid the human body in defending against other pathogenic strains. [What other functions do the bacteria in the gut have?[65]] Due to their close relationship with their host cells, these bacteria often have smaller genomes with a more limited number of cellular products that are made, since the host cells can provide some of what the bacteria need. This can often mean that the symbiotic bacteria do not survive long outside of the host environment.

---

[63] Archaea would need to use separate strategies to increase their genetic diversity, just like eubacteria. The ability to become more genetically diverse would not be built into reproduction as it is in humans, in part because meiosis is not occurring.

[64] Viruses are obligate intracellular parasites. They do not have the option to replicate outside of a host cell, but must also balance the damage that is done to the host cell against what is needed for more virus to be made.

[65] The gut flora is responsible for the production of vitamin K, which is necessary for blood clotting and in feeding off of undigested material from what humans have consumed; they are one of the final stages in processing our solid waste for excretion.

Chapter 5 Summary

- All viruses are made up of nucleic acids (either RNA or DNA) surrounded by a protein coat (capsid). They are obligate intracellular parasites and must rely on other cells to reproduce.

- Animal viruses may also have an envelope (lipid bilayer) surrounding the capsid. The envelope is derived from the host cell and is acquired by budding through the host cell membrane.

- Viral infection is specific; molecules on the viral surface determine which type of host cell it will infect.

- Viruses replicate via two major life cycles, the lytic cycle (in which more virus is made very quickly) and the lysogenic cycle (in which the virus goes dormant by integrating into the host cell genome). Viruses in the lysogenic cycle can excise from the genome and enter the lytic cycle.

- Animal viruses can also participate in a third life cycle, the productive cycle. This is very similar to the lytic cycle, but the new viruses escape by budding instead of by lysing the host.

- Lysogenic viruses can take pieces of the host DNA with them when they excise and transfer it to the next host. This is called transduction.

- RNA viruses require special virus-derived enzymes (RNA dependent RNA polymerases) in order to replicate their genomes.

- Prions and viroids are subviral particles that can cause disease and infection. They are unique in that prions are simply abnormal proteins (with no genetic material) and viroids are small pieces of RNA with no associated capsid, that do not code for proteins.

- The primary difference between prokaryotes and eukaryotes is that prokaryotes have no membrane-bound organelles (e.g., nucleus, mitochondria, etc.), thus all cellular processes occur in the cytosol.

- The shapes of bacteria can be used to classify them (round = coccus, rod = bacillus, spiral = spirochete).

- Bacteria have cell walls made out of peptidoglycan that can bind crystal violet (a purple stain used in Gram stain). Gram-positive bacteria have thick cell walls and stain a dark purple. Gram-negative bacteria have thinner cell walls and an outer membrane; they stain a light pink.

- Some bacteria can be classified by the presence or absence of flagella. Bacterial flagella are used for motility and are distinct from eukaryotic flagella in structure.

- Preferred growth temperature, nutrition, and oxygen use/tolerance are means of characterizing bacteria and can be used to select for growth of a particular bacteria.

- Binary fission is a means of asexual bacterial reproduction that increases the population size exponentially, but it does not increase the genetic diversity of the population.

- Conjugation is a means of increasing genetic diversity in a bacterial population by exchanging DNA (plasmid or genomic) via a conjugation bridge.

- Bacteria in Domain Archaea are sometimes classified as extremophiles because they can live in harsh, extreme environments, like hot springs, thermal vents, extreme acids/bases, and hyper-saline environments.

- Parasitic bacteria can live inside or outside of host cells and harm the host cells. Symbiotic bacteria coexist with host cells, but provide the host cells with a benefit; for example, the gut bacteria provide us with vitamin K.

CHAPTER 5 FREESTANDING PRACTICE QUESTIONS

1. A researcher has an agar plate covered with a lawn of *E. coli*. She adds a drop of a substance, and the next day there is a clear spot on the plate where the substance was added. This substance could be:

    I. a virus undergoing the lytic cycle.
    II. a virus undergoing the productive cycle.
    III. a chemical that is toxic to prokaryotes.

A) I only
B) III only
C) I and III
D) I, II, and III

2. A lab technician grows a liquid bacterial culture overnight, in media without any antibiotics. The next morning, the culture is cloudy. She takes a small amount of this culture and puts it into new media containing tetracycline. The next day, she checks the culture and the media is not cloudy. What happened?

A) The bacterial culture grew the first night but not the second night.
B) The bacteria were resistant to the antibiotic tetracycline.
C) The bacteria were in the lag phase after the first night of growth.
D) The bacteria were in the stationary phase after the second night of growth.

3. Which of the following is associated with prokaryotes and does NOT introduce new genetic material?

A) Mitosis
B) Binary fission
C) Transformation
D) Transduction

4. Which of the following statements concerning viruses is true?

A) The productive cycle is the most efficient infective cycle for phages.
B) Viruses that infect human cells must have an envelope.
C) Genetic information can be transferred between hosts via transfection.
D) A lytic virus with an RNA genome must code for an RNA-dependent RNA polymerase.

5. A researcher is trying to characterize a novel prokaryotic organism that has been found in the Indian Ocean. When Gram stained, the cells are a light pink color under the microscope. When exposed to antibiotics commonly used in the lab, the bacteria are able to enter the log growth phase in a manner similar to *E. coli* grown in media lacking ampicillin. A reasonable explanation is that:

A) this is a Gram-positive bacterium with an additional lipopolysaccharide layer that increases their resistance to antibiotics.
B) this is a Gram-positive bacterium with a cell membrane outside its peptidoglycan layer that increases their resistance to antibiotics.
C) this is a Gram-negative bacterium with an additional lipopolysaccharide layer that increases their resistance to antibiotics.
D) this is a Gram-negative bacterium with a peptidoglycan layer outside the cell membrane that increases their resistance to antibiotics.

6. Which of the following is true regarding prokaryotic flagella?

A) It is the predominant form of bacterial locomotion.
B) It is made of microtubules connected by dynein proteins.
C) It allows viruses to maneuver between host cells.
D) It can only be located on one end of a bacterium and this defines the polarity of the cell.

7. In prion diseases like Creutzfeldt-Jakob disease (CJD), the characteristic misfolded proteins are notoriously resistant to degradation. As a result, abnormal proteins accumulate in the endosomes and lysosomes of the cell, eventually leading to cellular dysfunction and death through a chronic, neurodegenerative process. Which of the following is the most likely explanation for the unusual resistance of these proteins to breakdown?

A) Accelerated rate of protein biosynthesis leads to early cell lysis
B) Excessive amount of protein accumulation results in cellular dysfunction
C) Aberrant protein function leads to disruption of normal cellular processes
D) Abnormal protein secondary structure results in poor binding with innate lysosomal proteases

CHAPTER 5 PRACTICE PASSAGE

Laboratory tests are a useful diagnostic tool for determining the cause of illness. One such test is the complete blood count or, CBC, as it is commonly called. In an infected individual, the white blood cell count can increase from a normal range of 4000–10,000 cells/µL to 15,000 to 20,000 cells/µL. Circulating neutrophils have a short lifespan upon release from the bone marrow (generally about ten hours); however, the demand for phagocytic cells during an infection increases markedly. The result is the release of immature neutrophils called band cells. In a differential white blood cell count, the presence of band cells is referred to as a *shift to the left*. A decrease in the number of neutrophils (neutropenia) can also occur as a result of inflammation or severe infection, when the removal of the neutrophils from the circulation outpaces their production. Neutropenia is also seen in certain blood cancers, such as leukemia and lymphomas, as the neutrophil precursor cells are crowded out by the cancerous cells.

The type of microorganism responsible for an infection can often be determined by changes identified in the population of white blood cells. For example, an increase in neutrophils is commonly seen in bacterial infections. An increase in eosinophils frequently accompanies parasitic infections, as well as allergic responses. A decrease in neutrophils with an increase in lymphocytes (lymphocytosis) can signify a viral infection. All types of infections can result in inflammation (fever, swelling, redness, pain).

An emergency room saw patients presenting with respiratory complaints and fever. One symptom was cough, either productive and mucus-producing, or non-productive. The fevers were mild to severe. A blood sample was obtained from each patient; a CBC was ordered on each and each sample was cultured for any infection-causing bacteria. Standard growth media providing sufficient nutrients for a wide range of bacteria was used. The following results were obtained:

Table 1   Bacterial Culture Results in Four Different Patients

Patient	Growth in culture
1	No
2	Yes
3	No
4	Yes

Table 2   WBC Counts in Four Different Patients

Patient	Elevated eosinophils	Elevated neutrophils	Elevated lymphocytes
1	Yes	No	No
2	No	No	Yes
3	No	No	Yes
4	No	Yes	No

1. If placed on a course of antibiotic therapy, which of the following patients would feel significantly improved after approximately 1–2 days?

A) Patient 1
B) Patient 2
C) Patient 3
D) Patient 4

2. Why did the culture performed on the sample obtained from Patient 3 not yield any growth?

A) The bacteria causing the infection in Patient 3 is a uracil auxotroph.
B) Patient 3 has a bacterial infection.
C) Patient 3 is suffering from allergic symptoms.
D) A different growth medium was required.

3. To determine the most appropriate type of antibiotic to prescribe, which of the following additional tests could be performed on a patient sample for classification purposes?

A) Phage-typing
B) Gram-staining
C) Fermentation
D) Transduction

4. Which of the following bacterial types are LEAST likely to cause a respiratory infection?

A) Tolerant anaerobe
B) Obligate aerobe
C) Facultative anaerobe
D) Obligate anaerobe

5. If a patient's symptoms included neutropenia and elevated lymphocyte counts, which of the following diagnoses could be possible?

   I. Allergies

   II. Leukemia/lymphoma

   III. Viral infection

A) I only
B) II only
C) I and III only
D) II and III only

6. An experimental therapy to treat patients with multiple antibiotic-resistant bacteria involves introduction of a highly specific bacteriophage to the infected patient's bloodstream. Which of the following bacteriophage types would be the LEAST useful for this type of therapy?

A) A lytic bacteriophage
B) A lysogenic bacteriophage
C) An RNA virus
D) An enveloped virus

SOLUTIONS TO CHAPTER 5 FREESTANDING PRACTICE QUESTIONS

1. **C** A clear spot on a plate (known as a *plaque*) indicates that the *E. coli* are dead. This could be due to the addition of a lytic virus (Item I is true, and choice B can be eliminated) or toxin (Item III is true, and choice A can be eliminated). However, only animal viruses can go through the productive cycle because viruses cannot bud out of a cell with a cell wall, such as bacteria (Item II is false; choice D can be eliminated, and choice C is correct).

2. **A** Cloudy cultures are usually in the stationary phase and clear cultures are either not growing or still in the lag phase. Since the culture was cloudy on the first morning, bacteria had grown overnight and were most likely in stationary phase (choice A is correct, and choice C is wrong). The culture on the second morning was clear, indicating minimal growth (choice D is wrong). Since the first overnight culture did not contain tetracycline and the second overnight culture did, it is possible that the strain was sensitive to tetracycline, not resistant (choice B is wrong).

3. **B** Binary fission is the means by which bacteria divide and reproduce. It produces two progeny cells that are genetically identical to the parent; no new genetic information is introduced (choice B is correct). Although mitosis also does not introduce new genetic information, it is a process undergone by eukaryotic cells, not prokaryotes (choice A is wrong). Both transformation and transduction are associated with prokaryotes, but both involve the introduction of new genetic material. Transformation is the uptake of genetic material (plasmids or chromosomal DNA) from the extracellular environment (choice C is wrong), and transduction is the transfer of genetic information from one bacteria to another via a lysogenic phage (choice D is wrong).

4. **D** In order to replicate its genome, a lytic RNA virus must code for an RNA-dependent RNA polymerase; this enzyme will create a new strand of RNA by reading a template strand of RNA. Viral host cells will not express these enzymes naturally; they have no need to make RNA by reading RNA. Host cells normally produce RNA using DNA as a template (choice D is correct). Note also that lysogenic RNA viruses do not need an RNA-dependent RNA polymerase either, because they are not replicating their RNA genome. They first convert it to DNA using an RNA-dependent DNA polymerase (reverse transcriptase), then insert the DNA version of their genome into the host genome. New copies of the viral RNA genome can be made by simply transcribing (using host RNA polymerases) new copies of the viral genome. Phages only infect bacteria and can only undergo the lytic and lysogenic cycles; the productive cycle involves budding through cell membrane and cannot occur in hosts with cell walls, such as bacteria (choice A is wrong). Although viruses with an envelope (lipid bilayer coating) are restricted to infecting animal cells, the outer membrane is not required (choice B is wrong). Genetic information can indeed be transferred between hosts, but this process is called *transduction*, not *transfection* (choice C is wrong).

5. **C** The answer options all start with Gram positive or Gram negative, and the light pink staining in the question stem indicates that this bacteria is Gram negative. Gram-positive bacteria have a peptidoglycan layer outside the cell membrane and therefore stain a dark purple (choices A and B are wrong). Gram-negative bacteria have a lipopolysaccharide layer outside

the peptidoglycan layer. This additional outer layer prevents dark staining (thus the light pink color) and increases resistance to antibiotics (choice C is correct, and choice D is wrong).

6. **A**   Prokaryotic flagella are the predominant means of bacterial locomotion (choice A is correct). Only eukaryotic flagella are made of microtubules and dynein; bacterial flagella have a different structure and are made of the protein flagellin (choice B is wrong). Viruses rely on diffusion to maneuver between host cells, not flagella (choice C is wrong). Bacteria can have flagella on one end (monotrichous), both ends (amphitrichous), or in multiple places (peritrichous; choice D is wrong).

7. **D**   Typically in a cell, abnormal proteins are targeted to proteasomes in the cytosol for degradation or to the lysosomes for digestion. The accumulation of the abnormal prions in the lysosomes suggests that they are somehow resistant to the lysosomal enzymes, and this could be due to their abnormal structure that prevents efficient binding at the active sites of the lysosomal digestive enzymes (choice D is correct). CJD and other prion diseases do not involve accelerated protein biosynthesis; normal prion proteins are produced at their typical rate, but are converted after translation into the abnormal prion version (choice A is wrong). While the accumulation of misfolded proteins likely contributes to cellular dysfunction, and while prions could (and likely do) lead to disruption of normal cellular processes, neither of these explain why the abnormal proteins are resistant to breakdown (choice D is a better choice than either B or C).

SOLUTIONS TO CHAPTER 5 PRACTICE PASSAGE

1. **D**   Antibiotics only treat bacterial infections. Table 1 shows that Patients 2 and 4 have positive cultures, confirming a bacterial infection (choices A and C can be eliminated). However, from Table 2, only Patient 4 has elevated neutrophils, which the passage states is indicative of a bacterial infection, making this patient a candidate for antibiotic therapy. Patient 2 has elevated lymphocytes (not neutrophils), which indicates a concomitant viral infection; the lack of elevated neutrophils in this patient is most likely the result of overwhelming infection. While the bacterial infection of Patient 2 would begin to subside by 1–2 days, the viral infection would take longer to eradicate, and therefore this patient would still be feeling poorly at this point (choice D is better than choice B).

2. **D**   From Table 2, Patient 3 has elevated lymphocytes, indicating a viral infection (choices A, B, and C can be eliminated); no growth would occur on standard growth media. Viruses are obligate intracellular parasites and require special growth media containing live cells for reproduction. According to the passage, standard growth media for bacterial culturing was used. Note that if the patient had elevated neutrophils and normal lymphocyte levels (indicating a bacterial infection), choice A would be the best answer, since uracil was not added to the culture media.

3. **B**   Determination of Gram status can aid in antibiotic selection. Phage typing applies to bacteriophage, not bacteria (choice A can be eliminated). Fermentation refers to metabolic activity (choice C can be eliminated). Transduction is not a classification method (choice D can be eliminated).

4. **D** The lungs are a high oxygen environment that is unfavorable to obligate anaerobes. Tolerant anaerobes, obligate aerobes, and facultative anaerobes can all survive in the presence of oxygen (choices A, B, and C can be eliminated).

5. **D** Item I is false: the passage states that elevated eosinophil counts (not lymphocytes) accompany allergic reactions (choices A and C can be eliminated). Note that both remaining answer choices include Item II, so it must be true: the passage states that neutropenia and elevated lymphocyte counts are seen in lymphoma and leukemia (blood cancers). Item III is true: neutropenia and lymphocytosis are seen in viral infections (choice B can be eliminated, and choice D is correct).

6. **D** Enveloped viruses infect only animal cells and would not be useful in eliminating bacteria from a human patient. The most useful type of virus would attack the infecting bacteria and cause the bacteria to lyse, eradicating the patient's infection (choice A would be useful and can be eliminated), and this virus could have either an RNA or a DNA genome (choice C could be useful and can be eliminated). A virus that incorporates itself into the bacterial genome and then goes dormant (a lysogenic virus) would not be as helpful as a lytic virus in eradicating an infection; however, it would still be more useful than a virus that cannot infect bacteria at all (choice B would be more useful than choice D).

Chapter 6
Eukaryotic Cells

The first cells were prokaryotes. They consisted of a cell membrane and a cell wall surrounding the cytoplasm or cell fluid. All of the structures necessary for survival and reproduction floated in the cytoplasm, including the double-stranded circular DNA genome, ribosomes, the enzymes of aerobic and anaerobic metabolism, etc. As evolution proceeded, cell complexity increased. The greatest landmark in the evolution of the cell was the development of membrane-bound compartments within the cytoplasm known as organelles. These served to organize the cytoplasm, with each membrane acting to seal its compartment. The most important organelle is the control center of the cell: the nucleus. In fact, *eukaryotic* is from the Greek *karyon*, meaning "kernel" or "nucleus," plus the prefix "eu," meaning "true." *Prokaryotic* means "before the nucleus" and also implies "before organelles." All true living organisms are either prokaryotes or eukaryotes. There are three well-defined kingdoms within Domain Eukarya (Plantae, Animalia, and Fungi), and one group of organisms for whom the kingdom classifications are under debate (single-celled eukaryotes—the Protists).

6.1 INTRODUCTION

It would be impossible to understand medicine without sound knowledge of the eukaryotic cell. In this chapter, we will examine each of the principal organelles, beginning with the nucleus. Next we will focus on the plasma membrane, then the cytoskeleton, and finally we will finish with a discussion of the cell cycle. You should be able to explain the function of each item labeled in Figure 1 below. Our discussion will be based on the animal cell; fungi, plants, and protists are not covered on the MCAT.

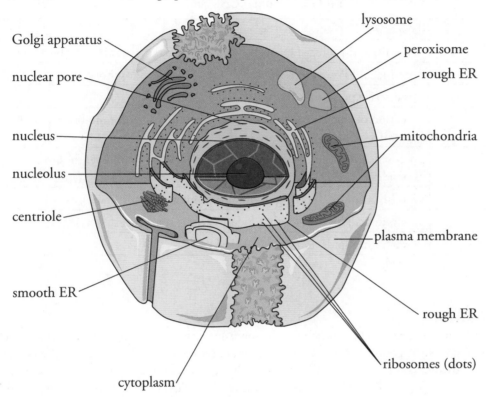

Figure 1 The Eukaryotic Cell

6.2 THE ORGANELLES

An **organelle** is a small structure within a cell that carries out specific cellular functions. Most organelles are bounded by their own lipid bilayer membrane. The membrane acts like a plastic bag to seal off the contents of the organelle from the rest of the cytoplasm and control what enters and exits. A summary of the major animal cell organelles is given in the table below:

Table 1 Animal Cell Organelles

Organelle	Function [number of membranes surrounding]
nucleus	contain and protect DNA; transcription; partial assembly of ribosomes (2)
mitochondria	produce ATP via the Krebs cycle and oxidative phosphorylation (2)
ribosomes	synthesize proteins (0)
RER	location of synthesis/modification of secretory, membrane-bound, and organelle proteins (1)
SER	detoxification and glycogen breakdown in liver; steroid synthesis in gonads (1)
Golgi apparatus	modification and sorting of protein, some synthesis (1)
lysosomes	contain acid hydrolases that digest various substances (1)
peroxisomes	metabolize lipids and toxins using H_2O_2 (1)

The Nucleus

One of the primary features of eukaryotic cells distinguishing them from prokaryotic cells is the **nucleus**. The nucleus contains the genome surrounded by the **nuclear envelope** that separates the contents of the nucleus into a distinct compartment, isolated from other organelles and from the cytoplasm. In prokaryotes the genome may be localized in the cell, but without a nuclear envelope to form a separate compartment, the genome remains accessible to the cytoplasm. In prokaryotes, replication, transcription and translation, and everything else all happens in the same compartment (the cytoplasm). In eukaryotes, replication, transcription, and splicing occur in the nucleus, while translation occurs in the cytoplasm.

- If an enzyme that degrades mRNA is injected into the cytoplasm of a cell and all translation ceases, is the cell prokaryotic or eukaryotic?[1]
- When an enzyme that degrades DNA (DNase) is incubated with intact DNA isolated from an organism, the DNA is degraded. But when DNase is injected into the cytoplasm of cells from the same organism, no effect on the genome is observed. Which one of the following is the best explanation for this?[2]
    - A) The cell is a prokaryote; therefore, the genome is inaccessible to cytoplasmic enzymes.
    - B) The cell is a prokaryote; therefore, the circular genome is resistant to DNase.
    - C) The cell is a eukaryote; therefore, the genome is inaccessible to cytoplasmic enzymes.
    - D) The cell is a eukaryote; therefore, the linear genome is resistant to DNase.

---

[1] It could be either. mRNA and translation are found in the cytoplasm of both prokaryotes and eukaryotes, so the cell could be either.

[2] The isolated genome and the genome in the cell respond differently, so the key is not the circular or linear nature of the genome (choices B and D are wrong). The key is that in prokaryotes the injected cytoplasmic DNase will have access to the genome to degrade since they are in the same compartment, while in eukaryotes the DNase will not have access to the genome unless it enters the nucleus (choice **C** is the best answer).

The Genome

The eukaryotic genome was discussed in Chapter 4, so we will not repeat that material. The large size of the typical eukaryotic genome appears to make it necessary to split the genome into pieces, each a separate linear DNA molecule, termed a **chromosome**. Yeast have 4 different chromosomes, while there are 23 different human chromosomes. Since humans and most adult animals are diploid, they have two copies of each chromosome (except for the sex chromosomes; see Chapter 7).

Within each chromosome is also a portion of the many thousands of genes in the genome as a whole. Genes can be mapped genetically and physically to the chromosome they reside on and to a specific location on that chromosome, a **locus**.

Finally, the nucleus is not a loose membrane bag with DNA floating inside. If nuclei are treated with DNase and with detergent, an insoluble mesh of protein, known as the **nuclear matrix** or **nuclear scaffold**, is left behind. The role of the nuclear matrix may be in part analogous to the role of the cytoskeleton in the cytoplasm: to support and provide overall structure. The matrix may also play a role in regulating gene expression. The DNA in chromosomes is attached to the matrix at specific sites, and these (in some cases) appear to be involved in regulating gene expression or in limiting the effects of promoters and enhancers to discrete chromosomal regions known as domains. The role of the nuclear matrix is an area of ongoing research.

The Nucleolus

The **nucleolus** ("little nucleus") is a region within the nucleus which functions as a ribosome factory. There is no membrane separating the nucleolus from the rest of the nucleus. It consists of loops of DNA, RNA polymerases, rRNA, and the protein components of the ribosome. [Would you expect the nucleolus to be larger in cells that are actively synthesizing protein, or in quiescent cells?[3] What role would the loops of DNA in the nucleolus play?[4]]

The nucleolus is the site of transcription of rRNA by RNA pol I. Transcription of mRNA and tRNA is performed by other polymerases in other areas of the nucleus. [Does a similar "division of labor" exist in the prokaryotic cell?[5]] The ribosome is partially assembled while still in the nucleolus. The protein components of the ribosome are not produced in the nucleolus; they are transported into the nucleus from the cytoplasm (remember that *all* translation takes place in the cytoplasm). After partial assembly, the ribosome is exported from the nucleus, remaining inactive until assembly is completed in the cytoplasm. This may serve to prevent translation of hnRNA.

---

[3] The nucleolus is largest in cells that are producing large amounts of protein. The increased size reflects increased synthesis of ribosomes.

[4] The DNA will serve as template for ribosomal RNA production.

[5] No. Bacteria have only a single kind of RNA pol which is responsible for all transcription.

The Nuclear Envelope

Surrounding the nucleus and separating it from the cytoplasm is the **nuclear envelope**, composed of two lipid bilayer membranes. The inner nuclear membrane is the surface of the envelope facing the nuclear interior, and the outer nuclear membrane faces the cytoplasm. The membrane of the endoplasmic reticulum is at points continuous with the outer nuclear membrane, making the interior of the ER (the **lumen** of the ER) contiguous with the space between the two nuclear membranes. [Is the space between the inner and outer membranes contiguous with the cytoplasm?[6]]

The nuclear envelope is punctuated with large **nuclear pores** that allow the passage of material into and out of the nucleus (see Figures 2 and 3). Molecules that are smaller than 60 kilodaltons, including small proteins, can freely diffuse from the cytoplasm into the nucleus through the nuclear pores. Larger proteins cannot pass freely through nuclear pores and are excluded from the nuclear interior unless they contain a sequence of basic amino acids called a **nuclear localization sequence**. Proteins with a nuclear localization sequence are translated on cytoplasmic ribosomes and then imported into the nucleus by specific transport mechanisms. It also appears likely that RNA is transported out of the nucleus by a specific transport system rather than freely diffusing into the cytoplasm. [If a 15 kD protein has a nuclear localization sequence that is then deleted from its gene, will the mutated protein still be found in the nucleus?[7]]

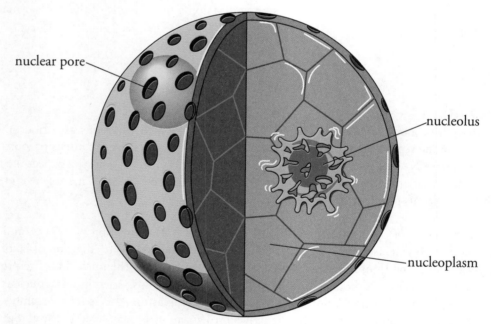

Figure 2 The Nucleus, Showing Pores

---

[6] No, it is not. The space between the nuclear membranes is contiguous with the ER lumen, which is isolated from the cytoplasm.

[7] Yes. The protein is small enough that it can still pass through the nuclear pores by diffusion even without a nuclear localization sequence.

Figure 3 A Nuclear Pore Close-Up

- Which one of the following proteins would NOT be found within the nucleus?[8]
  - A) A protein component of the large ribosomal subunit
  - B) A factor required for splicing
  - C) A histone
  - D) An aminoacyl tRNA synthetase

- A researcher injects tiny gold beads into a cell and waits an hour. Then she examines the cell and finds gold beads in the cytoplasm and in the nucleus. When she injects larger gold beads, they are not found in the nucleus. However, when she binds the larger beads to a nuclear localization sequence, she finds that they end up in the nucleus. One can conclude that:[9]
  - A) the nuclear localization sequence is lysine-rich.
  - B) gold beads have an inherent import signal.
  - C) the nuclear localization mechanism is nonspecific enough to confer nuclear import on gold beads.
  - D) nuclear import relies primarily on simple diffusion.

Mitochondria

Mitochondria are the site of oxidative phosphorylation. The interior of mitochondria, the **matrix**, is bounded by the inner and outer mitochondrial membranes (see Figure 4, next page). The matrix contains pyruvate dehydrogenase and the enzymes of the Krebs cycle. The inner membrane is the location of the electron transport chain and ATP synthase and is the site of the proton gradient used to drive ATP synthesis by ATP synthase. The inner membrane is impermeable to the free diffusion of polar substances,

---

[8] Aminoacyl tRNA synthetases are enzymes that function in the cytoplasm to attach amino acids to their respective tRNAs. They are never needed in the nucleus and would not be found there (choice **D** is correct). The protein components of ribosomes are synthesized in the cytoplasm and then imported into the nucleus to be assembled in the nucleolus (choice A would be found in the nucleus and can be eliminated). Splicing occurs in the nucleus, so anything involved in splicing would be found there (choice B can be eliminated). Histones are used for DNA packaging and would be found in the nucleus (choice C can be eliminated).

[9] Gold beads are not normally found in cells, so there cannot be an existing mechanism for moving them. However, since the cell is capable of moving them when the localization signal is attached, the localization signal must be somewhat nonspecific (choice **C** is correct). It is true that the nuclear localization signal is lysine-rich, but this cannot be concluded based on the given information (true, but it doesn't answer the question; choice A is wrong). If gold beads had an inherent import signal, then they would be transported into the nucleus on their own, without the researcher having to bind them to the localization sequence (choice B is wrong). If simple diffusion were the primary means of moving things into the nucleus, no import signal would be needed (choice D is wrong).

like protons, and is folded into the matrix in projections called **cristae**. The outer membrane is smooth and contains large pores that allow free passage of small molecules. The space between the membranes is called the intermembrane space. ATP produced within mitochondria is transported out into the cytoplasm to drive a great variety of cellular processes. [Why is the inner membrane folded into cristae?[10] Are the enzymes of glycolysis found in the matrix?[11] If the inner membrane is impermeable, how does pyruvate get into the matrix where pyruvate dehydrogenase is located?[12]]

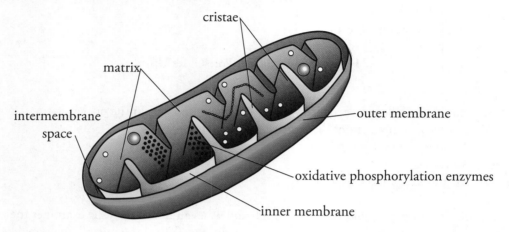

Figure 4   The Mitochondrion

Mitochondria possess their own genome which is far smaller than the cellular genome and consists of a single circular DNA molecule. (Sound familiar?) It encodes rRNA, tRNA, and several proteins, including some components of the electron transport chain and parts of the ATP synthase complex although most mitochondrial proteins are encoded by nuclear genes. Even more curious, mitochondria use a different system of transcription and translation than nuclear genes do. This includes a unique genetic code and unique RNA polymerases, DNA replication machinery, ribosomes, and aminoacyl-tRNA synthetases. In order to explain the fact that mitochondria possess a second system of inheritance, investigators have postulated that mitochondria originated as independent unicellular organisms living within larger cells. This is known as the **endosymbiotic theory** of mitochondrial evolution (*endo* = within; *symbiotic* = living together). In fact, if you compare a mitochondrion to a Gram-negative bacterium, you'll note that they look pretty similar. Pay attention to where the enzymes of electron transport are located and the genome shape.[13] Because many unique mitochondrial polypeptides are encoded by the cellular genome and not the mitochondrial genome, it has been suggested that the genes coding for these proteins may have been transferred to the nuclear genome over time. [What difficulty may be encountered in translation of a mitochondrial gene moved to the nucleus?[14]]

---

[10]   The folding of the membrane increases its surface area and allows for increased electron transport and ATP synthesis per mitochondrion. (Folding is used elsewhere to increase surface area, such as in the kidney tubules and the lining of the small intestine.)

[11]   No, in the cytoplasm.

[12]   Pyruvate is transported through the inner mitochondrial membrane by a specific protein in the membrane.

[13]   Remember that bacterial electron transport depends on a proton gradient across the cell membrane. In a Gram-negative bacterium, this membrane would correspond to the mitochondrial inner membrane.

[14]   The coding system of the cellular genome is different from that of the mitochondrial genome. One might wonder how our transcription and translation machinery could sensibly produce mitochondrial gene products.

Mitochondria exhibit **maternal inheritance**. This means that mitochondria are inherited only from the mother, since the cytoplasm of the egg becomes the cytoplasm of the zygote. (The sperm contributes only genomic [nuclear] DNA.) Maternal inheritance departs from the rules of Mendelian genetics, which state that traits are inherited from both parents (see Chapter 7). If a woman has a disease caused by an abnormality in her mitochondrial genome, what are the chances that her children will have the disease (assuming her mate does not have the disease)?[15]

Endoplasmic Reticulum (ER)

The **endoplasmic reticulum** (**ER**) is a large system of folded membrane accounting for over half of the membrane of some cells. There are two types of ER (see Figure 5): **rough ER** and **smooth ER**, each with distinct functions. The rough ER is called rough due to the large number of ribosomes bound to its surface; it is the site of protein synthesis for proteins targeted to enter the secretory pathway. The smooth ER is not actively involved in protein processing but can contain enzymes involved in steroid hormone biosynthesis (gonads) or in the degradation of environmental toxins (liver). The membrane of the endoplasmic reticulum is joined with the outer nuclear membrane in places, meaning that the space within the nuclear membranes is continuous with the interior of the ER (the ER **lumen**). The rough ER plays a key role directing protein traffic to different parts of the cell.

Figure 5 The ER

The Rough ER and the Secretory Pathway

There are two sites of protein synthesis in the eukaryotic cell: either on ribosomes free in the cytoplasm or on ribosomes bound to the surface of the rough ER. Proteins translated on free cytoplasmic ribosomes

---

[15] All of her children will have it, since they will inherit mitochondria exclusively from her. For a maternally inherited trait, it doesn't matter whether the father has it or not.

are headed toward peroxisomes, mitochondria, the nucleus, or will remain in the cytoplasm. Proteins synthesized on the rough ER will end up either 1) secreted into the extracellular environment, 2) as integral plasma membrane proteins, or 3) in the membrane or interior of the ER, Golgi apparatus, or lysosomes. Membrane-bound vesicles pass between these cellular compartments. Since the membranes of these organelles communicate through the traffic of vesicles, the interior of the ER, the Golgi apparatus, lysosomes, and the extracellular environment are in a sense contiguous. Proteins synthesized on the rough ER are transported in vesicles that bud from the ER to the Golgi apparatus, then to the plasma membrane or lysosome. A secreted protein that enters the ER lumen is separated by a membrane from the cytoplasm until the protein leaves the cell.

Whether a protein is translated on the rough ER is determined by the sequence of the protein itself. All proteins start translation in the cytoplasm; however, some proteins (secreted proteins and lysosomal proteins) have an amino acid sequence at their N-terminus called a **signal sequence.** The signal sequence of a nascent polypeptide is recognized by the **signal recognition particle** (**SRP**), which binds to the ribosome. The rough ER has SRP receptors that dock the ribosome-SRP complex on the cytoplasmic surface (along with the nascent polypeptide and mRNA). Translation then pushes the polypeptide, signal peptide first, into the ER lumen. After translation is complete, the signal peptide is removed from the polypeptide by a signal peptidase in the ER lumen. For secreted proteins, once the signal sequence is removed, the protein is transported in the interior of vesicles through the Golgi apparatus to the plasma membrane, where it is released by exocytosis into the extracellular environment.

- The mRNA for a secreted protein encodes a longer protein than is actually observed in the cellular exterior. Why?[16]
  - A) The protein was cleaved by a cytoplasmic protease.
  - B) The mRNA was not spliced properly.
  - C) The gene encoding the protein contained a nonsense mutation.
  - D) The signal sequence of the protein was removed in the rough ER.

Integral membrane proteins are processed slightly differently. Integral membrane proteins have sections of hydrophobic amino acid residues called **transmembrane domains** that pass through lipid bilayer membranes. The transmembrane domains are essentially signal sequences that are found in the interior of the protein (that is, not at the N-terminus). They are *not* removed after translation. A single polypeptide can have several transmembrane domains passing back and forth through a membrane. During translation, the transmembrane domains are threaded through the ER membrane. The protein is then transported in vesicles to the Golgi apparatus and plasma membrane in the same manner as a secreted protein (see Figure 6). [For a protein in the plasma membrane, does the portion of the protein in the ER lumen end up facing the cytoplasm or the cellular exterior?[17]]

Additional functions of the rough ER include the initial post-translational modification of proteins. Although glycosylation (the addition of saccharides to proteins) is usually associated with the Golgi apparatus, some glycosylation occurs in the lumen of the ER. Disulfide bond formation also occurs in the ER lumen.

---

[16] The only way a protein can be smaller than would be expected from its mRNA would be if some post-translational modification were to occur (choice **D** is correct). Choices B and C are pre-translational modifications and would not account for a size difference between mRNA and protein, and since secreted proteins are synthesized on the rough ER, they are inaccessible to cytoplasmic proteases (so choice A is wrong).

[17] The cellular exterior

Two last notes about protein traffic throughout the cell: First, the default target for proteins that go through the secretory path is the plasma membrane. **Targeting signals** are needed if a protein going through that path needs to end up elsewhere (e.g., the Golgi, the ER, the lysosome). Second, proteins that are made in the cytoplasm but need to be sent to an organelle that is not part of the secretory path (e.g., the nucleus, mitochondria, or peroxisomes) require sequences called **localization signals**. Table 2 summarizes protein traffic.

Table 2   Summary of Cellular Protein Traffic

Protein Final Destination	Signal Sequence?	Localization Signal?	Transmembrane Domains?	Targeting Signal?	Example
Secreted	Yes	No	No	No	Antibodies, neurotransmitters, peptide hormones
Plasma Membrane	Yes	No	Yes	No	Receptors, channels
Lysosome	Yes	No	No	Yes	Acid hydrolases
Rough ER	Yes	No	No	Yes	Enzymes required for protein modification
Smooth ER	Yes	No	No	Yes	Enzymes required for lipid synthesis
Golgi Apparatus	Yes	No	No	Yes	Enzymes required for protein modification
Cytoplasm	No	No	No	No	Glycolysis enzymes
Nucleus	No	Yes	No	No	Histones, DNA/RNA polymerase
Mitochondria	No	Yes	No	No	PDC/Krebs cycle enzymes
Peroxisome	No	Yes	No	No	Catalase

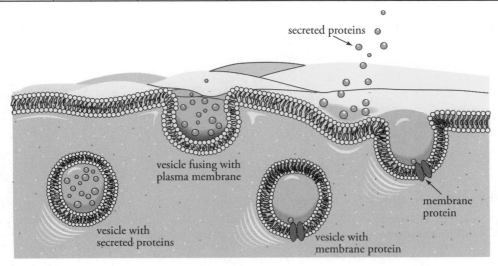

Figure 6   The Secretory Pathway—Secreted Proteins and Integral Membrane Proteins

- Disulfide bridges are found in extracellular proteins because the cytoplasm is a reducing environment that changes cystine to two cysteines. Given this fact, does it make sense that disulfide bridges are formed in the ER lumen?[18]
- Can mRNA coding for a protein destined to be embedded in the plasma membrane associate with rough ER prior to the initiation of translation?[19]

The Golgi Apparatus

The Golgi apparatus is a group of membranous sacs stacked together like collapsed basketballs (see Figure 7). It has the following functions: 1) Modification of proteins made in the RER; especially important is the modification of oligosaccharide chains. 2) Sorting and sending proteins to their correct destinations. 3) The Golgi also synthesizes certain macromolecules, such as polysaccharides, to be secreted.

The vesicle traffic to and from the Golgi apparatus is mostly unidirectional; the membrane-bound or secreted proteins which are to be sorted and modified enter at one defined region and exit at another. (Traffic is said to be *mostly* unidirectional because on occasion, proteins that are supposed to reside in the ER accidentally escape, and must be returned to the ER from the Golgi. This is called "retrograde traffic.") Each region of the Golgi has different enzymes and a different microscopic appearance. The portion of the Golgi nearest the rough ER is called the *cis* stack, and the part farthest from the rough ER is the *trans* stack. The *medial* stack is in the middle.[20] Vesicles from the ER fuse with the *cis* stack. The proteins in these vesicles are then modified and transferred to the *medial* stack, where they are further modified before passing to the *trans* stack. Proteins leave the Golgi at the *trans* face in transport vesicles. [If vesicle fusion with the *cis* Golgi was inhibited, could plasma membrane proteins still reach the cell surface?[21]] The route taken by a protein is determined by signals within the protein that determine which vesicle a protein is sorted into in the *trans* Golgi.

---

[18] Yes. Remember, the ER lumen is equivalent to (contiguous with) the extracellular space.

[19] No. It is the signal peptide in the nascent polypeptide that is recognized and bound by SRP and taken to receptors on the surface of the rough ER. The signal is an amino acid sequence on the nascent polypeptide, not a nucleotide sequence on mRNA.

[20] Note that *cis* means "near," as in a *cis* double bond. *Trans* means "far." *Medial* means "in the middle." Also note that the order is alphabetical: *cis-medial-trans*.

[21] No. Secretory proteins must proceed via a specific path: from the ER to the *cis* Golgi to the medial and *trans* Golgi and from there to the cell surface.

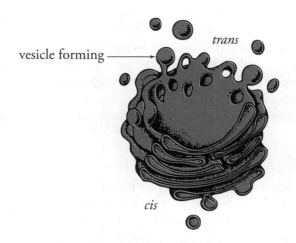

vesicle forming ⟶

trans

cis

Figure 7   The Golgi Apparatus

When a vesicle moves from the *trans* Golgi toward the cell surface, it fuses with the cell membrane. As a result, the contents of the vesicle are released into the extracellular environment in a process termed *exocytosis*. Alternatively, if the vesicle contains proteins anchored to its membrane, these proteins will remain attached to the cell as cell-surface proteins. Some proteins are sent in vesicles from the Golgi immediately to the cell surface, in the **constitutive secretory pathway**. *Constitutive* connotes *continuous* or *unregulated*. In contrast, specialized secretory cells (such as pancreatic cells, B cells of the immune system, etc.) store secretory proteins in **secretory vesicles** and release them only at certain times, usually in response to a change in (or signal from) the extracellular environment. This is a **regulated secretory pathway**.

Lysosomes

Lyse means cut. The **lysosome** is a membrane-bound organelle that is responsible for the degradation of biological macromolecules by hydrolysis. Lysosome proteins are made in the RER, modified in the Golgi, and released in their final form from the *trans* face of the Golgi. Organelles such as mitochondria that have been damaged or are no longer functional may be degraded in lysosomes in a process termed **autophagy** (self-eating). Lysosomes also degrade large particulate matter engulfed by the cell by **phagocytosis** (cell eating). For example, **macrophages** of the immune system engulf bacteria and viruses. The particle or microorganism ends up in a **phagocytic vesicle**, which will fuse with a lysosome. Finally, **crinophagy** refers to lysosomal digestion of unneeded (excess) secretory products. After hydrolysis, the lysosome will release molecular building blocks into the cytoplasm for reuse.

The enzymes responsible for degradation in lysosomes are called **acid hydrolases**. This name reflects the fact that these enzymes only hydrolyze substrates when they are in an acidic environment. This is a safety mechanism. The pH of the lysosome is around 5, so the acid hydrolases are active. But the pH of the cytoplasm is 7.4. If a lysosome ruptures, its enzymes will not damage the cell because the acidic fluid will be diluted, and the acid hydrolases will be inactivated. However, if many lysosomes rupture at once, the cell may be destroyed.

Peroxisomes

Peroxisomes are small organelles that perform a variety of metabolic tasks. The peroxisome contains enzymes that produce hydrogen peroxide (H_2O_2) as a by-product. They are essential for lipid breakdown in many cell types. In the liver they assist in detoxification of drugs and chemicals. H_2O_2 is a dangerous chemical, but peroxisomes contain an enzyme called **catalase** which converts it to $H_2O + O_2$. Separating these activities into the peroxisomes protects the rest of the cell from damage by peroxides or oxygen radicals.

6.3   THE PLASMA MEMBRANE

The evolution of life most likely began with a separation of "inside" from "outside." Once this had occurred, processes in the cell could increase their orderliness despite the entropic chaos of the surroundings. An alternate hypothesis is that life began with self-replicating RNA floating free in the ocean. As it grew more complex, this early genome would require protection. In any case, the separation of the cytoplasm from the extracellular environment was a major milestone in evolution. Bacteria, plants, and fungi accomplish this by forming a cell membrane and a cell wall (made of peptidoglycan, cellulose, and chitin, respectively). Eukaryotic animal cells have no cell wall and thus rely on the cell membrane as the only boundary between inside and outside. And they must devise another means of structural support: just as chordates have a bony endoskeleton instead of the primitive exoskeleton arthropods have, animal cells rely on an internal cytoskeleton instead of an external cell wall. Further problems arise in multicellular eukaryotes. Not only must each cell maintain its structural integrity, but it must also interact with its neighbors in an organized fashion. In the following discussion, we will study how each of these goals is accomplished.

Membrane Structure

All of the membranes of the cell are composed of **lipid bilayer** membranes. The three most common lipids in eukaryotic membranes are **phospholipids**, **glycolipids**, and **cholesterol**, of which phospholipids are the most abundant. An example of a phospholipid is *phosphatidyl choline* (see Figure 8) with two long hydrophobic fatty acids esterified to glycerol, along with a charged phosphoryl choline group. Thus, phospholipids have portions that are distinctly hydrophilic and hydrophobic. Glycolipids, with fatty acids groups and carbohydrate side chains, also have hydrophilic and hydrophobic regions. When fatty acids or phospholipids are mixed with water, they spontaneously arrange themselves with the hydrophobic tails facing the interior to avoid contact with water and the hydrophilic regions facing outward toward water (see Figure 9). Fatty acids form small micelles, but, due to steric hindrance, phospholipids arrange themselves spontaneously into **lipid bilayer membranes**. Since the lipid bilayer is the lowest energy state for these molecules, the bilayer membrane can reseal and repair itself if a small portion of membrane is removed. [Does the formation of a lipid bilayer when phospholipids are mixed with water have a positive or a negative ΔG (change in free energy)?[22]]

The interior of the lipid bilayer membrane is very hydrophobic, with water largely excluded. Hydrophilic molecules such as ions, carbohydrates, and amino acids are not soluble in this environment, making the membrane a barrier to the passage of these molecules. Nonpolar molecules such as CO_2, O_2, and steroid hormones can cross the membrane easily. Water can also pass through the membrane but does so through specialized protein channels.

---

[22] Lipid bilayers form spontaneously, as the lowest energy state, without external energy input. This describes a process with a negative ΔG.

Figure 8 Phosphatidyl Choline, a Phospholipid

• Which one of the following statements best describes the physical characteristics of phospholipids?[23]

A) Negatively charged at pH 7 and therefore entirely hydrophilic
B) Hydrophobic
C) Partially hydrophilic and partially hydrophobic
D) Positively charged at pH 7 and therefore entirely hydrophilic

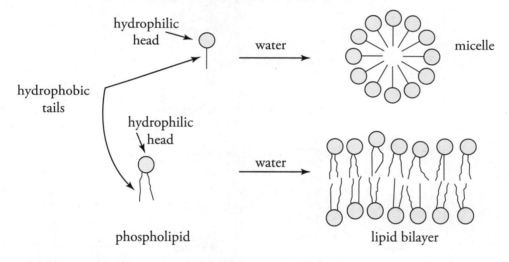

Figure 9 Lipid Behavior in an Aqueous Solvent

In addition to lipids, proteins are a major component of membranes. In some cases, such as the mitochondrial inner membrane, there is a higher protein than lipid concentration. Some proteins act to mediate interactions of the cell with other cells. Other proteins called **cell-surface receptors** bind extracellular signaling molecules such as hormones and relay these signals into the cell so that it can respond accordingly. **Channel proteins** selectively allow ions or molecules to cross the membrane. Each of these types of membrane protein is discussed below.

---

[23] Choice **C.** Phospholipids have hydrophobic components (fatty acid acyl chains) and hydrophilic components (phosphate and choline, for example, in phosphatidyl choline).

6.3

In general, membrane proteins are classified as peripheral or integral (see Figure 10). **Integral membrane proteins** are actually embedded in the membrane, held there by hydrophobic interactions. Membrane-crossing regions are called **transmembrane domains** (see Figure 11). Integral membrane proteins may have a complex pattern of transmembrane domains and portions not within the membrane. [At which point in the secretory pathway would the insertion of transmembrane domains into the membrane occur?[24]] **Peripheral membrane proteins** are not embedded in the membrane at all, but rather are stuck to integral membrane proteins, held there by hydrogen bonding and electrostatic interactions.

Figure 10 Membrane Proteins

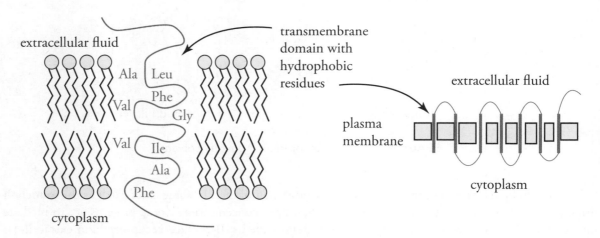

Figure 11 Transmembrane Domains

The current understanding of membrane dynamics is termed the **fluid mosaic model**, because the membrane is seen as a mosaic of lipids and proteins that are free to move back and forth fluidly. According to

---

[24] It occurs in the rough ER as the protein is translated and threaded across the ER membrane.

this model, lipids and proteins are free to diffuse laterally, in two dimensions, but are **not free to flip-flop**. Phospholipid head groups and hydrophilic protein domains are restricted from entering the hydrophobic membrane interior just as hydrophilic molecules in the extracellular space are. Thus, the membrane is said to have **polarity**. This just means that the inside face and the outside face remain different. We have already discussed one such difference: all glycosylations are found on the extracellular face. So the "fluid" in "fluid mosaic" means that things are free to move back and forth, but in two dimensions only. One exception is that some proteins are anchored to the cytoskeleton and thus cannot move in any direction.

- Phospholipids can be covalently attached to a fluorescent tag and then integrated into a lipid bilayer. If one cell has a red fluorescent tagged lipid in its plasma membrane and another cell has a green fluorescent tagged lipid in its membrane, what will happen if the two cells are fused together?[25]

The fluidity of a membrane is affected by the composition of lipids in the membrane (see Figure 12). The hydrophobic van der Waals interactions between the fatty acid side chains are a major determinant of membrane fluidity. Saturated fatty acids, lacking any double bonds, have a very straight structure and pack tightly in the membrane, with strong van der Waals forces between side chains. Unsaturated fatty acids, with one or more double bonds, have a kinked structure and pack in the membrane interior more loosely. Cholesterol also plays a key role in maintaining optimal membrane fluidity by fitting into the membrane interior. [If the percentage of unsaturated fatty acids in a membrane is increased, will membrane fluidity increase or decrease at body temperature?[26]]

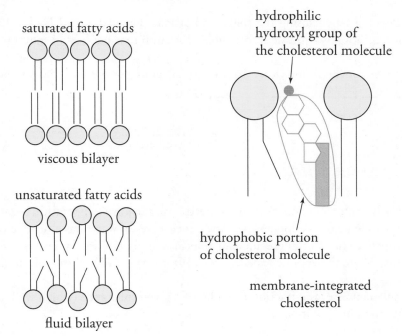

saturated fatty acids

viscous bilayer

unsaturated fatty acids

fluid bilayer

hydrophilic hydroxyl group of the cholesterol molecule

hydrophobic portion of cholesterol molecule

membrane-integrated cholesterol

Figure 12   Factors Affecting Membrane Fluidity

---

[25] After a short period of time, the red and green tagged lipids will diffuse laterally and mix. An even distribution of the tags will be seen across the surface of the new hybrid cell.

[26] Unsaturated fatty acids, with a kinked structure, have fewer van der Waals interactions, and therefore allow a more fluid membrane structure. Increasing the unsaturated fatty acids will increase membrane fluidity.

6.4 TRANSMEMBRANE TRANSPORT

The cell requires membranes to act as barriers to diffusion but also requires the transport of many different substances across membranes. Integral membrane proteins transport material through membranes that cannot diffuse on their own across membranes. Transport across a membrane can be either **passive** (does not require cellular energy) or **active** (requires cellular energy). Before we discuss movements across membranes, let's review basic rules about concentration, ionizability, colligative properties, and diffusion and osmosis.

Concentration Measurements

Molarity (*M*) expresses the concentration of a solution in terms of moles of solute per volume (in liters) of solution:

$$\text{Molarity } (M) = \frac{\text{\# moles of solute}}{\text{\# liters of solution}}$$

Concentration is denoted by enclosing the solute in brackets. For instance, "$[Na^+] = 1.0\ M$" indicates a solution whose concentration is equivalent to 1 mole of sodium ions per liter of solution.

Molality (*m*) expresses concentration in terms of moles of solute per *mass* (in kilograms) of solvent:

$$\text{Molality } (m) = \frac{\text{\# moles of solute}}{\text{\# kg of solvent}}$$

Molality is particularly useful when measuring properties that involve temperature because, unlike molarity, molality does not change with temperature. And, since a liter of water has a mass of one kilogram, the molar and molal concentrations of dilute aqueous solutions are nearly the same. This is particularly true in biological systems, where the volume (essentially a cell) is very small and the solvent is always water.

Mole fraction simply expresses the fraction of moles of a given substance (which we'll denote here by S) relative to the total moles in a solution:

$$\text{mole fraction of S} = X_S = \frac{\text{\# moles of substance S}}{\text{total \# moles in solution}}$$

Mole fraction is a useful way to express concentration when more than one solute is present.

Electrolytes

When ionic substances dissolve, they **dissociate** into ions. Free ions in a solution are called **electrolytes** because the solution can conduct electricity. Some salts dissociate completely into individual ions, while others only partially dissociate (that is, a certain percentage of the ions will remain paired, sticking close to each other rather than being independent and fully surrounded by solvent). Solutes that dissociate completely (like ionic substances) are called **strong electrolytes**, and those that remain ion-paired to some extent are called **weak electrolytes**. (Covalent compounds that don't dissociate into ions are **non-electrolytes**.) Solutions of strong electrolytes are better conductors of electricity than those of weak electrolytes.

Different ionic compounds will dissociate into different numbers of particles. Some won't dissociate at all, and others will break up into several ions. The **van't Hoff** (or **ionizability**) **factor** (**i**) tells us how many ions one unit of a substance will produce in a solution. For example,

- $C_6H_{12}O_6$ is non-ionic, so it does not dissociate. Therefore, $i = 1$.
  (Note: The van't Hoff factor for almost all biomolecules—hormones, proteins, steroids, etc.—is 1.)
- NaCl dissociates into Na^+ and Cl^-. Therefore, $i = 2$.
- HNO_3 dissociates into H^+ and NO_3^-. Therefore, $i = 2$.
- $CaCl_2$ dissociates into Ca^{2+} and $2Cl^-$. Therefore, $i = 3$.

Colligative Properties

Colligative properties depend on the *number* of solute particles in the solution rather than the *type* of particle. For example, when any solute is dissolved into a solvent, the boiling point, freezing point, and vapor pressure of the solution will be different from those of the pure solvent. For colligative properties, *the identity of the particle is not important.* That is, for a 1 *M* solution of *any* solute, the change in a colligative property will be the same no matter what the size, type, or charge of the solute particles. Remember to consider the van't Hoff factor when accounting for particles: one mole of sucrose ($i = 1$) will have the same number of particles *in solution* as 0.5 mol of NaCl ($i = 2$), and therefore will have the same effect on a colligative property. Thus, we can consider the effective concentration to be the product iM (or im); this is the concentration of particles present.

The four colligative properties we'll study for the MCAT are vapor-pressure depression, boiling-point elevation, freezing-point depression, and osmotic pressure.

Vapor-Pressure Depression

Think about being at the ocean or a lake in the summer. The air is always more humid (moist) than in the middle of a parking lot. Why? Because some of the water molecules gain enough energy to get into the gas phase, so we see a dynamic equilibrium setup between the molecules in the liquid phase and the molecules in the gas (vapor) phase.

Vapor pressure is the pressure exerted by the gaseous phase of a liquid that evaporated from the exposed surface of the liquid. The weaker a substance's intermolecular forces, the higher its vapor pressure and the more easily it evaporates. For example, if we compare diethyl ether, $H_5C_2OC_2H_5$, and water, we notice that while water undergoes hydrogen bonding, diethyl ether does not, so despite its greater molecular mass, diethyl ether will vaporize more easily and have a higher vapor pressure than water. Easily vaporized liquids—liquids with *high* vapor pressure—like diethyl ether are said to be **volatile.**

Now let's think about what happens to vapor pressure when the liquid contains a dissolved solute. The solute molecules are attached to solvent molecules and act as "anchors." As a result, more energy is required to enter the gas phase since the solvent molecules need to break away from their interactions with the solute before they can enter the gas phase. In fact, the boiling point of a liquid is defined as the temperature at which the vapor pressure of the solution is equal to the atmospheric pressure over the solution. Thus, at sea level, where the atmospheric pressure is 760 torr, the solution must have a vapor pressure of 760 torr in order to boil. Adding more solute to the same solution will decrease its vapor pressure. Boiling will still take place when vapor pressure is 760 torr, but more heat will have to be supplied to reach this vapor pressure, and thus the solution will boil at a higher temperature. For example, salted water (say, for cooking spaghetti) boils at a higher temperature than unsalted water.

Boiling-Point Elevation

When a liquid boils, the molecules in the liquid acquire enough energy to overcome the intermolecular forces and break free into the gas phase. The liquid molecules escape as a vapor at the surface between the liquid and air. But what happens when a non-volatile solute is added to the liquid? As described before, the solute particles are attached to solvent molecules and act as "anchors." As a result, more energy is required since you not only have to convert the solvent into the gas phase, but you first have to break the interaction with the solute. What happens to the boiling point? In order for the molecules to escape, they need more energy than they did without the solute. This translates into an elevation of the boiling point. The increase in boiling point is directly related to the number of particles in solution and the type of solvent. For a given solvent (again, in biological systems this is always water), the more solute particles, the greater the boiling-point elevation. Also, you have to consider that some compounds dissociate when they dissolve, so the equation for boiling-point elevation includes the van't Hoff factor, i:

Boiling-Point Elevation
$$\Delta T_b = k_b i m$$

In this equation, k_b is the solvent's boiling-point elevation constant, i is the solute's van't Hoff factor, and m is the molal concentration of the solution. For water, $k_b \approx 0.5°C / m$.

Freezing-Point Depression

What happens when we add a solute to a liquid, then try to freeze the solution? Solids are held together by attractive intermolecular forces. During freezing, the molecules in a liquid will assemble into an orderly, tightly packed array. However, the presence of solute particles will interfere with efficient arrangement of the solvent molecules into a solid lattice. As a result, a liquid will be less able to achieve a solid state when a solute is present, and the freezing point of the solution will decrease. (Or, equivalently, the melting point of a solid containing a solute is decreased.) The good news is that the formula for freezing-point depression has exactly the same form as the formula for boiling-point elevation, except that the temperature is going down instead of up (that is, the equation for freezing-point *depression* has a *minus* sign whereas the equation for boiling-point *elevation* has a *plus* sign).

> **Freezing-Point Depression**
>
> $$\Delta T_f = -k_f i m$$

In this equation, k_f is the solvent's freezing-point depression constant, i is the solute's van't Hoff factor, and m is the molal concentration of the solution. For water, $k_f \approx 1.9°C/m$.

- Addition of concentrated sulfuric acid to pure water will result in:[27]
  - A) vapor-pressure depression.
  - B) boiling-point elevation.
  - C) freezing-point depression.
  - D) all of the above.

Review of Diffusion and Osmosis

Diffusion is the tendency for liquids and gases to fully occupy the available volume (Figure 13, next page). Particles in the liquid or gas phase are in constant motion, depending on temperature. If all particles are concentrated in one portion of a container, we have an orderly situation, which is unfavorable according to the second law of thermodynamics (law of entropy). The constant thermal motion of particles in the cell leads to their spreading out to occupy all available space, which maximizes entropy.[28] A solute will always diffuse *down its concentration gradient*, which means *from high to low concentration*. Diffusion continues until the solute is evenly distributed throughout the available volume. At this point, movement of solute back and forth continues, but no net movement occurs.

Osmosis is a special type of diffusion in which solvent diffuses rather than solute (Figure 13). For example, if a chamber containing water and a chamber containing a solution of sucrose are connected directly, sucrose will diffuse throughout the entire volume until a uniform concentration is reached. However, if the two chambers are separated by a **semipermeable membrane** that allows water but not sucrose to cross, then diffusion of sucrose between the chambers cannot occur. In this case, osmosis draws water into the sucrose chamber to reduce the sucrose concentration as well as the volume in the water chamber. Ignoring

---

[27] The addition of a solute to a liquid always results in the effects of all the colligative properties simultaneously. Therefore, choice **D** is the answer.

[28] Remember, $\Delta G = \Delta H - T\Delta S$, so increasing ΔS decreases ΔG, indicating a thermodynamically favorable process.

gravity, water will flow into the sucrose chamber until the concentration is the same across the membrane. The plasma membrane of the cell is a semipermeable membrane that allows water—but not most polar solutes—to cross by osmosis. [If a cell is placed in a hypotonic solution (solute concentration lower than in the cell), what will happen to the cell?[29]]

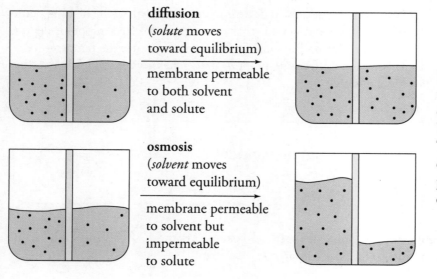

Figure 13 Diffusion and Osmosis

In both diffusion and osmosis, the final result is that solute concentrations are the same on both sides of the membrane. The only difference is that in diffusion the membrane is permeable to solute and in osmosis it is not.

The term **tonicity** is used to describe osmotic gradients. If the environment is **isotonic** to the cell, the solute concentration is the same inside and outside. A **hypertonic** solution has more total dissolved solutes than the cell, a **hypotonic** solution has less. You may also hear the terms **isoosmotic**, **hyperosmotic**, and **hypoosmotic**. The tendency of water to move down its concentration gradient (into cells) can be a powerful force, able to cause cells to explode. This tendency (of water to move to where there are more particles), along with the inability of those particles to cross the membrane, is what accounts for the difference in fluid levels in the beaker at the bottom right-hand corner of Figure 13. The large difference in fluid levels may be a rather extreme example, but it is conceptually accurate: just as osmotic forces can cause a cell to rupture, they can overcome gravity, as shown.

Osmotic Pressure

Osmosis describes the net movement of water across a semipermeable membrane from a region of low solute concentration to a region of higher solute concentration in an effort to dilute the higher concentration solution. The semipermeable membrane prohibits the transfer of solutes, but allows water to transverse through it. In the following figure, the net movement of water will be to the right.

---

[29] Water will flow into the cell through the plasma membrane until the cell volume increases to the point that the cell bursts.

Osmotic pressure (∏) can be defined as the pressure it would take to *stop* osmosis from occurring. If a pressure gauge were added to the same system, osmotic pressure could be measured.

external pressure = ∏

osmosis stopped

The osmotic pressure of a solution is given by the **van't Hoff equation**:

$$\Pi = MiRT$$

where Π is osmotic pressure in atm, M is the molarity of the solution, i is the van't Hoff factor, R is the universal gas constant (0.0821 L-atm/K-mol), and T is the temperature in kelvins.

Again, changes in osmotic pressure are affected only by the number of particles in solution (taking into account the van't Hoff factor), not by the identity of those particles.

Now, let's continue the discussion on movements across the cell membrane.

Passive Transport

Passive transport is a biochemical term that means diffusion. It refers to *any thermodynamically favorable movement of solute across a membrane.* Another way to phrase this is to say that passive transport is any movement of solute *down a gradient.* No energy is required since the concentration gradient drives movement of the solute. There are two types of passive transport: simple diffusion and facilitated diffusion.

Simple Diffusion

Simple diffusion is diffusion of a solute through a membrane without help from a protein. For example, steroid hormones are free to move back and forth across the membrane by simple diffusion as pushed by concentration gradients, thanks to their ___.[30]

However, lipid bilayer membranes are impermeable to most solutes; that is one of the main functions of membranes. The plasma membrane is a barrier to the free movement of all large and/or hydrophilic solutes. **Facilitated diffusion** is the movement of a solute across a membrane, down a gradient, when the membrane itself (the pure lipid bilayer) is intrinsically impermeable to that solute. Specific integral membrane proteins allow material to cross the plasma membrane down a gradient in facilitated diffusion. For example, red blood cells require glucose, which they get from the bloodstream. However, glucose is a bulky hydrophilic molecule that cannot cross the RBC lipid bilayer. Instead, it must be shuttled across by a particular protein in the RBC plasma membrane. There are two well-characterized types of proteins that serve this sort of function: **channel proteins** and **carrier proteins**. Channels and carriers give the membrane its essential feature of **selective permeability**: permeability to *some* things despite impermeability to *most* things.

Facilitated Diffusion: Channels

Channel proteins in the plasma membrane allow material that cannot pass through the membrane by simple diffusion to flow through the plasma membrane down a concentration gradient. Channels do this by forming a narrow opening in the membrane surrounded by the protein. Channels are very selective in what passes through the opening in the membrane. There are many kinds of ion channels, each of which allows the passage of only one type of ion through the channel down a gradient (see Figure 14). All cells have potassium ion channels, for example, that allow only potassium (and not sodium) to flow through the plasma membrane down a gradient. Ion channels are said to be **gated** if the channel is open in response to specific environmental stimuli. A channel that opens in response to a change in the electrical potential across the membrane is called a **voltage-gated** ion channel. One that opens in response to binding of a specific molecule like a neurotransmitter is called a **ligand-gated** ion channel. The regulation of membrane potential by gated ion channels plays a key role in the nervous system. [Can ion channels move ions against an electrochemical gradient?[31]]

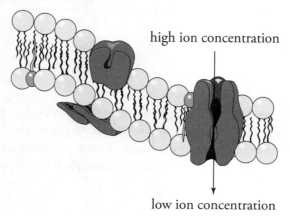

high ion concentration

low ion concentration

Figure 14   An Ion Channel

---

[30] hydrophobicity

[31] No. Ion channels are only involved in facilitated diffusion, the movement of molecules down an electrochemical gradient with the help of a protein.

Facilitated Diffusion: Carriers

Carrier proteins also can transport molecules through membranes by facilitated diffusion, but they do so by a mechanism different from that of ion channels. Carrier proteins do not form a tunnel through membranes like ion channels do. Instead, carriers appear to bind the molecule to be transported at one side of the membrane and then undergo a conformational change to move the molecule to the other side of the membrane. Some carriers, called **uniports**, transport only one molecule across the membrane at a time (see Figure 15). Other carriers termed **symports** carry two substances across a membrane in the same direction. **Antiports**, on the other hand, carry two substances in opposite directions.

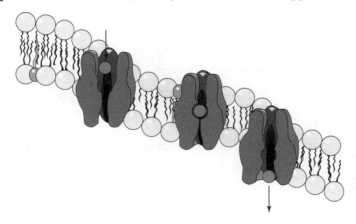

Figure 15 A Uniport

Pores and Porins

A **pore** is a tube through the membrane which is so large that it is *not selective* for any particular molecule. Rather, all molecules below a certain size may pass. (Also, a molecule which is just barely small enough to cross may not cross if it has the wrong charge on its surface.) Pores are formed by polypeptides known as **porins**. You are already familiar with several examples of pores. We have studied pores in the double nuclear membrane, the outer mitochondrial membrane, and the Gram-negative bacterial outer membrane. The eukaryotic plasma membrane does not have pores, because pores destroy the barrier function of the membrane, allowing solutes in the cytoplasm to freely diffuse out of the cell. [Are porins and ion channels found in the same membranes?[32]]

Kinetic Concerns

Simple diffusion can be distinguished from all forms of facilitated diffusion by the kinetics of the process. The rate of simple diffusion is limited only by the surface area of the membrane and the size of the driving force (gradient). Facilitated diffusion, however, depends on a finite number of integral membrane proteins. Hence, it exhibits saturation kinetics. Increasing the driving force for facilitated diffusion increases the rate of diffusion (the **flux**), but only to a point. Then all the transport proteins become saturated, and no further increase in flux is possible (Figure 16 on the following page).

---

[32] No. Porins are large holes, and ion channels are small, usually regulated channels. If porins and ion channels were found in the same membrane, the ion channels would be useless, because ions would flow in an unregulated manner through the pores.

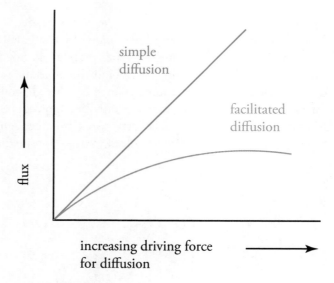

Figure 16 Saturation Kinetics of Facilitated Diffusion

Active Transport

Active transport is the movement of molecules through the plasma membrane against a gradient. Active transport requires energy input, since it is working against a gradient, and always involves a protein. Another way of saying that active transport requires energy input is to say that the transport process is coupled to a process which is thermodynamically favorable ($\Delta G < 0$). The gradient being pumped against is not necessarily just a concentration gradient, but for charged molecules, like ions, it can also involve electric potentials that form a combined electrochemical gradient that must be pumped against. The form of energy input used to drive movement of molecules against an electrochemical gradient varies. In **primary active transport**, the transport of a molecule is coupled to ATP hydrolysis. In **secondary active transport**, the transport process is not coupled *directly* to ATP hydrolysis. Instead, ATP is first used to create a gradient, then the potential energy in that gradient is used to drive the transport of some other molecule across the membrane. Since ATP is not used in the actual transport of the "other" molecule, the ATP use is described as *indirect*. For example, the transport of glucose into some cells is driven *against the glucose* concentration gradient by the cotransport of sodium ions *down the sodium* electrochemical gradient, previously established by an ATPase pump (see below). A common mechanism driving secondary active transport of many different molecules involves coupling transport to the flow of sodium ions down a gradient.

- If a protein moves sodium ions across the plasma membrane down an electrochemical gradient, what form of transport is this?[33]
    A) Simple diffusion
    B) Facilitated diffusion
    C) Primary active transport
    D) Secondary active transport

---

[33] Facilitated diffusion is the movement of molecules down a gradient with the help of a protein (choice **B** is correct). Membrane proteins are not required for simple diffusion (choice A is wrong), and active transport involves moving things *against* their gradients (choices C and D are wrong). Note also that in secondary active transport, the ion movement down its gradient must be coupled to the movement of some other molecule against *its* gradient.

The Na⁺/K⁺ ATPase and the Resting Membrane Potential

The Na⁺/K⁺ ATPase is a transmembrane protein in the plasma membrane of all cells in the body. The activity provided by this protein is to pump 3 Na⁺ out of the cell, 2 K⁺ into the cell, and to hydrolyze one ATP to drive the pumping of these ions against their gradients (Figure 17. next page). [The pumping of sodium and potassium by the Na⁺/K⁺ ATPase is an example of what form of transport?[34]] The sodium that is pumped out of the cell stays outside, since the plasma membrane is impermeable to sodium ions. Some of the potassium ions which are pumped into the cell are able to leak back out, however, through **potassium leak channels**. Potassium flows down its concentration gradient out of the cell through leak channels. The movement of ions out of the cell helps the cell to maintain osmotic balance with its surroundings. As potassium leaves the cell through the leak channels, the movement of positive charge out of the cell creates an electric potential across the plasma membrane with a net negative charge on the interior of the cell. This potential created by the Na⁺/K⁺ ATPase is known as the **resting membrane potential**. (The resting membrane potential will be examined again in Chapter 8 in relation to action potentials in neurons). The concentration gradient of high sodium outside of the cell established by the Na⁺/K⁺ ATPase is the driving force behind **secondary active transport** of many different molecules, including sugars and amino acids. To summarize, the activity of the Na⁺/K⁺ ATPase is important in three ways:

1) To maintain osmotic balance between the cellular interior and exterior
2) To establish the resting membrane potential
3) To provide the sodium concentration gradient used to drive secondary active transport

- If an inhibitor of Na⁺/K⁺ ATPase is added to cells, which of the following may occur?[35]
  - A) The cell will shrink and lose water.
  - B) The interior of the cell will become less negatively charged.
  - C) Secondary active transport processes will compensate for the loss of primary active transport.
  - D) The cell will begin to proliferate.

---

[34] The pumping of ions against a gradient which is coupled to ATP hydrolysis is primary active transport.

[35] The Na⁺/K⁺ ATPase is required to establish the resting membrane potential in which the cellular interior has a negative charge. It pumps out one net positive ion. If this net positive ion stays inside the cell, the resting potential becomes less negative (choice **B** is correct). Since the interior of the cell is now more charged, the cell will have a tendency to take on water by osmosis and will swell (choice A is wrong). Secondary active transport depends on the gradient established by primary active transport (the Na⁺/K⁺ pump). If the pump is shut down, the gradient won't be established, and secondary active transport will also stop (choice C is wrong). The Na⁺/K⁺ ATPase has nothing to do with cellular proliferation (choice D is wrong).

Figure 17 The Na⁺/K⁺ ATPase

How do we know exactly how the resting membrane potential is generated? For instance, how can we state with confidence that the electrogenicity of the Na⁺/K⁺ pump is far less important than the passive efflux of potassium in the generation of the RMP? The answer, given in the next two paragraphs, is not core MCAT material for memorization, but it is just the sort of thing that could show up in a passage.

The answers were determined using experiments. An artificial cell with no pumps and no channels in its membrane would have identical concentrations and charges inside and outside. An artificial cell with potassium leak channels but no active transporters would also obviously have no gradients across its membrane.

What about an artificial cell with Na⁺/K⁺ ATPase pumps and normal cellular concentrations of ATP and ADP + P_i but no potassium leak channels? Here is where experimentation was necessary. In this situation, the resting membrane potential is determined only by the electrogenicity of the Na⁺/K⁺ pump. The RMP in such a system turns out to be about −10 mV. [Why is it necessary to specify normal cellular concentrations of ATP and ADP + P_i? For example, what would happen if there were much, much more ADP + P_i

than ATP, as well as very high extracellular Na^+ concentration and very high intracellular K^+ concentration, in the artificial cell?[36]]

When K^+ leak channels are added to the membrane (in addition to the Na^+/K^+ ATPase pumps and normal cellular concentrations of ATP and ADP + P_i), the RMP is measured at the normal cellular level, around –70 mV.

The following table gives the concentrations of Na^+, K^+, and Cl^- inside and outside the cell. (Know trends; don't memorize numbers.) You already know why the Na^+ and K^+ concentrations are as they are. [Why is chloride so concentrated outside the cell?[37]] A useful mnemonic is to remember that life evolved in the ocean, which has very high concentrations of NaCl; thus the concentrations of Na^+ and Cl^- are high outside the cell and low inside.

Table 3 Concentrations of Ions Inside/Outside Cell

Ion	Intracellular Conc. (mM)	Extracellular Conc. (mM)
Na^+	10	142
K^+	140	4
Cl^-	4	110
Ca^{2+}	0.0001	2.4

Endocytosis and Exocytosis

Another mechanism used to transport material through the plasma membrane is within membrane-bound vesicles that fuse with the membrane (see Figure 18 on the next page). **Exocytosis** is a process to transport material outside of the cell in which a vesicle in the cytoplasm fuses with the plasma membrane, and the contents of the vesicle are expelled into the extracellular space. The materials released are products secreted by the cell, such as hormones and digestive enzymes.

Endocytosis is the opposite of exocytosis: generally, materials are taken into the cell by an invagination of a piece of the cell membrane to form a vesicle. Again, the cytoplasm is not allowed to mix with the extracellular environment. The new vesicle which is formed is called an **endosome**. There are three types of endocytosis:

1) Phagocytosis
2) Pinocytosis
3) Receptor-mediated endocytosis

---

[36] The pump would run backward! Remember: all active transporters are reversible.

[37] The cell contains millions of negative charges on macromolecules (e.g., nucleic acids). For the charge to be "approximately" balanced on both sides of the membrane, some negatively charged substance must be more concentrated outside. Chloride serves this role. Why did we say "approximately" balanced? Remember: the cell is a bit more negative on the inside; that's the RMP.

exocytosis   endocytosis

Figure 18   Endo- and Exocytosis

Phagocytosis means "cell eating." It refers to the nonspecific uptake of large particulate matter into a phagocytic vesicle, which later merges with a lysosome. Thus, the phagocytosed material will be broken down. The prime example of phagocytic human cells are macrophages ("big eaters") of the immune system, which engulf and destroy viruses and bacteria. (*Note*: This is *not* an invagination.)

Pinocytosis ("cell drinking") is the nonspecific uptake of small molecules and extracellular fluid via invagination. Primitive eukaryotic cells obtain nutrition in this manner, but virtually all eukaryotic cells participate in pinocytosis.

Receptor-mediated endocytosis, on the other hand, is very specific. The site of endocytosis is marked by pits coated with the molecule **clathrin** (inside the cell) and with **receptors** that bind to a specific molecule (outside the cell). An important example is the uptake of cholesterol from the blood. Cholesterol is transported in the blood in large particles called lipoproteins. Cells obtain some of the cholesterol they require by receptor-mediated endocytosis of these lipoproteins. If they are not removed from the blood, cholesterol accumulates in the bloodstream, sticking to the inner walls of arteries. This results in **atherosclerosis** (a buildup of plaque on the walls of the arteries). [Does clathrin recognize and bind to lipoproteins?[38]] When the receptor-lipoprotein complex internalizes, it is taken into a vesicle that is termed an endosome. Lipoproteins are taken from the endosome to a lysosome where the cholesterol is released from the lipoprotein and the lipoprotein is degraded. The lipoprotein receptor is returned to the cell surface where it may again bind a lipoprotein. [How is receptor-mediated endocytosis similar to and different from active transport?[39]]

---

[38] No. Clathrin is a fibrous protein inside the cell that associates with the cytoplasmic portions of the cell-surface receptors that bind lipoproteins.

[39] Both import a particular substance. One difference is that in endocytosis the substance ends up sealed in an endosome, whereas in active transport the substance is just dumped into the cytoplasm.

6.5   OTHER STRUCTURAL ELEMENTS OF THE CELL

Cell-Surface Receptors

Receptors form an important class of integral membrane proteins that transmit signals from the extracellular space into the cytoplasm. Each receptor binds a particular molecule in a highly specific lock-and-key interaction. The molecule that serves as the key for a given receptor is termed the **ligand**. The ligand is generally a hormone or a neurotransmitter. The binding of a ligand to its receptor on the extracellular surface of the plasma membrane triggers a response within the cell, a process termed **signal transduction**. Many cancers result from mutant cell-surface receptors which constitutively relay their signal to the cytoplasm, whether ligand is present or absent. For example, a growth factor exerts its effects by binding to a cell-surface receptor, and constitutive activity of a receptor for the growth factor causes uncontrolled growth of the cell. There are three main types of signal-transducing cell-surface receptors: ligand-gated ion channels, catalytic receptors, and G-protein-linked receptors.

Ligand-gated ion channels in the plasma membrane open an ion channel upon binding a particular neurotransmitter. An example is the ligand-gated sodium channel on the surface of the muscle cell at the neuromuscular junction. When the neurotransmitter acetylcholine binds to this receptor, the receptor undergoes a conformational change and becomes an open Na^+ channel. The result is a massive influx of sodium down its electrochemical gradient, which depolarizes the muscle cell and causes it to contract.

Catalytic receptors have an enzymatic active site on the cytoplasmic side of the membrane. Enzyme activity is initiated by ligand binding at the extracellular surface. Generally, the catalytic role is that of a protein **kinase**, which is an enzyme that covalently attaches phosphate groups to proteins. Proteins can be modified with phosphate on the side chain hydroxyl of serine, threonine, or tyrosine. The insulin receptor is an example of a tyrosine kinase. Modification of proteins with phosphates regulates their activity.

A **G-protein-linked receptor** does not directly transduce its signal, but transmits it into the cell with the aid of a **second messenger**. This is a chemical signal that relays instructions from the cell surface to enzymes in the cytoplasm. The most important second messenger is **cyclic AMP (cAMP)**. It is known as a "universal hunger signal" because it is the second messenger of the hormones epinephrine and glucagon, which cause energy mobilization (glycogen and fat breakdown). Second messengers such as cAMP allow a much greater signal than receptor alone produces (see Figure 19, next page). An epinephrine molecule activates one G-protein-linked receptor which activates many G-proteins, each G-protein activates many adenylyl cyclase enzymes, each adenylyl cyclase makes lots of cAMP from ATP, each cAMP activates many cAMP-dPK, and each cAMP-dPK phosphorylates many enzymes. Some of these enzymes will be activated, and others inactivated by phosphorylation, with the end result that the entire cell harmoniously works toward the same goal: energy mobilization.

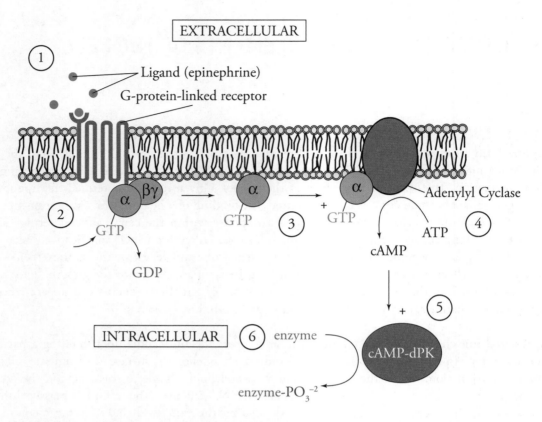

Figure 19   G-Protein Mediated Signal Transduction Stimulated by Epinephrine

1) Epinephrine arrives at the cell surface and binds to a specific G-protein-linked receptor.
2) The cytoplasmic portion of the receptor activates G-proteins, causing GDP to dissociate and GTP to bind in its place.
3) The activated G-proteins diffuse through the membrane and activate adenylyl cyclase.
4) Adenylyl cyclase makes cAMP from ATP.
5) cAMP activates cAMP-dependent protein kinases (cAMP-dPK) in the cytoplasm.
6) cAMP-dPK phosphorylates certain enzymes, with the end result being mobilization of energy. For example, enzymes necessary for glycogen breakdown will be activated, while enzymes necessary for glycogen synthesis will be inactivated, by cAMP-dPK phosphorylation.

There are different types of G-protein-linked receptors. The one depicted above is a **s**timulatory one. Its G-protein would be denoted **G$_s$**. Inhibitory G-protein-linked receptors activate **i**nhibitory G-proteins (**G$_i$**) which serve to *inactivate* adenylyl cyclase instead of activating it. In this way different hormones can modulate each other's effects.

There are also G-protein-linked receptors which have nothing to do with cAMP. Instead, their G-proteins activate an enzyme called phospholipase C, initiating a different second messenger cascade, which results in an increase in cytoplasmic Ca^{2+} levels. The common theme shared by all G-protein-based signal transduction systems is their reliance on a G-protein, which is a signaling molecule that binds GTP. You should understand these key notions: cAMP as a second messenger, signal transduction, and signal amplification. The remaining details are not important for the MCAT; read for concepts, not memory.

The Cytoskeleton

The animal cell **cytoskeleton** provides the structural support supplied by the cell wall in bacteria, plants, and fungi. It also allows movement of the cell and its appendages (cilia and flagella) and transport of substances within the cell. Animal cells have an internal cytoskeleton composed of three types of proteins: **microtubules**, **intermediate filaments**, and **microfilaments** (see Figure 20). Microtubules are the thickest, microfilaments the thinnest. All three are composed of noncovalently polymerized proteins; in other words, they are a massive example of quaternary protein structure.

a) individual cytoskeleton filaments

microtubules
25-nm diameter

microfilaments
7-nm diameter

intermediate filaments
10-nm diameter

plasma membrane

ribosomes

rough ER

microfilaments

intermediate filaments

mitochondrion

microtubules

b) a portion of a cell showing
the cytoskeleton

Figure 20   Cytoskeleton

Microtubules

The **microtubule** is a hollow rod composed of two globular proteins: α-tubulin and β-tubulin, polymerized noncovalently. First, α-tubulin and β-tubulin form an αβ-tubulin dimer. Then many dimers stick to one another noncovalently to form a sheet, which rolls into a tube. Once formed, the microtubule can elongate by adding αβ-tubulin dimers to one end. The other end cannot elongate, because it is anchored to the **microtubule organizing center** (**MTOC**), located near the nucleus. Microtubules are dynamic and can get longer or shorter by adding or removing tubulin monomers from the end.

Within the MTOC is a pair of **centrioles** (see Figure 21, next page). Each centriole is composed of a ring of nine microtubule triplets. When cell division occurs, the centrioles duplicate themselves, and then one pair moves to each end of the cell. During mitosis, microtubules radiating out from the centrioles attach to the replicated chromosomes and pull them apart so that one copy of each chromosome (one chromatid) moves to each end of the cell. The resulting daughter cells each get a full copy of the genome plus a centriole pair. The microtubules that radiate out from the centrioles during mitosis are called the **aster**, because they are star-shaped. The microtubules connecting the chromosomes to the aster are **polar fibers**. The whole assembly is called the **mitotic spindle**. The centromere of each chromosome contains a **kinetochore** which is attached to the spindle by tiny microtubules called **kinetochore fibers**. Refer to the figure in the upcoming section on mitosis.

individual microtubules

centrioles

Figure 21   A Pair of Centrioles

In mitosis, the MTOC is essential, but the centrioles are not. There are two major pieces of evidence for this: 1) Plant cells lack centrioles but still undergo mitosis; 2) Experimenters have succeeded in removing the centrioles from animal cells, and the cells were still able to undergo mitosis.

Microtubules also mediate transport of substances within the cell. In nerve cells, materials are transported from the cell body to the axon terminus on a microtubule railroad. The transport process is driven by proteins that hydrolyze ATP and act as molecular motors along the microtubule.

Eukaryotic Cilia and Flagella

Cilia are small "hairs" on the cell surface which move fluids past the cell surface. For example, cilia on lining cells of the human respiratory tract continually sweep mucus toward the mouth in a mechanism termed the **mucociliary escalator**. A **flagellum** is a large "tail" which moves the cell by wiggling. The only human cell which has a flagellum is the __.[40] Cilia are small and flagella are long, but they have the same structure, with a "**9 + 2**" arrangement of microtubules (see Figure 22). Nine pairs of microtubules form a ring around two lone microtubules in the center. Each microtubule is bound to its neighbor by a contractile protein called **dynein** which causes movement of the filaments past one another. The cilium or flagellum is anchored to the plasma membrane by a **basal body**, which has the same structure as a centriole (a ring of nine triplets of microtubules). Remember that the prokaryotic flagellum is different in structure, and its motion is driven by a different mechanism.

---

[40] sperm

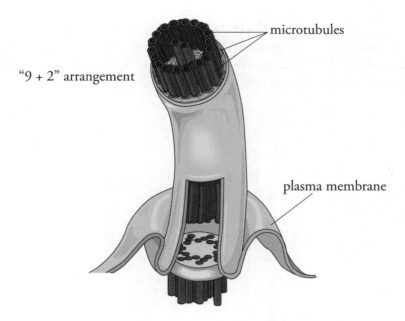

microtubules

"9 + 2" arrangement

plasma membrane

Figure 22   The Base of a Cilium or Flagellum

Microfilaments

Microfilaments are rods formed in the cytoplasm from polymerization of the globular protein **actin**. Actin monomers form a chain, and then two chains wrap around each other to form an actin filament. Microfilaments are dynamic and are responsible for gross movements of the entire cell, such as pinching the dividing parent cell into two daughters during cell division, and **amoeboid movement**. Amoeboid movement involves changes in the cytoplasmic structure which cause cytoplasm and the rest of the cell to flow in one direction.

Intermediate Filaments

Intermediate filaments are named for their thickness, which is between that of microtubules and microfilaments. Unlike microtubules and microfilaments, intermediate filaments are heterogeneous, composed of a wide range of polypeptides. Another difference is that intermediate filaments are more permanent, whereas microfilaments and microtubules are often disassembled and reassembled as needed by the cell. Intermediate filaments appear to be involved in providing strong cell structure, such as in resisting mechanical stress.

Cell Adhesion and Cell Junctions

In some tissues, cells are tightly bound to one another. For example, the intestinal wall is lined with a type of tissue called **epithelium**.[41] The layer of epithelial cells in the gut forms a tight seal, preventing items from moving freely between the intestinal lumen and the body; this is accomplished by **tight**

---

[41] An epithelial cell layer is a layer of cells which lies "upon nipples" of a type of extracellular connective tissue called *basement membrane* (*epi*- means "upon," and -*thele* means "nipple," in the sense of small bump). The basement membrane is a strong molecular sheet made of collagen. Under the microscope the basement membrane under epithelial cells has "bumps" which make epithelial cell layers easy to recognize.

junctions. Epithelial cells in the skin are held together tightly but do not form a complete seal; this is accomplished by **desmosomes**. Some specialized cell types, such as heart muscle cells, are connected by holes called **gap junctions** that allow ions to flow back and forth between them. We discuss each of these structures (see Figure 23) in the following paragraphs.

Figure 23   Cell Junctions

Tight junctions are also termed *occluding junctions* because they do not just join cells at one point, but form a seal between the membranes of adjacent cells that blocks the flow of molecules across the entire cell layer. They are not spots where cells are stuck together, but rather bands running all the way around the cells. Intestinal epithelial cells are involved in the active transport of glucose and other molecules from one side of epithelium to the other. A tight seal between these cells is required to prevent the two compartments from mixing. Tight junctions also block the flow of molecules within the plane of the plasma membrane. For example, the surface of the plasma membrane facing the intestinal lumen, termed the **apical** surface, has different membrane proteins than the plasma membrane on the other side of the cell facing the tissues beneath, called the **basolateral** surface. [Will a transmembrane protein inserted into the apical surface of an intestinal epithelial cell diffuse in the plane of the plasma membrane to reach the basolateral surface of the cell?[42]]

Desmosomes do not form a seal, but merely hold cells together; they are also known as *spot desmosomes* because they are concise points, not bands all the way around the cell. The desmosome is composed of fibers that span the plasma membranes of two cells. Inside each cell, the desmosome is anchored to the plasma membrane by a plaque formed by the protein **keratin**. Intermediate filaments of the cytoplasm attach to the inside of the desmosome. Desmosomes do not freely diffuse in the plane of the plasma membrane, as suggested by the fluid mosaic model, because they are anchored in place by intermediate filaments of the cytoskeleton. As you can see, the fluid mosaic model is an idealization describing the plasma membrane in pure form. In the real cell membrane, things are highly organized.

Gap junctions form pore-like connections between adjacent cells, allowing the two cells' cytoplasms to mix. The connection is large enough to permit the exchange of solutes such as ions, amino acids, and carbohydrates, but not polypeptides and organelles. Gap junctions in smooth muscle and cardiac muscle allow the membrane depolarization of an action potential to pass directly from one cell to another.

—

[42] No. It is free to move around on the apical surface, but the tight junctions prevent it from diffusing to the basolateral surface.

6.6 THE CELL CYCLE AND MITOSIS

Our cells must reproduce themselves in order to replace lost or damaged cells and so that tissues can grow. Cells reproduce themselves by first doubling everything in the cytoplasm and the genome and then splitting in half. Some cells continually go through a cycle of growth and division, which is traditionally discussed in four phases (see Figure 24). **S (synthesis)** phase is when the cell actively replicates its genome, as described in Chapter 7. **M phase** includes **mitosis** and **cytokinesis**. Mitosis is the partitioning of cellular components (genes, organelles, etc.) into two halves. Cytokinesis is the physical process of cell division. Between M phase and S phase, there are two "gap" phases, G_1 and G_2. The gap phases plus S phase together form the part of the cell cycle between divisions, known as *interphase*.

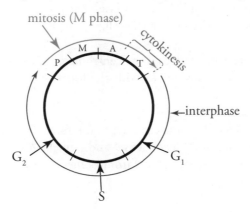

Figure 24   The Cell Cycle

The cell spends most of its time in interphase, busily metabolizing and synthesizing materials. Some cells are permanently stuck in interphase (G_0). In fact, the more specialized a cell becomes, the less likely it is to remain capable of reproducing itself. Examples are neurons, blood cells, and cells on the surface of the skin. They must be replenished by reproduction of less specialized precursor cells called **stem cells**. All the blood cells, for example, are derived from a single type of stem cell found in the bone marrow.

During interphase, the genome is spread out in a form that is not visible with a light microscope without special stains, and DNA is accessible to the enzymes of replication. By the end of S phase, the nucleus contains two complete copies of the genome. The cell now has twice the normal amount of DNA.

Mitosis is divided into four phases: **prophase, metaphase, anaphase**, and **telophase**.[43] The first sign of prophase is that the genome becomes visible upon condensing into densely packed chromosomes, instead of diffuse chromatin. [Why do the chromosomes condense?[44]] Observing a human cell under the light microscope at the beginning of prophase, one can see 46 differently shaped chromosomes. Upon closer observation, one notes that each chromosome actually consists of two identical particles joined at a centromere. These two particles are the two copies of a chromosome, known as **sister chromatids**. When mitosis is complete, each new daughter cell will have 46 chromosomes, each consisting of a single chromatid, separated from its sister. Spending a little more time staring at the nucleus, you might notice that the jumble of 46 chromatid pairs actually consists of 23 **homologous pairs** of identical-appearing sister chromatid pairs (23 pairs of pairs). Homologous chromosomes are different copies of the same chromosome, one from your mother and the other from your father. (Also refer to Chapter 7.) To repeat:

---

[43] A mnemonic is "I Pee on the MAT," where I is for interphase.

[44] Presumably so that they can be separated without tangling.

Sister chromatids are identical copies of a chromosome, attached to each other at the centromere. Homologous chromosomes are equivalent but nonidentical and do not come anywhere near each other during mitosis.

Other important events occur during prophase. The nucleolus disappears, the spindle and kinetochore fibers appear, and the centriole pairs begin to move to opposite ends of the cell. So now the cell has two MTOCs, called **asters** (stars) because of the star-like appearance of microtubules radiating out. Also at the end of prophase, the nuclear envelope converts itself into many tiny vesicles.[45]

Metaphase is simple: all the chromosomes line up at the center of the cell, forming the **metaphase plate**. The chromosomes line up in the center of the cell because the kinetochore of each sister chromatid is attached to spindle fibers that attach to MTOC at opposite ends of the cell. So each member of a pair of chromatids is pulled toward the opposite pole of the cell.

During anaphase, the spindle fibers shorten, and the centromeres of each sister chromatid pair are pulled apart. The cell elongates, and cytokinesis begins with the formation of a **cleavage furrow**, which is accomplished by __.[46]

In telophase (*telos* is Greek for "end"), a nuclear membrane forms around the bunch of chromosomes at each end of the cell, the chromosomes decondense, and a nucleolus becomes visible within each new daughter nucleus. Each daughter nucleus has $2n$ chromosomes. Cytokinesis is complete, and the cell is split in two (see Figure 25).

interphase G_1 interphase S phase   prophase

metaphase   anaphase   telophase and cytokinesis   two new cells in interphase

Figure 25   The Phases of Mitosis

---

[45] This stage of prophase is also referred to as **prometaphase.** It is the last event in prophase and is rather dramatic; once the nuclear membrane is disintegrated into vesicles, the spindle fibers can attach to the centromeres of the chromosomes and the cell can enter metaphase.

[46] a ring of microfilaments encircling the cell and contracting

6.6

The **karyotype** is a display of an organism's genome (see Figure 26). A cell is frozen during metaphase, its chromosomes are stained, and a photograph is taken. The micrograph is enlarged, and each chromosome is cut out of the picture with an artist's blade. Then all homologues are paired, and the entire genome is examined for abnormalities.

Figure 26   A Genetic Karyotype

- Eukaryotic chromosomes generally have only one of which of the following?[47]
    A) Reading frame
    B) Origins of replication
    C) Promoter
    D) Centromere

---

[47] If a chromosome had more than one centromere, it could be pulled toward different ends of the cell simultaneously and be torn (choice **D** is correct). Each eukaryotic gene has only one reading frame, but since there are many genes per chromosome there are different reading frames too. Note that the total number of possible reading frames is only 3, since a codon is only 3 nucleotides long (choice A is wrong). Eukaryotic chromosomes are so large that they must have more than one origin of replication to finish replication of the genome in a reasonable time period (choice B is wrong), and each gene has its own promoter, and there are many genes per chromosome (choice C is wrong).

6.7 CANCER, ONCOGENES, AND TUMOR SUPPRESSORS

Inappropriate cell division (i.e., cells that have lost control of the cell cycle) can have disastrous consequences. A mutation in a protein that is normally involved in regulating progression through the cell cycle can result in unregulated cell division and cancer. Cancer means "crab," as in the zodiac sign. The name derives from the observation that malignant tumors grow into the surrounding tissue, embedding themselves like clawed crabs.

- In normal eukaryotic cells, mitosis will not begin until the entire genome is replicated. If this inhibition is removed so that mitosis begins during S-phase, which one of the following would occur?[48]
  A) The cells would grow more quickly.
  B) The genome would become fragmented and incomplete.
  C) The cells would display unregulated, cancerous growth.
  D) The genome would be temporarily incomplete in each daughter cell, but DNA repair will fill in the missing gaps.

Cancers can present as malignant solid tumors or in a more diffuse cellular state, such as leukemia, a cancer occurring in the bone marrow where improper leukocytes are formed and circulated.

Mutated genes that induce cancer are termed **oncogenes** ("onco-" is a prefix denoting cancer). Normally, these genes are required for proper growth of the cell and regulation of the cell cycle. Oncogenes, then, are genes that can convert normal cells into cancerous cells. Sometimes these are abnormal versions of standard cellular growth genes. Sometimes the genes enter the cell because of a viral infection. In fact, the first identified oncogene, labeled *src*, was isolated from a retrovirus found in chickens; the oncogene contributes to sarcomas, cancers of the bone, cartilage, adipose, muscular, vascular, or hematopoietic tissues. [*Teratomas* are tumors with formed tissues from multiple germ layers. What steps might lead to their formation?[49]]

Protooncogenes are the normal versions of the genes that allow for regular growth patterns, but can be converted into oncogenes under the right circumstances. Conversion may be due to mutation or because of exposure to a mutagen. Ultraviolet radiation (such as sunlight or light from tanning booths) and various chemicals (such as benzene) are both examples of common mutagens.

Tumor suppressor genes produce proteins that are the inherent defense system to prevent the conversion of cells into cancer cells. The two primary means of cancer prevention are to (a) detect damage to the genome and halt cell growth and division until the damage can be repaired, or (b) to trigger programmed cell death if the damage is too severe to be repaired. **p53** is an example of a product of a common tumor suppressor gene. Though normally at low levels in cells, its production is scaled up when genetic damage or oncogene activity is detected, and if sufficient repair is not possible, p53 will cause the cell to die in a process referred to as **apoptosis**.

---

[48] If the genome is not completely replicated and condensed prior to mitosis, it will be torn during cell division. Each daughter cell will receive only pieces of the genome rather than the complete genome and will not be able to survive (choice **B** is correct, and choice A and C are wrong). DNA repair systems can only repair sequence errors or minor structural problems; this problem would be too large to fix (choice D is wrong).

[49] Teratomas form when oncogenes cause certain tissues to dedifferentiate (lose their specific function and regress), and then redifferentiate to become something different. This is why teratomas can contain tissues such as teeth and hair.

Figure 27   Representation of p53 triggering apoptosis

Apoptosis

Apoptosis, or programmed cell death, allows a cell to shrink and die while simultaneously minimizing damage to neighboring cells and limiting the exposure of other cells to its cytosolic contents. The death of a cell is triggered by a stressor which may be external (such as nitric oxide, a toxin, or cytokines) or internal (such as when the level of the p53 tumor suppressor protein reaches a critical level).

The process of apoptosis begins with the shrinking of the cell and the disassembly of the cytoskeleton. While the cellular infrastructure is taken apart, the nuclear envelope breaks down and the genome is broken into pieces. A different profile of cell surface proteins emerges, thus signaling various phagocytic cells, including macrophages, to finish deconstructing and clearing away the dead cell.

A family of proteases, referred to as **caspases**, is responsible for carrying out the events of apoptosis. They have a cysteine in their active site and they cleave their target proteins at aspartic acid sites, hence their name (*c-asp*-ases). Caspases, like all potentially damaging enzymes, are produced in their inactive form as *procaspases*. Twelve different caspases have been identified in humans, and they are generally grouped into two categories, initiators and effectors. **Initiator caspases** respond to extra- or intracellular death signals by clustering together; this clustering allows them to activate each other. The activation of the initiators leads to the activation of the effector caspases in a cascade of activation. **Effector caspases** then cleave a variety of cellular proteins to trigger apoptosis.

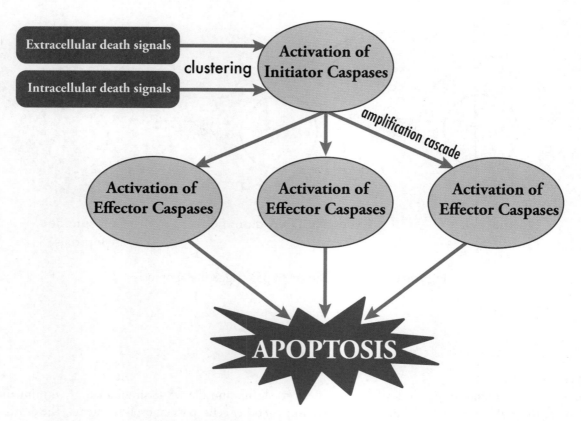

Figure 28   Caspase Activation and Cascade

Oxidative Stress

Oxidative stress occurs when the level of production of reactive oxygen species outstrips the cell's ability to detoxify them. This can include increased levels of peroxides or free oxygen, which then generates radicals. While reactive oxygen species are normally produced as part of metabolism, at high untreated levels they can damage DNA, cellular proteins, and even lipid bilayers. As such, oxidative stress is linked to cancer, since the damage it can cause sets up conditions in the cell to allow oncogenes to become active and cell growth to be impacted.

Though the potential for damage exists, creating oxidative stress is also a component of the immune system. Activated phagocytes may produce nitric oxide or superoxide (O_2^-) in order to broadly kill pathogens. The effect on foreign cells needs to be balanced against the damage being caused to host tissues.

Regenerative Capacity

The ability to restore damaged tissues is an important survival strategy, and depends on how stem cells are maintained in the body of an organism. Planarians (simple flatworms) have collections of stem cells throughout their bodies that can migrate to areas of damage and rebuild necessary tissues. Newts or lizards that lose a limb have cells that dedifferentiate and then redifferentiate to grow back all the components of that limb. Within mammals, however, the regenerative capacity is considerably more limited. The multipotent stem cells within the bone marrow are constantly regenerating the cellular components of the blood and immune system. Hepatocytes in the liver divide to produce more cells, but this process is much slower; these cells are described as being unipotent. Some cells, like neurons, do not regenerate, though inducing them to do so is an active area of research so as to better address injuries and damage caused by neurological degrading illnesses. [The benefits of having regenerative capacity are clear, but if it does not proceed properly, what could be the outcome?[50]]

Senescence

Senescence describes the process of biological aging which occurs at both the cellular and the organismal level. For eukaryotic cells, the length of the telomeres on the ends of chromosomes are a measure of cellular age; the longer the telomeres, the younger the cell. These sequences are meant to be maintained by the enzyme telomerase (Chapter 4). Research is being pursued as to whether the biological age of a cell can be reset if telomerases are manipulated to maintain the length of the telomeres. Additionally, as cells age they become prone to apoptosis. Though stressors can induce apoptosis earlier than expected, this mechanism of programmed cell death is also how organisms destroy and disassemble cells that need to be removed due to age.

The cumulative effects of cellular senescence lead to the aging of the entire organism. The functioning of organs is affected to the point where the body stops working and death occurs. These effects can be hastened based on environmental exposures and behavioral factors, but even without additional stressors, senescence is inevitable for organisms.

---

[50] Since regenerative capacity involves cell growth, dedifferentiation and redifferentiation, the possibility exists for the process to go awry and for cancerous growth to then be stimulated. Regeneration needs to be tightly regulated in order for it to proceed correctly.

Chapter 6 Summary

- For the MCAT, you should know the structures and functions of the following key eukaryotic organelles: nucleus, mitochondria, ribosomes, rough ER, smooth ER, Golgi apparatus, lysosomes, and peroxisomes.

- The rough ER is the site of translation of proteins to be either secreted from the cell, inserted into the membrane, or targeted to the lysosomes, ER, or Golgi apparatus.

- Signal sequences are specific amino acid sequences that direct proteins in translation to the rough ER and the secretory pathway (rough ER → Golgi apparatus → final location).

- Post-translational modification can occur in the rough ER or in the Golgi apparatus.

- All cellular membranes are composed of lipid bilayers with distinct hydrophobic and hydrophilic regions. The membranes act as selective barriers that regulate which molecules can cross.

- An electrolyte is a solute that produces free ions in solution. Strong electrolytes produce more ions in solution than weak electrolytes.

- The van't Hoff (or ionizability) factor, i, tells us how many ions one unit of a substance will produce in solution.

- Colligative properties depend on the number of particles in solution. Colligative properties include vapor pressure depression, boiling point elevation, freezing point depression, and osmotic pressure.

- Molecules naturally want to move from regions of higher concentration to regions of lower concentration (with respect to that particular molecule). Diffusion is the movement of particles down their concentration gradient, and osmosis is the movement of water down *its* concentration gradient.

- Hydrophobic molecules (e.g., O_2, CO_2, and steroids) cross the membrane by simple diffusion, while hydrophilic, polar molecules (e.g., ions, glucose, and water) must cross the membrane with the help of a special membrane protein (a channel or a carrier). This is called facilitated diffusion.

- Active transport uses energy to move molecules against their concentration gradients (from low concentration areas to higher concentration areas). Primary active transport uses ATP directly, while secondary active transport relies on gradients previously established by a primary active transporter.

- The Na^+/K^+ ATPase is a primary active transporter that moves three Na^+ ions out of the cell for every two K^+ ions it moves into the cell. This helps establish the resting membrane potential of the cell, helps maintain osmotic balance in the cell, and sets up a Na^+ gradient that can be used for secondary active transport.

- G-proteins help transduce signals from extracellular ligands across the membrane. They change the level of cAMP or calcium (second messengers) in the cell, which changes the metabolic enzyme pathways active in the cell.

- Microtubules form centrioles, cilia, and eukaryotic flagella, while microfilaments participate in contractile activity.

- Tight junctions help form a seal between cells so that the flow of molecules across the entire cell layer is regulated. Desmosomes form general adhesions between cells. Gap junctions form connections between cells that allow the flow of cytoplasm from cell to cell.

- During the cell cycle, DNA replication occurs during the S-phase of interphase, and cell division occurs during mitosis (M-phase).

- Mitosis is comprised of four major phases (prophase, metaphase, anaphase, and telophase) and results in two daughter cells that are identical to each other and identical to the original parent cell.

- Protooncogenes can be mutated to form oncogenes, which can lead to cancer. Tumor suppressor genes can prevent cancer by halting the cell cycle until damaged DNA is repaired or by inducing apoptosis (cell suicide).

- Apoptosis is triggered by a cascade of activation of enzymes called caspases. Caspases can be activated by extracellular or intracellular signals.

CHAPTER 6 FREESTANDING PRACTICE QUESTIONS

1. *Kartegener's syndrome* is a rare genetic disorder that results in immotile cilia. The immotile cilia cause infertility, bronchiectasis (permanent dilation of the bronchi) and recurrent sinusitis (due to the inability to "push out" bacteria and particles from the sinuses). The genetic defect causes a deficiency of a protein primarily involved in which of the following structures?

A) Microfilament
B) Intermediate filament
C) Microtubule
D) Plasma membrane

2. Different proteins have been found to be involved in vesicular trafficking. Specific proteins are responsible for specific pathways; for instance, COP-I is responsible for retrograde transmission of vesicles, while COP-II is involved in anterograde transmission. Clathrin is involved in receptor-mediated endocytosis. Vesicles on which of the following pathways would be expected to have COP-I proteins on its surface?

A) RER → *cis* Golgi
B) RER → *trans* Golgi
C) *cis* Golgi → RER
D) Nucleus → RER

3. The steroid hormones produced by the smooth endoplasmic reticulum would be stored in which of the following organelles?

A) Secretory vesicles, so the hormones could be released when needed.
B) Peroxisomes, so the hormones could aid in lipid breakdown.
C) Lysosomes, so the hormones could aid in the destruction of excess secretory products.
D) Steroid hormones are not stored, as they are able to diffuse through lipid bilayers.

4. Which of the following gives the correct order for the signals leading to the formation of cyclic AMP? (GPCR = G-Protein Coupled Receptor)

A) Epinephrine → G-proteins → GPCR → adenylyl cyclase → cAMP
B) Epinephrine → GPCR → G-proteins → adenylyl cyclase → cAMP
C) Epinephrine → GPCR → adenylyl cyclase → G-proteins → cAMP
D) Epinephrine → adenylyl cyclase → cAMP → GPCR → G-proteins

5. The nuclear membrane is absent in which of the following phases of mitosis?

   I. Anaphase
   II. Telophase
   III. Metaphase

A) I
B) I and II
C) I and III
D) II and III

6. Both the Golgi complex and rough endoplasmic reticulum contribute to protein modification through all of the following EXCEPT:

A) phosphorylation.
B) creation of disulfide bridges.
C) glycosylation.
D) creation of peptide bonds.

7. Tumor suppressor genes like *BRCA1/2* promote anticancer processes like DNA repair. When these genes are disabled via mutation, the risk for developing cancer later in life increases dramatically. A female who inherits a single mutation in *BRCA2* has a 50% and 20% chance of developing breast and ovarian cancer, respectively. Which of the following best explains why these respective chances are not 100%?

A) Individuals who are homozygous for the *BRCA2* mutation do not have a functional allele.
B) Individuals who are homozygous for the *BRCA2* mutation can still rely on other DNA repair mechanisms.
C) Individuals who are heterozygous for the *BRCA2* mutation still have a functional allele.
D) Individuals who are heterozygous for the *BRCA2* mutation can still rely on other DNA repair mechanisms.

CHAPTER 6 PRACTICE PASSAGE

Apoptosis is the most studied form of programmed cell death. It is limited to multicellular organisms and is a process that involves cells being dismantled from within. When a cell is undergoing apoptosis, it has several characteristic morphological traits; for example, the cells retract and become rounded as they detach from the extracellular matrix and neighboring cells. In addition, the plasma membrane starts blebbing, and apoptotic bodies (similar to vesicles) are pinched off the plasma membrane.

There are several stimuli that could induce apoptotic pathways in a cell. For example, there are receptor-mediated or extrinsic signals that trigger a cell to initiate apoptosis (Figure 1).

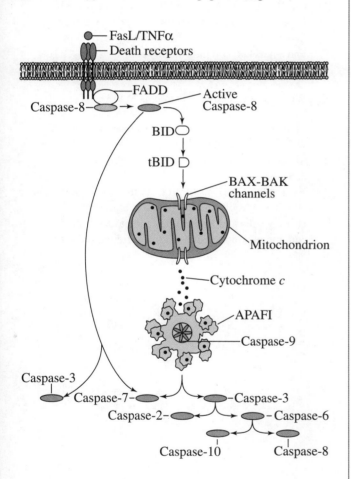

Figure 1   The Extrinsic Apoptosis Pathway

In this case, a death receptor ligand such as FasL or TNFα binds to a death receptor on the surface of the cell. This causes recruitment of adaptor proteins to the plasma membrane. The adaptor proteins serve as docking sites for other proteins, most commonly caspase 8, which is recruited to the plasma

membrane and activated. Active caspase 8 is a protease and cleaves other members of the caspase family along with a protein called BID. The cleaved form of BID (tBID) promotes the release of cytochrome c from mitochondria, and downstream activation of other caspase family members. These proteins dismantle the cytoskeleton and cause nuclear fragmentation, detachment from the surrounding environment, genome degradation, and fragmentation of organelles. After termination of the demolition phase, phagocytes are recruited to the apoptotic cell to clean up the cellular debris.

Autophagy is also a self-destructive process, but does not necessarily lead to cell death. When cells are under stress, parts of the cytoplasm and intracellular organelles are sequestered in specialized double-membrane organelles called autophagosomes. These vacuoles ultimately fuse with lysosomes and the acid hydrolases in the lysosome degrade the contents, which are then recycled to the cell to provide the missing or limited nutrients.

If the degradation of cellular material does not alleviate the stress that induced autophagy, the cell will switch to apoptosis. It is known that autophagy protein Atg5 is essential to autophagy induction and in the regulation of apoptosis. For example, Atg5 generally induces autophagy by promoting autophagosome and autolysosome formation. Atg5 also enhances the susceptibility of cancer cells to apoptosis. It has been found that the full-length Atg5 protein induces autophagy, but with lethal stress, the full-length Atg5 is proteolytically cleaved to generate a 24 kDa pro-apoptotic protein that promotes cytochrome c release and mitochondrial permeabilization.

1. p53 is a tumor suppressor protein that is commonly mutated or deleted in aberrantly growing cancer cells. Which of the following is the most likely function of p53?

   A) It is a transcription factor that induces expression of pro-apoptotic proteins.
   B) It indirectly induces autophagy to supply the cell with biomacromolecules.
   C) It stimulates phospholipid synthesis in the smooth ER.
   D) It induces cell cycle progression in response to genome stability, as part of the G_2-M checkpoint pathway.

2. Which of the following are NOT examples of enzymes found in lysosomes?

   A) Phosphatases and nucleases
   B) Phospholipase C and adenylyl cyclase
   C) Proteases and peptidases
   D) Glucosidases and lipases

3. Which of the following would NOT induce autophagy?

   A) Increase in inner mitochondrial membrane permeability
   B) Accumulation of incorrectly folded proteins in the ER lumen
   C) Incomplete genome replication
   D) Decreased intracellular metabolite concentrations

4. A researcher adds the BAX-BAC channel inhibitor Bci1 to a plate of cells in the lab. Which of the following is observed?

   A) Retention of cytochrome c in the inner mitochondrial membrane
   B) Inhibition of BAX-BAC channel formation in the inner mitochondrial membrane
   C) Rounded cells and blebbing of the plasma membrane
   D) A rapid increase in the amount of cellular autophagy

5. Monophosphate Atg13 initiates autophagosome formation and mTOR phosphorylates three amino acids on Atg13 simultaneously. Which of the following is true?

   A) mTOR is anti-autophagic and functions as a kinase.
   B) mTOR activates Atg13 and functions as a phosphatase.
   C) Rapamycin, an mTOR inhibitor, represses autophagy.
   D) In cells that are undergoing autophagy, Atg13 is phosphorylated on three amino acids.

6. Which of the following is true of Atg5?

   A) Southern blot analysis of proteins from healthy cells would show a 24 kDa Atg5.
   B) Calpain, the protease that cleaves Atg5, is activated in cells that have bound FasL.
   C) Western blot analysis of proteins from cells undergoing autophagy would show a 19 kDa Atg5.
   D) Healthy cells and autophagic cells have alternative splicing of Atg5 to generate two different proteins.

SOLUTIONS TO CHAPTER 6 FREESTANDING PRACTICE QUESTIONS

1. **C** Cilia and flagella are both made up of microtubules; thus, a defect causing immotile cilia would likely involve a protein associated with microtubules (choice C is correct). In fact, *Kartegener's syndrome* is a defect in the dynein protein, which is an ATPase that links the peripheral 9 doublets of the cilium (remember that eukaryotic cilia and flagella both have a 9 + 2 arrangement of microtubules) and causes bending (motion) of the cilium by differential sliding of the doublets. Microfilaments are composed of the protein actin and are responsible for contractile motility and changing of cell shape, specifically, muscle contraction, leukocyte motility, and cytokinesis (choice A is wrong). Intermediate filaments are primarily responsible for the cytoskeletal structure of cells (choice B is wrong). The plasma membrane is composed of phospholipids and cholesterol, although it does include many different proteins. However, the proteins of the plasma membrane are not responsible for cilia motility (choice D is wrong).

2. **C** The question stem states that COP-I proteins are involved in retrograde, or "backward," vesicular trafficking. Therefore, these vesicles would be traveling in the reverse pathway. Choice C (*cis* Golgi to RER) is the only correct option listed. The anterograde, or "forward," pathway in cells involves vesicles traveling from the RER to the cis Golgi (choice A is wrong), the *medial* Golgi, the *trans* Golgi and then to the cell membrane or other target site within the cell. Vesicles do not normally travel from the RER to the *trans* Golgi (choice B is wrong). Also vesicles are not involved in transport from the nucleus (choice D is wrong).

3. **D** Because steroid hormones are made from cholesterol as lipid derivatives, they cannot be stored by lipid bilayers. Since secretory vesicles, peroxisomes, and lysosomes are membrane-bound, they cannot store steroids (choices A, B, and C are wrong). Note also that peptide hormones are stored in secretory vesicles (choice A would be true of a peptide hormone, but not of a steroid hormone). Be careful to differentiate between answer choices that are simply true versus answer choices that actually address the question. Though choices A, B, and C all describe the general function of their particular organelle, only choice D addresses the issue specific to steroids.

4. **B** Since the question is asking about the formation of cAMP, it should be the last step in the sequence (choice D can be eliminated). G-protein coupled receptors receive the signal from ligand binding (in this example, epinephrine), and affect G-proteins. Therefore, GPCR must come before G-protein in the sequence (choice A can be eliminated). GPCRs activate G-proteins, which then affect the enzyme adenylyl cyclase (choice B is correct, and choice C is wrong). Remember also that some GPCRs activate adenylyl cyclase and others inhibit it. This depends on the cell, the ligand, and many other factors.

5. **C** Item I is true: the nuclear membrane is degraded by the end of prophase so that the chromosomes can be appropriately separated into the daughter cells. It is therefore absent in anaphase (choice D can be eliminated). Item II is false: the nuclear membrane reforms after cytokinesis in telophase (choice B can be eliminated). Item III is true: since the membrane does not reform until telophase, it must be absent in metaphase (choice A can be eliminated).

6. **D** Phosphorylation, formation of disulfide bridges, and glycosylation are all types of protein modification and can occur in both the Golgi apparatus and the rough ER (choices A, B, and C can be eliminated). Peptide bond formation occurs during translation, prior to any protein modification (choice D is not a type of protein modification and is the correct answer choice).

7. **C** A female who inherits a single mutation still has an allele which can produce functional proteins (choice C is correct) and is heterozygous, not homozygous (choices A and B are wrong). While an individual who is heterozygous for the mutation can rely on other DNA repair mechanisms, this is not the primary reason why these individuals will not have a 100% chance of developing breast or ovarian cancer (choice C is better than choice D).

SOLUTIONS TO CHAPTER 6 PRACTICE PASSAGE

1. **A** The key to answering this question is decoding the question stem: *If p53 is commonly defective in cancer cells, it must normally have some sort of protective role.* In other words, p53 loss is beneficial for cancer cells. If p53 normally induces apoptosis and becomes mutant or lost, then it would no longer cause cell death in aberrant conditions. This could be a benefit for cancer cells, and in fact could lead to the rapid cell proliferation and tumor growth that is typically seen in cancer (choice A is correct). The passage says that autophagy can help the cell deal with times of stress, including nutrient deprivation. Since cancer cells grow quickly, they have high metabolic demands, which are accommodated in part using autophagy to supply macromolecules. If p53 normally helped the cell supply macromolecules, p53 loss would not help the growth of cancer cells (choice B can be eliminated). Similarly, if cancer cells are growing quickly, they will need lots of phospholipids. If p53 normally stimulated phospholipid synthesis, its loss would not be beneficial for the cancer cell (choice C can be eliminated). Finally, if p53 normally pushed the cell cycle forward, its loss would arrest the cell cycle. This is clearly not the case in "aberrantly growing cancer cells" (choice D is wrong).

2. **B** The passage says that the lysosome contains acid hydrolases, which degrade the contents of the autophagosomes. Since the autophagosomes contain cellular and organelle material, it is possible that they would contain proteins (which would be broken down by proteases and peptidases; choice C can be eliminated), nucleic acids (which would be broken down by nucleases; choice A can be eliminated), carbohydrates (which would be broken down by glucosidases), and lipids (which would be broken down by lipases; choice D can be eliminated). However, phospholipase C and adenylyl cyclase are both involved in cell signaling pathways, downstream of ligands binding receptors. Neither of these would function in macromolecule degradation (choice B would not be found in lysosomes and is the correct answer choice). Note that phosphatases remove the phosphate group from molecules, and in many cases, this is part of degradation.

3. **C** The passage says that autophagy is induced when cells are under nutrient stress, reactive oxygen stress, or organelle stress. Decreased intracellular metabolite concentrations would be an example of nutrient stress (choice D would induce autophagy and can be eliminated). An increase in mitochondrial permeability and an accumulation of incorrectly folded proteins in the ER lumen are examples of organelle stress (autophagy degrades broken or sickly organelles; choices A and B could induce autophagy and can be eliminated). While incomplete genome replication in the S phase is a problem for cells, there is no information to indicate that this would induce autophagy. Also, the effects of autophagy as described in the passage (break down of cytoplasmic and organelle material) would not solve this problem since the genome cannot be degraded (there is only one, after all). In fact, incomplete genome replication is detected by cell cycle checkpoint pathways to halt cell cycle progression and allow time for DNA replication and repair (choice C would not induce autophagy and is the correct answer choice).

4. **A** According to the figure, BAX proteins form channels in the mitochondrial membrane and this facilitates cytochrome c release. If Bci1 inhibits these channels, it would cause cytochrome c to remain in the inner mitochondrial membrane (choice A is correct). This would prevent apoptosis (and thus rounded cells and blebbing; choice C is wrong). While choice B might be tempting, just because Bci1 inhibits BAX channels doesn't mean it has to inhibit channel formation (although this is certainly possible). We can be sure about the end result, though (retention of cytochrome c), even if we aren't sure of the mechanism (choice A is better than choice B). Note that BAX functions in apoptosis, not autophagy (choice D is wrong).

5. **A** Note that there is no information about Atg13 in the passage, so this question must be answered based entirely on information in the question. The question text states that when Atg13 is phosphorylated on one amino acid, it initiates autophagy by inducing autophagosome formation (choice D is wrong). If mTOR phosphorylates Atg13 on three amino acids, it is acting as a kinase and is inhibiting Atg13 function and autophagy (choice A is correct, and choice B is wrong). If rapamycin inhibits mTOR, it is inhibiting an inhibitor of autophagy. In other words, rapamycin would induce autophagy (choice C is wrong).

6. **B** The passage says that Atg5 cleavage (from a longer precursor protein to a shorter 24 kDa protein) is involved in the switch from autophagy to apoptosis. If cells have bound FasL (a death receptor ligand), they are undergoing apoptosis, or will be soon. Since Atg5 cleavage induces apoptosis, choice B is very likely. Southern blot analysis is a lab technique used to study DNA, not proteins (choice A is wrong). While western blot analysis is the correct lab technique to study proteins, in cells undergoing autophagy (not apoptosis), Atg5 would be in the longer, nontruncated form (the 24 kDa protein, not the 19 kDa protein; choice C is wrong). The passage describes proteolytic cleavage as the mechanism for generating differently sized Atg5, not alternative splicing (choice D is wrong).

GUT MICROBIOME FERMENTATION DETERMINES THE EFFICACY OF EXERCISE FOR DIABETES PREVENTION

Yan Liu, Yao Wang, Yueqiong Ni, Cynthia K. Y. Cheung, Karen S. L. Lam, Yu Wang, Zhengyuan Xia, Dewei Ye, Jiao Guo, Michael Andrew Tse, Gianni Panagiotou, and Aimin Xu

Cell Metabolism 31, 77-91 January 7, 2020 © 2019 Elsevier Inc. https://doi.org/10.1016/j.cmet.2019.11.001

INTRODUCTION

Exercise is a cost-effective lifestyle intervention for the prevention and treatment of obesity, type 2 diabetes (T2D) and its complications, which are the leading causes of morbidity and mortality worldwide. Despite the well-recognized benefits of exercise on metabolic homeostasis, the biomarkers and molecular transducers conferring its pleotropic effects remain poorly understood. Clinical implementation of exercise for diabetes management is still in its infancy, in part due to the high variability in physiological response to standardized exercise regimen. A large proportion of individuals, ranging from 7% to 69%, do not respond (non-responders) or even respond adversely to exercise in terms of insulin sensitivity and glucose homeostasis. Though genetic predispositions and epigenetic modifications have been proposed to be potential contributors, neither the pathomechanisms nor potential predictors for the heterogeneity of exercise responsiveness have been clarified so far.

A growing body of evidence suggests that dysbiosis of gut microbiota plays an important role in the pathogenesis of insulin resistance and T2D through multiple mechanisms. Compositional and functional changes of gut microbiota have been observed in individuals with T2D and prediabetes, whereas fecal microbial transplantation from healthy donors into patients with metabolic syndrome results in increased microbial diversity and improved glycemic control, as well as insulin sensitivity.

Recently, a modulatory effect of exercise on gut microbiota in both humans and animals has been observed. The microbiome of professional athletes exhibits higher diversity and more favorable metabolic capacity compared to sedentary counterparts. Mice receiving exercise training also display favorable changes in the composition of gut microbiota, including reduced *Bacteroidetes*, but augmented *Firmicutes* and *Proteobacteria*. However, whether and how alterations in gut microbiota are functionally involved in the metabolic benefits of exercise remain obscure.

To address the above questions, we conducted a well-controlled exercise intervention in medication-naive overweight men with prediabetes, followed by comprehensive metagenomics and metabolomics analysis, and a functional interrogation in mice using fecal microbial transplantation to explore the roles of differentially shaped gut microbiota by exercise in glucose metabolism and insulin sensitivity.

RESULTS AND DISCUSSION

Heterogeneous Glycemic Responses of Individuals with Prediabetes to High-Intensity Training

Eligible participants were randomized to either sedentary control or 12-week supervised exercise training, in which exercise responsiveness was further evaluated (Figure 1A). All participants were recommended to maintain their diet routine during the study period, which was closely monitored to ensure that no significant difference existed among all these subjects (Table S1).

After exercise intervention, a modest but significant reduction in body weight and adiposity, together with obvious improvements in insulin sensitivity, lipid profiles, cardiorespiratory fitness, and levels of adipokines functionally related to insulin sensitivity had been achieved in the whole exercise group (Table S1). However, in contrast to a homogenous change in body compositions (Figures 1B–1D), a high interpersonal variability in the alterations of fasting glucose, insulin, and the homeostatic model assessment of insulin resistance (HOMA-IR) was observed (Figures 1E–1G), suggesting a highly heterogeneous response of the cohort with respect to glucose homeostasis and insulin sensitivity. Therefore, we

Figure 1 High Interpersonal Variability in the Improvement of Insulin Sensitivity

(A) Schematic diagram of the study design. (B–G) Boxplots (with median) showing the dynamic changes of (B) body weight and (C) fat mass and (D) lean mass body compositions at 0, 6, and 12 weeks of exercise intervention, as well as (E) fasting glucose, (F) fasting insulin and (G) HOMA-IR at 0, 4, 8, and 12 weeks of exercise, respectively. Lines connect the same subject at different time points. #$p < 0.05$ and ###$p < 0.001$ by repeated-measures ANOVA within Responders or non-responders; and *$p < 0.05$, **$p < 0.01$ and ***$p < 0.001$ by repeated-measures ANOVA within all subjects. (H–M) The relative change of (H) body weight, (I) fat mass and (J) lean mass body compositions, (K) fasting glucose, (L) fasting insulin, and (M) HOMA-IR over 12 weeks of exercise intervention. Data were shown as mean ± SEM. *$p < 0.05$ by repeated-measures two-way ANOVA.

Table S1 Summary of clinical characteristics of the exercise group and sedentary control, Related to Figure 1

Variables	Sedentary control			Exercise group			Between group difference (p value)	
	0-week	12-week	p value[*]	0-week	12-week	p value[*]	0-week[#]	12-week[§]
Age (years)	44.94 ± 2.43	NA	NA	42.80 ± 2.55	NA	NA	0.549	NA
Weight (kg)	83.63 ± 1.96	83.46 ± 1.85	0.965	85.50 ± 3.16	84.22 ± 3.21	0.003	0.760	0.897
BMI (Kg/m^2)	29.40 ± 0.72	29.32 ± 0.85	0.807	29.09 ± 0.90	28.95 ± 0.91	0.192	0.625	0.623
WHR	0.92 ± 0.02	0.91 ± 0.02	0.852	0.95 ± 0.01	0.93 ± 0.01	2.00E-06	0.157	0.276
Fat mass%	34.79 ± 1.28	34.64 ± 0.78	0.742	35.95 ± 0.98	33.74 ± 0.91	1.00E-06	0.470	0.855
Lean mass%	61.79 ± 1.50	60.53 ± 1.48	0.745	61.22 ± 0.91	63.38 ± 0.83	1.88E-06	0.736	0.612
Fasting glucose (mM)	5.79 ± 0.25	5.94 ± 0.28	0.758	5.61 ± 0.08	4.99 ± 0.09	3.00E-06	0.943	0.022
2h glucose (mM)	8.79 ± 0.42	9.12 ± 0.46	0.182	8.30 ± 0.32	6.30 ± 0.30	1.00E-06	0.376	1.70E-05
Fasting insulin (μU/mL)	9.83 ± 1.04	8.86 ± 0.81	0.393	12.10 ± 2.17	9.10 ± 2.19	0.026	0.474	0.806
HOMA-IR	2.86 ± 0.31	2.58 ± 0.19	0.464	2.98 ± 0.49	1.99 ± 0.45	0.031	0.847	0.042
Triglycerides (mM)	2.53 ± 0.44	2.40 ± 0.39	0.992	2.33 ± 0.17	1.90 ± 0.14	0.016	0.803	0.741
Total cholesterol (mM)	5.10 ± 0.25	4.68 ± 0.25	0.256	5.37 ± 0.23	4.98 ± 0.21	0.027	0.434	0.349
HDL-c (mM)	1.15 ± 0.06	1.08 ± 0.56	0.429	1.16 ± 0.04	1.21 ± 0.43	0.301	0.859	0.260
LDL-c (mM)	3.57 ± 0.20	3.68 ± 0.20	0.669	3.55 ± 0.20	3.29 ± 0.17	0.054	0.926	0.425
Systolic blood pressure (mmHg)	133.75 ± 5.10	132.28 ± 4.39	0.790	130.79 ± 3.64	128.37 ± 3.12	0.375	0.632	0.493
Diastolic blood pressure (mmHg)	83.75 ± 2.03	85.88 ± 2.95	0.587	80.42 ± 1.93	77.37 ± 2.22	0.131	0.245	0.025
Resting heart rate (bpm)	76.83 ± 2.65	77.83 ± 3.72	0.475	77.53 ± 2.18	73.74 ± 2.04	0.028	0.743	0.711
hs-CRP (mg/L)	3.59 ± 0.75	3.72 ± 0.82	0.912	3.60 ± 0.41	2.55 ± 0.29	0.002	0.662	0.440
Total energy (Kcal/d)	1648 ± 90.05	1646.97 ± 59.86	0.988	1656.67 ± 49.45	1655.32 ± 43.61	0.983	0.935	0.904
Carbohydrate (g)	267.15 ± 14.92	257.96 ± 11.26	0.625	266.02 ± 7.16	260.08 ± 7.69	0.483	0.945	0.965
% of Energy intake	63.21 ± 1.25	61.11 ± 1.11	0.215	64.40 ± 1.05	63.55 ± 1.03	0.601	0.469	0.098

Table 2 Changes in Clinical Parameters of Prediabetic Individuals in Response to 12-Week Exercise Intervention

Characteristics	0-Week			12-Week			p Value$_c$
	Responders	Non-responders	p Value$_a$	Responders	Non-responders	p Value$_b$	Between Group Difference in Relative Change
Age (years)	43.29 ± 3.27	36.00 ± 4.55	0.228	—	—	—	—
BMI	28.78 ± 1.08	29.82 ± 1.75	0.603	28.65 ± 1.09	29.66 ± 1.78	0.850	0.613
Fat mass%	36.13 ± 1.33	35.78 ± 1.22	0.878	33.82 ± 1.22	33.53 ± 1.22	0.888	0.882
Lean mass%	60.98 ± 1.24	61.57 ± 1.10	0.776	63.26 ± 1.11	63.67 ± 1.09	0.856	0.799
WHR	0.95 ± 0.02	0.94 ± 0.01	0.730	0.93 ± 0.02	0.92 ± 0.01	0.761	0.702
Fasting glucose (mM)	5.65 ± 0.09	5.51 ± 0.13	0.426	4.95 ± 0.11	5.08 ± 0.21	0.311	0.980
2-h glucose (mM)	8.24 ± 0.33	8.46 ± 0.81	0.757	6.15 ± 0.39	6.64 ± 0.45	0.520	0.578
Fasting insulin (μU/mL)	10.37 ± 1.31	16.12 ± 6.67	0.522	5.70 ± 0.77	17.04 ± 6.26	3.84E−04	0.030
Matsuda index	5.83 ± 1.09	3.24 ± 0.78	0.097	11.01 ± 1.91	3.81 ± 0.78	0.002	0.017
Triglycerides (mM)	2.30 ± 0.21	2.41 ± 0.30	0.690	1.91 ± 0.19	1.86 ± 0.21	0.859	0.807
Total cholesterol (mM)	5.26 ± 0.31	5.60 ± 0.27	0.524	4.76 ± 0.26	5.49 ± 0.24	0.103	0.247
Systolic blood pressure (MmHg)	130.54 ± 4.74	131.33 ± 5.84	0.923	128.31 ± 4.47	128.50 ± 2.67	0.956	0.944
Diastolic blood pressure (MmHg)	80.00 ± 2.71	81.33 ± 2.04	0.759	78.08 ± 2.77	75.83 ± 3.94	0.452	0.912
Resting heart rate (bpm)	75.00 ± 2.02	83.00 ± 4.91	0.087	70.46 ± 1.92	80.83 ± 3.65	0.081	0.024
VO$_{2\,Max}$ (mL/kg/min)	25.27 ± 1.30	26.83 ± 1.38	0.485	31.42 ± 1.20	31.03 ± 1.85	0.861	0.755
Leg press (kg)	239.23 ± 11.79	226.67 ± 15.85	0.547	282.69 ± 17.97	270.83 ± 14.52	0.894	0.608
Chest press (kg)	32.46 ± 2.17	34.40 ± 3.41	0.642	38.92 ± 2.30	39.50 ± 2.97	0.886	0.546
hs-CRP (mg/L)	3.68 ± 0.46	3.39 ± 0.94	0.565	2.53 ± 0.32	2.59 ± 0.67	0.461	0.880
Total energy (Kcal/d)	1,694.74 ± 59.99	1,567.84 ± 82.97	0.250	1,685.20 ± 51.93	1,585.59 ± 79.62	0.308	0.137
Carbohydrate (g)	270.21 ± 8.94	256.26 ± 11.69	0.386	266.96 ± 9.64	244.04 ± 10.55	0.178	0.177
Protein (g)	70.51 ± 3.57	69.01 ± 4.52	0.813	70.24 ± 2.30	71.81 ± 4.65	0.738	0.933
Fat (g)	35.76 ± 3.00	33.31 ± 2.86	0.629	39.86 ± 2.63	37.43 ± 5.80	0.663	0.490
Fiber (g)	9.30 ± 0.85	8.23 ± 1.32	0.500	9.25 ± 0.56	8.10 ± 0.54	0.235	0.238

BMI, body mass index; HDL-c, high-density lipoprotein cholesterol; hs-CRP, high-sensitive C-reactive protein; LDL-c, low-density lipoprotein cholesterol; WHR, waist-hip ratio. Responders ($n = 14$) and Non-responders ($n = 6$). Data are shown as means ± SEM.
a   Determined by independent Student's t test.
b   Determined by ANCOVA model controlling for baseline measurements.
c   Determined by repeated-measures two-way ANOVA.

further classified the participants into responders (n = 14) and non-responders (n = 6), depending on whether they could demonstrate a decrease of HOMA-IR greater than 2-fold technical error, which is a threshold for true physiological adaptation. Notably, despite a homogeneous baseline characteristic (Table 1) and a similar degree of reduction in body weight and fat percentage between these two sub-groups (Figures 1H–1J), responders showed a remarkable 42.70% and 49.60% decrease in fasting insulin and HOMA-IR index, respectively (Figures 1L and 1M), as well as a striking 116.29% increase of Matsuda index (a comprehensive evaluation of both hepatic and peripheral insulin sensitivity derived from oral glucose tolerance test), whereas no obvious improvement or even deterioration in glucose homeostasis and insulin sensitivity was observed in non-responders (Table 1; Figures 1K–1M). Considering the important role of the gut microbiota in regulating glucose homeostasis and insulin sensitivity, we next explored whether it was involved in the heterogeneous metabolic effects of exercise in our cohort.

A Modest but Distinguishable Change of Gut Microbiota by Exercise Intervention in All Participants

We performed shotgun metagenome sequencing of fecal samples collected before and after the 12-week exercise regimen. We performed a compositional analysis and found that the relative abundances of 6 species, belonging to *Firmicutes*, *Bacteroidetes*, and *Proteobacteria*, respectively, were significantly altered after exercise (Figure 2A). Moreover, species falling into the *Bacteroides* genus and *Clostridiales* order, most of which are involved in the production of SCFAs, underwent a significant strain-level genomic variation by exercise (Figure 2B). Importantly, none of the alterations observed above could be detected in sedentary controls sharing similar metabolic characteristics (Table S1; Figure 3). In addition, the number of positive connections among those butyrate-producing genera within *Firmicutes* was obviously promoted, the decreased abundance of which is reported to be associated with obesity and T2D.

Figure 2 Exercise Promotes Differential Alteration of Gut Microbiota in Responders and Non-responders
(A and B) Participants were further classified into responders (R, blue) and non-responders (NR, red) based on the relative improvement of HOMA-IR. (A) Non-metric multidimensional scaling analysis plot of taxonomic variation induced by exercise training in R and NR, respectively. p = 0.008 by ADONIS test between R and NR. (B) Significantly altered species (p < 0.05) caused by exercise intervention in R and NR, respectively. Fold change was defined as the ratio of relative microbial abundance after exercise to those at baseline and the log fold changes were set to zero if not statistically significant.

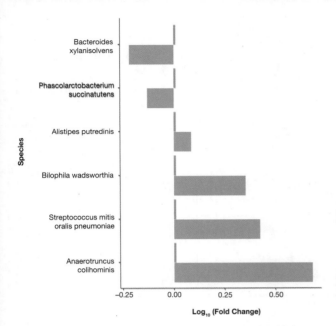

Figure 3 None of the exercise-induced microbial alterations can be detected in sedentary controls, Related to Figure 2. Green and purple indicate exercise and sedentary control respectively. Fold change was defined as the ratio of relative microbial abundance at 12-week to that at baseline (0-week).

Differential Alterations of Gut Microbiota between Exercise Responders and Non-responders

As there was a high interpersonal variability in the alteration of gut, we next interrogated whether the heterogeneous responses to exercise in glucose homeostasis and insulin sensitivity were related to differential changes in gut microbiota between responders and non-responders. We observed a significant segregation of dynamic alterations of gut microbiota between the two sub-groups (Figure 2D). Compared to responders, the microbial profiles of non-responders after 12-week exercise training shared more similarity with those of the sedentary controls (p < 0.0 01), suggesting a maladaptation of gut microbiota in non-responders. Notably, we observed that the significant decrease of *Bacteroides xylanisolvens* and increase of *Streptococcus mitis* group found in all participants only occurred in responders, but not non-responders. Contrary

to an increase of *Alistipes putredinis* in the whole group, this bacterium was found to be reduced in responders (Figure 2E). In addition, responders were characterized by a 3.5-fold increase of *Lanchospiraceae bacterium* (a butyrate-producer), whereas non-responders were featured by nearly a 70% decrease in *Ruminococcus gnavus*, which has been reported to alleviate growth and metabolic impairments caused by transplanting microbiota from undernourished donors. Moreover, *Alistipes shahii*, previously reported to be associated with inflammation and enriched in obese Japanese, decreased by 43% in responders, but increased by 3.88-fold in non-responders (Figure 2E). When taking the growth dynamics of bacteria into consideration, responders were characterized by a decreased replication rate of *Prevotella copri*, a main bacterium responsible for the production of BCAAs and a contributor to insulin resistance, as well as an increased growth rate of several species in *Bacteroides* genus, most of which are propionate producers. Collectively, these findings suggest that exercise intervention exerts differential modulatory effects on microbial compositions in responders and non-responders.

Exercise-Conditioned Microbiota from Responders Ameliorate Glucose Intolerance and Insulin Resistance in Obese Mice

To further examine the causal relationship between differentially shaped microbiota and changes in glucose metabolism and insulin sensitivity by exercise intervention, conventional antibiotics-treated mice were transplanted with microbiota from two responders and two non-responders collected at both baseline and after exercise intervention (Figure 4A). A number of microbial species, such as *Alistipes shahii*, *Alistipes putredinis* and *Ruminococcus gnavus*, demonstrated a similar trend of changes between recipient mice and human donors (Figure S7). Mice colonized with microbiota from responders and non-responders after exercise displayed a similar trend of changes in body composition, oxygen consumption, and respiratory exchange ratio compared to those receiving microbiota from the same donors taken at baseline (Figures 4B–4D). On the other hand, significant reductions in glucose and insulin levels were observed only in mice transplanted with microbiota from responders, but not non-responders after exercise training (Figures 4E–4F).

Figure 4 Transplantation of Human Fecal Microbiota into Mice Mimics the Effect of Exercise on Glucose Homeostasis and Insulin Sensitivity

(A) Schematic diagram showing the study design for fecal microbial transplantation. (B) Relative changes of body compositions. (C and D) Recipient mice were subjected to indirect calorimetry analysis for the determination of (C) oxygen consumption and (D) respiratory exchange ratio after 4 weeks of microbial colonization. (E and F) Glucose (E) and insulin (F) levels at both fasting and fed status. Data were expressed as mean ± SEM ($n = 6$ mice/group). $*p < 0.05$, $**p < 0.01$, and $***p < 0.001$ between R-FMT-0w and R-FMT-12w; $\#p < 0.05$ between NR-FMT-0w and NR-FMT-12w by unpaired Student's t test. Dots with different colors represent individual mice receiving FMT from different human donors.

In this well-controlled interventional study conducted in medication-naïve individuals with prediabetes, we showed that gut microbiota was an important mediator conferring the effect of exercise on glucose metabolism and insulin sensitivity. The high interpersonal variability in the adaptive changes upon exercise intervention was attributed to divergent functional alterations of gut microbiota, leading to production of distinct sets of microbial metabolites. These findings were further strengthened by animal studies showing that exercise-induced differential changes in glucose homeostasis, insulin sensitivity, and metabolites in responders and non-responders can be transferred into mice by FMT.

Although there was no obvious difference in baseline microbial structures between responders and non-responders, we were able to establish a model based on the microbiome signatures before exercise to accurately predict the exercise outcomes with respect to glycemic control and insulin sensitivity, raising the possibility of screening for individuals with high likelihood of exercise resistance using gut microbiota, so that personalized adjustments can be implemented in time to maximize the efficacy of exercise intervention. These findings uncover the diversity of gut microbiota as a key determinant for the variability of glycemic control after dietary and exercise intervention. However, how exercise imposes such a differential impact on the composition and function of gut microbiota remains unclear and warrants further investigation. We speculate that exercise may amplify subtle difference of gut microbiota at baseline by remodeling the intestinal microenvironment (such as inflammatory and oxidative status and local immunity) critical for microbial growth and interaction, which ultimately lead to a divergent response of glycemic control to exercise intervention.

In conclusion, our study uncovers gut microbiota and its metabolism as key molecular transducers to the heterogeneous adaption to exercise intervention on glucose metabolism and insulin sensitivity. This finding, together with our demonstration of the predictive value of baseline microbial signatures for individualized responsiveness to exercise, may facilitate clinical implementation of personalized lifestyle intervention for diabetes management.

Limitations of Study

The main limitation of the current study is a relatively small sample size and rigid inclusion criteria for our study participants, which constrains the applicability of this result. Though limited only to Chinese males, these results demonstrate the adequacy of this non-invasive proxy measurement in the prediction of exercise responsiveness. Considering the regional and ethnic variations in gut microbiota, the wide applicability of our findings and prediction model needs further validation in larger and more diverse populations.

MATERIALS AND METHODS

Study Participants

Inclusion criteria were: (i) non-smoking and male Chinese aged between 20 and 60 years; (ii) weight stable (<5% weight change over last 3 months) and overweight/obese as defined by Asian criteria BMI>23 kg/m^2; (iii) pre-diabetes as defined by impaired glucose tolerance (7.8 mmol/L ≤ 2-h blood glucose ≤ 11.0 mmol/L after a 75-g oral glucose challenge) and/or impaired fasting glucose (5.6 mmol/L ≤ fasting blood glucose ≤ 6.9 mmol/L) following the American Diabetes Association practice guidelines; (iv) absence of any systemic, metabolic and cardiovascular diseases, as well as infections within the previous month; and (v) absence of any diet or medication that might interfere with glucose homeostasis and gut microbiota, especially antibiotics and probiotics.

Exclusion criteria were: (i) acute illness or current evidence of acute or chronic inflammatory or infective diseases; (ii) any neurological, musculoskeletal or cardio-respiratory conditions, which will put them at risk during exercise or inhibit their ability to adapt to an exercise program; (iii) participation in regular exercise and/or diet program more than 2 times per week in the latest 3 months prior to recruitment; and (iv) mental illness rendering them unable to understand the nature, scope, and possible consequences of the study.

Subject Recruitment and General Design

Overweight/obese subjects were recruited from our local community. Oral glucose tolerance test (OGTT) was used to screen for potential participants who met the inclusion criterion of prediabetes. Eligible subjects were randomly assigned to exercise or sedentary group. Aside from exercise training, all participants recruited were instructed to continue their normal routine and not make any changes to their habitual physical activity and diet. One-to-one interview with a validated questionnaire including nutritional intakes and physical activity was conducted every month to assess their adherence. Fecal samples were collected at baseline and 12 weeks after exercise training while fasting plasma samples were collected every 4 weeks. All examinations were conducted at 48-72 h from the final exercise session to control for the acute effects of exercise.

High-Intensity Exercise Training Protocol

The 12-week exercise program consisted of three sessions per week on non-consecutive days at the Active Health Clinic, supervised by certified exercise specialists in a one-to-one manner. Compliance in the exercise session was highly encouraged and participants were required to take part in at least 85% of all the exercise sessions for inclusion into the analysis for responsiveness. The exercise program consisted of a combination of aerobic and strength training, which was selected for its superior effectiveness in the alleviation of insulin resistance. The 70-min high-intensity combined aerobic and resistance interval training sessions including high-intensity treadmill intervals, high-intensity resistance and calisthenics exercises intervals, and high-intensity stationary bike intervals, with 3–4 min recovery. Participants wore a wireless heart rate telemetry sensor to monitor their heart rate (HR) and to ensure that they were working at the appropriate intensity level. The intensity was adjusted according to the real-time HR telemetry and the subjects were encouraged to work at 80-95% HR_{max}. The intensity of this resistance and calisthenics intervals was progressed during the 12-week training to keep the exercises challenging and also to provide adequate work to rest ratio to stimulate high intensity interval training-based resistance intervals.

Collection of Dietary and Clinical Data

Dietary data were collected by means of food frequency questionnaire administered by a nutritionist.

Definition of Responders and Non-responders

The distribution of exercise responsiveness in our cohort exhibits a two-sided shape, ranging from high responders to adverse responders with respect to changes in insulin sensitivity (data not shown). According to previous interventional surveys, the inter-individual variability in response was evaluated by technical error (TE), a parameter that captures the totality of the variance among laboratories or laboratory technicians and the normal day-to-day biological variation of a trait. It is defined as the within-subject standard deviation as derived from repeated measures (or assays) over a given period of time. A change greater than 2 times the TE means that there is a high probability that this response is a true physiological adaptation rather than a technical and/or biological variability. Therefore, non-response to exercise intervention was defined as a failure to demonstrate a decrease of HOMA-IR (levels at 12-week against those at 0-week) that was greater than 2-fold TE from zero.

Fecal Microbial Transplantation in Mice

500 mg of fresh stools obtained from donors before and after 12-week exercise intervention were suspended in 5 mL of PBS buffer containing 0.5 g/L cysteine as reducing agent. Two donors from exercise responders and non-responders respectively were randomly selected from each subgroup to perform fecal microbial transplantation. Fecal slurry from each donor was transferred into 3 conventional antibiotics-treated mice. Mice were randomized to receive fecal slurry from the same responder donors or non-responder donors collected at both baseline and after exercise training. Mice receiving FMT from responders after exercise with sterile tap water and mice receiving sterile PBS were included as controls. All the mice were fed with high fat diet (40% kcal fat) for 6 weeks to induce obesity before and during the 4-week period of colonization.

JOURNAL ARTICLE EXERCISE 1

The science sections on the MCAT include a significant number of passages with experiments. Questions for these passages often ask you to analyze data, read charts and graphs, and come to some reasonable conclusion based on the information they give you. If you don't know how to extract information efficiently and analyze data effectively, you will be at a distinct disadvantage.

There are three "Journal Article Exercises" in this book. In this first exercise, we'll show you the type of information you should be able to extract from the article and the sorts of things to pay attention to in the data. In subsequent exercises, you'll do more of that on your own, and in the final exercise we'll show you how that article might get turned into an MCAT-style passage.

When analyzing an experiment, you should be able to:

- identify the control group(s)
- extract information from graphs and data tables
- determine how the experimental group(s) change relative to the control
- determine if the results are statistically significant
- come to a reasonable conclusion about WHY the results were observed
- consider potential weaknesses in the study
- determine how to increase the power of the study
- decide what the next most logical experiment or study should be

The goal of these exercises is NOT to learn content from the articles, just to get a little more comfortable reading and extracting information from them.

For the (abridged) article on pages 219–226, try to summarize the purpose of the experiment and the methods in 4–5 sentences. Consider the following mnemonic: Oh ouR Car Won't Start (ORCWS).

- O = Organism and Organization: Is the research being conducted on humans or on animals or on bacteria in a petri dish, or something else? What is being done to these organisms? Are there any unique qualities to these organisms? Are there multiple groups? Is the study conducted over a long period of time with multiple data points, or is it a short-term study? Does it have a large or small n?
- R = Results: Where and how are the results presented? Is it a graph? A data table? Figures and images? What is/are the independent variable(s)? What is/are the dependent variable(s)? What are the results? Do the results show correlation or cause and effect, or both? Describe.
- C = Control and Comparison: Is there a control group? How does it differ from the experimental group? Is it given a placebo or nothing at all? Is it held under different conditions? If there are multiple experimental groups, how do they differ from one another? Is it a blinded study? If so, double blind or single blind?
- W = Weirdness: Does anything or do any of the results stand out as unexpected?
- S = Statistics: Was any sort of statistical analysis done? How is it presented? Are there error bars on a graph? Standard errors around a mean? Are there p-values? Is there an asterisk indicating statistical significance? Is there any data that is not statistically significant?

Try interpreting the data on your own before reading the results/discussion section. When you do read the discussion, consider:

- What are the conclusions of the study?
- How are the conclusions supported by the data?
- What potential weaknesses or flaws do you see in the experimental design? Are these addressed in the discussion section?
- How might this study be potentially biased?
- How might this study be improved?
- What would be the next most logical experiment?

Let's answer the above questions for the article on pages 219–226.

SOLUTIONS TO JOURNAL ARTICLE EXERCISE 1

1. O = Organism and Organization:
   - Is the research being conducted on humans or on animals or on bacteria in a petri dish, or something else? *Humans.*
   - What is being done to these organisms? *They are subjected to 12 weeks of exercise and gut microbiome assessed.*
   - Are there any unique qualities to these organisms? *All volunteers were diabetic men, no medication.*
   - Are there multiple groups? *Not initially, but they were ultimately divided into two groups.*
   - Is the study conducted over a long period of time with multiple data points, or is it a short-term study? *Long time (12 weeks) with multiple data points over that 12-week period.*
   - Does it have a large or small *n*? *Small n: 39 total subjects, 19 control, 20 experimental (6 non-responders and 14 responders).*

2. R = Results:
   - Where and how are the results presented? Is it a graph? A data table? Figures and images? *Graphs and data tables.*
   - What is/are the independent variable(s)? *Time and exercise regimen, gut microbes.*
   - What is/are the dependent variable(s)? *Body weight, fat mass, lean mass, fasting glucose, fasting insulin, insulin resistance.*
   - What are the results of the study? *As a whole, the exercise group showed reduction in body weight, fat mass, lean mass, fasting glucose, fasting insulin, and insulin resistance compared to controls. Within that group there were significant differences in fasting insulin and insulin resistance in "responders" and "nonresponders." There were also significant differences in gut microbiomes between responders and nonresponders. Obese mice transplanted with fecal samples from responders showed similar microbiomes and results as responders, whereas mice transplanted with fecal samples from nonresponders did not show these results.*
   - Do the results show correlation or cause and effect, or both? Describe. *Both. Correlation: exercise responders show gut microbe populations similar to that of professional athletes and different from those of sedentary controls; exercise non-responders show gut microbe populations similar to sedentary controls. Cause and effect: fecal transplant of responder gut microbes into obese mice result in the same types of changes in mice as seen in the humans.*

3. C = Control and Comparison:
   - Is there a control group? *Yes.*
   - How does it differ from the experimental group? Is it given a placebo or nothing at all? Is it held under different conditions? *Control group did not participate in the exercise regimen.*
   - If there are multiple experimental groups, how do they differ from one another? *Only one experimental group.*
   - Is it a blinded study? If so, double blind or single blind? *Not a blinded study.*

4. W = Weirdness:
   - Does anything or do any of the results stand out as unexpected? *I found the fact that some people responded differently to exercise unexpected.*

5. S = Statistics:
   - Was any sort of statistical analysis done? *Yes.*
   - How is it presented? Are there error bars on a graph? Standard errors around a mean? Are there *p*-values? Is there an asterisk indicating statistical significance? *P-values, error bars, asterisks.*
   - Is there any data that is not statistically significant? *Yes, initial characteristics of the responders and non-responders (weight, age, etc.) are not statistically different. Changes in body weight, fat mass, lean mass, and fasting glucose are not statistically significant.*

6. Interpreting the data:
   - What are the conclusions of the study? *Some individuals respond better to exercise (in terms of insulin levels and sensitivity) than others, and this is likely due to differences in their gut microbiomes.*
   - How are the conclusions supported by the data? *Data on fasting insulin and insulin resistance show significant differences between responders and nonresponders. These two groups also show significant differences in the makeup of their gut bacteria. Transplantation of fecal bacteria from responders into obese mice produced similar changes.*
   - What potential weaknesses or flaws do you see in the experimental design? Are these addressed in the discussion section? *Small, very select group of subjects. Maybe dietary intake. The small sample size was discussed.*
   - How might this study be potentially biased? *Sample bias: it was only conducted on Chinese males.*
   - How might this study be improved? *Bigger sample size, more diversity in subjects, include women.*
   - What would be the next most logical experiment? *Repeat the exercise intervention using different groups (women, non-Chinese origin).*

7. Final Summary of Experiment and Results:
   - *In this study a group of approximately 40 overweight diabetic Chinese men were divided into two groups, one sedentary control group and one exercise experimental group. Some of the exercisers showed significant changes in insulin sensitivity and other markers associated with a reduction in diabetic symptoms (called responders), and some of them did not (called nonresponders). The gut microbes of the responders were significantly different than those of the nonresponders, and matched the gut microbes of professional athletes. Transplantation of responder microbes into obese mice produced similar changes in insulin sensitivity and other markers.*

Chapter 7
Genetics and Evolution

The nature of the fundamental unit of inheritance, the gene, has been agreed upon by scientists only since the mid-nineteenth century. Aristotle believed that traits were passed on in the form of "pangenes," particles derived from all parts of the body and distilled into eggs and sperm. In the seventeenth century, different theorists believed that all genetic information was passed by either the father or the mother. Finally, early in the nineteenth century, people began to see that characteristics are passed from both parents; this led to the idea that parental characteristics were evenly mixed in offspring, in a process termed "blending." The notion that some characteristics were inherited in an either-or fashion, while others were in fact blended, remained unconceived.

The proponents of these early theories cannot be faulted for their lack of electron microscopes and other modern tools and techniques. But one is tempted to criticize their ideas for their obvious irrelevance to reality. One didn't need a Cray supercomputer to figure out that both parents contributed to a child's makeup. Why did researchers fail to arrive at this seemingly obvious hypothesis? Probably for two reasons: methods and dogma.

First, their approach to discovery was not empirical, but rather *a priori*. They believed knowledge could be derived by speculation alone, and that to perform experiments in the physical world was to dirty one's hands. And second, the prevailing religious dogma strongly censored empirical exploration, since it threatened the metaphysical tenets of the church.

What is different today is the approach to discovery known as the scientific method. Modern scientists know that only through careful, sober consideration of a question, formulation of a tentative answer, and testing of that hypothesis can new knowledge be uncovered. In this chapter, we will examine what is now considered to be the truth about genetics and evolution, all the way back to the origin of life.

We challenge you to attack this knowledge in the way its discoverers did. This is difficult material. Spend time thinking about the in-text questions before reading the answers. If you have trouble with a topic, stop and take out a fresh piece of paper. Write down all the facets of your current understanding, and look for internal inconsistencies and fallacies. Make up your own Punnett squares, pedigrees, and sketches of chromosomes during meiosis if the ones we present aren't sufficient. And finally, as you review, ask yourself which of the modern "truths" will one day be looked back on as preposterous ponderings of blindfolded pseudo-scientists.

7.1 INTRODUCTION TO GENETICS

Genetics is the science that describes the inheritance of traits from one generation to another. At the origin of genetics, patterns of inheritance were observed to follow certain predictable patterns, as described by Mendel's laws. The reasons for these patterns of inheritance were to remain a mystery until the nature of DNA as the genetic material was known. Today we can use our knowledge of DNA and the cell to understand Mendel's laws at the molecular level.

DNA as the Genetic Information of the Cell

Gregor Mendel described the basic principles of heredity (see Section 7.3), but not the molecular foundations. It wasn't until years later that DNA was shown to be the building block of cellular genetics. Mitosis and meiosis were actively studied in the late nineteenth century, and this paved the way for the chromosome theory of inheritance, which indicated that genes are located on chromosomes. Thomas Hunt Morgan associated a specific gene and its subsequent phenotype (eye color in the fruit fly) with a specific chromosome (the X chromosome). However, chromosomes are composed of both DNA and protein. It wasn't until an important series of experiments, which started in the 1920s, that DNA was accepted as the genetic material of the cell.

First, Frederick Griffith showed that cell extracts can transform bacteria, indicating biological macromolecules carry hereditary information. This work made use of two strains of *Streptococcus pneumoniae*. One strain is lethal in mice and is characterized by a smooth (S) appearance under the microscope due to the presence of a polysaccharide capsule. The other strain is less virulent and does not kill mice. It lacks the capsule and so has a rough (R) appearance under the microscope. When heat-killed S bacteria were injected into mice, the animals survived. However, when heat-killed S strain was mixed with live R strain and then injected together, the mice died. This suggested that the cell extract of dead S strain was capable of conferring virulence to the R strain. In addition, it was found that live S strain *S. pneumoniae* could be isolated from the dead mice (Figure 1).

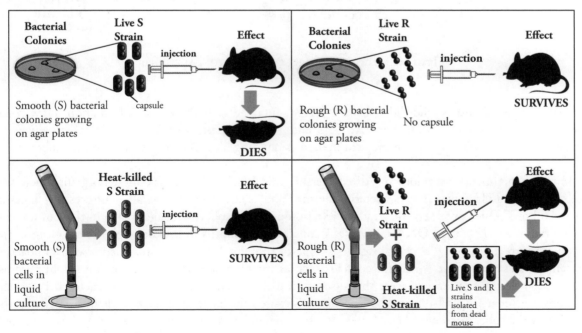

Figure 1 The Griffith Experiment

However, it still wasn't clear how the R strain was obtaining virulence. To figure this out, Oswald Avery, Colin MacLeod, and Maclyn McCarty systematically and chemically destroyed each biological macromolecule in the extracts from dead S strain *S. pneumoniae*. These treated extracts were then injected into mice with live R strain. Since the two strains were phenotypically different because of a polysaccharide coat, an obvious hypothesis was that virulence was being transferred via a polysaccharide. However, when polysaccharides were destroyed, virulence was still transferred from the dead S bacteria to the live R bacteria. Indeed, this was the case for all macromolecules save one: DNA (Figure 2). When DNase was added to S strain extracts, virulence was not conferred to the R strain. This suggested that DNA was able to transform bacteria, and was the molecule of heritability that scientists had been looking for.

Figure 2   The Avery-MacLeod-McCarty Experiment

Still, there were scientists who didn't believe DNA contained cellular genetic information. How could a molecule with only four monomers (A, C, G and T) be the basis of such extensive genetic diversity? Wouldn't proteins (with twenty amino acid monomer building blocks) be more suited to this job?

Definitive experiments were done by Alfred Hershey and Martha Chase. The model organism here was the phage T2, a virus that infects bacteria. Hershey and Chase grew two parallel cultures of phages in bacterial hosts. One contained ^{32}P, a radioactive isotope of phosphorus. Phages made in this culture contained radioactively labeled DNA, since DNA contains phosphorus in backbone phosphate groups. The second culture contained ^{35}S, a radioactive isotope of sulphur. In this culture, phages with radioactive protein capsids were made (since amino acids such as methionine and cysteine contain sulphur atoms). The two labeled phage samples were then used to infect new cultures of unlabeled bacteria. Later, the cultures were centrifuged (spun at high speeds); this caused the bacterial cells to settle into a pellet at the bottom of the tube. The liquid layer (called the supernatant) contained growth media and phage ghosts (capsid particles without internal nucleic acids). Hershey and Chase found that for phages grown in ^{32}P, the radioactive label was transferred to bacteria host cells in the pellet. This confirmed that DNA was being transferred and was therefore the hereditary material. ^{35}S was not transferred to the bacterial cells, indicating that capsid proteins remained outside the host cell (in the supernatant) and therefore do not contribute to heritability.

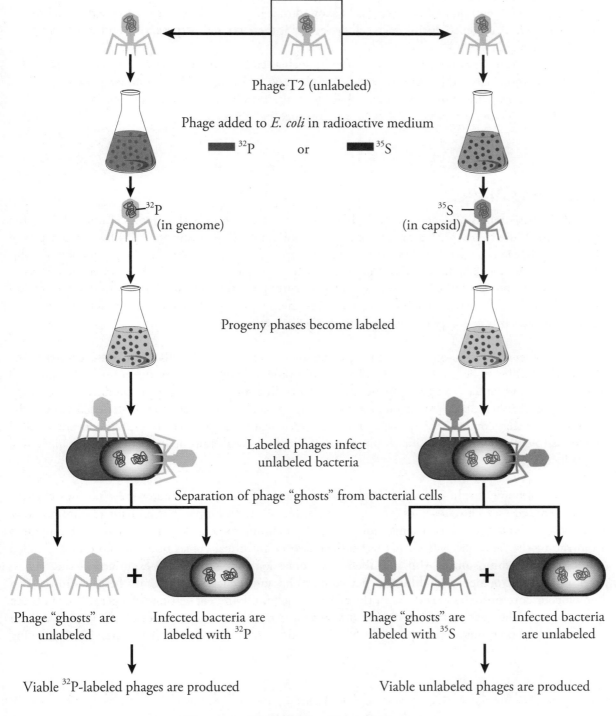

Figure 3 The Hershey-Chase Experiment

In addition to these three seminal projects, some additional evidence supports the fact that DNA carries genetic information of the cell:

- The total amount of DNA in a given cell (and species) is constant, and work by Erwin Chargaff suggested that each species has a consistent make-up of DNA; human DNA for example is 30.9% adenine, 29.4% thymine, 19.9% guanine, and 19.8% cytosine.
- Matthew Meselson and Franklin Stahl showed that DNA replication is semiconservative; cellular DNA is copied during each cell cycle, and is therefore self-perpetuating and consistent (see Chapter 4).
- In quiescent (resting) cells, macromolecules such as carbohydrates and proteins have a relatively short half-life and are constantly recycled and replaced. DNA is not broken down.
- Studies involving mutagens showed that DNA-altering chemicals induce phenotypic mutations, as do wavelengths of light that are absorbed by DNA.

Genes and Alleles

One of the basic tenets of genetics is that children inherit traits from both parents. Humans have a life cycle in which life begins with a diploid cell, the zygote. Diploid organisms (or cells) have two copies of the genome in each cell, while haploid cells have one copy of the genome. In sexual reproduction, the diploid zygote is produced by fusion of two haploid gametes: a haploid ovum from the mother and a haploid spermatozoon from the father. The zygote then goes through many mitotic divisions to develop into an adult, with half of the genetic material in each cell from each parent. The adult, male or female, produces haploid gametes by meiotic cell division to repeat the life cycle once again.

The development of a zygote into an adult and the maintenance of adult cells and tissues requires many thousands of different gene products. All of these gene products are encoded in the genome and inherited from mother and father. The **gene**, a length of DNA coding for a particular gene product, is the fundamental unit of inheritance. [Are gene products always proteins?[1]] The genes are distributed among the chromosomes that compose the genome, and every gene can be pinpointed to a specific location called the **locus** (plural: **loci**) on a specific chromosome. [Can all physical traits of an organism be mapped to a single locus?[2]]

The human genome is split into 24 different chromosomes: 22 of these are autosomes (non-sex chromosomes) and 2 are sex chromosomes (or allosomes, X and Y). Each human has 23 pairs of chromosomes (22 autosomes and a sex chromosome), for a total of 46 chromosomes. One chromosome of each pair is from the mother and one is from the father. The two nonidentical copies of a chromosome are called **homologous chromosomes**. Although these two copies look the same when examined at the crudest level under a microscope, and although they contain the same genes, the copies of the genes in the two homologous chromosomes may differ in their DNA sequence. Different versions of a gene, called **alleles**, may carry out the gene's function differently. Since a person carries two copies of every gene, one on each homologous chromosome, a person could potentially carry two different alleles. Individuals carrying

---

[1] No. tRNA and rRNA genes, as well as other small nuclear RNA genes, do not encode polypeptides.

[2] No. Every gene is located at a specific locus, but physical traits, particularly complex traits, like weight or height, can be controlled by many different genes and therefore do not map to a single locus, but to many.

different alleles of a gene will often have traits that allow the inheritance of alleles to be followed. [Is it possible for there to be more than two different alleles of a specific gene?[3]]

- Which one of the following is true if an individual has two different alleles at a given locus?[4]
  A) The individual has two phenotypes, e.g., one brown eye and one blue.
  B) There are two alleles in one place on one particular chromosome.
  C) Two siblings have different appearances.
  D) There is a different allele on each of the two members of a homologous pair.

Genotype vs. Phenotype

The **genotype** is the DNA sequence of the alleles a person carries. A person carrying two different alleles at a given locus is called a **heterozygote**, while an individual carrying two identical alleles is called a **homozygote**. The expression of alleles often is different in heterozygotes and homozygotes.

The **phenotype** is the physical expression of the genotype. For example, the phenotype of a gene involved in hair color may be brown or blond. Since there are many different kinds of alleles, there are different ways these alleles can be expressed in the phenotype. If an allele is the one expressed in the phenotype, regardless of what the second allele carried is, the expressed allele is referred to as **dominant**. An allele that is not expressed in the heterozygous state is referred to as **recessive**. For example, consider a heterozygous organism in which one allele encodes the functional version of an enzyme, while the second allele encodes an inactive version of that enzyme. Upon observation, it is noted that the organism's enzymes are all functional; then the functional-enzyme allele is *dominant* and the inactive-enzyme allele is *recessive*. Since recessive alleles are not expressed in heterozygotes, it is not always possible to tell the genotype of an individual based solely on the phenotype. [Can a haploid organism like an adult fungus have recessive alleles?[5]]

There are certain conventions used in denoting genotypes in genetics that are useful to know. The alleles of a gene are usually denoted by letters. For example, for a gene called "curly," a dominant allele may be denoted by the capital letter *C* and a recessive allele may be denoted by the lower case letter *c*. A heterozygote is referred to as *Cc*, while homozygotes would be either *CC* or *cc*. More complex situations require more complex conventions, but most questions probably only involve two alleles at a locus. [If the dominant allele for curly (*C*) results in curly hair and the recessive allele (*c*) causes straight hair, what are the phenotypes of *CC*, *Cc* and *cc* individuals?[6]]

---

[3] Yes, there can be many versions (alleles) of a particular gene. Under normal circumstances, however, one individual cannot have more than two of those different alleles, since they have only two copies of a gene (one on each homologous chromosome). An exception is when an individual is polyploid for a certain chromosome (i.e., they have more than two homologous chromosomes, for example, in Down syndrome and Klinefelter syndrome).

[4] An individual with two different alleles at a given locus has one allele on one chromosome and the other allele on its homologous partner (so choice **D** is correct and choice B is not possible). While choice A may be possible, it is an exceedingly complex phenomenon and not discernible from the information given. The question discusses a single individual, not a pair of siblings (eliminating choice C).

[5] No. If there is only one copy of a gene, then that is the copy which determines the phenotype.

[6] *CC* and *Cc* individuals have curly hair, and *cc* individuals have straight hair. Only homozygous recessive individuals express recessive traits. In the heterozygote, the presence of the recessive allele is masked by the dominant allele, so there are only two different phenotypes, although there are three different genotypes. This type of interaction between alleles is called **classical dominance**.

7.2 MEIOSIS

Mitotic cell division produces two daughter cells that are identical to the parent. However, the production of haploid cells such as gametes from a diploid cell requires a type of cell division that reduces the number of copies of each chromosome from two to one; this method of cell division is called **meiosis**. In males, meiosis occurs in the testes with haploid spermatozoa as the end result; in females, meiosis in the ovaries produces ova. (*Note*: This is not always the case, and while meiosis begins in the ovaries, it is completed only after fertilization; see Chapter 13 for a further discussion on oogenesis.) Specialized cells termed **spermatogonia** in males and **oogonia** in females undergo meiosis. Spermatogenesis and oogenesis share the same basic features of meiosis but differ in many of the specific features of gamete production. Meiosis itself will be discussed in this chapter, while the specifics of spermatogenesis and oogenesis will be discussed in Chapter 13.

Mitosis and meiosis are similar in many respects. Mitosis and meiosis are both preceded by one round of replication of the genome (S phase), leaving a diploid cell with four copies of the genome (Figure 4). The different phases in cell division are referred to by the same names (prophase, metaphase, anaphase, and telophase) in both meiosis and mitosis and are mechanistically very similar. The primary difference between meiosis and mitosis is that replication of the genome is followed by one round of cell division in mitosis and two rounds of cell division in meiosis, **meiosis I** and **meiosis II** (Figure 5). Another important difference is that in meiosis, recombination occurs between homologous chromosomes.

Figure 4 S Phase

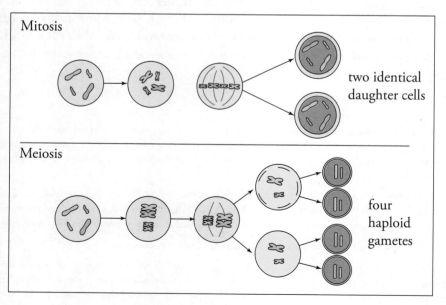

Figure 5 Mitosis vs. Meiosis

The first step in meiosis is **prophase I** (Figure 6). To depict meiosis, we will use a hypothetical model organism with a diploid genome with two different (nonhomologous) chromosomes (Figures 6–10).

- How many chromosomes are present in a cell from this organism during prophase I of meiosis?[7]

As in mitotic prophase, chromosomes condense in meiotic prophase I, and then the nuclear envelope breaks down. Unlike mitosis, however, homologous chromosomes pair with each other during meiotic prophase I in **synapsis**. Homologous chromosomes align themselves very precisely with each other in synapsis, with the two copies of each gene on two different chromosomes brought closely together. The paired homologous chromosomes are called a **bivalent** or **tetrad**.

When the DNA is aligned properly, it can then be cut precisely at the same location on homologous chromosomes. Genes are then swapped between the pair, and the chromosomes are religated (Figure 6). This process is known as **crossing over** or **recombination** (Figure 7, next page). Due to the extreme complexity of crossing over, meiotic prophase takes the most time in meiosis, days sometimes. Recombination during meiosis is an important source of genetic variation during sexual reproduction.

- Does crossing over change the number of genes on a chromosome?[8]
- Does recombination create combinations of alleles on a chromosome that are not found in the parent?[9]

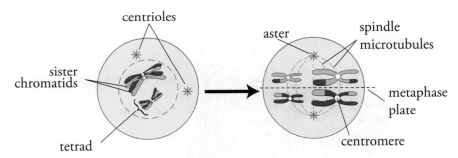

Figure 6 Prophase I and Metaphase I

---

[7] The organism is diploid normally, with two copies of two chromosomes, or four chromosomes total. After DNA synthesis, during prophase I, the cell still has four chromosomes; however, the chromosomes are replicated and held together at the centromere. Thus, each chromosome consists of two sister chromatids, and the cell has a total of eight sister chromatids.

[8] Not if it is done correctly. Error-free recombination involves a one-for-one swap of DNA between homologous chromosomes.

[9] Yes. Although each chromosome contains the same genes after crossing over, it may contain different alleles of some genes that were not present on the same chromosome previously.

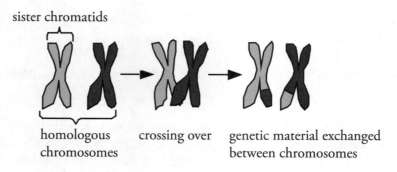

Figure 7   Crossing Over (Recombination)

Since precision is crucial in chromosome swapping, formation of the tetrad is highly regulated. Synapsis is mediated by a protein structure called the **synaptonemal complex** (SC). This structure starts to form early in meiotic prophase I. First, proteins named SYCP2 and SYCP3 attach to each of the two homologous chromatin structures that are to be paired (Figure 8). This makes up the lateral elements of the SC. The lateral regions then align and attach via a central region (made of SYCP1 and many other proteins). Both the lateral and central regions together form the SC, and essentially work like a zipper to connect homologous chromosomes.

Figure 8   The Synaptonemal Complex

While no physical connection has yet been shown between the synaptonemal complex and recombination machinery, it's been demonstrated that SC formation and recombination are interdependent. Both happen around the same time of meiosis, and work on mice with defective synaptonemal complex formation or recombination shows that these two processes rely on one another. When synaptonemal complex formation is inhibited, recombination is disturbed, and vice versa.

After prophase I is **metaphase I**. In meiotic metaphase I, alignment along the metaphase plate occurs, as in mitosis. The difference is that in meiotic metaphase I, the *tetrads* are aligned at the center of the cell (the metaphase plate), whereas in mitosis, *sister chromatids* are aligned on the metaphase plate. In **anaphase I**, homologous chromosomes separate, and sister chromatids remain together (Figure 9). The cell then divides into two cells during **telophase I** (Figure 10). *It is important to note that at this point the cells are considered to be haploid.* Each cell has a single set of chromosomes. The chromosomes, however, are still replicated (still exist as a pair of sister chromatids). The whole point to the second set of meiotic divisions is to separate the sister chromatids so that each cell has a single set of unreplicated chromosomes.

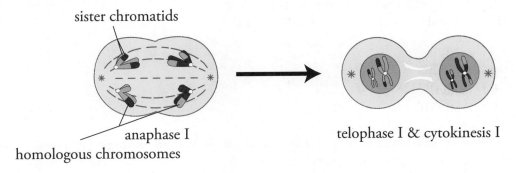

Figure 9   Anaphase I, Telophase I, and Cytokinesis I

In some species, meiosis II begins immediately after telophase I, while in other species there is a period of time before meiosis II begins. In either case, there is no further replication of the DNA before the second set of divisions. The movements of the chromosomes during meiosis II are identical to the movements in mitosis, with the sole difference being that in meiosis II there is a haploid number of chromosomes, while in mitosis there is a diploid number. The sister chromatids are separated during anaphase II, and after telophase II is complete, four haploid cells have been produced from a single diploid parent cell (Figure 10).

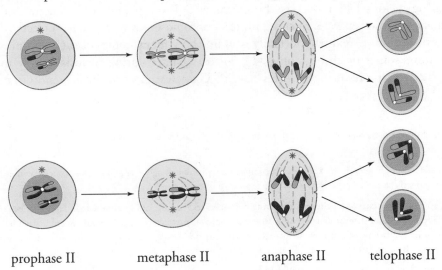

prophase II   metaphase II   anaphase II   telophase II

Figure 10   Meiosis II

- When homologous chromosomes separate, do all paternal and maternal chromosomes stay together in the daughter cells?[10]

- Are the sister chromatids that separate during meiotic anaphase II identical in their DNA sequence?[11]

- Which of the following occur in meiosis but NOT in mitosis?[12]
    I.   Separation of sister chromatids on microtubules
    II.   Pairing of homologous chromosomes
    III. Recombination between sister chromatids

    A) I only
    B) II only
    C) I and II
    D) II and III

- If cells are blocked in meiotic metaphase II and prevented from moving on in meiosis, which one of the following will be prevented?[13]
    A) Crossing over
    B) Separation of homologous chromosomes
    C) Separation of sister chromatids
    D) Breakdown of the nuclear envelope

Nondisjunction

Sometimes during meiosis I homologous chromosomes fail to separate, and sometimes during meiosis II sister chromatids fail to separate. Such a failure of chromosomes to separate correctly during meiosis is called **nondisjunction**. [A gamete normally contains how many copies of each chromosome?[14] If two homologous chromosomes of chromosome #12 fail to separate during meiosis I, how many copies of chromosome #12 will the resulting gametes have?[15]] Gametes resulting from nondisjunction will have

---

[10] No. Homologous chromosomes separate (segregate) randomly. This is one aspect of meiosis that increases genetic variation during sexual reproduction.

[11] The sister chromatids *would* be identical, except that recombination with homologous chromosomes occurred earlier in meiosis, during prophase I, altering the sister chromatids.

[12] Item I is false: the spindle separates sister chromatids during both (choices A and C can be eliminated). Note that both remaining answer choices include Item II, so Item II must be true. **Item II is true**: only meiosis involves pairing and recombination between homologous chromosomes. Item III is false: meiotic recombination occurs between homologous chromosomes, not sister chromatids (choice D can be eliminated, and choice **B** is correct).

[13] Crossing over occurs during prophase I, separation of homologous chromosomes occurs during anaphase I, and nuclear envelope breakdown occurs during prophase I and sometimes prophase II (choices A, B, and D are false). Only separation of sister chromatids occurs after metaphase II, in anaphase II. Answer: **C**.

[14] Normal gametes have one copy of each chromosome; this is the definition of haploid.

[15] If the homologous chromosomes do not separate in meiosis I, then one daughter cell from this division will have four copies of this chromosome and the other cell will have none. In meiosis II, sister chromatids will separate, leaving two gametes with two copies of the chromosome and two gametes with no copies of the chromosome.

two copies or no copies of a given chromosome. Such a gamete can fuse with a normal gamete to create a zygote with either three copies of a chromosome (**trisomy**) or one copy of a chromosome (**monosomy**).

The genetic defect caused when an entire chromosome is either added or removed is usually so great that a zygote with either trisomy or monosomy cannot develop into a normal individual. There are examples in which nondisjunction is not lethal in humans, although it results in significant developmental abnormalities. Trisomy of chromosome #21 results in Down syndrome, with intellectual disability and abnormal growth. Nondisjunction of the sex chromosomes is also generally not lethal during development. Individuals who have only one X chromosome and no Y, for example, have Turner syndrome, with external female appearance but underdeveloped ovaries and sterility. Individuals with nondisjunction of the sex chromosomes will develop to have male appearance if they have at least one Y, no matter how many X chromosomes are present, and will have female genitalia if only X chromosomes are present. Most will be sterile, however, and many will suffer intellectual disability. [In an individual with Down syndrome, are the defects in development caused by an absence of genetic information?[16] If not, why does trisomy of this chromosome or other chromosomes have such dramatic effects?[17]]

7.3 MENDELIAN GENETICS

Gregor Mendel described the statistical behavior of the inheritance of traits in pea plants long before the nature of DNA and chromosomes was known. Unlike Mendel, however, we are now familiar with the molecular basis of genetics in meiosis and genes, and the laws of genetics that Mendel formulated can now be presented with insight based on this knowledge. Although Mendelian genetics generally only involves the simplest patterns of inheritance, it forms the foundation for understanding more complicated situations.

Mendel observed that traits were governed by pairs of hereditary material (alleles). The first of Mendel's laws, the **law of segregation**, states that the two alleles of an individual are separated and passed on to the next generation singly. [At what stage during meiosis are different alleles of a gene separated?[18]] Mendel's second law, the **law of independent assortment**, states that the alleles of one gene will separate into gametes independently of alleles for another gene. We will illustrate these principles using the garden pea plant, but the principles apply equally well to humans.

A trait that can be studied in the pea plant is the color of the pea. We can call *G* the allele for green color, while *g* is the allele for yellow pea color. Mating between plants, a **cross**, is used as a tool in genetics to discern genotypes by looking at the phenotypes of progeny from a cross. A **pure-breeding strain** of yellow or green peas consistently yields progeny of the same color when mated within the strain. For example, if mating yellow plants with yellow plants always produces yellow progeny, yellow is a pure-breeding

---

16 There is no information missing in a person with trisomy. All of the chromosomes are present, and there is no reason to believe that any of the genes on these chromosomes are deleted or mutated to render them inactive.

17 The problem with trisomy appears not to be that genetic information is missing, but that there is *too much* present. A mechanism involved might be gene dosage. Genes are regulated to produce the right amount of each gene product. In trisomy, many genes are present in one more copy than usual, resulting in greater quantities of the gene products encoded on this chromosome. The extra quantities of so many gene products, even if they are normal in sequence, can have dramatic consequences.

18 During meiosis I, at the time when homologous chromosomes separate.

strain. [Can anything be deduced about the genotype of the pure-breeding strain of yellow peas?[19] If a pure-breeding yellow and pure-breeding green strain are crossed, and all of the progeny are green, what does this indicate about the expression of the yellow and green alleles?[20]] Let's assume that G is the dominant allele of the color gene, and g is the recessive allele. [Is it possible to deduce the genotype of a pea plant at the color gene if it is green?[21]] If a green plant is encountered, a **testcross** can be performed to deduce the genotype of the plant. A testcross is when one individual is crossed to another individual that has a homozygous (or pure-breeding) recessive genotype. The presence of all recessive alleles in one parent allows alleles from the other parent to be displayed phenotypically. The progeny of a testcross are called the F_1 **generation**. [If a green plant is testcrossed with a pure-breeding yellow strain, and some of the F_1 generation are yellow while others are green, what is the genotype of the original green plant?[22]] The results of a testcross are dependent on statistics and follow Mendel's laws.

The principle of segregation can be illustrated with the color gene described above for the pea. If a pea is heterozygous Gg, its gametes will contain either the G allele or the g allele, but never both. [If a gamete contained both G and g, what occurred during meiosis?[23]] The probability that a gamete in the heterozygote will contain one allele or the other is 50%, completely random. [Would the principle of segregation apply to a gene on the X chromosome in a woman?[24]] To illustrate the law of independent assortment, we need to introduce a second gene, one that controls the shape of the pea. W is the dominant allele, resulting in wrinkled peas, while w is the recessive allele, resulting in smooth peas in homozygous ww plants. According to the law of independent assortment, the genes for the color of peas and the shape of peas are passed from one generation to another independently. [If the color gene and the shape gene are right next to each other on a chromosome, will they display independent assortment?[25]] The nature of the shape gene in a given gamete does not depend on and is not influenced by the color gene, if independent assortment is true. [If an individual is heterozygous at the color gene, Gg, and heterozygous at the shape gene, Ww, what are the chances that a gamete containing the G allele will also contain the W allele?[26]]

The Punnett Square

It is possible to predict the results of a cross between two individuals using the laws of segregation and independent assortment. Determining the result can be complex, however, so a visual tool called the **Punnett square** is often employed to make the process simpler. Let's use a simple square first, with only one trait involved (Figure 11); we will then tackle a more complicated problem with two different traits (Figure 12, page 246).

---

[19] If a strain always produces the same trait when mated with itself, it is likely to be homozygous for the trait. The pure-breeding yellow pea is homozygous for the yellow allele g of the color gene.

[20] The two strains were both pure-breeding and could only produce gametes containing one type of allele. All of the progeny would be the Gg genotype. If all progeny are green, then the green allele is dominant and the yellow allele is recessive.

[21] No. A green plant could either be heterozygous Gg or homozygous GG.

[22] The original pea is heterozygous Gg.

[23] The gamete must be the result of nondisjunction.

[24] Yes. The principles are the same for human genes as for pea genes, as long as an organism is diploid and goes through sexual reproduction.

[25] No, they would not. They would display an important exception to independent assortment, linkage, which is discussed later.

[26] According to independent assortment, the segregation of one gene does not depend on segregation of another. The chances of a gamete containing the W allele are 50%, regardless of the identity of the color allele.

Possible gametes: Male (*Gg*)

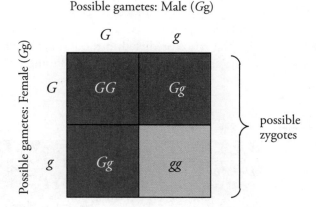

Figure 11   A Punnett Square Involving One Gene

In Figure 11, a Punnett square depicts a cross between two pea plants that are heterozygous for the color gene, with *G* the dominant green allele and *g* the recessive yellow allele. To draw a Punnett square, the following steps are involved:

Step 1: Determine the gametes that are possible from each parent in the cross.
Step 2: Draw a square with the possible gametes from each parent on two sides.
Step 3: Fill in the square with the zygote genotypes that would result from each possible combination of gamete.
Step 4: Determine the phenotype of each genotype.
Step 5: Find the probability of each genotype and each phenotype.

- In the situation shown in Figure 11, which one of the following will be true?[27]
  A) 25% of the offspring will be green, and 75% will be yellow.
  B) 50% of the offspring will be green, and 50% will be yellow.
  C) 75% of the offspring will be green, and 25% will be yellow.
  D) 100% of the offspring will be green.

A more complicated Punnett square is needed to look at two traits during a cross. In Figure 12, a cross is performed between Plant 1, heterozygous at the color gene (*Gg*), and Plant 2, also heterozygous at the color gene. Plant 1 is also homozygous for the dominant allele of the shape gene (wrinkled peas) while Plant 2 is homozygous for the recessive allele (smooth). [What are the phenotypes of the plants being crossed?[28]] The same steps are followed to construct the Punnett square in Figure 12 as the one in Figure 11. First, determine the possible gametes for each pea plant being crossed. (In this case, there are really two possible gamete types from each parent, so the box could be simplified to have only two gametes on a side). Then, determine the possible combinations of gametes that could join to form zygotes and the phenotypes and frequencies of the F$_1$ generation. [What percentage of the F$_1$ generation will have smooth

---

[27] If *G* (green allele) is dominant, then both *GG* homozygotes and *Gg* heterozygotes will be green, while only *gg* homozygotes will be yellow. 25% of the offspring in Figure 11 will be *GG* homozygotes, and 50% will be *Gg* heterozygotes, so a total of 75% of the offspring will be green (choice **C**).

[28] Plant 1 has green wrinkled peas, while Plant 2 has green smooth peas.

peas?[29] What percentage of peas will be green and wrinkled?[30] Yellow and wrinkled?[31] The cross depicted in Figure 12 was performed and produced 77 green wrinkled plants and 20 yellow wrinkled plants; why do these results not agree exactly with the ratios predicted in the Punnett square?[32]] Independent assortment and the principle of segregation are assumptions built into this Punnett square.

Plant 1: *GgWW*

Gametes	*GW*	*GW*	*gW*	*gW*
Gw	*GGWw*	*GGWw*	*GgWw*	*GgWw*
Gw	*GGWw*	*GGWw*	*GgWw*	*GgWw*
gw	*GgWw*	*GgWw*	*ggWw*	*ggWw*
gw	*GgWw*	*GgWw*	*ggWw*	*ggWw*

Plant 2: *Ggww*

Figure 12   A Punnett Square Depicting a Cross with Two Traits Involved

- In the cross depicted in Figure 12, how does the shape gene affect inheritance of the alleles for the color gene?[33]
    A) The percentage of green peas is increased by the shape gene.
    B) The shape has no effect on the inheritance of the alleles for the color gene.
    C) The percentage of green peas is decreased by the shape gene.
    D) The shape gene prevents segregation of the alleles for the color gene.

---

[29] All peas receive one *w* allele and one *W* allele, so all are wrinkled *Ww* heterozygotes (i.e., 0% are smooth).

[30] All F_1 peas are wrinkled and 75% are green, so 75% are green and wrinkled.

[31] All F_1 peas are wrinkled and 25% are yellow, so 25% are yellow and wrinkled.

[32] The results obtained in reality rarely agree exactly with the predicted result. If the results differ slightly from the prediction, the most likely explanation is statistical variability. The more progeny from the cross, the closer the result should be to the prediction.

[33] Independent assortment and the principle of segregation are inherent in the Punnett square. There is no reason to believe that these are not followed, making choice **B** the best response. Choices A, C, and D all assume that either independent assortment or segregation did not occur.

- If a green wrinkled plant from the F_1 generation in Figure 12 is crossed with a pure-breeding yellow smooth pea plant, what phenotypes are possible?[34]
- If any yellow smooth progeny are observed in this testcross, what does this indicate about the genotype of the F_1 plant?[35]

The Rules of Probability

Punnett squares are only one way to determine the probability of an outcome in a cross. Another way involves using statistical rules called the *rule of multiplication* and the *rule of addition*. The **rule of multiplication** states that the probability of both of two independent events happening can be found by multiplying the odds of either event alone. For example, if the probability of being struck by lightning is 1 in a million (10^{-6}) and the probability of winning the lottery is 10^{-7}, then the probability of both happening is the product: $10^{-6} \times 10^{-7} = 10^{-13}$.

The **rule of addition** can be used to calculate the chances of *either* of two events happening. The chance of either A or B happening is equal to the probability of A added to the probability of B, minus the probability of A and B occurring together. For example, the chance of either getting hit by lightning *or* winning the lottery is $10^{-6} + 10^{-7} = 1.1 \times 10^{-6}$. (*Note:* The product of 10^{-6} and 10^{-7} is so small that it can be neglected from the equation.) These rules can be a shortcut to using a Punnett square in some problems.

- A man that is homozygous for eye color, *bb*, is married to a woman who is heterozygous at the same gene: *Bb*. What are the chances that a child will have the *Bb* genotype and be a boy?[36]

Other Biostatistical Methods

Biologists use many other statistical methods in genetics, and many other areas. The chi-square test is used to compare observed and expected data, and *t*-tests are used to compare two data sets. Data is often summarized using mean, median and mode. Finally, standard deviation and standard error give an indication of how spread out a dataset is. Each of these is reviewed in an appendix of our *MCAT Physics and Math Review* book.

---

[34] There are two different genotypes possible for the green wrinkled phenotype in the F_1 generation: *GGWw* or *GgWw*. The best way to determine all possible phenotypes in the cross is to draw a Punnett square for both of these potential genotypes:

If the F_1 plant is *GGWw*:

	GW	GW	Gw	Gw
gw	GgWw	GgWw	Ggww	Ggww

Two genotypes are produced in equal ratios:
50% *GgWw* = green wrinkled phenotype
50% *Ggww* = green smooth

If the F_1 plant is *GgWw*:

	GW	Gw	gW	gw
gw	GgWw	Ggww	ggWw	ggww

Four genotypes are produced:
25% *GgWw* = green wrinkled phenotype
25% *Ggww* = green smooth
25% *ggWw* = yellow wrinkled
25% *ggww* = yellow smooth

[35] If yellow smooth progeny are observed, the F_1 plant must be *GgWw*.

[36] Without drawing a Punnett square, it is possible to see that all children must receive at least one *b* allele (from the father), and that 50% of the children will receive the *B* allele from the mother; thus, 50% of the children will be *Bb*. The odds of a boy are 50%. Therefore, the odds a child is both a boy and has the *Bb* genotype are, by the rule of multiplication, $0.5 \times 0.5 = 0.25$, or 25%.

7.4 EXTENDING MENDELIAN GENETICS

Mendel first started his work using mice, but abandoned rodents (either because of the mess involved, or because of the questionable ethics of a monk studying breeding schemes). In picking pea plants instead, he made a fortuitous decision. The traits he chose to study are (for the most part) controlled by a single gene with two alleles each. These two alleles have one completely dominant to the other, and therefore a simple relationship between genotype and phenotype. Although Mendel's peas all displayed very simple patterns of inheritance, the inheritance of traits is often more complicated.

Incomplete Dominance

Some alleles of genes display neither dominant nor recessive patterns of expression. If the phenotype of a heterozygote is a blended mix of both alleles, this is called **incomplete dominance**, and the alleles for that trait are given different, upper-case letters. For example, if a gene for flower color has two incompletely dominant alleles, R could be used to indicate the allele for red color and W to indicate the allele for white color. [If a gene for flower color has two alleles, R (red) and r (white), and R is dominant while r is recessive, what is the phenotype of Rr heterozygotes?[37] If R and W display incomplete dominance, what is the phenotype of RW heterozygotes?[38] How many phenotypes are possible if R and W display incomplete dominance?[39]]

Codominance

Codominance is a slightly different situation, in which two alleles are both expressed but are not blended. For example, the alleles of the gene for ABO blood group antigens that are found on the surface of red blood cells display codominance. Each of the alleles is expressed on red blood cells, regardless of the second allele in the cell. There are three alleles for the ABO blood group antigens: I^A, I^B, and i. The alleles I^A and I^B are codominant and will be expressed regardless of the second allele, while i is recessive to both I^A and I^B. The alleles I^A and I^B cause type A or type B antigens to be expressed, while i does not cause antigen expression.

- What is the phenotype of an individual heterozygous for the I^A and I^B alleles?[40]
- What is the phenotype of an individual heterozygous for I^B and i?[41]
- If a woman heterozygous for type A blood marries a man who is heterozygous for type B blood, what are the possible genotypes (and blood types) of their children?[42]

---

[37] Rr heterozygotes will have the phenotype of the dominant allele: red.

[38] In this case, RW heterozygotes will be neither red nor white, but a blend of the two: pink.

[39] Three phenotypes and three genotypes: RR (red), RW (pink), and WW (white).

[40] The red blood cells will express both type A and type B antigens, so the blood type will be AB.

[41] The red blood cells will express type B antigen only, and the blood type will be B.

[42] Because they are both heterozygous, the woman's genotype is $I^A i$ and the man's genotype is $I^B i$. Thus, their children could be $I^A I^B$ (type AB), $I^A i$ (type A), $I^B i$ (type B), or ii (type O).

The other main antigen used in blood typing is the Rh (rhesus) factor. The expression of this antigen follows a classically dominant pattern; Rh^DRh^D and Rh^DRh^d (also seen as *RR* and *Rr*) genotypes lead to the expression of this protein on the surface of the red cell (Rh positive), and the Rh^dRh^d (or *rr*) genotype leads to the absence of the protein (Rh negative).

Although Mendel's peas all displayed very simple patterns of inheritance, there are often many complications in the inheritance of traits. For example:

Pleiotropism: A gene is said to have pleiotropic effects if its expression alters many different, seemingly unrelated aspects of the organism's total phenotype. For example, a mutation in a gene may cause altered development of heart, bone, and inner ears.

Polygenism: Complex traits that are influenced by many different genes are called polygenic. These traits tend to display a range of phenotypes in a continuous distribution. For example, height is polygenic and is influenced by genes for growth factors, receptors, hormones, bone deposition, muscle development, energy utilization, and so on. As a consequence, there is a wide range of normal heights for adult humans; we are not just "tall" and "short," like Mendel's peas. Skin color and mouse fur color are additional examples of mammalian polygenic traits.

Penetrance: Penetrance describes the likelihood that a person with a given genotype will express the expected phenotype. While many traits are completely penetrant (all individuals with a given allele or mutation display the phenotype), there is a spectrum of options: alleles or mutations can also have high, incomplete, or low penetrance. The root cause of penetrance depends on the allele. Some have age-related penetrance, where the phenotype is displayed more frequently in mutation-carrying individuals as they age. The penetrance of other alleles depends on environmental and lifestyle modifiers. For example, women who carry a certain mutation that increases their risk of breast cancer display variable rates of breast cancer, depending on their diet, if they smoke, if they have had children and breast fed, etc. Finally, many alleles have genetic modifiers that affect penetrance; since several human traits are polygenic, alleles at different loci can affect penetrance.

Epistasis: This refers to a situation where expression of alleles for one gene is dependent on a different gene. For example, a gene for curly hair cannot be expressed if a different gene causes baldness.

Recessive Lethal Alleles: Some mutant alleles can cause death of an organism when present in a homozygous manner. These are called **recessive lethal alleles**, and they typically code for essential gene products. In diploid organisms, these alleles can be studied by maintaining heterozygous stocks, which are then mated together to form a homozygous recessive offspring. Embryonic development studies can shed light on when this organism dies and possibly why. Studying recessive lethal alleles in haploid organisms is much harder. Here, a conditional system is usually used where the allele is normal (or permissive) under certain conditions, allowing survival of the organism. The mutant allele can be induced under different conditions (such as a different temperature), to study effects of the allele.

- 100 people are homozygous for an allele that is implicated in cancer, but only 20 develop cancer. What are potential explanations for why only some people express a gene out of a broader population with the same genotype?[43]
- In one strain of mouse, homozygotes for an allele of a gene develop heart defects, while in another strain of mouse, homozygotes with the same allele develop normally. Heterozygotes develop normally in both strains. What is the most likely explanation for the difference between the two strains?[44]
    - A) The allele is recessive.
    - B) The development of the heart defect is influenced by more than one locus.
    - C) The allele has pleiotropic effects on development.
    - D) The allele is codominant.

The Sex Chromosomes

Early in the twentieth century it was observed that women have 23 pairs of chromosomes that are homologous, while men have only 22 pairs of chromosomes that match in appearance. The two chromosomes in men that did not match each other were termed the **X** and the **Y chromosomes** because of their appearance during mitosis (Figure 13). Males have an X and a Y, while females have two X chromosomes. The presence of a Y chromosome in humans (genotype XY) is a key factor in the determination of the gender of an embryo, and subsequent development into a male. The absence of a Y (genotype XX) results in a female as the default developmental pathway. During meiosis, females generate gametes that contain an X chromosome; males generate gametes with either an X or a Y chromosome, meaning that it is the *male* gamete that determines the sex of an embryo (Figure 14).

This is an X chromosome during interphase. (Note that it doesn't look like an "X" at all.)

This is a condensed X chromosome after S phase (replication). The X is formed by the two sister chromatids.

This is a Y chromosome after S phase.

Figure 13 The Sex Chromosomes

[43] The trait of cancer development is probably polygenic, so it does not display simple patterns of inheritance. Cancer development is also influenced by the environment, such as exposure to carcinogens, further complicating the penetrance of the genotype.

[44] The key variable must not lie within the allele itself, since this remains the same (so choices A and D are wrong). The genetic background of the two different strains of mice must affect whether or not the heart defect phenotype is expressed. Further, only one defect is observed (so it can't be pleiotropic; choice C is wrong). Therefore, the heart defect phenotype must be influenced by some other locus that is different in the two strains of mice, making choice **B** the best answer.

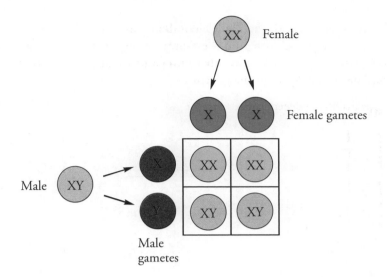

Figure 14   Determination of the Zygote's Sexual Genotype

The sex chromosomes also play a key role in the inheritance of other traits that are not directly involved in sexual development. Much of what has been discussed about inheritance was dependent on the assumption that there are two copies of every chromosome and therefore two copies of every gene in each cell. This is true for genes found on every pair of chromosomes except for one pair: the sex chromosomes. Genes that lie on the X chromosome will be present in two copies in females but only in one copy in males. [What pattern of expression will a recessive allele on the X chromosome display in males?[45]] Traits that are determined by genes on the X or Y chromosome are called **sex-linked traits** because of their unique patterns of expression and inheritance. The inheritance of traits coded by genes on sex chromosomes will be covered in Section 7.6.

7.5   LINKAGE

The traits that Mendel studied and based the law of independent assortment on were located on separate chromosomes. Genes that are located on the *same* chromosome may not display independent assortment, however. The failure of genes to display independent assortment is called **linkage**.

- If eye color is controlled by a gene on chromosome #11 and the hair color locus is located on chromosome #14, do these genes assort independently?[46]
- If the portion of chromosome #14 containing the hair color gene is translocated onto chromosome #11, will these genes still assort independently?[47]

If genes are located very close to each other on the same chromosome, then they will probably *not* be inherited independently of each other. Let's illustrate this with a pea gene for height and two alleles of the

---

[45]   In males, recessive alleles on the X chromosome are always expressed, since no other allele is present that can mask the recessive allele.

[46]   Yes, they will. Assortment of nonhomologous chromosomes into gametes is random during meiosis.

[47]   A translocation occurs when a piece of one chromosome is moved onto another chromosome. The two genes are then found on the same chromosome and may not assort independently.

height gene, tall (*T*) and short (*t*), with the *T* allele dominant and the *t* allele recessive. If the height gene and the color gene are very near each other on the same chromosome, then the alleles of these genes on a specific chromosome will probably assort together into gametes during meiosis (Figure 15). This limits the possible combinations of the alleles in the gametes.

Figure 15   Linkage of Alleles during Meiosis

- If the color gene and the height gene display linkage, is it possible to predict the possible gametes of a *TTgg* individual?[48] Of a *TtGg* individual?[49]

To know how alleles that display linkage assort during meiosis, it may be necessary to know which alleles were on a chromosome together. As seen in Figure 15, there are two possible ways the height and color genes could be linked. The dominant alleles of two different genes can be linked together on the same chromosome (*TG*), the recessive alleles of two different genes can be linked (*tg*), or one dominant and one recessive allele can be linked (*Tg* and *tG*).

With genes that are found on the same chromosome, the design of a Punnett square is slightly different. The possible gametes are limited since they cannot assort independently. Consider a cross between a homozygous *ttgg* pea plant and a double-heterozygous plant with both dominant alleles on one

---

[48] Yes. A *TTgg* individual can only make *Tg* gametes, regardless of whether the genes are on the same chromosome or not.

[49] No. To predict how these traits will assort, it is necessary to know which alleles are present together on the same chromosome.

chromosome and both recessive alleles located together on another chromosome. They can only make a limited number of different gametes, not the four possible combinations of alleles that would be found if the genes were on different chromosomes. A Punnett square will help to illustrate linkage in this example (Figure 16).

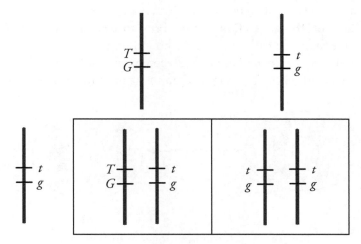

Figure 16   Assortment of Linked Genes

- What are the phenotypes of the F$_1$ progeny in the cross in Figure 16?[50]
- If a tall green pea from the F$_1$ progeny is crossed with a pure-breeding short yellow plant, what phenotypes will be observed and in what ratios?[51]
- If height and color genes were not linked, what ratios of phenotypes would be observed in a cross between a *TtGg* and a *ttgg* individual?[52]
- Assume all of the characteristics already introduced for the height, color, and shape pea genes that have been used as examples. The height and color genes are located near each other on the same chromosome and display complete linkage, but the shape gene is located on a different chromosome. If an individual with a *TtGgWw* genotype and the *T* and *g* alleles on the same chromosome is crossed with a *ttGgWw* individual, what result will be observed?[53]
    - A) All tall peas will be wrinkled.
    - B) All wrinkled peas will be tall.
    - C) All yellow peas will be tall.
    - D) All tall peas will be yellow.

---

[50] There are only two phenotypes: 50% tall green and 50% short yellow.

[51] The pure-breeding short yellow plant can only have *tg* gametes. The tall green plant can make only two types of alleles, the same gametes shown for its parent. The results of the backcross will be the same as for the original cross in Figure 16, with 50% tall green and 50% short yellow plants.

[52] The *ttgg* individual can make only *tg* gametes. The *TtGg* individual can make four different types of gametes if the genes are not linked: *TG*, *Tg*, *tG*, and *tg*. The genotypes and phenotypes of the cross will be 25% *TtGg* (tall green), 25% *Ttgg* (tall yellow), 25% *ttGg* (short green), and 25% *ttgg* (short yellow).

[53] The gene for shape (wrinkled versus smooth) is on a different chromosome than the other two genes, so there is no correlation between the wrinkled trait and the other traits (eliminating choices A and B). To be yellow, a pea must be homozygous *gg*. One of the *g* alleles must come from the chromosome with *T* and *g* together, making all yellow plants tall (choice **C** is correct). Some of the *Tg* gametes will join with *tG* gametes from the *ttGg* individual, meaning that some plants are tall and green (choice D is wrong). Drawing a Punnett Square can help to solve this problem.

Linkage and Recombination

Linkage is the exception to the law of independent assortment. When genes are located on the same chromosome, they will display linkage and will not assort independently. Meiotic recombination provides the exception to linkage. During the formation of gametes, meiotic recombination between homologous chromosomes can separate alleles that were located on the same chromosome. In the example in Figure 17, three genes are located on the same chromosome. Prior to recombination, *ABC* were found on one chromosome and *abc* were found on the homologous chromosome. [What combinations of alleles will be found in gametes in the absence of recombination?[54]] Recombination produces new combinations of alleles not found in the parent and also allows genes located on the same chromosome to assort independently.

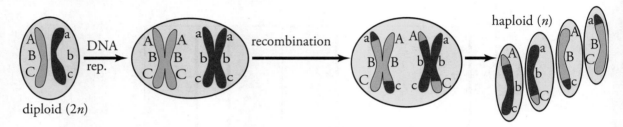

Figure 17   Recombination—Another Look

The example of the height and color genes in pea plants will help to illustrate linkage and the effects of recombination on patterns of inheritance. As before, the height and color genes are located on the same chromosome. There are two alleles of the height gene, dominant *T* (tall) and recessive *t* (short) and two alleles of the color gene, dominant *G* (green) and recessive *g* (yellow). The following cross is performed: a pure-breeding tall green plant is crossed with a pure-breeding short yellow plant. [What phenotypes are predicted in this cross if linkage is complete?[55]] A pea plant from this cross is then self-pollinated (crossed with itself) to produce an F_2 generation. [If linkage is complete, what genotypes and phenotypes will be observed in the F_2 generation?[56] If the genes assort completely randomly, what genotypes and phenotypes will be observed in the F_2 generation?[57]] The F_2 generation in this cross was observed to have the following plants: 30 tall green plants, 9 short yellow plants, 2 tall yellow plants, and 1 short green plant. [Which of these phenotypes are recombinant phenotypes?[58]] Often in a cross involving genes on the same chromosome, the result will be intermediate between independent assortment and complete linkage. The reason for this is that recombination occurs between the genes during meiosis of *some* of the gametes but not *all* of the gametes. [If it is known that two genes are located on the same chromosome but during a cross they assort completely randomly, how can this be?[59]]

---

[54] *ABC* or *abc* genotypes

[55] Only one phenotype. The F_1 generation will all receive a *TG* chromosome from the pure-breeding tall green parent and a *tg* chromosome from the pure-breeding short yellow parent.

[56] 75% tall green and 25% short yellow. Try a Punnett square to verify this result, remembering to assort alleles together into gametes.

[57] 9:3:3:1 of tall green, tall yellow, short green, and short yellow, respectively. This is a classical Mendelian ratio observed when heterozygotes at two alleles are crossed.

[58] The tall yellow and short green phenotypes would not be observed if linkage was complete (as in #56). The only way to produce these phenotypes is if a small number of gametes received chromosomes in which the *TG* and *tg* alleles were separated from each other by recombination, so these are the recombinant phenotypes.

[59] If the genes are on the same chromosome, but are far apart from one another, then recombination occurs frequently. The genes will assort randomly during meiosis and will not display any linkage even though they are on the same chromosome.

The frequency of recombination between two genes on a chromosome is proportional to the physical distance between the genes along the linear length of the DNA molecule. [Does recombination occur between genes more frequently if they are near each other or far apart?[60]] The farther apart two genes are on a chromosome, the more likely recombination will occur between the genes during meiosis. If the genes are located far enough apart, recombination will occur so frequently between the genes that they will no longer display linkage and will assort as independently as if they were on separate chromosomes. The **frequency of recombination** is given as the *number of recombinant phenotypes* resulting from a cross *divided by the total number of progeny.*

$$RF = \text{recombination frequency} = \frac{\text{number of recombinants}}{\text{total number of offspring}}$$

Since the frequency of recombination is proportional to the physical distance of genes from each other, it can be used as a tool to map genes in relation to each other on chromosomes.

Example: The height and color gene in pea plants are on the same chromosome as a third gene for big or small flowers. The alleles of flower size are a dominant B (big) and a recessive b (small). The color gene (G, green or g, yellow) is studied in relation to the flower size gene. In the first cross, pure-breeding homozygous $BBGG$ plants are crossed with $bbgg$ plants. [What is the phenotype of the F_1 progeny?[61] If a small flower green plant is observed in the F_1 generation, was recombination responsible?[62]] An F_1 progeny is then crossed with a $bbgg$ plant and the following phenotypes observed: 44 big flower green plants, 40 small flower yellow plants, 8 big flower yellow plants, and 8 small flower green plants.

- Which of these are recombinant phenotypes?[63]
- What is the frequency of recombination between the genes?[64]
- What is the maximal frequency of recombination?[65]
- In another cross, the frequency of recombination between the flower size and height genes is examined and found to be 10 recombinant plants out of 100 progeny. Is the height gene or the color gene closer to the flower size gene?[66]
- If the recombination frequencies are 0.16 between the height and color genes, 0.10 between the height and flower size genes, and 0.26 between the flower size and color genes, what is the order of the genes on the chromosome?[67]

---

[60] The farther two genes are away from each other, the greater the odds that recombination will occur between them.

[61] The F_1 progeny are all $BbGg$ genotype and therefore are big flower green plants.

[62] The small flower green phenotype could not be produced by recombination. These alleles do not exist together in either parent and so could not be recombined together in the gametes. This must be the result of mutation.

[63] Big flower yellow plants and small flower green plants can only be produced through recombination between the flower size and color genes.

[64] The frequency of recombination is 16 recombinant phenotypes out of 100 progeny = 16%.

[65] The maximal frequency of recombination would be when there was no linkage and the genes assorted independently. In this case, there would be 25% big flower yellow plants and 25% small flower green plants, or 50% maximal frequency of recombination.

[66] There is less recombination between the height and flower size genes (10% frequency) than between the color and flower size genes (16%), so the height gene is closer to the flower size gene than the color gene is.

[67] The flower size and color genes have the most recombination between them, so they must be farthest apart, with the height gene in the middle.

- Is it possible to map the distance between genes on the same chromosome even if they are so far apart that they assort independently?[68]
- Assume that hair color in humans is determined by a gene for which there are two alleles: *B* or brown, which is dominant, and *b* or blond, which is recessive. The hair color gene is located on the same chromosome as another gene that determines the strength of bones, and the two genes are very close together. The alleles of the bone strength gene are *S*, the dominant sturdy bone allele, and *s*, the recessive fragile bone allele. Jose and Tonya have dark hair and sturdy bones. One of their children has brown hair and fragile bones. One grandparent of Jose and one grandparent of Tonya had fragile bones and blond hair, while the remaining grandparents were homozygous for brown hair and sturdy bones. Which of the following is/are true?[69]

    I.   The child of Jose and Tonya represents a recombinant phenotype.

    II. All of the children of Jose and Tonya must have fragile bones.

    III. Jose and Tonya may have other children with blond hair and fragile bones.

    A) I only
    B) II only
    C) I and III only
    D) II and III only

7.6 INHERITANCE PATTERNS

There are six inheritance patterns that you should be familiar with: autosomal recessive, autosomal dominant, mitochondrial, Y-linked, X-linked recessive, and X-linked dominant. In this section, each will be described and then a summary table will be presented.

Autosomal traits are caused by genetic variation on the autosomes (the 22 pairs of non-sex chromosomes in humans). These traits can be **autosomal dominant** (in which case a single copy of the allele will confer the trait or disease phenotype) or **autosomal recessive** (in which case two copies of the allele are required for the affected phenotype). Both tend to affect males and females equally; in other words, there is no sex bias for these traits.

There is a small, haploid DNA genome inside the mitochondria and humans inherit this genome from their mothers. This is because the sperm contributes only nuclear chromosomes to the zygote; the ovum contributes nuclear chromosomes and the rest of the cellular material including the organelles. There are some traits that are inherited via the mitochondrial genome, although these **mitochondrial traits** are rare. Luckily, they are fairly easy to spot because affected females have all affected offspring (sons and daughters). Affected individuals must have an affected mother, and affected males cannot have any

---

[68] Yes, but it requires one or more genes located between the two genes. The distance between the two genes could not be mapped directly by measuring the frequency of recombination between them, but if the distance from both of them to a gene in the middle can be mapped, then the overall distance between the genes can be mapped. Whole chromosomes can be mapped this way.

[69] **Item I is true:** the simplest explanation is that the grandparent on each side passed on the fragile allele and the blond allele, but recombination occurred, so that the fragile and blond alleles assorted independently. Item II is false: Jose and Tonya both have the dominant sturdy bone gene in at least one copy, so some children are likely to have sturdy bones. **Item III is true:** both Jose and Tonya may have one chromosome with the blond allele and the fragile bone allele linked. If so, a nonrecombinant phenotype would be blond/fragile. The answer is choice **C**.

affected offspring. An individual cannot inherit mitochondrial traits from their father. Mitochondrial traits (like Y-linked traits and X-linked traits in human males) are an example of **hemizygosity**; the individual only has one copy of the chromosome in a diploid organism. Because of this, there is only one allele to keep track of for each individual. Genes encoded by the mitochondrial genome are usually given the prefix **mt** (for example, mt-*Atp6* is encoded in the mitochondrial genome and codes for a subunit of the ATP synthase). When working with inheritance patterns though, it is best to define the allele letters you are going to use and then use one letter per individual. For example, you could assign "*a*" as a normal individual and "*A*" as an affected individual. The assignment here is arbitrary since one allele is not dominant to the other (they are mutually exclusive since humans only have one mitochondrial genome). The key is to be consistent.

Traits that are determined by genes located on the X or Y chromosome are called **sex-linked traits** and display unusual patterns of inheritance. Traits encoded by genes on the Y chromosome (Y-linked traits) would only be passed from male parents to male children. [Would it be possible for a father to pass a Y-linked trait to female children?[70] Can males be carriers of recessive Y-linked traits without expressing them?[71]] Y-linked traits are quite rare, because the Y chromosome is small and contains a relatively small number of genes. Many of the genes on the Y-chromosome function in sex determination.

X-linked traits are observed quite frequently and can be X-linked recessive or X-linked dominant. There are several well-studied examples of X-linked recessive traits that are common in the human population; hemophilia is an example. Women are often carriers of X-linked recessive alleles but will only express recessive X-linked traits when they are homozygous. Men are hemizygous for X-linked traits; they have only one copy of genes on the X chromosome. As a result, males *always* express recessive X-linked alleles. [From which parent do males receive X-linked traits?[72]] These traits tend to affect males more than females.

Red-green colorblindness, an X-linked trait, is caused by a defect in a visual pigment gene on the X chromosome. The allele that is responsible for colorblindness is a pigment gene that does not produce functional protein. [Is the colorblindness allele recessive or dominant?[73]] The colorblindness allele, like many recessive traits carried in the population, is not expressed in heterozygotes. Colorblindness is unusual in women but fairly common in men. Females have two copies of the gene, so will not express the trait if they are heterozygotes, while males have only one X chromosome and so will always express the allele whenever they receive it. [A man is colorblind, and his wife is homozygous normal for genes encoding visual pigment proteins. What will be the phenotypes and genotypes of sons and of daughters of this couple?[74]]

X-linked dominant traits are harder to identify. A female will display an X-linked dominant phenotype if she has one or two copies of the allele on her X chromosomes. A male will express the phenotype if

---

[70] No. Females never have a Y chromosome and so can never carry or express a Y-linked trait.

[71] No. Y-linked traits are carried in only one copy, since there is only one Y chromosome per cell. If a male carries a recessive Y-linked trait, he will express it.

[72] Since males receive their X chromosome from their mother (and their Y chromosome from their father), they receive X-linked traits from their mother.

[73] An allele that encodes inactive protein or no protein is generally recessive, since the gene's function can be compensated for by the remaining normal copy of the gene.

[74] Sons will have a normal phenotype and carry one copy of the normal gene. Daughters will carry one normal gene and one recessive colorblindness allele and will have the normal phenotype.

7.6

he inherited the affected allele from his mother. While these traits still tend to affect males more than females, this trend is less obvious than for X-linked recessive traits.

Table 1 summarizes the six inheritance patterns you should be familiar with, and lists some strategies you can use to distinguish between them.

Inheritance Pattern	Identification Techniques	Unaffected Genotypes	Affected Genotypes
Autosomal recessive	• Can skip generations (affected individuals can have unaffected parents) • Number of affected males is usually equal to the number of affected females	AA Aa	aa
Autosomal dominant	• Does not skip generations (affected individuals must have an affected parent) • Number of affected males is usually equal to number of affected females • An affected parent passes the trait to either all or half of offspring	aa	AA Aa
Mitochondrial	• Maternal inheritance • Affected female has all affected children • Affected male cannot pass the trait onto his children • Unaffected female cannot have affected children	a	A
Y-linked	• Affects male only; females never have the trait • Affected father has all affected sons • Unaffected father cannot have an affected son	XY^a	XY^A
X-linked recessive	• Can skip generations (affected individuals can have unaffected parents) • Tend to affect males more than females • Unaffected females can have affected sons • Affected female has all affected sons, but can have both affected and unaffected daughters	$X^A X^A$ $X^A X^a$ $X^A Y$	$X^a X^a$ $X^a Y$
X-linked dominant	• Hardest to identify • Does not skip generations (affected individuals must have an affected parent) • Usually affects males more than females • Affected fathers have all affected daughters • Affected mothers can have unaffected sons (and unaffected daughters), and pass the trait equally to sons and daughters	$X^a X^a$ $X^a Y$	$X^A X^A$ $X^A X^a$ $X^A Y$

Table 1 Summary of Inheritance Patterns

7.6

- Two mouse genes located on the X chromosome are being studied. The alleles of the genes are:

Fuzzy hair: *F*, dominant (normal hair) and *f*, recessive (fuzzy hair)

Extra toes: *E*, dominant (extra toes), and *e*, recessive (normal toes)

A female with normal hair and extra toes is crossed with a male with normal hair and extra toes. The progeny have the following phenotypes:

Phenotype	Male	Female
Normal hair, extra toes	46	100
Normal hair, normal toes	4	0
Fuzzy hair, extra toes	5	0
Fuzzy hair, normal toes	45	0

Which one of the following is true concerning this experiment?[75]

- A) Males have a higher rate of recombination than females do.
- B) In the absence of recombination, all males would have normal hair and extra toes.
- C) The rate of recombination on the X chromosome is the same in males and females.
- D) Both males and females have recombinant genotypes, but only males have recombinant phenotypes.

7.7 POPULATION GENETICS

Mendelian genetics describes the inheritance of traits in the progeny of specific individuals. For the purposes of large topics such as natural selection and evolution, however, the more relevant issue is not the inheritance of traits from individuals but in a whole population from one generation to another. **Population genetics** describes the inheritance of traits in populations over time. The word *population* has a specific meaning in this setting: *a population consists of members of a species that mate and reproduce with each other.* [If a group of sea turtles lives most of the year dispersed over a large area of ocean without contact with one another but congregate once a year to reproduce, is this group a population?[76]] To a population geneticist, each individual is merely a temporary carrier of the alleles in a population.

In population genetics, the units of genetic inheritance are alleles of genes, just as in Mendelian genetics. However, in population genetics alleles are examined across the entire population rather than in individuals. The sum total of all genetic information in a population is called the **gene pool**. [For an autosomal

---

[75] The genotype of the male parent must be X^{FE} Y. The predominance of the normal hair-extra toes and fuzzy hair-normal toes phenotypes in the F$_1$ generation indicates that the female parent must have one X chromosome with both dominant alleles together, and one X chromosome with both recessive alleles together, in other words, her genotype must be X^{FE} X^{fe}. The fuzzy hair-extra toes and normal hair-normal toes phenotypes are much less common and must be the result of recombination in the female parent, producing X^{Fe} and X^{fE} chromosomes. Note that recombination between the X and Y chromosomes in males is not possible due to the fact that the X and Y carry different genes (choices A and C are wrong). If recombination had not occurred in the female parent, all F$_1$ males would have received either X^{FE} or X^{fe}, giving both normal hair-extra toes and fuzzy hair-normal toes phenotypes (choice B is wrong). Choice **D** is the correct answer: the F$_1$ females must also have recombinant genotypes on the X chromosomes they received from their mother, but every F$_1$ female also received both dominant alleles on the X chromosome they received from their father. Thus, only the dominant phenotypes are seen in the F$_1$ females.

[76] Yes. A population does not need to live with one another, only to reproduce sexually with one another.

gene in a population of 2,000 individuals, how many copies of the gene are present in the gene pool?[77]] The frequency of an allele in a population is a key variable used to describe the gene pool. [If there are 5,000 hippos in a population, out of which there are 100 homozygotes of an autosomal allele *h* and 400 heterozygotes, what is the frequency of the *h* allele in the population?[78] If 20% of the population is heterozygous for an allele *Q* and 10% is homozygous, what will be the frequency of the allele in the population?[79]]

Hardy-Weinberg in Population Genetics

Population genetics does not simply describe the gene pool of a population but attempts to predict the gene pool of a population in the future. The **Hardy-Weinberg law** states that the *frequencies of alleles in the gene pool of a population will not change over time*, provided that a number of assumptions are true:

1) There is no mutation.
2) There is no migration.
3) There is no natural selection.
4) There is random mating.
5) The population is sufficiently large to prevent random drift in allele frequencies.

What Hardy-Weinberg means at the molecular level is that segregation of alleles, independent assortment, and recombination during meiosis can alter the combinations of alleles in gametes but cannot increase or decrease the frequency of an allele in the gametes of one individual or the gametes of the population as a whole.

- If 100 homozygous green pea plants and 100 homozygous yellow pea plants are crossed, 1,000 green pea plants are produced. Does this mean that the yellow alleles disappeared from the population?[80]
- What is the frequency of the yellow allele in the gene pool of the progeny?[81]
- If the green peas from the F_1 generation are allowed to mate randomly within the population, and there is no mutation, migration, natural selection, or random drift, what will be the frequency of the yellow allele in the population after four generations?[82]
- If two genes are closely linked on the same chromosome, will Hardy-Weinberg still apply to these genes?[83]

---

[77] There are two copies of the gene in each of the 2,000 individuals, for a total of 4,000 copies in the gene pool.

[78] The allele frequency is the number of copies of a specific allele divided by the total number of copies of the gene in the population. If there are 5,000 hippos, and each has 2 copies of the gene, there are 10,000 copies of the gene in the population. There are 100 homozygotes of the *h* allele, each with 2 copies of it, and 400 heterozygotes with one *h* allele, for a total of 600 *h* alleles in the population. Thus, the frequency of the *h* allele is 600/10,000 = 0.06.

[79] In this case, the number of individuals in the population is not provided, but it is not needed. The total number of alleles is 100%. The frequency of the allele is 0.5 × (20% heterozygotes) + 10% homozygotes = 20%.

[80] The yellow alleles are still there (but in the heterozygous state), so they do not appear in the phenotype.

[81] The frequency of the yellow allele will be 50%, just as it was in the parents. None of the alleles in a population were destroyed, so the frequency is the same as in the parental generation.

[82] According to Hardy-Weinberg, there will be no change in the frequency of the allele. The frequency of the yellow allele will still be 50% after four generations.

[83] Yes. Independent assortment is not a requirement of Hardy-Weinberg. Allele frequencies for the genes will still remain constant, regardless of the extent of recombination between the genes, as long as the assumptions of Hardy-Weinberg hold true.

- According to Hardy-Weinberg, what will happen to the frequency of the yellow allele if predation occurs on yellow plants, but yellow plants attract bees more successfully?[84]

The Hardy-Weinberg law has also been translated into mathematical terms. Assuming that there are two alleles of a gene in a population, the letter p is used to represent the frequency of the dominant allele, and the letter q is used to represent the frequency of the recessive allele. Since there are only two alleles, the following fundamental equation must be true:

$$p + q = 1$$

Based on allele frequency, it is possible to calculate the proportion of genotypes in a population. Take a situation where the frequency of a dominant allele, G, equals p and the frequency of a recessive allele, g, equals q. If the equation above is squared on both sides, it becomes:

$$(p + q)^2 = 1$$

$$p^2 + 2pq + q^2 = 1$$

where

$$p^2 = \text{the frequency of the } GG \text{ genotype}$$

$$2pq = \text{the frequency of the } Gg \text{ genotype}$$

$$q^2 = \text{the frequency of the } gg \text{ genotype}$$

- If the frequency of the G allele is 0.25 in a population of 1,000 mice, determine the number of individuals who are Gg heterozygotes if there is random mating but no migration, mutation, random drift, or natural selection.[85]
- If allele frequencies in a population are constant, and genotype frequencies can be calculated from allele frequencies, how will genotype frequencies vary over time?[86]

After one generation, a population will reach **Hardy-Weinberg equilibrium**, in which allele frequencies no longer change. Since allele frequencies do not change, and genotype frequencies can be calculated from allele frequencies, it follows that genotype frequencies also do not change over time. [If 100 green peas (GG) and 100 yellow peas (gg) are allowed to mate randomly, will the genotype frequencies in the next generation (F_1) be the same?[87] If not, why not?[88] If the plants are allowed to mate randomly for another generation (F_2), will the genotype frequencies in the F_1 and F_2 generations be the same?[89]]

---

[84] Hardy-Weinberg says nothing about this situation. Once the assumptions no longer hold true, Hardy-Weinberg no longer applies.

[85] If the frequency of the G allele (p) is 0.25, then the frequency of the g allele (q) must be 0.75, since $p + q = 1$. The frequency of the heterozygotes in the population will be $2pq = 2(0.25)(0.75) = 0.375$. Therefore, the number of individuals in this population who are heterozygotes will be $0.375 \times 1000 = 375$.

[86] Genotype frequencies as well as allele frequencies will remain constant according to Hardy-Weinberg.

[87] No. The next generation will include GG, Gg, and gg genotypes.

[88] The population was not at Hardy-Weinberg equilibrium to start out.

[89] Yes. A population reaches Hardy-Weinberg equilibrium after one generation. The F_2 generation (and all generations after that) will have the same genotype frequencies as the F_1 generation.

Hardy-Weinberg in the Real World

Hardy-Weinberg requires a number of assumptions in order to be true. The assumptions, as presented earlier, are that in a population there is random mating and no mutation, migration, natural selection, or random drift. Thus, Hardy-Weinberg describes a highly idealized set of conditions required to prevent alleles from being added or removed from a population. In reality, it is not possible for a population to meet all of the conditions required by Hardy-Weinberg.

1) **Mutation**: Mutation is inevitable in a population. Even if there are no chemical mutagens or radiation, inherent errors by DNA polymerase would over time cause mutations and introduce new alleles in a population.

2) **Migration**: If migration occurs, animals leaving or entering the population will carry alleles with them and disturb the Hardy-Weinberg equilibrium.

3) **Natural Selection**: For there to be no natural selection, there would have to be unlimited resources, no predation, no disease, and so on. This is not a set of conditions encountered in the real world.

4) **Non-random Mating**: If individuals pick their mates preferentially based on one or more traits, alleles that cause those traits will be passed on preferentially from one generation to another.

5) **Random Drift**: If a population becomes very small, it cannot contain as great a variety of alleles. In a very small population, random events can alter allele frequencies significantly and have a large influence on future generations.

7.8 EVOLUTION BY NATURAL SELECTION

At one time, life on Earth was generally viewed as static and unchanging, but we now know that this is not the case. Over the geologic span of Earth's history, many species have arisen, changed over millions of years, given rise to new species, and died out. These changes in life on Earth are called **evolution**. Although he did not arrive at his theory alone, Charles Darwin played an important role in shaping modern thought by proposing natural selection as the mechanism that drives evolution. **Natural selection** is an interaction between organisms and their environment that causes differential reproduction of different phenotypes and thereby alters the gene pool of a population. In essence, the theory of evolution by natural selection is this:

1) In a population, there are heritable differences between individuals.
2) Heritable traits (alleles of genes) produce traits (phenotypes) that affect the ability of an organism to survive and have offspring.
3) Some individuals have phenotypes that allow them to survive longer, be healthier, and have more offspring than others.
4) Individuals with phenotypes that allow them to have more offspring will pass on their alleles more frequently than those with phenotypes that have fewer offspring.
5) Over time, those alleles that lead to more offspring are passed on more frequently and become more abundant, while other alleles become less abundant in the gene pool.
6) Changes in allele frequency are the basis of evolution in species and populations.

To put it simply, evolution occurs when natural selection acts on genetic variation to drive changes in the genetic composition of a population. A key term in evolution is **fitness**. In evolutionary terms, fitness is not how well an animal is physically adapted to a niche in the environment, or how well it can feed itself, but how successful it is in passing on its alleles to future generations. The way to have greater fitness is by having more offspring that pass on their alleles to future generations of the population. Some species achieve greater fitness through sheer numbers of progeny produced, who are then left to fend for themselves. Other species have fewer progeny, but protect and nurture the young to maturity.

- If an allele of a gene causes cancer in elderly polar bears after their reproductive years have passed, how will it affect the fitness of bears carrying the allele?[90]
- If a recessive allele causes sterility in homozygotes, how will it affect the fitness of heterozygotes?[91]
- A group of mice are infected with recombinant virus in bone marrow cells that allows the mice to live longer. The mice are then released into a wild population. Will natural selection act to increase the life span of the population?[92]
- Which of the following will have greater fitness: A fish that has two offspring and protects and nurtures its young to maturity, or a fish that has 10 offspring and abandons them, resulting in the death of 8 young fish before maturity?[93]
- The recessive allele that causes cystic fibrosis is strongly selected against in modern society, since individuals with this disease often die before sexual maturity. However, the frequency of the allele takes many generations to decrease in the population. Why?[94]
- A certain genetic disease is caused by a recessive allele. In the absence of effective therapy, homozygous individuals with this allele generally die before reaching sexual maturity. The allele also protects heterozygous individuals against several life-threatening viral diseases. If a medicine is found that provides a complete remedy for the disease, allowing individuals with the disease to live an entirely normal life, which of the following statements describes what will happen to the frequency of the allele in the population after that time?[95]
  - A) The frequency of the allele will decrease.
  - B) The frequency of the allele will remain constant.
  - C) The frequency of the allele will increase.
  - D) It is not possible to predict the future frequency of the allele.

7.8

Sources of Genetic Diversity

Natural selection acts on the genetic diversity in a population to alter allele frequencies, causing evolution. Genetic diversity in a population is a requirement for natural selection to occur. [If a population of sea otters contains only one allele of a gene that protects against cold, can natural selection drive evolution of

---

[90] The allele will not affect fitness. The bears will only be affected at a time when they can no longer have offspring, so it will not affect the ability of bears to transmit their alleles to future generations.

[91] If the allele is truly recessive, it will not affect fitness at all. Natural selection can act only on phenotypes, not genotypes.

[92] No. Natural selection only acts on heritable traits. Infected bone marrow cells will not be passed on in the germ line to the next generation and so the long life span of these mice is not a heritable trait.

[93] The fish will technically have the same fitness, since both will contribute to the gene pool of future generations equally.

[94] Natural selection acts on phenotypes, not genotypes. Even if the allele is lethal in homozygotes, heterozygotes will not be selected against if the allele is not expressed. It takes many generations for deleterious recessive alleles to decrease in frequency in a population.

[95] The correct answer is choice **C**. Homozygotes have low fitness in the absence of medicine, while heterozygotes have increased fitness due to their resistance to viral disease. In the absence of the medicine, natural selection tends to reduce the frequency of the allele by removing individuals who are homozygous but tends to increase the frequency of the allele through the higher fitness of heterozygotes. Over time these opposing selection pressures can be balanced to keep the allele at a relatively constant frequency. If medicine removes the selection against homozygotes, then the heterozygotes with the increased fitness cause to allele frequency to increase over time.

this trait?[96] Can natural selection cause new alleles to appear in the population?[97]] Natural selection does not introduce genetic diversity, however; it can act only on existing diversity to alter allele frequencies.

There are two sources of genetic variation in a population: *new alleles* and *new combinations of existing alleles*. New alleles are the result of mutations in the genome. New combinations of alleles are generated during sexual reproduction as a result of independent assortment, recombination and segregation during meiosis. By increasing and maintaining genetic variation in a population, sexual reproduction allows for greater capacity for adaptation of a population to changing environmental conditions.

- Do new alleles in a population generally confer greater or lesser fitness on an individual carrying them?[98]
- If a mutation occurs in a muscle cell of an individual who then has many progeny, does this mutation increase genetic variation in the population?[99]
- Does mitosis contribute to the genetic variation in a population?[100]
- If a population of flowers loses the ability to reproduce sexually and reproduces only asexually, how will this affect natural selection in the population?[101]
- Plants that are pollinated by insects sometimes have physical features of the flower that prevent self-pollination. What is the advantage to the plant of preventing self-pollination?[102]
- Which one of the following can create new alleles in a population?[103]
  A) Non-random mating
  B) Random drift
  C) Recombination
  D) Deletion

---

[96] If there is only one allele, then there is no variability that natural selection can act on, and no way that allele frequencies can change to cause evolution.

[97] No. Natural selection can only alter the frequency of existing alleles, not create new alleles.

[98] New alleles caused by mutation generally render gene products less active or even inactive. Animals have adapted over long periods of time to have most gene products function in the optimal manner, so most changes are harmful rather than beneficial.

[99] No. Mutation must occur in the germ line to introduce a new allele into a population. A mutation in a somatic cell cannot be passed on to the next generation.

[100] No. Mitosis can only copy a cell into an identical cell; it is not involved in creating new combinations of alleles in the same manner as meiosis.

[101] If the flowers can only reproduce asexually, then they have lost the ability of meiosis to generate new combinations of alleles and new genetic variation for natural selection to act on.

[102] Self-pollination reduces genetic variability. More variability is maintained in the population if different individuals mate, making new combinations of alleles.

[103] Nonrandom mating and random drift will alter allele frequencies but do not create new alleles (choices A and B are incorrect). Recombination will not alter allele frequencies or create new alleles, but create new combinations of alleles (choice C is wrong). The correct answer is choice **D**. Only mutation of the genome can create new alleles. A deletion can create a new allele, even if the new allele is a truncated gene product or does not express any gene product at all.

Modes of Natural Selection

Natural selection can occur in many different manners and have different effects in a population. The following are a few examples:

1) **Directional Selection:** Polygenic traits often follow a bell-shaped curve of expression, with most individuals clustered around the average and some members of a population trailing off in either direction away from the average. If natural selection removes those at one extreme, the population average over time will move in the other direction. Example: Giraffes get taller as all short giraffes die for lack of food.

2) **Divergent Selection:** Rather than removing the extreme members in the distribution of a trait in a population, natural selection removes the members near the average, leaving those at either end. Over time divergent selection will split the population in two and perhaps lead to a new species. Example: Small deer are selected for because they can hide, and large deer are selected because they can fight, but mid-sized deer are too big to hide and too small to fight.

3) **Stabilizing Selection:** Both extremes of a trait are selected against, driving the population closer to the average. Example: Birds that are too large or too small are eliminated from a population because they cannot mate.

4) **Artificial Selection:** Humans intervene in the mating of many animals and plants, using artificial selection to achieve desired traits through controlled mating. Example: The pets and crop plants we have are the result of many generations of artificial selection.

5) **Sexual Selection:** Animals often do not choose mates randomly, but have evolved elaborate rituals and physical displays that play a key role in attracting and choosing a mate. Example: Some birds have bright plumage to attract a mate, even at the cost of increased predation.

6) **Kin Selection:** Natural selection does not always act on individuals. Animals that live socially often share alleles with other individuals and will sacrifice themselves for the sake of the alleles they share with another individual. Example: A female lion sacrifices herself to save her sister's children.

7.9 THE SPECIES CONCEPT AND SPECIATION

A **species** is a group of organisms which are capable of reproducing with each other sexually. (Other criteria, such as morphology, are used to classify species that only reproduce asexually.) [What's the difference between a population and a species?[104]] Two individuals are not members of the same biological species if they cannot mate and produce fit offspring. [When a horse mates with a donkey a mule is born. Mules are healthy animals with long life spans, but they are sterile. Are horses and donkeys members of the same species?[105]] **Reproductive isolation** keeps existing species separate. There are two types of reproductive isolation: **prezygotic** and **postzygotic**.

Prezygotic barriers prevent the formation of a hybrid zygote. Such barriers may be:

- Ecological: individuals who could otherwise mate live in different habitats, and thus cannot access each other

---

[104] Members of a species *can* mate and produce fit offspring. Members of a population *do*. Remember it this way: a population is a subset of a species.

[105] No, since their offspring are unfit (unable to reproduce).

- Temporal: individuals mate at different times of the day, season, or year
- Behavioral: some species require special rituals or courtship behaviors before mating can occur
- Mechanical: reproductive structures or genital organs of two individuals are not compatible (even if they court and attempt copulation)
- Gametic: sperm from one species cannot fertilize the egg of a different species due incompatibilities in the sperm-egg recognition system, discussed in Chapter 13

Postzygotic barriers to hybridization prevent the development, survival, or reproduction of hybrid individuals (those that arise from a mating between two different species), and thus prevent gene flow if fertilization between two different species does occur. There are three types of postzygotic barriers:

- Hybrid inviability: hybrid offspring do not develop or mature normally, and normally die in the embryonic stage
- Hybrid sterility: a hybrid individual is born and develops normally, but does not produce normal gametes, and thus is incapable of breeding (e.g., a mule, offspring of a mating between a horse and a donkey, is sterile)
- Hybrid breakdown: when two hybrids mate successfully to produce a hybrid offspring, but this second generation hybrid is somehow biologically defective

The creation of new species is known as **speciation**. An important premise in modern biology is that all species come from pre-existing species. *Cladogenesis* is branching speciation (*clado* is from the Greek for branch), where one species diversifies and becomes two or more new species. *Anagenesis* is when one biological species simply becomes another by changing so much that if an individual were to go back in time, it would be unable to reproduce sexually with its ancestors. One type of cladogenesis, *allopatric isolation*, is initiated by geographical isolation. Over time, geographical isolation leads to reproductive isolation. *Sympatric* speciation occurs when a species gives rise to a new species in the same geographical area, such as through divergent selection.

Cladogenesis has left traces which taxonomists use to classify organisms. **Homologous structures** are physical features shared by two different species as a result of a common ancestor. For example, bird wings have five bony supports which resemble distorted human fingers, and dog paws also resemble distorted human hands. The explanation is that dogs, birds, and people all have a common ancestor which had five-toed feet. **Analogous structures** serve the same function in two different species, but *not* due to common ancestry. The flagellum of the human sperm and bacterial flagella are an example; they have entirely different structures from different organisms yet play the same role in motility. **Convergent evolution** is when two different species come to possess many analogous structures due to similar selective pressures. For example, bats and birds appear very similar even though bats are mammals. The opposite of convergent evolution is **divergent evolution**, in which divergent selection causes cladogenesis. **Parallel evolution** describes the situation in which two species go through similar evolutionary changes due to similar selective pressures. For example, in an ice age, all organisms would be selected for their ability to tolerate cold.

7.10 TAXONOMY

Taxonomy is the science of biological classification, originated by Carolus Linnaeus in the eighteenth century. He devised the **binomial classification** system we use today, in which each organism is given two names: genus and species. The binomial name of an organism is written in italics (or is underlined) with the genus capitalized and the species not, as in *Homo sapiens* (man the wise). There are eight principal taxonomic categories: **domain**, **kingdom**, **phylum**, **class**, **order**, **family**, **genus**, and **species**.[106] You should know how humans are classified and the defining characteristics of each kingdom. Table 2 below provides a general summary.

Domain	Bacteria	Archaea	Eukarya			
Kingdom	Eubacteria	Archaea	Protista	Fungi	Plantae	Animalia
Cell wall	peptidoglycan	polysaccharides and proteins, but no peptidoglycan	optional and varied	chitin	cellulose	none
Organelles	none	none	Typical eukaryotic organelles such as: nucleus, RER, SER, Golgi, peroxisome, lysosomes, chloroplasts, vacuoles, mitochondria, etc.			
Chromosomes	1 circular ds DNA	1 circular ds DNA	several linear ds DNA chromosomes			
Life cycle	asexual repro. (binary fission)	asexual repro. (binary fission)	varied (sexual and asexual)	varied (sexual and asexual)	mostly sexual reproduction	mostly sexual reproduction
Ploidy and Cellularity	Unicellular	Unicellular	Mostly unicellular	Mostly multicellular and mostly haploid	Multicellular, alternates between haploid and diploid	Multicellular and diploid
Cellular motility	flagella	flagella	amoeboid or flagellar	non-motile	some flagellated sperm	amoeboid or flagellar
Cilia/flagella	unique structure	unique structure	characteristic 9 + 2 arrangement of microtubules			
Nutrition	varied, absorptive	varied, absorptive	varied	chemohetero., absorptive	most photo-auto. w/chlorophyll	chemohetero., ingestive
Glycolysis/ ATP	All living organisms perform glycolysis and use ATP. All kingdoms contain at least some members which perform oxidative phosphorylation.					
Examples	bacteria and blue-green algae	Archaea (extremophiles)	*Plasmodium* plankton, algae, kelp, seaweed	yeasts, molds, mushrooms, truffles	trees, flowers, mosses, ferns	sponges, worms, mollusks, insects, reptiles, birds, mammals

Table 2 Taxonomic Characteristics

[106] A mnemonic goes: "Dumb King Philip Came Over From Greece Sunday" (or "Dumb King Phil Came Over For Great…").

Domain Bacteria and Domain Archaea were both previously classified into Kingdom Monera. Because of huge diversity in these organisms, they have since been separated into two domains, and for these organisms, the kingdom and domain are the same.

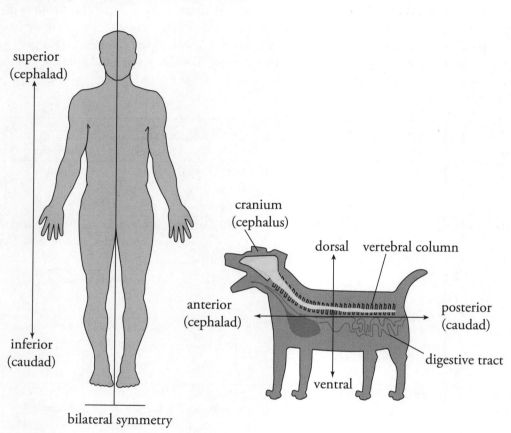

Figure 18   Bilateral Symmetry and the Anatomical Axes

Anatomists describe bodies with reference to axes such as the dorsal-ventral axis and the anterior-posterior axis (Figure 18). These are imaginary planes through the body. **Anterior** means "front-facing"; **posterior** is the opposite. **Dorsal** means "on top." A shark has a "dorsal fin," and the spines of dogs and humans are considered dorsal as well. **Ventral** is the opposite of dorsal. The belly button is a ventral structure in dogs and humans. In humans, **superior** is used to indicate "toward the head." **Inferior** means "toward the feet." Another way to say "toward the head" is **cephalad**. (Cephalus is Latin for head.) The opposite is **caudad**, meaning "toward the tail." [Does the axis of bilateral symmetry in vertebrates run parallel or perpendicular to the dorsal-ventral axis?[107]]

---

[107] The dorsal-ventral axis slices the body in half, separating front from back. The axis of symmetry separates left from right. So the two axes are perpendicular. Remember, the axes are planes, not lines.

7.11   THE ORIGIN OF LIFE

Based on radioisotope dating, the Earth is thought to be 4.5 billion years old. All life evolved from pro-karyotes. The oldest fossils are 3.5 billion-year-old outlines of primitive prokaryotic cell walls found in stromatolites (layered mats formed by colonies of prokaryotes). Even older life forms certainly existed, but lacked cell walls and thus left no fossil record (at least none have yet been discovered). Therefore, life on Earth is older than 3.5 billion years, nearly as old as the planet itself.

The atmosphere of the young Earth was different from today's atmosphere. The predominant gases then were probably H_2O, CO, CO_2, and N_2. The most important thing to note here is the absence of O_2. It is thought that the early atmosphere was a **reducing environment**, where electron donors were prevalent (see Chapter 3). Oxygen is an electron acceptor, and as such tends to break organic bonds. In this early world, simple organic molecules, or monomers ("single units") could form spontaneously. The energy for this synthesis was provided by lightning, radioactive decay, volcanic activity, or the Sun's radiation, which was more intense than it is today due to the thinner atmosphere. Laboratory recreations of the early envi-ronment result in the spontaneous formation of amino acids, carbohydrates, lipids, and ribonucleotides, as well as other organic compounds.

Spontaneous polymerization of these monomers can also be observed in the lab (including spontaneous polymerization of ribonucleotides). No enzymes were present when this was occurring for the first time in nature, but it is thought that metal ions on the surface of rocks and especially clay acted as catalysts. This is known as **abiotic synthesis**. Polypeptides made in this way are called **proteinoids**.

Proteinoids in water spontaneously form droplets called **microspheres**. When lipids are added to the solution **liposomes** form, with lipids forming a layer on the surface of proteins. A more complex particle known as a **coacervate** includes polypeptides, nucleic acids, and polysaccharides. Coacervates made with pre-existing enzymes are capable of catalyzing reactions. Microspheres, liposomes, and coacervates are collectively referred to as **protobionts**.

Protobionts resemble cells in that they contain a protected inner environment and perform chemical reactions. They can also reproduce to a certain extent: when they grow too large they split in half. What is lacking, however, is an organized mechanism of heredity. This was first provided by RNA. As noted previously, RNA chains form spontaneously in the appropriate solution. Even more interesting is the observation that single-stranded RNA chains can be self-replicating. A daughter chain lines up on the parent by base pairing and then spontaneously polymerizes with a surprisingly low error rate. A non-specific catalyst such as a metal ion can further increase the efficiency of RNA self-replication. Further-more, it is now known that RNA has catalytic activity in modern cells. For example, in primitive eukary-otes, introns are spliced out of the mRNA by **ribozymes**, which are RNA enzymes.

Somehow a mechanism evolved for polypeptides to be copied from early RNA genes. You already know about the inherent tendency for phospholipids to form lipid bilayers. Given all this information, it's not too hard to imagine true cells evolving from a primordial soup at the dawn of time. The last step in the evolution of the earliest cells would have been the switch from RNA to DNA as the genetic material. DNA is more stable due to its 2'-deoxy structure and also due to the fact that it spontaneously forms a compact double-stranded helix.

Chapter 7 Summary

- Organisms express phenotypes (physical characteristics) according to their genotypes (combinations of alleles).

- From a single diploid precursor cell, meiosis generates four haploid cells (gametes) with a random mix of alleles. This is due to crossing over in prophase I and separation of homologous chromosomes in anaphase I. Nondisjunction is a failure to separate the DNA properly during meiosis, and it can result in gametes with improper numbers of chromosomes.

- The Punnett square or the rules of probability can be used to determine the genotypes and phenotypes of offspring from given crosses, or the probability of having offspring with certain traits.

- The rule of multiplication states that the probability of A and B occurring is equal to the probability of A multiplied by the probability of B.

- The rule of addition states that the probability of A or B occurring is equal to the probability of A plus the probability of B, minus the probability of A and B together.

- Classical dominance occurs when a phenotype or trait is determined by one gene with two alleles, and one allele is dominant (expressed) and the other is recessive (silent). There are several exceptions to classical dominance, including incomplete dominance, codominance, epistasis, pleiotropism, polygenism, and penetrance.

- Incomplete dominance occurs when two different alleles for a single trait result in a blended phenotype. Codominance occurs when two different alleles for a single trait are expressed simultaneously, but independently (no blending).

- Epistasis occurs when the expression of one gene depends on the expression of another.

- Pleitropic genes affect many different aspects of the overall phenotype, while polygenic traits are affected by many different genes.

- Penetrance refers to the likelihood that a particular genotype will result in a given phenotype. Penetrance can be affected by several factors including age, environment, and lifestyle.

- Linkage occurs when two genes are close together on the same chromosome; it leads to alleles being inherited together (less recombination) instead of independently.

- The Hardy-Weinberg law can be used to study population genetics. It assumes classical dominance with only two alleles and unchanging allele frequencies. It is based on five assumptions: no mutation, no natural selection, no migration, large populations, and totally random mating.

- Natural selection drives evolution by allowing individuals with random, beneficial mutations to survive and pass those beneficial mutations on to their offspring.

- Homologous structures are the result of divergent evolution to form new species, and analogous structures are the result of convergent evolution, in which different start species must meet similar environmental challenges.

CHAPTER 7 FREESTANDING PRACTICE QUESTIONS

1. A woman is phenotypically normal but had a brother who had an autosomal recessive disorder that resulted in death during infancy. What is the probability that this woman is a carrier for the disorder that afflicted her brother?

   A) 1/4
   B) 1/3
   C) 1/2
   D) 2/3

2. A set of inherited traits show a phenotypic ratio of 9:3:3:1 among offspring of a given mating. A possible explanation for this observation is a two locus–two allele system where each locus exhibits:

   A) independent assortment.
   B) linkage.
   C) epistasis.
   D) incomplete dominance.

3. If a woman is a carrier for an X-linked recessive disorder and mates with a normal, unaffected male, what is the probability her grandson has the disorder? Assume she has a normal son and a daughter, and they both have homozygous normal partners.

   A) 0
   B) 1/4
   C) 1/2
   D) 3/4

4. In fruit flies, the gene that produces white eyes is X-linked recessive (red eyes are dominant to white). Two autosomal genes determine body color and leg length; a brown body is dominant to ebony and long legs are dominant to short. Assume dominant alleles are considered wild-type. A white-eyed male is mated to an ebony colored, short-legged female. The resulting F_1 males are all wild type. If these males are backcrossed to the female parent, what is the probability that an F_2 offspring will be a wild-type male?

   A) 0
   B) 1/2
   C) 1/4
   D) 1/8

5. A geneticist is analyzing a family tree, where mothers affected by the trait under study pass the trait on to 100% of their offspring, both sons and daughters. Fathers affected by the trait pass it on to 0% of their offspring. All affected individuals have an affected mother. What is the inheritance pattern of this trait?

   A) Y-linked
   B) Autosomal dominant
   C) Autosomal recessive
   D) Mitochondrial

6. A purebred long-tailed cat with long whiskers (*TTww*) is mated to a purebred short-tailed cat with short whiskers (*ttWW*). The kittens will be:

   A) 100% long-tailed with long whiskers.
   B) 100% long-tailed with short whiskers.
   C) 100% short-tailed with short whiskers.
   D) 50% long-tailed cat with long whiskers, 50% short-tailed cat with short whiskers.

7. A homozygous white bull is mated to a homozygous cow with a red coat. The offspring all have a roan coat color, which is composed of a mix of white hairs and red hairs. Which of the following is true?

   A) Coat color in cattle is an example of codominance.
   B) White hair is recessive to red hair.
   C) Coat color in cattle is an example of incomplete dominance.
   D) White hair is dominant over red hair.

8. If the genes for ear size (*E* or *e*) and aggressiveness (*A* or *a*) in mice are linked and 25 mu apart, what is the probability of getting a large-eared aggressive pup (*EeAa*) from a mating between a small-eared aggressive female (*eeAA*) and a large-eared nonaggressive male (*EEaa*)?

   A) 12.5%
   B) 25%
   C) 75%
   D) 100%

CHAPTER 7 PRACTICE PASSAGE

The fruit fly, *Drosophila melanogaster*, is an ideal organism on which to study genetic mechanisms. This organism has simple food requirements, occupies little space, and the reproductive life cycle is complete in about 12 days at room temperature, allowing for quick analysis of test crosses. In addition, fruit flies produce large numbers of offspring, which allows for sufficient data to be collected quickly. Many *Drosophila* genes are homologous to human genes, and are studied to gain a better understanding of what role these proteins have in humans.

To understand the inheritance patterns of certain genes in *Drosophila*, the following experiments were carried out. Assume that the alleles for red eyes, brown body, and normal wings are dominant and the alleles for white eyes, ebony body, and vestigial wings are recessive.

Experiment 1:

A red-eyed female and a white-eye male were crossed. The subsequent generation of flies was also crossed. The phenotypic results of both generations are shown below:

Generation	Red-eyed female	White-eyed female	Red-eyed male	White-eyed male
Parental	1	0	0	1
F_1	9	0	13	0
F_2	27	0	12	14

Experiment 2:

Five of the red-eyed female *Drosophila* from the F_1 generation of Experiment 1 were crossed with white-eyed males. The result of this cross is shown below:

Generation	Red-eyed female	White-eyed female	Red-eyed male	White-eyed male
F_1	5	0	0	10
F_2	8	8	9	8

Experiment 3:

The white-eyed females from Experiment 2 were crossed with red-eyed males. The result of this cross is shown below:

Generation	Red-eyed female	White-eyed female	Red-eyed male	White-eyed male
Parental	0	8	7	0
F_1	9	0	0	10

Experiment 4:

A male heterozygous for body color and wing type is crossed with an ebony, vestigial-winged female. The results of the cross are shown below:

Phenotype	Male	Female
Brown body, normal wings	32	30
Brown body, vestigial wings	2	1
Ebony body, normal wings	1	3
Ebony body, vestigial wings	28	33

1. What is the most likely mode of inheritance for white eye color?

A) X-linked recessive
B) X-linked dominant
C) Autosomal recessive
D) Autosomal dominant

2. What ratio of white-eyed to red-eyed females would be expected if the F_1 generation of Experiment 3 were crossed?

A) White-eyed females would not be present.
B) Red-eyed females would not be present.
C) 1:1
D) 1:2

3. Approximately how many of the red-eyed females of the F_2 generation of Experiment 2 are homozygous dominant?

A) 0
B) 2
C) 4
D) 8

4. Which of the following statements is/are true with regard to the results obtained from Experiment 4?

   I. The genes for body color and wing type are on the same chromosome.
   II. Recombination occurred.
   III. The heterozygous male had a dominant and recessive allele on each homologous chromosome.

A) I only
B) I and II
C) I and III
D) II only

5. What is the recombination frequency shown by the results of Experiment 4?

A) Recombination did not occur.
B) 5%
C) 50%
D) 95%

6. If the frequency of vestigial wings in a population of *Drosophila* ($n = 1500$) is 4%, how many flies would be heterozygous with regard to wing type? Assume random mating, but no migration, mutation, random drift, or natural selection.

A) 60
B) 240
C) 480
D) 960

SOLUTIONS TO CHAPTER 7 FREESTANDING PRACTICE QUESTIONS

1. **D** If the woman's brother was affected with this autosomal recessive disorder, both of her parents must have been carriers for the trait. Since it is lethal in infancy, you know both parents must have been heterozygous. The mating between two heterozygotes produces the following genotypic ratio in their offspring: 25% homozygous recessive, 50% heterozygous, 25% homozygous dominant. Since the woman is phenotypically normal, she must not have the disorder, so she is not in the 25% homozygous recessive group. She is either in the 25% homozygous dominant group or the 50% heterozygous group, so the chance she is a carrier is 2/3 (choice D is correct).

2. **A** If two heterozygous parents are mated (for example, $AaBb \times AaBb$), the expected F_1 phenotype ratio if the two traits are assorting independently is 9:3:3:1 (choice A is correct). If linkage were occurring, this ratio would be skewed after the mating of two double heterozygotes, since alleles would be preferentially inherited together. Since the ratio is not skewed, linkage is not occurring (choice B can be eliminated). This is not a case where one gene is silencing another, or controlling the expression of the other, as this would also lead to a skewed ratio (choice C can be eliminated). Incomplete dominance of two alleles leads to a blended heterozygous phenotype; thus, if it occurs at a single locus, it produces three different phenotypes. If it were to occur at two different loci (as in this case), there would be nine possible phenotypes (3 possible phenotypes at the first locus times 3 possible phenotypes at the second locus = $3^2 = 9$). In this case there are only four different phenotypes (choice D can be eliminated).

3. **B** If we assign "A" as the normal allele and "a" as the affected allele, the woman is $X^A X^a$ and her mate is $X^A Y$. The question stem says that she has a normal son, who must have the genotype $X^A Y$; he received the X^A from his mother and his Y chromosome from his father. There is no probability associated with this that must be factored into the solution, because this is the only way the couple could have a normal son. If this son mates with a homozygous normal female, he will pass his Y chromosome onto his son(s), which means there is zero chance of having an affected son. In other words, an $X^A Y \times X^A X^A$ mating cannot generate $X^a Y$ sons. Next, let's work with the daughter of the woman in the question stem. The question says she has a normal phenotype. She must receive an X^A from her father. There is a 50% probability she will receive an X^a from her mother. If the daughter is $X^A X^a$ (remember there is a 50% chance of this) and her mate is $X^A Y$, there is a 50% chance their son will be affected. Overall, then, the probability that a grandson is affected is $0 + (1/2)(1/2)$, or 1/4. Therefore, choice B is correct.

4. **D** Assign X^R = red eyes (dominant and wild-type), X^r = white eyes, B = brown body color (dominant and wild-type), b = ebony body color, S = long legs (dominant and wild-type), and s = short legs. Since all the male offspring from the first cross are wild-type, then the male parent must have been homozygous for body color and leg length, and the female parent must have been homozygous for eye color; thus, the first cross is $X^r YBBSS \times X^R X^R bbss$. The male F_1 offspring will be $X^R YBbSs$. Next, this male was backcrossed to the female parent ($X^R YBbSs \times X^R X^R bbss$), and you are asked for the probability of a wild-type male. This is equal to the probability of a male (1/2), multiplied by the probability that it will have brown

body color (1/2), multiplied by the probability that it will have long legs (1/2). Therefore, the probability of a wild-type male is = $1/2 \times 1/2 \times 1/2 = 1/8$ (choice D is correct). Notice that you do not have to factor in the probability of the F_2 being red-eyed because this is guaranteed given the genotype of their mother.

5. **D** Females are not affected by Y-linked traits (choice A is wrong). If the trait was autosomal dominant, affected fathers would pass the trait to at least some of their offspring (choice B is wrong). Autosomal recessive traits do not demonstrate the sex bias that is described in the question stem (choice C is incorrect). By Process of Elimination, this trait must be inherited via the mitochondrial genome. All humans inherit their mitochondrial genome from their mothers; during fertilization, the sperm only contributes 23 chromosomes but the ovum contributes 23 chromosomes along with all other cellular organelles and cytoplasm (choice D is correct).

6. **B** The offspring will be 100% *TtWw* and will display the dominant phenotype for each trait. Since each parent has a dominant and a recessive phenotype, the kittens will not have the phenotype of either parent (choice B is correct, and choices A, C, and D are wrong).

7. **A** Since the offspring are neither red nor white, this trait is not inherited via simple Mendelian genetics, and neither trait is dominant or recessive (choices B and D are wrong). The individual hairs on the F_1 cattle are either red or white, which means that both alleles are being expressed. This best matches the definition of codominance (choice A is correct). If the individual hairs were a blend of white and red, the best answer would have been incomplete dominance (choice C is wrong).

8. **D** The pups will get *eA* from their mom and *Ea* from their dad. All the pups will be *eA/Ea*, so the answer must be choice D. Note that the linkage information was not useful in answering this question.

SOLUTIONS TO CHAPTER 7 PRACTICE PASSAGE

1. **A** The passage states that the allele for red eyes is dominant and the allele for white eyes is recessive (choices B and D are wrong). The results from Experiment 1 suggest that the gene for eye color is X-linked. If it were autosomal, all F_1 flies from that experiment would be heterozygous, and there would be an equal distribution of both genders and colors in the F_2 generation. Remember that a gender bias in the phenotype of a trait usually indicates that you're working with a sex-linked trait.

2. **C** The passage states that the red allele is dominant and the white allele is recessive; further eye color is a sex-linked trait (see the explanation for Question 1). For Experiment 3, the female parental genotype must be homozygous recessive (X^cX^c), and the male parental genotype must be X^cY. Thus, the F_1 generation consists of heterozygous females (X^CX^c) and males with the recessive white-eyed allele (X^cY). If these two were mated with each other, the female progeny of this generation would consist of homozygous recessive (X^cX^c) and heterozygous (X^CX^c) females in an approximate 1:1 ratio (choice C is correct).

3. **A** Experiment 2 is a cross between an F_1 female and a white-eyed male. The genotype of the F_1 females from Experiment 1 is $X^C X^c$; they have red eyes, so they must have X^C, and they are female, so they inherited X^c from their white-eyed father. If these $X^C X^c$ females are crossed with $X^c Y$ (white-eyed) males, the females generated in the F_2 must be 50% $X^C X^c$ (red-eyed) and 50% $X^c X^c$ (white-eyed). If the father has white eyes, it is impossible to generate homozygous red-eyed females in the F_2 (choice A is correct).

4. **B** There is no sex bias in the results from Experiment 4, so you can assume the alleles are autosomal. The passage states that the alleles for brown bodies and normal wings are dominant, and the alleles for ebony bodies and vestigial wings are recessive. Let's assign B = brown and b = ebony for body color, and W = normal and w = vestigial for wing phenotype. Thus, the cross in Experiment 4 is $BbWw \times bbww$. Item I is true: if the genes for body color and wing type were on separate chromosomes, one would expect the law of independent assortment to hold true and the phenotypic ratio of the progeny would be expected to be 1:1:1:1. However, this is not the case. Two of the phenotypes predominate, indicating that the genes are close together on the same chromosome, or are linked (choice D can be eliminated). Item II is also true: the recombinant phenotypes, although rare, are nonetheless seen. Recombination between homologous chromosomes is the best explanation for this observation (choices A and C can be eliminated, and choice B is correct). Note that Item III is false: the double heterozygous *Drosophila* must have both dominant alleles on one chromosome and both recessive alleles on the other to account for the results seen. In other words, the cross performed was $BW/bw \times bw/bw$. The parental combinations of alleles are BW and bw (more frequent), and the recombinant combinations of alleles (less frequent) are Bw and bW.

5. **B** Recombination did in fact occur (see explanation for Question 4; choice A is wrong). Recombination frequency = number of recombinants/total number of offspring. In this case, the total number of recombinants is 7 and the total number of offspring is 130. 7/130 = 0.05 or 5% recombination frequency (choice B is correct, and choices C and D are wrong). Note that choice D is the frequency of non-recombination, and choice C would be correct if the genes were not linked.

6. **C** Using the Hardy-Weinberg equations for allele frequency and genotype, the frequency of the vestigial wing allele (q) must be equal to $\sqrt{0.04}$, or 0.20. Therefore, the frequency of the normal wing allele (p) is 0.80 and the frequency of the heterozygous genotype (pq and qp) is equal to $2 \times 0.2 \times 0.8$, or 0.32. The actual number of *Drosophila* that would have this genotype would be 480 (0.32×1500).

Chapter 8
The Nervous and
Endocrine Systems

The nervous and endocrine systems are presented in the same chapter since their functions are related: they both provide communication, integrating, and coordinating the activities of the tissues and organs of the body. The means of communication by the two systems are quite different (although complementary) in many ways. The nervous system communicates through electrochemical signals (action potentials), while the endocrine system uses chemical messengers carried in the blood (hormones). The nervous system in general regulates rapid responses such as those of skeletal muscle or smooth muscle, while the endocrine system takes longer to have an effect and regulates longer-term responses such as metabolism and homeostasis. The two systems are interconnected, with two of the primary endocrine glands—the pituitary and the adrenals—regulated by the nervous system, and with the endocrine system feeding back to modulate the nervous system.

8.1 NEURONAL STRUCTURE AND FUNCTION

Neurons are specialized cells that transmit and process information from one part of the body to another. This information takes the form of electrochemical impulses known as **action potentials**. The action potential is a localized area of depolarization of the plasma membrane that travels in a wave-like manner along an axon. When an action potential reaches the end of an axon at a synapse, the signal is transformed into a chemical signal with the release of neurotransmitter into the synaptic cleft, a process called **synaptic transmission** (Section 8.2). The information of many synapses feeding into a neuron is integrated to determine whether that neuron will in turn fire an action potential. In this way the action of many individual neurons is integrated to work together in the nervous system as a whole.

Structure of the Neuron

The basic functional and structural unit of the nervous system is the **neuron** (Figure 1 on the next page). The structure of these cells is highly specialized to transmit and process **action potentials**, the electrochemical signals of the nervous system (Figure 3, page 283). Neurons have a central cell body, the **soma**, which contains the nucleus and is where most of the biosynthetic activity of the cell takes place. Slender projections, termed **axons** and **dendrites**, extend from the cell body. Neurons have only one axon (as long as a meter in some cases), but most possess many dendrites. Neurons with one dendrite are termed **bipolar**; those with many dendrites are **multipolar**. Neurons generally carry action potentials in one direction, with dendrites receiving signals and axons carrying action potentials away from the cell body. Axons can branch multiple times and terminate in **synaptic knobs** that form connections with target cells. When action potentials travel down an axon and reach the synaptic knob, chemical messengers are released and travel across a very small gap called the **synaptic cleft** to the target cell. The nature of the action potential and the transmission of signals across the synaptic cleft are key aspects of nervous system function. [In Figure 1, in what direction does an action potential travel in the axon shown?[1] What's the difference between a neuron and a nerve?[2]]

---

[1] Action potentials travel from the cell body down the axon, or from left to right in Figure 1.

[2] A neuron is a single cell. A nerve is a large bundle of many different axons from different neurons.

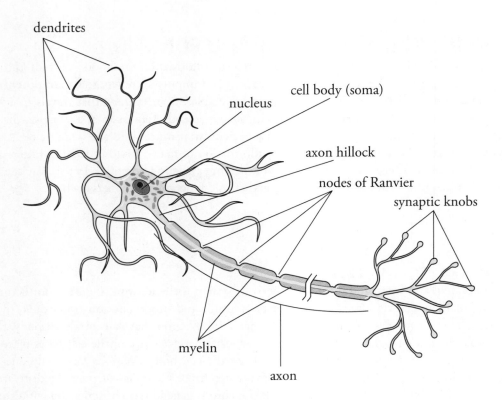

Figure 1   A Multipolar Neuron

- A motor protein called *kinesin* is one of several different proteins that drive movement of vesicles and organelles along microtubules in axons. Kinesin specifically drives anterograde movement (movement from the soma toward the axon terminus). If a kinesin inhibitor is added to neurons in culture, what is the likely result?[3]
    A) Spontaneous action potentials
    B) Cell division
    C) Accumulation of material in the synaptic knob
    D) Atrophy of axons

The Action Potential

The Resting Membrane Potential

The **resting membrane potential** is an electric potential across the plasma membrane of approximately –70 millivolts (mV), with the interior of the cell negatively charged with respect to the exterior of the cell.

—

[3] A large amount of biosynthetic activity takes place in the cell body, and materials are transported from the cell body down the axon to its end by kinesin. The correct answer is choice **D**. If material cannot be transported through the axon from the cell body, the axon will atrophy. Note that although this may not immediately be apparent, choices A, B, and C should have been easily eliminated; kinesin has nothing to do with action potentials, neurons in general do not divide (and inhibiting kinesin should not change this), and the inhibition of kinesin would prevent materials from accumulating at the synaptic knobs.

Two primary membrane proteins are required to establish the resting membrane potential: the Na⁺/K⁺ ATPase and the potassium leak channels. The **Na⁺/K⁺ ATPase** pumps three sodium ions out of the cell and two potassium ions into the cell with the hydrolysis of one ATP molecule. [What form of transport is carried out by the Na⁺/K⁺ ATPase?[4]] The result is a sodium gradient with high sodium outside of the cell and a potassium gradient with high potassium inside the cell. **Leak channels** are channels that are open all the time, and that simply allow ions to "leak" across the membrane according to their gradient. Potassium leak channels allow potassium, but no other ions, to flow down their gradient out of the cell. The combined loss of many positive ions through Na⁺/K⁺ ATPases and the potassium leak channels leaves the interior of the cell with a net negative charge, approximately 70 mV more negative than the exterior of the cell; this difference is the resting membrane potential. Note that there are very few sodium leak channels in the membrane (the ratio of K⁺ leak channels to Na⁺ leak channels is about 100:1), so the cell membrane is virtually impermeable to sodium.

- Are neurons the only cells with a resting membrane potential?[5]
- If the potassium leak channels are blocked, what will happen to the membrane potential?[6]
- What would happen to the membrane potential if sodium ions were allowed to flow down their concentration gradient?[7]

The resting membrane potential establishes a negative charge along the interior of axons (along with the rest of the neuronal interior). Thus, the cells can be described as **polarized**; negative on the inside and positive on the outside. An action potential is a disturbance in this membrane potential, a wave of **depolarization** of the plasma membrane that travels along an axon. Depolarization is a change in the membrane potential from the resting membrane potential of approximately –70 mV to a less negative, or even positive, potential. After depolarization, **repolarization** returns the membrane potential to normal. The change in membrane potential during the passage of an action potential is caused by movement of ions into and out of the neuron through ion channels. The action potential is therefore not strictly an electrical impulse, like electrons moving in a copper telephone wire, but an electro*chemical* impulse.

Depolarization

Key proteins in the propagation of action potentials are the **voltage-gated sodium channels** located in the plasma membrane of the axon. In response to a change in the membrane potential, these ion channels open to allow sodium ions to flow down their gradient into the cell and depolarize that section of membrane. [What is the effect of opening the voltage-gated sodium channels on the membrane potential?[8]] These channels are opened by depolarization of the membrane from the resting potential of –70 mV to a **threshold potential** of approximately –50 mV. Once this threshold is reached, the channels are opened fully, but below the threshold they are closed and do not allow the passage of any ions through the channel. When the channels open, sodium flows into the cell, down its concentration gradient, depolarizing that

---

[4] The Na⁺/K⁺ ATPase uses ATP to drive transport against a gradient; this is primary active transport.

[5] No. All cells have the resting membrane potential. Neurons and muscle tissue are unique in using the resting membrane potential to generate action potentials.

[6] The flow of potassium out of the cell makes the interior of the cell more negatively charged. Blocking the potassium leak channels would reduce the magnitude of the resting membrane potential, making the interior of the cell less negative.

[7] Sodium ions would flow into the cell and reduce the potential across the plasma membrane, making the interior of the cell less negative and even relatively positive if enough ions flow into the cell.

[8] Sodium (positively charged) flows into the cell, down its concentration gradient, making the interior of the cell less negatively charged, or even positively charged.

section of the membrane to about +35 mV before inactivating. Some of the sodium ions flow down the interior of the axon, slightly depolarizing the neighboring section of membrane. When the depolarization in the next section of membrane reaches threshold, those voltage-gated sodium channels open as well, passing the depolarization down the axon (Figure 2). [If an action potential starts at one end of an axon, can it run out of energy and not reach the other end?[9]]

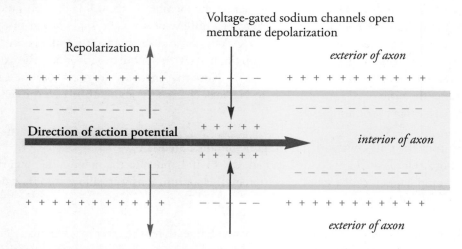

Figure 2   The Action Potential is a Wave of Membrane Depolarization

- Which one of the following can cause the interior of the neuron to have a momentary positive charge?[10]
    A) Opening of potassium leak channels
    B) Activity of the Na+/K+ ATPase
    C) Opening of voltage-gated sodium channels
    D) Opening of voltage-gated potassium channels

- Given the above description, which of the following best describes the response of voltage-gated sodium channels to a membrane depolarization from −70 mV to −60 mV?[11]
    A) All of the channels open fully.
    B) 50% of the channels open fully.
    C) All of the channels open 50%.
    D) None of the channels open.

---

[9] No, it cannot. Action potentials are continually renewed at each point in the axon as they travel. Assuming there are enough voltage-gated channels, once an action potential starts, it will propagate without a change in amplitude (size) until it reaches a synapse.

[10] Choices A, B, and D all make the interior of the cell more negative. Choice **C** is the answer. Voltage-gated sodium channels can make the interior of the cell momentarily positive during passage of an action potential.

[11] Voltage-gated sodium channels require a threshold depolarization to open. A depolarization below the threshold will produce essentially no response, while a depolarization greater than or equal to the threshold will cause all of the channels to open fully. This is called an **all-or-none** response. The correct answer is choice **D**. The depolarization is less than the threshold, so there is no response.

Repolarization

With the opening of voltage-gated sodium channels, sodium flows into the cell and depolarizes the membrane to positive values. As the wave of depolarization passes through a region of membrane, however, the membrane does not remain depolarized (Figure 3).

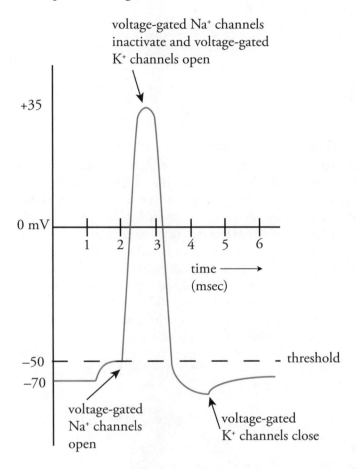

Figure 3   The Action Potential at a Single Location

After depolarization, the membrane is **repolarized**, re-establishing the original resting membrane potential. A number of factors combine to produce this effect:

1) Voltage-gated sodium channels **inactivate** very quickly after they open, shutting off the flow of sodium into the cell. The channels remain inactivated until the membrane potential nears resting values again.

2) Voltage-gated potassium channels open more slowly than the voltage-gated sodium channels and stay open longer. Voltage-gated potassium channels open in response to membrane depolarization. As potassium leaves the cell down its concentration gradient, the membrane potential returns to negative values, actually overshooting the resting potential by about 20 mV (to about −90 mV). At this point the voltage-gated potassium channels close.

3) Potassium leak channels and the Na^+/K^+ ATPase continue to function (as they always do) to bring the membrane back to resting potential. These factors alone would repolarize the membrane potential even without the voltage-gated potassium channels, but it would take a lot longer.

- If a toxin prevents voltage-gated sodium channels from closing, which of the following will occur?[12]
  - I. Voltage-gated potassium channels will open but not close.
  - II. The membrane will not repolarize to the normal resting membrane potential.
  - III. The Na⁺/K⁺ ATPase will be inactivated.

  A) I only
  B) II only
  C) I and II only
  D) II and III only

Saltatory Conduction

The axons of many neurons are wrapped in an insulating sheath called **myelin** (Figure 4). The myelin sheath is not created by the neuron itself, but by cells called **Schwann cells**[13], a type of glial cell, that exist in conjunction with neurons, wrapping layers of specialized membrane around the axons. No ions can enter or exit a neuron where the axonal membrane is covered with myelin. [Would an axon be able to conduct action potentials if its entire length were wrapped in myelin?[14]] There is no membrane depolarization and no voltage-gated sodium channels in regions of the axonal plasma membrane that are wrapped in myelin. There are periodic gaps in the myelin sheath however, called **nodes of Ranvier** (Figures 1, 4, and 5). Voltage-gated sodium and potassium channels are concentrated in the nodes of Ranvier in myelinated axons. Rather than impeding action potentials, the myelin sheath dramatically speeds the movement of action potentials by forcing the action potential to jump from node to node. This rapid jumping conduction in myelinated axons is termed **saltatory conduction**.

myelin (Schwann cell)

axon

nodes of Ranvier

Figure 4   A Schwann Cell Wrapping an Axon with Myelin

---

[12] **Item I is true:** voltage-gated potassium channels are normally closed by the repolarization of the membrane, so if the membrane is not repolarized, they will not close. **Item II is true:** sodium ions will continue to flow into the cell, even as the Na⁺/K⁺ ATPase works to pump them out. This will prevent the repolarization of the membrane. Item III is false: the Na⁺/K⁺ ATPase will work harder than ever. The answer is choice **C**.

[13] Schwann cells are found in the peripheral nervous system (PNS). In the central nervous system (CNS) myelination of axons is accomplished via similar cells called oligodendrocytes.

[14] No. The action potential requires the movement of ions across the plasma membrane to create a wave of depolarization.

- Which one of the following is true concerning myelinated and unmyelinated axons?[15]
  A) The amount of energy consumed by the Na⁺/K⁺ ATPase is much less in myelinated axons than in unmyelinated axons.
  B) Myelinated axons can conduct many more action potentials per second than can unmyelinated axons.
  C) The size of action potential depolarization is much greater in myelinated axons than in unmyelinated axons.
  D) Voltage-gated potassium channels do not play a role in repolarization in unmyelinated axons.

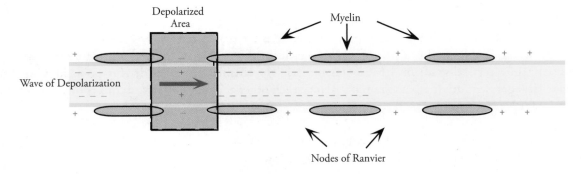

Figure 5 Propagation of the AP in a Myelinated Axon (cross section)

Glial Cells

As mentioned above, the myelin sheath is formed by a type of glial cell called a Schwann cell. However, Schwann cells are not the only type of glial cell. **Glial cells** are specialized, non-neuronal cells that typically provide structural and metabolic support to neurons (Table 1). Glia maintain a resting membrane potential but do not generate action potentials.

Table 1 Types of Glial Cells and Their Functions

Cell Type	Location	Primary Functions
Schwann cells	PNS	Form myelin—increase speed of conduction of APs along axon
Oligodendrocytes	CNS	Form myelin—increase speed of conduction of APs along axon
Astrocytes	CNS	Guide neuronal development Regulate synaptic communication via regulation of neurotransmitter levels
Microglia	CNS	Remove dead cells and debris
Ependymal cells	CNS	Produce and circulate cerebrospinal fluid

---

[15] Since the area of membrane that is conducting is much less in myelinated axons, Na⁺/K⁺ ATPase only works to maintain the resting potential in the nodes of Ranvier, whereas in unmyelinated axons the Na⁺/K⁺ ATPase hydrolyzes ATP to maintain the resting potential across the entire membrane (choice A is correct). The length of the refractory period (and hence the frequency of action potentials) is based on the characteristics of the voltage-gated sodium and potassium channels, which do not change (choice B is false). The size of depolarization in an action potential does not vary greatly; action potentials are an all-or-nothing response (choice C is false). Voltage-gated potassium channels are the same in both neurons (choice D is false).

Equilibrium Potentials

During the action potential, the movement of Na$^+$ and K$^+$ ions across the membrane through the voltage-gated channels is *passive*; driven by gradients. The **equilibrium potential** is the membrane potential at which this driving force (the gradient) does not exist; in other words, there would be no net movement of ions across the membrane. Note that the equilibrium potential is specific for a particular ion. For example, the Na$^+$ equilibrium potential is *positive*, approximately +50 mV. Na$^+$ ions are driven inward by their concentration gradient. However, if the interior of the cell is too positive, the positively charged ions are repelled; in other words, the *electrical* gradient would drive sodium *out*. These forces, the chemical gradient driving sodium in and the electrical gradient driving sodium out balance each other at about +50 mV, so this is the equilibrium potential for Na$^+$.

K$^+$, however, has a *negative* equilibrium potential. K$^+$ ions are driven outward by their concentration gradient. However, if the interior of the cell is too negative, the positively charged ions cannot escape the attraction; the electrical gradient drives potassium *in*. The chemical gradient driving potassium out and the electrical gradient driving potassium in balance each other at about –90 mV, so this is the equilibrium potential for K$^+$.

The equilibrium potential for any ion is based on the electrochemical gradient for that ion across the membrane, and can be predicted by the **Nernst equation**:

$$E_{ion} = \frac{RT}{zF} \ln \frac{[X]_{outside}}{[X]_{inside}}$$

where E_{ion} is the equilibrium potential for the ion, R is the universal gas constant, T is the temperature (in Kelvin), z is the valence of the ion, F is Faraday's constant, and [X] is the concentration of the ion on each side of the plasma membrane. Note that the relative concentrations of the ion on each side of the membrane create the *chemical* gradient, while the valence (charge of the ion) helps determine the electrical gradient.

Note that the fact that the resting membrane potential is –70 mV reflects both the differences in the equilibrium potentials for Na$^+$ and K$^+$, and also the relative numbers of leak channels for these two ions. If the cell were completely permeable to K$^+$, the resting potential would be about –90 mV. The fact that the resting potential is *very close* to the K$^+$ equilibrium potential indicates that there are a large number of K$^+$ leak channels in the membrane; the cell at rest is almost completely permeable to potassium. However, the resting potential is slightly more positive than –90 mV, indicating that there are a few Na$^+$ leak channels allowing Na$^+$ in. Not very many Na$^+$ leak channels, though, or the resting potential would be much more positive; closer to the Na$^+$ equilibrium potential. (This is in fact what we see when the cell *does* become completely permeable to Na$^+$ at the beginning of the action potential; the membrane potential shoots upward to +35 mV.)

The Refractory Period

Action potentials can pass through a neuron extremely rapidly, thousands each second, but there is an upper limit to how soon a neuron can conduct an action potential after another has passed. The passage of one action potential makes the neuron nonresponsive to membrane depolarization and unable to transmit another action potential, or **refractory**, for a short period of time. There are two phases of the refractory period, caused by two different factors. During the **absolute refractory period**, a neuron will not fire another action potential no matter how strong a membrane depolarization is induced. During this time, the voltage-gated sodium channels have been *inactivated* (not the same as *closed*) after depolarization. They will not be able to be opened again until the membrane potential reaches the resting potential and the Na+ channels have returned to their "closed" state. During the **relative refractory period**, a neuron can be induced to transmit an action potential, but the depolarization required is greater than normal because the membrane is **hyperpolarized**. When repolarization occurs, there is a brief period in which the membrane potential is more negative than the resting potential (Figure 3), caused by voltage-gated potassium channels that have not closed yet. Because it is further from threshold, a greater stimulus is required to open the voltage-gated sodium channels to start an action potential. [If a fruit fly mutant is found that has voltage-gated potassium channels that shut more quickly after repolarization, how would this affect the refractory period in the fly?[16]]

8.2 SYNAPTIC TRANSMISSION

A **synapse** is a junction between the axon terminus of a neuron and the dendrites, soma, or axon of a second neuron. It can also be a junction between the axon terminus of a neuron and an organ. There are two types of synapses: electrical and chemical. **Electrical synapses** occur when the cytoplasms of two cells are joined by gap junctions. If two cells are joined by an electrical synapse, an action potential will spread directly from one cell to the other. Electrical synapses are not common in the nervous system although they are quite important in propagating action potentials in smooth muscle and cardiac muscle. In the nervous system, **chemical synapses** are found at the ends of axons where they meet their target cell; here, an action potential is converted into a chemical signal. The following steps are involved in the transmission of a signal across a chemical synapse in the nervous system (Figure 6 on the next page), as well as at the junctions of neurons with other cell types, such as skeletal muscle cells:

1) An action potential reaches the end of an axon, the synaptic knob.
2) Depolarization of the presynaptic membrane opens voltage-gated calcium channels.
3) Calcium influx into the presynaptic cell causes exocytosis of neurotransmitter stored in secretory vesicles.
4) Neurotransmitter molecules diffuse across the narrow synaptic cleft (small space between cells).
5) Neurotransmitter binds to receptor proteins in the postsynaptic membrane. These receptors are ligand-gated ion channels.
6) The opening of these ion channels in the postsynaptic cell alters the membrane polarization.
7) If the membrane depolarization of the postsynaptic cell reaches the threshold of voltage-gated sodium channels, an action potential is initiated.
8) Neurotransmitter in the synaptic cleft is degraded and/or removed to terminate the signal.

---

[16] The absolute refractory period would not be altered, since this is due to the inability of voltage-gated sodium channels to open. However, the relative refractory period would be decreased.

8.2

Presynaptic Neuron
1. Voltage-gated calcium channels open
2. Influx of calcium
3. Exocytosis of secretory vesicle
4. Release of neurotransmitter into synaptic cleft

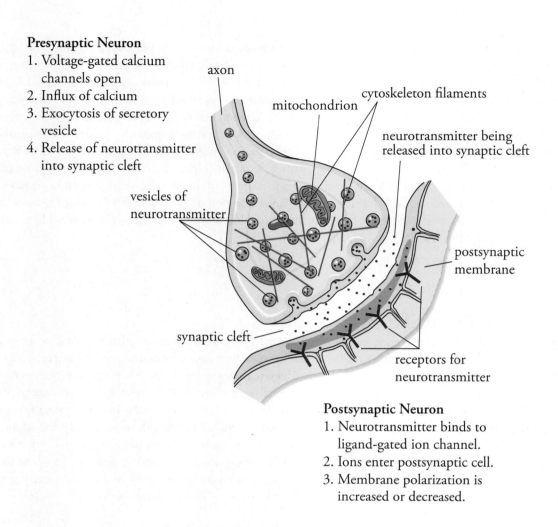

Postsynaptic Neuron
1. Neurotransmitter binds to ligand-gated ion channel.
2. Ions enter postsynaptic cell.
3. Membrane polarization is increased or decreased.

Figure 6   A Typical Synapse

An example of a chemical synapse that is commonly used is the **neuromuscular junction** between neurons and skeletal muscle. The neurotransmitter that is released at the neuromuscular junction is **acetylcholine (ACh)**. When an action potential reaches such a synapse, acetylcholine is released into the synaptic cleft. The acetylcholine binds to the acetylcholine receptor on the surface of the postsynaptic cell membrane. When acetylcholine binds to its receptor, the receptor opens its associated sodium channel, allowing sodium to flow down a gradient into the cell, depolarizing the postsynaptic cell membrane. Meanwhile, acetylcholine in the synaptic cleft is degraded by the enzyme **acetylcholinesterase (AChE)**.

There are several different neurotransmitters and neurotransmitter receptors. Some of the other neurotransmitters are **gamma-aminobutyric acid (GABA)**, **serotonin**, **dopamine**, and **norepinephrine**. If a neurotransmitter, such as acetylcholine, opens a channel that depolarizes the postsynaptic membrane, the neurotransmitter is termed **excitatory**. Other neurotransmitters, however, have the opposite effect, making the postsynaptic membrane potential more negative than the resting potential, or hyperpolarized. Neurotransmitters that induce hyperpolarization of the postsynaptic membrane are termed **inhibitory**. (Note, however, that ultimately it is not the *neurotransmitter* that determines the effect on the postsynaptic cell, it is the *receptor* for that neurotransmitter and its associated ion channel. The same neurotransmitter can be excitatory in some cases and inhibitory in others.) Postsynaptic neurons may have many different receptors, allowing them to respond to many different neurotransmitters.

- If a neurotransmitter causes the entry of chloride into the postsynaptic cell, is the neurotransmitter excitatory or inhibitory?[17]

- If an inhibitor of acetylcholinesterase is added to a neuromuscular junction, then the postsynaptic membrane will:[18]
    - A) be depolarized by action potentials more frequently.
    - B) be depolarized longer with each action potential.
    - C) be resistant to depolarization.
    - D) spontaneously depolarize.

- Signals can be sent in only one direction through synapses such as the neuromuscular junction. Which of the following best explains unidirectional signaling at synapses between neurons?[19]
    - A) The neurotransmitter is always degraded by the postsynaptic cell or in the synaptic cleft.
    - B) Only the presynaptic cell has vesicles of neurotransmitter.
    - C) Axons can propagate action potentials in only one direction.
    - D) Only the postsynaptic cell has a resting membrane potential.

Summation

Once an action potential is initiated in a neuron, it will propagate to the end of the axon at a speed and magnitude of depolarization that do not vary from one action potential to another. The action potential is an "**all-or-nothing**" event. The key regulated step in the nervous system is whether or not a neuron will fire an action potential. Action potentials are initiated when the postsynaptic membrane reaches the threshold depolarization (about −50 mV) required to open voltage-gated sodium channels. The postsynaptic depolarization caused by the release of neurotransmitter by one action potential at one synapse is not generally sufficient to induce this degree of depolarization. A postsynaptic neuron has many different neurons with synapses leading to it, however, and each of these synapses can release neurotransmitter many times per second. The "decision" by a postsynaptic neuron whether to fire an action potential is determined by adding the effect of all of the synapses impinging on a neuron, both excitatory and inhibitory. This addition of stimuli is termed **summation**.

---

[17] Chloride ions are negatively charged. The entry of chloride ions into the cell will make the postsynaptic potential more negative, or hyperpolarized, so the neurotransmitter is inhibitory.

[18] Choice **B** is the correct answer. If acetylcholinesterase is inhibited, acetylcholine will remain in the synaptic cleft longer, and acetylcholine-gated sodium channels will remain open longer with each action potential that reaches the synapse. If the sodium channels are open longer, the depolarization of the postsynaptic membrane will last longer.

[19] Signaling is unidirectional because only the presynaptic cell has vesicles of neurotransmitter that are released in response to action potentials, and only the postsynaptic neuron has receptors that bind neurotransmitter to either depolarize or hyperpolarize the cell (choice **B** is correct). The degradation of neurotransmitter is irrelevant to the direction of signal propagation (choice A is wrong), axons are capable of propagating action potentials in both directions (even though this is not what they normally do; choice C is wrong), and all cells have a resting membrane potential (choice D is wrong).

Excitatory neurotransmitters cause postsynaptic depolarization, or **excitatory postsynaptic potentials (EPSPs)**, while inhibitory neurotransmitters cause **inhibitory postsynaptic potentials (IPSPs)**. One form of summation is **temporal summation**, in which a presynaptic neuron fires action potentials so rapidly that the EPSPs or IPSPs pile up on top of one another. If they are EPSPs, the additive effect might be enough to reach the threshold depolarization required to start a postsynaptic action potential. If they are IPSPs, the postsynaptic cell will hyperpolarize, moving further and further away from threshold, effectively becoming inhibited. The other form of summation is **spatial summation**, in which the EPSPs and IPSPs from all of the synapses on the postsynaptic membrane are summed at a given moment in time. If the total of all EPSPs and IPSPs causes the postsynaptic membrane to reach the threshold voltage, an action potential will be fired.

- In which one of the following ways can a presynaptic neuron increase the intensity of signal it transmits?[20]
    - A) Increase the size of presynaptic action potentials
    - B) Increase the frequency of action potentials
    - C) Change the type of neurotransmitter it releases
    - D) Change the speed of action potential propagation

8.3 FUNCTIONAL ORGANIZATION OF THE HUMAN NERVOUS SYSTEM

The nervous system must receive information, decide what to do with it, and cause muscles or glands to act upon that decision. Receiving information is the **sensory** function of the nervous system (carried out by the peripheral nervous system, or **PNS**), processing the information is the **integrative** function (carried out by the central nervous system, or **CNS**), and acting on it is the **motor** function (also carried out by the PNS).[21] **Motor neurons** carry information from the nervous system toward organs which can act upon that information, known as **effectors**. [What are the two types of effectors?[22]] Notice that "motor" neurons do not lead only "to muscle." Motor neurons, which carry information away from the central nervous system and innervate effectors, are called **efferent** neurons (remember, efferents go to effectors). **Sensory neurons**, which carry information toward the central nervous system, are called **afferent** neurons.

---

[20] A neuron cannot change the size of action potentials it transmits, but it can increase the *number* of action potentials it transmits in a given amount of time (the *frequency* of action potentials). The increased frequency of action potentials will add up through temporal summation in the postsynaptic cell to produce an increased response (choice **B** is correct). Action potentials are all-or-nothing once they are started. The magnitude of membrane depolarization during propagation of the action potential does not change (choice A is wrong). A neuron does not change the neurotransmitter it releases (choice C is wrong), and the speed of propagation cannot be varied from one action potential to the next (choice D is wrong).

[21] More detailed information about the anatomy and functions of the CNS and PNS will be presented later in this chapter.

[22] Muscles and glands

Reflexes

The simplest example of nervous system activity is the **reflex**. This is a direct motor response to sensory input which occurs without conscious thought. In fact, it usually occurs without any involvement of the brain at all. In the simplest example, a sensory neuron transmits an action potential to a synapse with a motor neuron in the spinal cord, which causes an action to occur. For example, in the **muscle stretch reflex**, a sensory neuron detects stretching of a muscle (Figure 7). The sensory neuron has a long dendrite and a long axon, which transmits an impulse to a motor neuron cell body in the spinal cord. The motor neuron's long axon synapses with the muscle that was stretched and causes it to contract. That is why the quadriceps (thigh) muscle contracts when the patellar tendon is stretched by tapping it with a reflex hammer. A reflex such as this one, involving only two neurons and one synapse, is known as a **monosynaptic reflex arc.**

Something else also happens when a physician taps the patellar tendon. Not only does the quadriceps *contract*, but the hamstring also *relaxes*. If it did not, the leg would not be able to extend (straighten). The sensory neuron (that detects stretch) synapses with not only a motor neuron for the quadriceps, but also with an **inhibitory interneuron**. This is a short neuron which forms an inhibitory synapse with a motor neuron innervating the hamstring muscle. When the sensory neuron is stimulated by stretch, it stimulates both the quadriceps motor neuron and the inhibitory interneuron to the hamstring motor neuron. The interneuron inhibits the motor neuron for the hamstring. As a result, the quadriceps contracts and the hamstring relaxes (note that the hamstring part of the reflex—sensory neuron to interneuron to hamstring motor neuron—involves three neurons and two synapses, hence it is known as a **disynaptic reflex arc**). An interneuron is the simplest example of the integrative role of the nervous system. Concurrent relaxation of the hamstring and contraction of the quadriceps is an example of **reciprocal inhibition**.

- If a reflex occurs without the involvement of the brain, how are we aware of the action?[23]

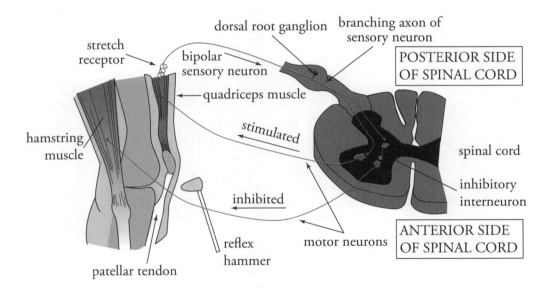

Figure 7 The Muscle Stretch Reflex

---

[23] Two ways: first, the sensory neuron also branches to form a synapse with a neuron leading to the brain. Second, other sensory information is received after the action is taken.

Large-Scale Functional Organization

The peripheral nervous system can be subdivided into several functional divisions (Figure 8). The portion of this system concerned with conscious sensation and deliberate, voluntary movement of skeletal muscle is the **somatic** division. The portion concerned with digestion, metabolism, circulation, perspiration, and other involuntary processes is the **autonomic** division. The somatic and autonomic divisions both include afferent and efferent functions, though the sources of sensory input and the target of efferent nerves are different. The efferent portion of the autonomic division is further split into two subdivisions: **sympathetic** and **parasympathetic**. When the sympathetic system is activated, the body is prepared for "fight or flight." When the parasympathetic system is activated, the body is prepared to "rest and digest." Table 2 summarizes the main effects of the autonomic system. Notice that many sympathetic effects result from release of epinephrine[24] into the bloodstream by the adrenal medulla. The parasympathetic system prepares you to rest and digest food.

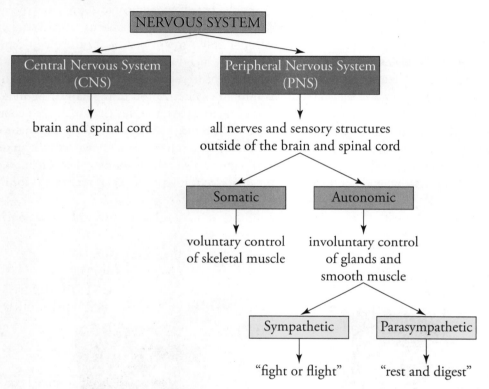

Figure 8 Overall Organization of the Nervous System

---

[24] In Greek, "epi" means upon or on top of, and "nephr" refers to the kidney (as in nephron, the microscopic functional unit of the kidney); thus epinephrine is "the hormone secreted by the gland on top of the kidney." Another name for epinephrine is adrenaline. In Latin, "ad" also means upon, and "renal" likewise refers to the kidney. The gland which secretes epinephrine is the adrenal gland.

Table 2 Effects of the Autonomic Nervous System

Organ or System	Parasympathetic: rest and digest	Sympathetic: fight or flight
digestive system: glands	stimulation	inhibition
motility	stimulation (stimulates digestion)	inhibition (inhibits digestion)
sphincters	relaxation	contraction
urinary system: bladder	contraction (stimulates urination)	relaxation (inhibits urination)
urethral sphincter	relaxation (stimulates urination)	contraction (inhibits urination)
bronchial smooth muscle	constriction (closes airways)	relaxation (opens airways)
cardiovascular system		
heart rate and contractility	decreased	increased
blood flow to skeletal muscle	—	increased
skin	—	sweating and general vasoconstriction
eye: pupil	constriction	dilation
muscles controlling lens	accommodation for near vision	accommodation for far vision
adrenal medulla	—	release of epinephrine
genitals	erection / lubrication	ejaculation / orgasm

8.4 ANATOMICAL ORGANIZATION OF THE NERVOUS SYSTEM

The main anatomical division of the nervous system is between the **central nervous system** (**CNS**) and the **peripheral nervous system** (**PNS**). The central nervous system is the brain and spinal cord. The peripheral nervous system includes all other axons, dendrites, and cell bodies. Bundles of myelinated axons in both the CNS and PNS is referred to as **white matter**; specifically, white matter in the brain is called a **tract**, white matter in the spinal cord is called a **tract** or a **column**, and white matter in the PNS is called a **nerve**. Unmyelinated neuronal cell bodies in both the CNS and PNS are referred to as **grey matter**; specifically, grey matter deep in the brain is called a **nucleus**, grey matter on the surface of the brain is called **cortex**, grey matter in the spinal cord is called a **horn**, and grey matter in the PNS is a **ganglion**.

CNS Anatomical Organization

The CNS includes the **spinal cord** and the brain. The brain has three subdivisions: the **hindbrain** (or the rhombencephalon), the **midbrain** (or the mesencephalon), and the **forebrain** (or the prosencephalon). These four regions of the CNS (which will be discussed individually below) perform increasingly complex functions. The entire CNS (brain and spinal cord) floats in **cerebrospinal fluid** (**CSF**), a clear liquid that serves various functions such as shock absorption and exchange of nutrients and waste with the CNS.

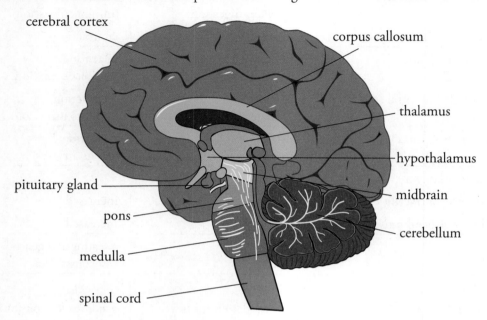

Figure 9   Organization of the CNS (cross-section of the brain)

1) The spinal cord is connected to the brain and is protected by the CSF and the vertebral column. It is a pathway for information to and from the brain. Most sensory data is relayed to the brain for integration, but the spinal cord is also a site for information integration and processing. The spinal cord is responsible for simple spinal reflexes (like the muscle stretch reflex) and is also involved in primitive processes such as walking, urination, and sex organ function.

2) The hindbrain includes the medulla, the pons, and the cerebellum.

   • The **medulla** (or medulla oblongata) is located below the pons and is the area of the brain that connects to the spinal cord. It functions in relaying information between other areas of the brain and regulates vital autonomic functions such as blood pressure and digestive functions (including vomiting). Also, the respiratory rhythmicity centers are found here.

   • The **pons** is located below the midbrain and above the medulla oblongata. It is the connection point between the brain stem and the cerebellum (see below). The pons controls some autonomic functions and coordinates movement; it plays a role in balance and antigravity posture.

   • The **cerebellum** (or "little brain") is located behind the pons and below the cerebral hemispheres. It is an integrating center where complex movements are coordinated. An instruction for movement from the forebrain must be sent to the cerebellum, where the billions of decisions necessary for smooth execution of the movement are made. Damage to the cerebellum results in poor hand-eye coordination and balance. Both the cerebellum and the pons receive information from the vestibular apparatus in the inner ear, which monitors acceleration and position relative to gravity.

3) The midbrain is a relay for visual and auditory information and contains much of the reticular activating system (RAS), which is responsible for arousal or wakefulness.

Another term you should be familiar with is **brainstem**. Together, the medulla, pons, and midbrain constitute the brainstem, which contains important processing centers and relays information to or from the cerebellum and cerebrum.

4) The forebrain includes the **diencephalon** and the **telencephalon**.
a) The diencephalon includes the thalamus and hypothalamus:
* The thalamus is located near the middle of the brain below the cerebral hemispheres and above the midbrain. It contains relay and processing centers for sensory information.
* The hypothalamus interacts directly with many parts of the brain. It contains centers for controlling emotions and autonomic functions, and has a major role in hormone production and release. It is the primary link between the nervous and the endocrine systems, and by controlling the pituitary gland is the fundamental control center for the endocrine system (discussed later in this chapter).
b) All parts of the CNS up to and including the diencephalon form a single symmetrical stalk, but the telencephalon consists of two separate cerebral hemispheres. Generally speaking, the areas of the left and right hemispheres have the same functions. However, the left hemisphere primarily controls the motor functions of the right side of the body, and the right hemisphere controls those of the left side. Also, in most people, the left side of the brain is said to be dominant. It is generally responsible for speech. The right hemisphere is more concerned with visual-spatial reasoning and music.
* The **cerebral hemispheres** are connected by a thick bundle of axons called the **corpus callosum**. A person with a cut corpus callosum has two independent cerebral cortices and to a certain extent two independent minds![25]
* The **cerebrum** is the largest region of the human brain and consists of the large, paired cerebral hemispheres. The hemispheres of the cerebrum consist of the **cerebral cortex** (an outer layer of gray matter) plus an inner core of white matter connecting the cortex to the diencephalon.[26] The gray matter is composed of trillions of somas; the white matter is composed of myelinated axons. (Most axons in the CNS and PNS are myelinated.) The cerebral hemispheres are responsible for conscious thought processes and intellectual functions. They also play a role in processing somatic sensory and motor information. The cerebral cortex is divided into four pairs of lobes, each of which is devoted to specific functions:
  i) The **frontal lobes** initiate all voluntary movement and are involved in complex reasoning skills and problem solving.
  ii) The **parietal lobes** are involved in general sensations (such as touch, temperature, pressure, vibration, etc.) and in gustation (taste).
  iii) The **temporal lobes** process auditory and olfactory sensation and are involved in short-term memory, language comprehension, and emotion.
  iv) The **occipital lobes** process visual sensation.

---

[25] Anyone interested in reading about jaw-dropping neurological cases should begin with Oliver Sacks' *The Man Who Mistook His Wife for a Hat*. You will *not* be sorry if you buy this book.

[26] The word *cortex* means "outside layer"; for example, an orange peel may be called the cortex of the orange; the outside layer of a gland is also known as its cortex.

Figure 10 shows some of the more important cortical areas.

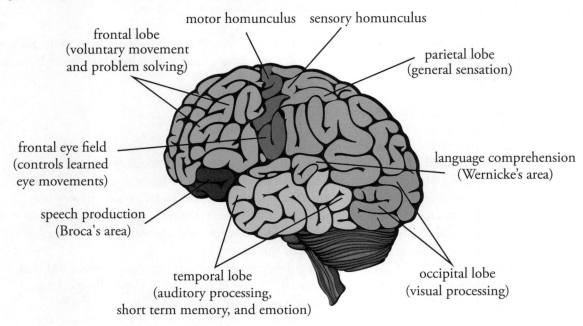

Figure 10 Principal Areas of the Cerebral Cortex

Two last regions of the brain deserve mention:

* The **basal nuclei** (also called the "cerebral nuclei," and previously known as the basal ganglia) are composed of gray matter and are located deep within the cerebral hemispheres. They include several functional subdivisions, but broadly function in voluntary motor control and procedural learning related to habits. The basal nuclei and cerebellum work together to process and coordinate movement initiated by the primary motor cortex; the basal nuclei are inhibitory (preventing excess movement), while the cerebellum is excitatory.

* The **limbic system** is located between the cerebrum and the diencephalon. It includes several substructures (such as the amygdala, the cingulate gyrus, and the hippocampus) and works closely with parts of the cerebrum, diencephalon, and midbrain. The limbic system is important in emotion and memory.

The information above describes the general functions of each region of the brain. Table 3 summarizes the brain functions and provides a little more specific detail for each region.

Table 3 Summary of Brain Functions

Structure	General Function	Specific Functions
Spinal cord	Simple reflexes	• controls simple stretch and tendon reflexes • controls primitive processes such as walking, urination, and sex organ function
Medulla	Involuntary functions	• controls autonomic processes such as blood pressure, blood flow, heart rate, respiratory rate, swallowing, vomiting • controls reflex reactions such as coughing or sneezing • relays sensory information to the cerebellum and the thalamus

Structure	General Function	Specific Functions
Pons	Relay station and balance	• controls antigravity posture and balance • connects spinal cord and medulla with upper regions of brain • relays information to the cerebellum and thalamus
Cerebellum	Movement coordination	• integrating center • coordination of complex movement, balance and posture, muscle tone, spatial equilibrium
Midbrain	Eye movement	• integration of visual and auditory information • visual and auditory reflexes • wakefulness and consciousness • coordinates information on posture and muscle tone
Thalamus	Integrating center and relay station	• relay center for somatic (conscious) sensation (except olfactory sensory input) • relays information between spinal cord and cerebral cortex
Hypo-thalamus	Homeostasis and behavior	• controls homeostatic functions (such as temperature regulation, fluid balance, appetite) through both neural and hormonal regulation • controls primitive emotions such as anger, rage, and sex drive • controls the pituitary gland
Basal nuclei	Movement	• regulate body movement and muscle tone • coordination of learned movement patterns • general pattern of rhythmic movements (such as controlling the cycle of arm and leg movements when walking) • subconscious adjustments of conscious movements
Limbic system	Emotion, memory, and learning	• controls emotional states • links conscious and unconscious portions of the brain • helps with memory storage and retrieval
Cerebral cortex	Perception, skeletal muscle movement, memory, attention, thought, language, and consciousness	• divided into four lobes (frontal, parietal, temporal, and occipital) with specialized subfunctions • perception and processing of the special senses (vision, hearing, smell, taste, touch) • conscious thought processes and planning, awareness, and sensation • intellectual function (intelligence, learning, reading, communication) • abstract thought and reasoning • memory storage and retrieval • initiation and coordination of voluntary movement • complex motor patterns • language (speech production and understanding) • personality
Corpus callosum	Connection	• connects the left and right cerebral hemispheres

8.4

The motor and sensory regions of the cortex are organized such that a particular small area of cortex controls a particular body part. A larger area is devoted to a body part which requires more motor control or more sensation (Figure 11). For example, more cortex is devoted to the lips than to the entire leg. The body parts represented on the cortex can be sketched. The drawing looks like a distorted person, known as a **homunculus** (little man).

Figure 11   The Sensory Homunculus

PNS Anatomical Organization

All neurons entering and exiting the CNS are carried by 12 pairs of **cranial nerves** and 31 pairs of **spinal nerves**. Cranial nerves convey sensory and motor information to and from the brainstem. Spinal nerves convey sensory and motor information to and from the spinal cord. The different functional divisions of the nervous system have different anatomical organizations (Figure 12).

The **vagus nerve** is an important example of a cranial nerve, and one that you should be familiar with for the MCAT. The effects of this nerve upon the heart and GI tract are to decrease the heart rate and increase GI activity; as such it is part of the *parasympathetic division* of the autonomic nervous system. It is a bundle of axons that end in ganglia on the surface of the heart, stomach, and other visceral organs. The many axons constituting the vagus nerve are preganglionic and come from cell bodies located in the CNS. On the surface of the heart and stomach they synapse with postganglionic neurons. The detailed terminology in this paragraph will make more sense to you as you read through the next couple of sections.

Somatic PNS Anatomy

The somatic system has a simple organization:

- *All* somatic motor neurons innervate skeletal muscle cells, use ACh as their neurotransmitter, and have their cell bodies in the brain stem or the ventral (front) portion of the spinal cord.

- *All* somatic sensory neurons have a long dendrite extending from a sensory receptor toward the soma, which is located just outside the CNS in a **dorsal root ganglion**. The dorsal root ganglion is a bunch of somatic (and autonomic) sensory neuron cell bodies located just dorsal to (to the back of) the spinal cord. There is a pair of dorsal root ganglia for every segment of the spinal cord, and thus the dorsal root ganglia form a chain along the dorsal (back) aspect of the vertebral column. The dorsal root ganglia are protected within the vertebral column but are outside the **meninges** (protective sheath of the brain and cord) and thus outside the CNS. An axon extends from the somatic sensory neuron's soma into the spinal cord. In all somatic sensory neurons, the first synapse is in the CNS; depending on the type of sensory information conveyed, the axon either synapses in the cord, or stretches all the way up to the brain stem before its first synapse!

Autonomic PNS Anatomy

Anatomical organization of autonomic efferents is a bit more complex.[27] The efferents of the sympathetic and parasympathetic systems consist of two neurons: a preganglionic and a postganglionic neuron. The **preganglionic neuron** has its cell body in the brainstem or spinal cord. It sends an axon to an autonomic ganglion, located outside the spinal column. In the ganglion, this axon synapses with a **postganglionic neuron**. The postganglionic neuron sends an axon to an effector (smooth muscle or gland). *All* autonomic preganglionic neurons release acetylcholine as their neurotransmitter. *All* parasympathetic postganglionic neurons also release acetylcholine. Nearly all sympathetic postganglionic neurons release norepinephrine (NE, also known as noradrenaline) as their neurotransmitter.

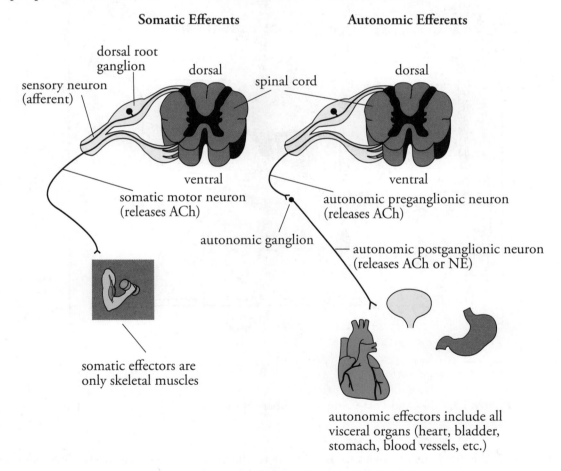

Figure 12 Anatomical Organization of PNS Efferents

---

[27] The anatomy of autonomic sensory neurons (afferents) is poorly defined and will not be on the MCAT.

All sympathetic preganglionic efferent neurons have their cell bodies in the thoracic (chest) or lumbar (lower back) regions of the spinal cord. Hence the sympathetic system is also referred to as the *thoraco-lumbar system*. The parasympathetic system is known as the *craniosacral system*, because all of its preganglionic neurons have cell bodies in the brainstem (which is in the head or cranium) or in the lowest portion of the spinal cord, the sacral portion. In the sympathetic system, the preganglionic axon is relatively short, and there are only a few ganglia; these sympathetic ganglia are quite large. The sympathetic postganglionic cell sends a long axon to the effector. In contrast, the parasympathetic preganglionic neuron sends a long axon to a small ganglion which is close to the effector. For example, parasympathetic ganglia controlling the intestines are located on the outer wall of the gut. The parasympathetic postganglionic neuron has a very short axon, since the cell body is close to the target.[28] These differences are visualized in Figure 13 and summarized in Table 4.

Figure 13 Pre- and Post-Ganglionic Fibers of the Autonomic Nervous System

The autonomic afferent (sensory) neurons are similar to the somatic afferent neurons with one exception: they can synapse in the PNS (at the autonomic ganglia) with autonomic efferent neurons in what is known as a "short reflex." (Recall that the first synapse of somatic afferent neurons is in the CNS.)

---

[28] The mnemonic "*p*ara long *p*re" will help you in med school.

Table 4 Sympathetic vs. Parasympathetic

	Sympathetic	Parasympathetic
General function	fight or flight, mobilize energy	rest and digest, store energy
Location of preganglionic soma	thoracolumbar = thoracic and lumbar spinal cord	craniosacral = brainstem ("cranial") and sacral spinal cord
Preganglionic axon neurotransmitter = acetylcholine (ACh)	short	long
Ganglia	close to cord, far from target	far from cord, close to target
Postganglionic axon (usual neurotransmitter)	long (norepinephrine [NE])	short (acetylcholine [ACh])

8.5

The Adrenal Medulla

The **adrenal gland** is named for its location: "Ad-" connotes "above," and "renal" refers to the kidney. There are two adrenal glands, one above each kidney. The adrenal has an inner portion known as the **medulla** and an outer portion known as the **cortex**. The cortex is an important endocrine gland, secreting **glucocorticoids** (the main one is cortisol), **mineralocorticoids** (the main one is aldosterone), and some sex hormones.

The adrenal medulla, however, is part of the sympathetic nervous system. It is embryologically derived from sympathetic postganglionic neurons and is directly innervated by sympathetic preganglionic neurons. Upon activation of the sympathetic system, the adrenal gland is stimulated to release **epinephrine**, also known as **adrenaline**. Epinephrine is a slightly modified version of *nor*epinephrine, the neurotransmitter released by sympathetic postganglionic neurons. Epinephrine is a hormone because it is released into the bloodstream by a ductless gland. But in many ways it behaves like a neurotransmitter. It elicits its effects very rapidly, and the effects are quite short-lived. Ongoing release of epinephrine from the adrenal medulla during fight-or-flight situations prolongs and enhances the effects of the sympathetic neurons. In general, epinephrine's effects are those listed in Table 2 for the sympathetic system. Stimulation of the heart is an especially important effect.

8.5 SENSATION AND PERCEPTION

Sensation is the process by which we receive information from the world around us. Sensory receptors detect data, both internally (from within the body) and externally (from the environment), and send this information to the central nervous system for processing. Sensation is the act of receiving information, while perception is the act of organizing, assimilating, and interpreting the sensory input into useful and meaningful information.

Types of Sensory Receptors

Sensory receptors are designed to detect one type of stimulus from either the interior of the body or the external environment. Each sensory receptor receives only one kind of information and transmits that information to sensory neurons, which can in turn convey it to the central nervous system. [How does the brain know the difference between stimulation of visual receptors and olfactory receptors?[29]] Sensory receptors that detect stimuli from the outside world are **exteroceptors** and receptors that respond to internal stimuli are **interoceptors**. A more important distinction between sensory receptors is based on the type of stimulus they detect. The types of sensory receptors are listed below.

1) **Mechanoreceptors** respond to mechanical disturbances. For example, **Pacinian corpuscles** are pressure sensors located deep in the skin. The Pacinian corpuscle is shaped like an onion. It is composed of concentric layers of specialized membranes. When the corpuscular membranes are distorted by firm pressure on the skin, the nerve ending becomes depolarized and the signal travels up the dendrite (note that these are graded potential changes—*not* action potentials). Another important mechanoreceptor is the **auditory hair cell**. This is a specialized cell found in the cochlea of the inner ear. It detects vibrations caused by sound waves. **Vestibular hair cells** are located within special organs called semicircular canals, also found in the inner ear. Their role is to detect acceleration and position relative to gravity. An example of an autonomic mechanoreceptor would be a receptor detecting stretch of the intestinal wall.

2) **Chemoreceptors** respond to particular chemicals. For example, **olfactory receptors** detect airborne chemicals and allow us to smell things. Taste buds are **gustatory receptors**. Autonomic chemoreceptors in the walls of the carotid and aortic arteries respond to changes in arterial pH, PCO_2, and PO_2 levels.

3) **Nociceptors** are pain receptors.[30] They are stimulated by tissue injury. Nociceptors are the simplest type of sensory receptor, generally consisting of a free nerve ending that detects chemical signs of tissue damage. (In that sense the nociceptor is a simple chemoreceptor.) Nociceptors may be somatic or autonomic. Autonomic pain receptors do not provide the conscious mind with clear pain information, but they frequently give a sensation of dull, aching pain. They may also create the illusion of pain on the skin, when their nerves cross paths with somatic afferents from the skin. This phenomenon is known as **referred pain**.

4) **Thermoreceptors** are stimulated by changes in temperature. There are autonomic and somatic examples. Peripheral thermoreceptors fall into three categories: cold-sensitive, warm-sensitive, and thermal nociceptors, which detect painfully hot stimuli.

5) **Electromagnetic receptors** are stimulated by electromagnetic waves. In humans, the only examples are the rod and cone cells of the retina of the eye (also termed **photoreceptors**). In other animals, electroreceptors and magnetoreceptors are separate. For example, some fish can detect electric fields with electroreceptors, and magnetoreceptors allow animals to sense the Earth's magnetic field, which can help them navigate during migration.

Encoding of Sensory Stimuli

All sensory receptors need to encode relevant information regarding the nature of the stimulus being detected. There are four properties that need to be communicated to the CNS:

1) Stimulus **modality** is the type of stimulus. As mentioned above, the CNS determines the stimulus modality based on which type of receptor is firing.

---

[29] Both signals are received in the brain as action potentials from sensory neurons. The brain distinguishes the sensory stimuli based on which sensory neurons are signaling.

[30] *Noci-* is from the Latin *nocuus*, meaning harmful, as in *noxious*.

2) Stimulus **location** is communicated by the receptive field of the sensory receptor sending the signal. Localization of a stimulus can be improved by overlapping receptive fields of neighboring receptors. This works like a Venn diagram, and allows the brain to localize a stimulus activating neighboring receptors to the area in which their receptive fields overlap. Discrimination between two separate stimuli can be improved by lateral inhibition of neighboring receptors.

3) Stimulus **intensity** is coded by the frequency of action potentials. The *dynamic range*, or range of intensities that can be detected by sensory receptors, can be expanded by range fractionation—including multiple groups of receptors with limited ranges to detect a wider range overall. One example of this phenomenon is human cone cells responding to different but overlapping ranges of wavelengths to detect the full visual spectrum of light.

4) Stimulus **duration** may or may not be coded explicitly. *Tonic receptors* fire action potentials as long as the stimulus continues. However, these receptors are subject to adaptation, and the frequency of action potentials decreases as the stimulus continues at the same level (see below). *Phasic receptors* only fire action potentials when the stimulus begins, and do not explicitly communicate the duration of the stimulus. These receptors are important for communicating changes in stimuli, and essentially adapt immediately if a stimulus continues at the same level.

The ability to adapt to a stimulus is an important property of sensory receptors. This allows the brain to tune out unimportant information from the environment. **Adaptation** is a decrease in firing frequency when the intensity of a stimulus remains constant. For example, if you walk into a kitchen where someone is baking bread, the bread odor molecules stimulate your olfactory receptors to a great degree and you smell the bread baking. But if you remain in the kitchen for a few minutes, you stop smelling the bread; the continuous input to the olfactory receptors causes them to stop firing even though the odor molecules are still present. This is what allows us to "get used to" certain environments and situations, for example, cold pool water, loud background noise, etc. The receptors don't stop being *able* to respond; they can be retriggered if the stimulus intensity increases. For example, if you open up the oven door, you will smell the bread again. Likewise, if you are used to the background noise in a restaurant, but someone drops a plate, you'll hear it. In other words: the nervous system is programmed to respond to *changing stimuli* and not so much to constant stimuli, because for the most part, constant stimuli are not a threat, whereas changing stimuli might need to be dealt with. (Note that nociceptors *do not adapt* under any circumstance. We can learn to ignore them, but pain is something that the nervous system wants us to *do* something about since it is an indication that something is wrong.)

Proprioceptors

This is a broad category including many different types of receptors. **Proprioception** refers to awareness of self (i.e., awareness of body part position) and is also known as your **kinesthetic sense**.[31] An important example of a proprioceptor is the **muscle spindle**, a mechanoreceptor. This is a sensory organ specialized to detect muscle stretch. You are already familiar with it because it is the receptor that senses muscle stretch in the deep tendon reflex. Other proprioceptors include **Golgi tendon organs**, which monitor tension in the tendons, and **joint capsule receptors**, which detect pressure, tension, and movement in the joints. By monitoring the activity of the musculoskeletal system, the proprioceptive component of the somatic sensory system allows us to know the positions of our body parts. This is most important during activity, when precise feedback is essential for coordinated motion. [What portion of the CNS would you expect to require input from proprioceptors?[32]]

---

[31] *Proprio-* means *of or pertaining to the self*, as in "proprietary."

[32] The cerebellum, which is responsible for motor coordination

Gustation and Olfaction

Taste and smell are senses that rely on chemoreceptors in the mouth and nasal passages. **Gustation** is taste, and **olfaction** is smell. Much of what is assumed to be taste is actually smell. (Try eating with a bad head cold.) In fact, taste receptors (known as **taste buds**) can only distinguish five flavors: sweet (glucose), salty (Na^+), bitter (basic), sour (acidic), and umami (amino acids and nucleotides). Each taste bud responds most strongly to one of these five stimuli. The taste bud is composed of a bunch of specialized epithelial cells, shaped roughly like an onion. In its center is a **taste pore**, with **taste hairs** that detect food chemicals. Information about taste is transmitted by cranial nerves to an area of the brain's parietal lobe.

Olfaction is accomplished by olfactory receptors in the roof of the **nasopharynx** (nasal cavity). The receptors detect airborne chemicals that dissolve in the mucus covering the nasal membrane. Humans can distinguish thousands of different smells. Olfactory nerves project directly to the **olfactory bulbs** of the brain. The olfactory bulbs are located in the temporal lobe of the brain near the limbic system, an area important for memory and emotion (which may explain why certain smells can bring back vivid memories and feelings).

Interestingly, the perception of a smell as "good" or "bad" is entirely learned, based on experiences with those smells. There is no smell that is universally noxious to people (though the military has tried to find one in order to develop a "stink" bomb), because different smells can be associated with good or bad experiences based on culture and upbringing.

Pheromones are chemical signals that cause a social response in members of the same species. Though not well understood in humans, pheromones have been studied extensively in insects, particularly those species with complex social structures (such as bees and ants). Pheromones are an important means of communicating information; for example, alarm pheromones will alert the rest of the beehive of danger, food-trail pheromones allow ants to follow a trail to a promising food source, and sex pheromones play an important role in mating between most species. In humans, pheromones are much harder to study.

Hearing and the Vestibular System

Structure of the Ear

The **auricle** or **pinna** and the external **auditory canal** comprise the **outer ear**. The **middle ear** is divided from the outer ear by the **tympanic membrane** or eardrum. The middle ear consists of the **ossicles**, three small bones called the **malleus** (hammer), the **incus** (anvil), and the **stapes** (stirrup). The stapes attaches to the **oval window**, a membrane that divides the middle and **inner ear**. Structures of the inner ear include the **cochlea**, the **semicircular canals**, the **utricle**, and the **saccule**. The semicircular canals together with the utricle and saccule are important to the sense of balance. The **round window** is a membrane-covered hole in the cochlea near the oval window. It releases excess pressure. The **Eustachian tube** (also known as the **auditory tube**) is a passageway from the back of the throat to the middle ear. It functions to equalize the pressure on both sides of the eardrum and is the cause of the "ear popping" one experiences at high altitudes or underwater.

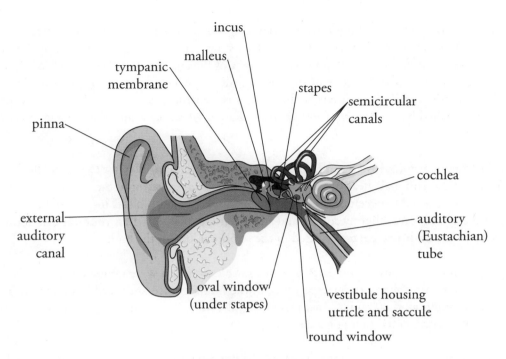

Figure 14   The Ear

Mechanism of Hearing

Sound waves enter the external ear to pass into the auditory canal, causing the eardrum to vibrate. The malleus attached to the eardrum receives the vibrations, which are passed on to the incus and then to the stapes. The bones of the middle ear are arranged in such a way that they amplify sound vibrations passing through the middle ear. The stapes is the innermost of the three middle-ear bones, contacting the oval window. Vibration of the oval window creates pressure waves in the **perilymph** and **endolymph**, the fluids in the cochlea. Note that sound vibrations are first conveyed through air, next through bone, and then through liquid before being sensed. The pressure waves in the endolymph cause vibration of the **basilar membrane**, a thin membrane extending throughout the coiled length of the cochlea. The basilar membrane is covered with the auditory receptor cells known as **hair cells**. These cells have **cilia** (hairs) projecting from their apical (top) surfaces (opposite the basilar membrane). The hairs contact the **tectorial membrane** (tectorial means "roof"), and when the basilar membrane moves, the hairs are dragged across the tectorial membrane and they bend. This displacement opens ion channels in the hair cells, which results in neurotransmitter release. Dendrites from bipolar auditory afferent neurons are stimulated by this neurotransmitter, and thus sound vibrations are converted to nerve impulses. The basilar membrane, hair cells, and tectorial membrane together are known as the **organ of Corti**. The outer ear and middle ear convey sound waves to the cochlea, and the organ of Corti in the cochlea is the primary site at which auditory stimuli are detected.

Summary: From Sound to Hearing

sound waves → auricle → external auditory canal → tympanic membrane → malleus → incus → stapes → oval window → perilymph → endolymph → basilar membrane → auditory hair cells → tectorial membrane → neurotransmitters stimulate bipolar auditory neurons → brain → perception

---

Pitch (frequency) of sound is distinguished by which *regions* of the basilar membrane vibrate, stimulating different auditory neurons. The basilar membrane is narrow, thick, and sturdy near the oval window and gradually becomes wider, thin, and floppy near the apex of the cochlea. Low frequency (long wavelength) sounds stimulate hair cells at the apex of the cochlear duct, farthest away from the oval window, while high-pitched sounds stimulate hair cells at the base of the cochlea, near the oval window. **Loudness** of sound is distinguished by the *amplitude* of vibration. Larger vibrations cause more frequent action potentials in auditory neurons.

Locating the source of sound is also an important adaptive function. Having two ears allows for stereo-phonic (or three-dimensional) hearing. The auditory system can determine the source of a sound based on the difference detected between the two ears. For example, if a horn blasts to your right, your right ear will receive the sound waves slightly sooner and slightly more intensely than your left ear. Sound stimuli are processed in the **auditory cortex**, located in the temporal lobe of the brain.

In humans, audition is highly adaptive. While we are able to hear a wide range of sounds, those sounds with frequencies within the range corresponding to the human voice are heard best, and we are able to differentiate variations among human voices. For example, when answering the phone, you will recognize your mom's voice within a fraction of a second.

- If a sensory neuron leading from the ear to the brain fires an action potential more rapidly, how will the brain perceive this change?[33]
- In some cases of deafness, sound can still be detected by conduction of vibration through the skull to the cochlea. If the auditory nerve is severed, can sound still be detected by conductance through bone?[34]
- If the bones of the middle ear are unable to move, would this impair the detection of sound by conductance through bone?[35]

Equilibrium and Balance

The vestibular complex is made up of the three **semicircular canals**, the **utricle**, the **saccule**, and the **ampullae**. All are essentially tubes filled with endolymph, and like the cochlea, they contain hair cells that detect motion. However, their function is to detect not sound, but rather rotational acceleration of the head. They are innervated by afferent neurons which send balance information to the pons, cerebellum, and other areas. The vestibular complex monitors both static equilibrium and linear acceleration, which contribute to your sense of balance.

Vision: Structure and Function

The eye is the structure designed to detect visual stimuli. The structures of the eye first form an image on the retina, which detects light and converts the stimuli into action potentials to send to the brain. Light enters the eye by passing through the **cornea**, the clear portion at the front of the eye. Light is bent or

---

[33] More rapid firing of a cochlear neuron indicates an increase in volume of sound. If the pitch changed, a different set of neurons would fire action potentials.

[34] Conductance through bone allows some hearing by causing the cochlea to vibrate, which stimulates action potentials that pass through the auditory nerve to the brain. However, if the auditory nerve is severed, no hearing of any kind is possible.

[35] The bones of the middle ear serve to conduct vibration from the outer ear to the liquid within the cochlea but are not involved directly in detecting sound. Bone conductance can still stimulate the cochlea and result in hearing if the middle ear is nonfunctional.

8.5

refracted as it passes through the cornea (which is highly curved and thus acts as a lens), since the refractive index of the cornea is higher than that of air. The cornea is continuous at its borders with the white of the eye, the **sclera**. Beneath the sclera is a layer called the **choroid**. It contains darkly pigmented cells; this pigmentation absorbs excess light within the eye. Beneath the choroid is the **retina**, the surface upon which light is focused.

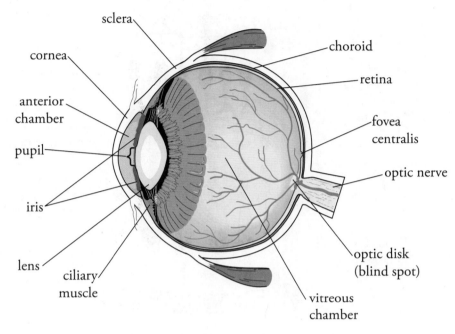

Figure 15   The Eye

Just inside the cornea is the **anterior chamber** (front chamber), which contains a fluid termed **aqueous humor**. At the back of the anterior chamber is a membrane called the **iris** with an opening called the **pupil**. The iris is the colored part of the eye, and muscles in the iris regulate the diameter of the pupil. Just behind the iris is the **posterior chamber**, also containing aqueous humor. In the back part of the posterior chamber is the **lens**. Its role is to fine-tune the angle of incoming light, so that the beams are perfectly focused upon the retina. The curvature of the lens (and thus its refractive power) is varied by the **ciliary muscle**.

Light passes through the **vitreous chamber** en route from the lens to the retina. This chamber contains a thick, jelly-like fluid called **vitreous humor**. The retina is located at the back of the eye. It contains electromagnetic receptor cells (photoreceptors) known as **rods** and **cones** which are responsible for detecting light. The rods and cones synapse with nerve cells called **bipolar cells**. In accordance with the name "bipolar," these cells have only one axon and one dendrite. The bipolar cells in turn synapse with **ganglion cells**, whose axons comprise the **optic nerve**, which travels from each eye toward the occipital lobe of the brain where complex analysis of a visual image occurs. In Figure 16 on the next page, you may notice that light has to pass through two layers of neurons before it can reach the rods and cones. The neurons are fine enough to not significantly obstruct incoming rays.

8.5

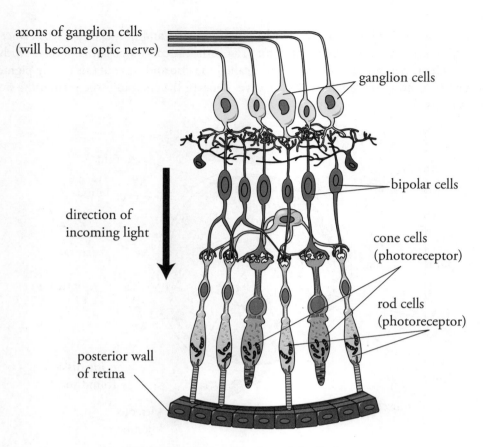

axons of ganglion cells
(will become optic nerve)

ganglion cells

bipolar cells

direction of
incoming light

cone cells
(photoreceptor)

rod cells
(photoreceptor)

posterior wall
of retina

Figure 16   Organization of the Retina

The point on the retina where many axons from ganglion cells converge to form the optic nerve is the **optic disk**. It is also known as the **blind spot** (Figure 17) because it contains no photoreceptors. Another special region of the retina is the **macula**. In the center of the macula is the **fovea centralis** (focal point), which contains only cones and is responsible for extreme visual acuity. When you stare directly at something, you focus its image on the fovea.

A   ●   ●   B

Cover your left eye and focus your right eye on dot A while holding the page about 5 inches away from your face. Move the page forward and back. You will find that at a certain distance, dot B becomes invisible. You are placing dot A on the fovea by focusing on it, and at the correct distance, dot B becomes focused on the blind spot.

Figure 17   Demonstrating the Blind Spot

The Photoreceptors: Rods and Cones

Rods and cones, named because of their shapes, contain special pigment proteins that change their tertiary structure upon absorbing light. Each protein, called an **opsin**, is bound to one molecule of **retinal**, which is derived from vitamin A. In the dark, when the rods and cones are resting, retinal has several *trans* double bonds and one *cis* double bond. In this conformation, retinal and its associated opsin keep a sodium channel open. The cell remains depolarized. Upon absorbing a photon of light, retinal is converted to the **all-trans form**. This triggers a series of reactions that ultimately closes the sodium channel, and the cell hyperpolarizes.

Rods and cones synapse on bipolar cells. Because of their depolarization in the dark, both types of photoreceptors release the neurotransmitter **glutamate** onto the bipolar cells. Upon the absorption of a photon of light and subsequent hyperpolarization, the photoreceptors release less glutamate, or stop releasing it altogether.

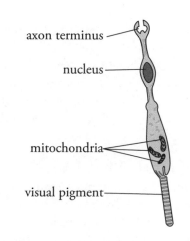

Figure 18   Rod Cell Structure

The effect on the bipolar cells varies. Some bipolar cells are "on center" and are inhibited by glutamate. This means that when the photoreceptor is in the dark and releasing glutamate, the on-center bipolar cell releases very little or no neurotransmitter. However, when the photoreceptor is in the light (light is ON the center), and stops releasing glutamate, the inhibition of the on-center bipolar cell stops, and the bipolar cell increases its release of neurotransmitter. "Off center" bipolar cells work in the opposite manner; they are stimulated by the glutamate released when the photoreceptor is in the dark, and inhibited when glutamate stops being released in the light.

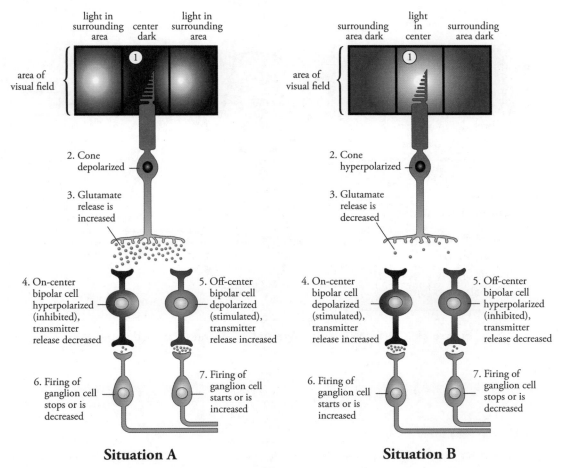

Figure 19   On-Center Off-Center Bipolar Cells

Night vision is accomplished by the rods, which are more sensitive to dim light and motion and are more concentrated in the periphery of the retina. Cones require abundant light and are responsible for color vision and high-acuity vision, and hence are more concentrated in the fovea.[36] Color vision depends on the presence of three different types of cones. One is specialized to absorb blue light, one absorbs green, and one absorbs red. [What physical difference allows this functional difference?[37]] The brain perceives hues by integrating the relative input of these three basic stimuli.

Defects in Visual Acuity

Normal vision is termed **emmetropia**. Too much or too little curvature of the cornea or lens results in visual defects. Too much curvature causes light to be bent too much and to be focused in front of the retina. The result is **myopia**, or nearsightedness. Myopia can be corrected by a concave (diverging) lens, which will cause the light rays to diverge slightly before they reach the cornea. **Hyperopia**, farsightedness, results from the focusing of light behind the retina. Hyperopia can be corrected by a convex (converging) lens, which causes light rays to converge before reaching the cornea. **Presbyopia** is an inability to **accommodate** (focus). It results from loss of flexibility of the lens, which occurs with aging.

Figure 20   Defects in Visual Acuity ("F" denotes the focal point)

---

[36]   Remember: *Cones—Color—aCuity.*

[37]   Each type of cone makes a particular pigment protein which is specialized to change conformation when light of the appropriate frequency strikes it.

Vision: Information Processing

For humans, vision is the primary sense; even if other information (such as sound or smell) counters visual information, we are more likely to "believe our eyes." The processing of visual information is extremely complex, and highly reliant on expectations and past experience. Neurons in the **visual cortex** fire in response to very specific information; feature detecting neurons are specific neurons in the brain that fire in response to particular visual features, such as lines, edges, angles, and movement. This information is then passed along to other neurons that begin to assimilate these distinct features into more complex objects, and so on. Therefore, **feature detection theory** explains why a certain area of the brain is activated when looking at a face, a different area is activated when looking at the letters on this page, etc. In order to process vast amounts of visual information quickly and effectively, our brain employs **parallel processing**, whereby many aspects of a visual stimulus (such as form, motion, color, and depth) are processed simultaneously instead of in a step-by-step or serial fashion. [Note: parallel processing is also employed for other stimuli as well.] The occipital lobe constructs a holistic image by integrating all of the separate elements of an object, in addition to accessing stored information. For example, the brain is simultaneously processing the individual features of an image, while also accessing stored information, to rapidly come to the conclusion that you are not only viewing a face, but you are specifically viewing your mom's face. All of this requires a tremendous amount of resources; in fact, the human brain dedicates approximately 30% of the cortex to processing visual information, while only 8% is devoted to processing touch information, and a mere 3% processes auditory information!

Table 5   Summary of Sensory Modalities

Modality	Receptor	Receptor type	Organ	Stimulus
Vision	• rods and cones	• electromagnetic	• retina	• light
Hearing	• auditory hair cells	• mechanoreceptor	• organ of Corti	• vibration
Olfaction	• olfactory nerve endings	• chemoreceptor	• individual neurons	• airborne chemicals
Taste	• taste cells	• chemoreceptor	• taste bud	• food chemicals
Touch (a few examples)	• Pacinian corpuscles • free nerve endings • temperature receptors	• mechanoreceptor • nociceptor • thermoreceptor	• skin	• pressure • pain • temperature
Interoception (two examples)	• aortic arch baroreceptors • pH receptors	• baroreceptor • chemoreceptor	• aortic arch • aortic arch / medulla oblongata	• blood pressure • pH

General Sensory Processing

Absolute Thresholds

We are very sensitive to certain types of stimuli. The minimum stimulus intensity required to activate a sensory receptor 50% of the time (and thus detect the sensation) is called the **absolute threshold**. In other words, for each special sense, the 50% recognition point defines the absolute threshold. (Note that this threshold can vary between individuals and different organisms—the absolute smell threshold for a human and a dog differs greatly.) Absolute thresholds also vary with age. For example, as we age, we gradually lose our ability to detect higher-pitched sounds. [What is the anatomical reason for this?[38]]

Difference Thresholds

8.5

Absolute thresholds are important for detecting the presence or absence of stimuli, but the ability to determine the change or difference in stimuli is also vital. The **difference threshold** (also called the *just noticeable difference*, or JND) is the minimum noticeable difference between any two sensory stimuli, 50% of the time. The magnitude of the initial stimulus influences the difference threshold; for example, if you lift a one pound weight and a two pound weight, the difference will be obvious, but if you lift a 100 pound weight and 101 pound weight, you probably won't be able to tell the difference. Indeed, **Weber's law** dictates that two stimuli must differ by a constant *proportion* in order for their difference to be perceptible. Interestingly, the exact proportion varies by stimulus; but for humans, two objects must differ in weight by 2% [in the weight example above, what is the minimum weight needed to detect a difference between it and the 100 pound weight?[39]], two lights must differ in intensity by 8%, and two tones must differ in frequency by 0.3%.

Signal Detection Theory

Detecting sensory stimuli not only depends on the information itself, but also on our psychological state, including alertness, expectation, motivation, and prior experience. **Signal detection theory** attempts to predict how and when someone will detect the presence of a given sensory stimulus (the "signal") amidst all of the other sensory stimuli in the background (considered the "noise"). There are four possible outcomes: a hit (the signal is present and was detected), a miss (the signal was present but not detected), a false alarm (the signal was not present but the person thought it was), and a correct rejection (the signal was not present and the person did not think it was). Signal detection can have important life-or-death consequences—imagine how crucial it is for doctors to be able to detect the signal (perhaps a tumor on a CT scan) from the noise.

Gestalt Psychology

Gestalt is the German word for "whole." Gestalt psychologists believe that the whole exceeds the sum of its parts; in other words, when humans perceive an object, rather than seeing lines, angles, colors, and shadows, they perceive the whole—a face or a table or a dog. Beyond merely registering the individual pieces, the human brain perceives the whole. **Bottom-up processing** begins with the sensory receptors and works up to the complex integration of information occurring in the brain. **Top-down processing** occurs when the brain applies experience and expectations to interpret sensory information; note that the brain in fact uses a combination of the two: information is received in a bottom-up fashion from sensory receptors while the brain is superimposing assumptions in a top-down manner.

---

[38] Loud sounds can mechanically harm the hair cells, causing them to die. When this occurs, the hair cell can no longer send sound signals to the brain. In people, once a hair cell dies, it will never regrow. The hair cells that detect higher frequency sounds are the smallest and the most easily damaged; therefore, as people age and more hair cells are damaged and lost, hearing loss occurs. Since the smallest hair cells are the ones most likely lost, loss of sensitivity to high-pitched sounds is common in older people.

[39] 102 pounds, which is 2% heavier than 100 pounds

8.6 THE ENDOCRINE SYSTEM

The nervous system and endocrine system represent the two major control systems of the body. The nervous system is fast-acting with relatively short-term effects, whereas the endocrine system takes longer to communicate signals but has generally longer lasting effects. These two control systems are interconnected, as neurons can signal the release of hormones from endocrine glands. [What is one such connection in the sympathetic nervous system?[40]] A primary connection between the nervous and endocrine systems is the *hypothalamic-pituitary axis*, which is described in more detail below.

Hormone Types: Transport and Mechanisms of Action

While the nervous system regulates cellular function from instant to instant, the endocrine system regulates physiology (especially metabolism) over a period of hours to days. The nervous system communicates via the extremely rapid action potential. The signal of the endocrine system is the **hormone**, defined as a molecule which is *secreted into the bloodstream* by an endocrine gland, and which has its effects upon *distant* target cells possessing the appropriate receptor. An **endocrine gland** is a *ductless* gland whose secretory products are picked up by capillaries supplying blood to the region. (In contrast, **exocrine glands** secrete their products into the external environment by way of ducts, which empty into the gastrointestinal lumen or the external world.) A **hormone receptor** is a polypeptide that possesses a ligand-specific binding site. Binding of ligand (hormone) to the site causes the receptor to modify target cell activity. *Tissue-specificity of hormone action is determined by whether the cells of a tissue have the appropriate receptor.*

Some signaling molecules modify the activity of the cell which secreted them; this is an **autocrine** activity (*auto-* means self). For example, a T cell secretes interleukin 2, which binds to receptors on the same T cell to stimulate increased activity.

Hormones can be grouped into one of two classes. *Hydrophilic* hormones, such as **peptides** and **amino-acid derivatives**, must bind to receptors on the cell surface, while *hydrophobic* hormones, such as the **steroid hormones**, bind to receptors in the cellular interior.

Peptide Hormones

Peptide hormones are synthesized into the rough ER and modified in the Golgi. Then they are stored in vesicles until needed, when they are released by exocytosis. In the bloodstream they dissolve in the plasma, since they are hydrophilic. Their hydrophilicity also means they cannot cross biological membranes and thus are required to communicate with the interior of the target cell by way of a ___,[41] discussed in Chapter 6. To briefly review, the peptide hormone is a first messenger which must bind to a cell-surface receptor. The receptor is a polypeptide with a domain on the inner surface of the plasma membrane that contains the ability to catalytically activate a second messenger. The end result of second messenger activation is that the function of proteins in the cytoplasm is changed. A key feature of second messenger cascades is signal amplification, which allows a few activated receptors to change the activity of many enzymes in the cytoplasm.

---

[40] The sympathetic nervous system directly innervates the adrenal medulla to stimulate the release of epinephrine.

[41] second messenger cascade

Because peptide hormones modify the activity of existing enzymes in the cytoplasm, their effects are exerted rapidly, minutes to hours from the time of secretion. Also, the duration of their effects is brief.

There are two subgroups within the peptide hormone category: polypeptides and amino acid derivatives. An example of a polypeptide hormone is insulin, which has a complex tertiary structure involving disulfide bridges. It is secreted by the β cells of the pancreatic islets of Langerhans in response to elevated blood glucose and binds to a cell-surface receptor with a cytoplasmic domain possessing protein kinase activity. Amino acid derivatives, as their name implies, are derived from single amino acids and contain no peptide bonds. For example, tyrosine is the parent amino acid for the catecholamines (which include epinephrine) and the thyroid hormones. Despite the fact that these two classes are derived from the same precursor molecule, they have different properties. The catecholamines act like peptide hormones, while the thyroid hormones behave more like steroid hormones. Epinephrine is a small cyclic molecule secreted by the adrenal medulla upon activation of the sympathetic nervous system. It binds to cell-surface receptors to trigger a cascade of events that produces the second messenger cyclic adenosine monophosphate (cAMP) and activates protein kinases in the cytoplasm. Thyroid hormones incorporate iodine into their structure. They enter cells, bind to DNA, and activate transcription of genes involved in energy mobilization.

Steroid Hormones

Steroids are hydrophobic molecules synthesized from cholesterol in the smooth endoplasmic reticulum. Due to their hydrophobicity, steroids can freely diffuse through biological membranes. Thus, they are not stored but rather diffuse into the bloodstream as soon as they are made. If a steroid hormone is not needed, it will not be made. Steroids' hydrophobicity also means they cannot be dissolved in the plasma. Instead they journey through the bloodstream stuck to proteins in the plasma, such as albumin. [What holds the steroid bound to a plasma protein?[42]] The small, hydrophobic steroid hormone exerts its effects upon target cells by *diffusing through the plasma membrane to bind with a receptor in the cytoplasm*. Once it has bound its ligand, the steroid hormone-receptor complex is transported into the nucleus, where it acts as a sequence-specific regulator of transcription. Because steroid hormones must modify transcription to change the *amount* and/or *type* of proteins in the cell, their effects are exerted slowly, over a period of days, and persist for days to weeks.

Steroids regulating sexuality, reproduction, and development are secreted by the testes, ovaries, and placenta. Steroids regulating water balance and other processes are secreted by the adrenal cortex. All other endocrine glands secrete peptide hormones. (Note that although thyroid hormone is derived from an amino acid, its mechanism of action more closely resembles that of the steroid hormones.)

---

[42] No bond—just hydrophobic interactions

Table 6 Peptide vs. Steroid Hormones

	Peptides	**Steroids**
Structure	hydrophilic, large (polypeptides) or small (amino acid derivatives)	hydrophobic, small
Site of synthesis	rough ER	smooth ER
Regulation of release	stored in vesicles until a signal for secretion is received	synthesized only when needed and then used immediately, not stored
Transport in bloodstream	free	stuck to protein carrier
Specificity	only target cells have appropriate surface receptors (exception: thyroxine = cytoplasmic)	only target cells have appropriate cytoplasmic receptors
Mechanism of effect	bind to receptors that generate second messengers which result in modification of *enzyme activity*	bind to receptors that alter *gene expression* by regulating DNA transcription
Timing of effect	rapid, short-lived	slow, long-lasting

8.6

Organization and Regulation of the Human Endocrine System

The endocrine system has many different roles. Hormones are essential for gamete synthesis, ovulation, pregnancy, growth, sexual development, and overall level of metabolic activity. Despite this diversity of function, endocrine activity is harmoniously orchestrated. Maintenance of order in such a complex system might seem impossible to accomplish in a preplanned manner. Regulation of the endocrine system is not preplanned or rigidly structured, but is instead generally automatic. Hormone levels rise and fall as dictated by physiological needs. The endocrine system is ordered yet dynamic. This flexible, automatic orderliness is attributable to feedback regulation. The amount of a hormone secreted is controlled not by a preformulated plan but rather by changes in the variable the hormone is responsible for controlling. Continuous circulation of blood exposes target cells to regulatory hormones and also exposes endocrine glands to serum concentrations of physiological variables that they regulate. Thus, *regulator* and that which is *regulated* are in continuous communication. Concentration of a species X in the aqueous portion of the bloodstream is denoted "serum [X]."

An example of feedback regulation is the interaction between the hormone calcitonin and serum $[Ca^{2+}]$. The function of calcitonin is to prevent serum $[Ca^{2+}]$ from peaking above normal levels, and the amount of calcitonin secreted is directly proportional to increases in serum $[Ca^{2+}]$ above normal. When serum $[Ca^{2+}]$ becomes elevated, calcitonin is secreted. Then when serum $[Ca^{2+}]$ levels fall, calcitonin secretion stops. The falling serum $[Ca^{2+}]$ level (*that which is regulated*) feeds back to the cells which secrete calcitonin (*regulators*). The serum $[Ca^{2+}]$ level is a **physiological endpoint** which must be maintained at constant levels. This demonstrates the role of the endocrine system in maintaining **homeostasis**, or physiological consistency.

An advantage of the endocrine system and its feedback regulation is that very complex arrays of variables can be controlled automatically. It's as if the variables controlled themselves. However, some integration (a central control mechanism) is necessary. Superimposed upon the hormonal regulation of physiological endpoints is another layer of regulation: hormones that regulate hormones. Such meta-regulators are known as **tropic hormones**.

For example, adrenocorticotropic hormone (ACTH) is secreted by the anterior pituitary. The role of ACTH is to stimulate increased activity of the portion of the adrenal gland called the **cortex**, which is responsible for secreting cortisol (among other steroid hormones). ACTH is a tropic hormone because it does not directly affect physiological endpoints, but merely regulates another regulator (cortisol). Cortisol regulates physiological endpoints, including cellular responses to stress and serum [glucose]. Feedback regulation applies to tropic hormones as well as to direct regulators of physiological endpoints; the level of ACTH is influenced by the level of cortisol. When cortisol is needed, ACTH is secreted, and when the serum [cortisol] increases sufficiently, ACTH secretion slows.

You may have noticed that in both of our examples the effect of feedback was *inhibitory*: the result of hormone secretion inhibits further secretion. Inhibitory feedback is called **negative feedback** or **feedback inhibition**. Most feedback in the endocrine system (and if you remember, most biochemical feedback) is negative. There are few examples of positive feedback, which we will not discuss here. A key example will be discussed in Chapter 13 with the reproductive systems.

There is yet another layer of control. Many of the functions of the endocrine system depend on instructions from the brain. The portion of the brain which controls much of the endocrine system is the **hypothalamus**, located at the center of the brain. The hypothalamus controls the endocrine system by releasing tropic hormones that regulate other tropic hormones, called **releasing and inhibiting factors** or **releasing and inhibiting hormones**.

For example (Figure 21), the hypothalamus secretes corticotropin releasing hormone (CRH, also known as CRF, where "F" stands for factor). The role of CRH is to cause increased secretion of ACTH. Just as ACTH secretion is regulated by feedback inhibition from cortisol, CRH secretion, too, is inhibited by cortisol. You begin to see that regulatory pathways in the endocrine system can get pretty complex.

Understanding that the hypothalamus controls the anterior pituitary and that the anterior pituitary controls most of the endocrine system is important. Damage to the connection between the hypothalamus and the pituitary is fatal, unless daily hormone replacement therapy is given.

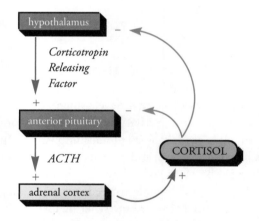

Figure 21   Feedback Regulation of Cortisol Secretion

This endocrine control center is given a special name: **hypothalamic-pituitary control axis** (Figure 22). The hypothalamus exerts its control of the pituitary by secreting its hormones into the bloodstream, just like any other endocrine gland; what's unique is that a special miniature circulatory system is provided for efficient transport of hypothalamic releasing and inhibiting factors to the anterior pituitary. This blood supply is known as the **hypothalamic-pituitary portal system**. You will also hear the term *hypothalamic-hypophysial portal system*. **Hypophysis** is another name for the pituitary gland.

A Note on Portal Systems: As a general rule, blood leaving the heart moves through only one capillary bed before returning to the heart, since the pressure drops substantially in capillaries. A portal system, however, consists of two capillary beds in sequence, allowing for direct communication between nearby structures. The two portal systems you need to understand are: the hypothalamic-pituitary portal system and the hepatic portal system (from the gastrointestinal tract to the liver, which you can read more about in Chapter 10).

8.6

One more bit of background information is necessary before we can delve into specific hormones. The pituitary gland has two halves: front (*anterior*) and back (*posterior*); see Figure 22. The **anterior pituitary** is also called the **adenohypophysis** and the **posterior pituitary** is also known as the **neurohypophysis**. It is important to understand the difference. The anterior pituitary is a normal endocrine gland, and it is controlled by hypothalamic releasing and inhibiting factors (essentially tropic hormones). The posterior pituitary is composed of axons which descend from the hypothalamus. These hypothalamic neurons that send axons down to the posterior pituitary are an example of **neuroendocrine cells**, neurons which secrete hormones into the bloodstream. The hormones released by the posterior pituitary are ADH (antidiuretic hormone or vasopressin), which causes the kidney to retain water during times of thirst, and oxytocin, which causes milk let-down for nursing as well as uterine contractions during labor. [Are these hormones made by axon termini in the posterior pituitary or by somas in the hypothalamus?[43]]

8.6

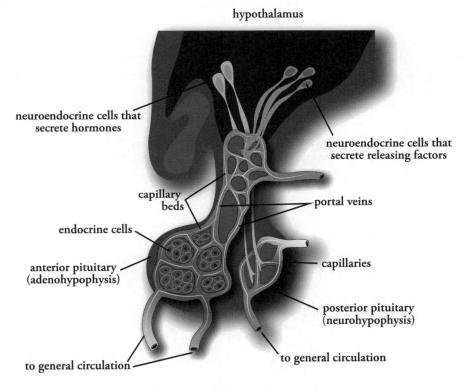

Figure 22   The Hypothalamic-Pituitary Control Axis

Major Glands and Their Hormones

The major hormones and glands of the endocrine system are listed in Table 7 on page 119. Many of these hormones will be discussed in detail in later chapters. Insulin and glucagon will be discussed in the chapter on digestion and energy metabolism (Chapter 10). Testosterone, estrogen, progesterone, FSH, and LH will be presented in the chapter on reproductive biology (Chapter 13). The function of epinephrine has already been presented as part of the sympathetic nervous system response. In general, the hormones are involved in development of the body and in maintenance of constant conditions, homeostasis, in the adult. [Is epinephrine secreted by a duct into the bloodstream?[44]]

---

[43] All hypothalamic and pituitary hormones are peptides, and there is no protein synthesis at axon termini. Thus, ADH and oxytocin must be made in nerve cell bodies in the hypothalamus and transported down the axons to the posterior pituitary. The posterior pituitary doesn't actually make any hormones, then, it just stores ADH and oxytocin for later release.

[44] No. Endocrine hormones are not secreted through ducts.

Thyroid hormone and **cortisol** have broad effects on metabolism and energy usage. Thyroid hormone is produced from the amino acid tyrosine in the thyroid gland and comes in two forms, with three or four iodine atoms per molecule. The production of thyroid hormone is increased by thyroid stimulating hormone (TSH) from the anterior pituitary, which is regulated by the hypothalamus and the central nervous system in turn. The mechanism of action of thyroid hormone is to bind to a receptor in the cytoplasm of cells that then regulates transcription in the nucleus. The effect of this regulation is to increase the overall metabolic rate and body temperature, and, in children, to stimulate growth. Exposure to cold can increase the production of thyroid hormone. Cortisol is secreted by the adrenal cortex in response to ACTH from the pituitary. In general, the effects of cortisol tend to help the body deal with stress. Cortisol helps to mobilize glycogen and fat stores to provide energy during stress and also increases the consumption of proteins for energy. These effects are essential, since removal of the adrenal cortex can result in the death of animals exposed to even a small stress. Long-term high levels of cortisol tend to have negative effects, however, including suppression of the immune system.

- Would an inhibitor of protein synthesis block the action of thyroid hormone?[45]
- Would the production of ATP by mitochondria be stimulated or repressed by thyroid hormone?[46]
- Would thyroid hormone affect isolated mitochondria directly?[47]

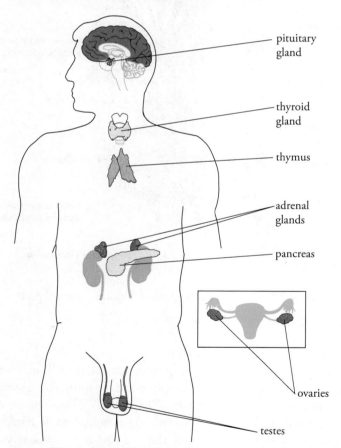

pituitary gland

thyroid gland

thymus

adrenal glands

pancreas

ovaries

testes

Figure 23   The Major Endocrine Glands

[45] Yes. Thyroid hormone binds to a receptor that regulates transcription. The mRNA stimulated by thyroid hormone receptor in the nucleus must be processed and translated before the effects of thyroid hormone can become evident.

[46] Thyroid hormone stimulates the basal metabolic rate throughout the body. More ATP will be consumed, so the mitochondria are stimulated to make more ATP.

[47] No. Thyroid hormone affects mitochondria *indirectly*, through the regulation of nuclear genes.

Table 7 Summary of the Hormones of the Endocrine System

Gland	Hormone (class)	Target/effect
Hypothalamus	releasing and inhibiting factors (peptides), posterior pituitary hormones	anterior pituitary/modify activity
Anterior pituitary	growth hormone (GH) (peptide)	↑ bone and muscle growth, ↑ cell turnover rate
	prolactin (peptide)	mammary gland/milk production
tropic	thyroid stimulating hormone (TSH) (peptide)	thyroid/↑ synthesis and release of TH
	adrenocorticotropic hormone (ACTH) (peptide)	↑ growth and secretory activity of adrenal cortex
gonadotropic	luteinizing hormone (LH) (peptide)	ovary/ovulation, testes/testosterone synth.
	follicle stimulating hormone (FSH) (peptide)	ovary/follicle development, testes/ spermatogenesis
Posterior pituitary	antidiuretic hormone (ADH, vasopressin) (peptide)	kidney/water retention
	oxytocin (peptide)	breast/milk letdown, uterus/contraction
Thyroid	thyroid hormone (TH, thyroxine) (modified amino acid)	child: necessary for physical and mental development; adult: ↑ metabolic rate and temp.
thyroid C cells	calcitonin (peptide)	bone, kidney; lowers serum $[Ca^{2+}]$
Parathyroids	parathyroid hormone (PTH) (peptide)	bone, kidney, small intestine/raises serum $[Ca^{2+}]$
Thymus	thymosin (children only) (peptide)	T cell development during childhood
Adrenal medulla	epinephrine (modified amino acid)	sympathetic stress response (rapid)
Adrenal cortex	cortisol ("glucocorticoid") (steroid)	longer-term stress response; ↑ blood [glucose]; ↑ protein catabolism; ↓ inflammation and immunity; many other
	aldosterone ("mineralocorticoid") (steroid)	kidney/↑ Na^+ reabsorption to ↑ b.p.
	sex steroids	not normally important, but an adrenal tumor can overproduce these, causing masculinization or feminization
Endocrine pancreas (islets of Langerhans)	insulin (β cells secrete) (peptide) —absent or ineffective in diabetes mellitus	↓ blood [glucose]/↑ glycogen and fat storage
	glucagon (α cells secrete) (peptide)	↑ blood [glucose]/↓ glycogen and fat storage
	somatostatin (SS—δ cells secrete) (peptide)	inhibits many digestive processes
Testes	testosterone (steroid)	male characteristics, spermatogenesis
Ovaries/placenta	estrogen (steroid)	female characteristics, endometrial growth
	progesterone (steroid)	endometrial secretion, pregnancy
Heart	atrial natriuretic factor (ANF) (peptide)	kidney/↑ urination to ↓ blood pressure
Kidney	erythropoietin (peptide)	bone marrow/↑ RBC synthesis

8.6

Chapter 8 Summary

- The neuron is the basic structural and functional unit of the nervous system. It has several specialized structures that allow it to transmit action potentials.

- Neurons receive incoming information via dendrites. Signals are summed by the axon hillock, and if the signal is greater than the threshold, an action potential is initiated.

- The action potential is an all-or-none signal that includes depolarization (via voltage-gated sodium channels) and repolarization (via voltage-gated potassium channels); it begins and ends at the cell's resting potential of −70 mV.

- Since action potentials are all-or-none events, intensity is coded by the frequency of the action potential.

- Neurons communicate with other neurons, organs, and glands at synapses. Most synapses are chemical in nature; an action potential causes the release of neurotransmitter into the synaptic cleft, and binding of the neurotransmitter to receptors on the postsynaptic cell triggers a change, either stimulatory or inhibitory, in that cell.

- The central nervous system includes the spinal cord and the brain; specialized areas control specific aspects of human behavior, movement, intelligence, emotion, and reflexes.

- The peripheral nervous system includes the somatic (voluntary) and autonomic (involuntary) subdivisions.

- The sympathetic branch of the autonomic system controls our fight-or-flight response; norepinephrine is the primary neurotransmitter of this system, and it is augmented by epinephrine from the adrenal medulla.

- The parasympathetic branch of the autonomic system controls our resting and digesting state; acetylcholine is the primary neurotransmitter of this system.

- Humans have several types of receptors (mechanoreceptors, chemoreceptors, nociceptors, thermoreceptors, electromagnetic receptors, and proprioceptors) that allow us to detect a variety of stimuli.

- The endocrine system controls our overall physiology and homeostasis by hormones that travel through the bloodstream. Hormones are released from endocrine glands, travel to distant target tissues via the blood, bind to receptors on target tissues, and exert effects on target cells.

- Peptide hormones are made from amino acids, bind to receptors on the cell surface, and typically affect target cells via second messenger pathways. Effects tend to be rapid and temporary.

- Steroid hormones are derived from cholesterol, bind to receptors in the cytoplasm or nucleus, and bind to DNA to alter transcription. Effects tend to occur more slowly and are more permanent.

CHAPTER 8 FREESTANDING PRACTICE QUESTIONS

1. Macular degeneration refers to the deterioration of the center portion of the retina, the macula, leading to vision loss. What type of receptor would you expect to see loss of in macular degeneration?

A) Deterioration of cone cells only
B) Deterioration of electromagnetic receptors found at the back of the eye
C) Deterioration of mechanoreceptors at the back of the eye
D) Deterioration of bipolar cells and ganglion cells, leading to loss of nociceptors

2. Which of the following is the correct order of events during synaptic transmission?

A) Depolarization of presynaptic membrane → Voltage-gated calcium channels open → Neurotransmitter binds to ligand-gated ion channels → Membrane depolarization of postsynaptic cell → Neurotransmitters cross the synaptic cleft
B) An action potential reaches the end of an axon at the synaptic knob → Depolarization of presynaptic membrane → Voltage-gated sodium channels open → Neurotransmitter binds to ligand-gated ion channels → Membrane depolarization of postsynaptic cell
C) Depolarization of presynaptic membrane → Neurotransmitter binds to ligand-gated ion channels → Neurotransmitter in the synaptic cleft is degraded and/or removed → An action potential reaches the end of an axon
D) An action potential reaches the end of an axon → Voltage-gated calcium channels open → Neurotransmitter binds to ligand-gated ion channels → Neurotransmitter in the synaptic cleft is degraded and/or removed

3. People who suffer from severe epilepsy are sometimes treated with a "split brain" procedure that prevents most communication between the left and right hemispheres of the brain. The structure that is most likely cut in this operation is the:

A) corpus callosum.
B) medulla.
C) thalamus.
D) pons.

4. Myasthenia gravis, an autoimmune disorder, results from the production of antibodies against acetylcholine receptors in the body. Which of the following statements is FALSE?

A) A patient may have difficulty opening his/her eyes.
B) Repeated injection of human acetylcholine receptor into an animal model will produce clinical symptoms in that animal.
C) The disease does not directly affect the release of neurotransmitter.
D) This disease only impacts the neuromuscular junction.

5. Which of the following is true about cortisol?

A) It is synthesized in the smooth ER and transported freely in the bloodstream.
B) It is synthesized in the rough ER and transported by a protein carrier in the bloodstream.
C) It is synthesized in the smooth ER and synthesized only when needed.
D) It is synthesized in the rough ER and stored in vesicles until signal for secretion is received.

6. Parathyroid adenomas are tumors that can lead to hyperparathyroidism. Which of the following can occur in a patient with a parathyroid adenoma?

    I.   Increased frequency of bone fractures
    II. Decreased reabsorption of calcium by the kidneys
    III. Increased serum calcium levels

    A) I only
    B) II only
    C) I and II
    D) I and III

7. All of the following hormones would activate second messenger systems to exert their effect on target cells, EXCEPT:

    A) insulin.
    B) glucagon.
    C) epinephrine.
    D) progesterone.

8. Blood levels of creatinine and urea nitrogen can be used to assess kidney function, with elevated values indicating possible kidney disease. Additionally, dehydration is known to reduce blood flow to the kidneys and elevate creatinine and urea nitrogen levels in the blood. A patient exhibits high levels of blood creatinine and blood urea nitrogen, but kidney disease is not suspected. The patient's blood pressure is also very low. Which of the following would you expect?

    I.   Increased release of ADH
    II. Decreased release of renin
    III. Decreased release of aldosterone

    A) I only
    B) II only
    C) II and III only
    D) I, II, and III

CHAPTER 8 PRACTICE PASSAGE

Mammalian nerve cells have on their outer surface a subtype of glutamate receptors called the *N*-methyl-D-aspartate (NMDA) receptor. The NMDA receptor binds glutamate, an amino acid neurotransmitter, which ultimately results in the inward flow of calcium ions.

The NMDA receptor has been studied by exposing nerve cells to ischemic conditions (a diminished flow of blood) which result in localized brain damage. The affected neurons demonstrate depleted energy reserves with decreased internal stores of ATP. Energy-driven Na^+/K^+ ATPase enzymes located in the cell membrane begin to fail. If the ischemic conditions continue, the neuronal cell membrane depolarizes, providing an excitatory stimulus for the release of excessive amounts of glutamate. Other nerve cells in close proximity experience sustained binding of glutamate to NMDA receptor sites, which can lead to further cell membrane depolarization.

Experiment 1:

Cultured nerve cells were exposed to normal or decreased oxygen concentrations. Differing concentrations of extracellular calcium or glutamate antagonists were also established. Intracellular calcium levels were measured after one minute. The results of this experiment are listed below:

Table 1

Extracellular environment			Intracellular calcium
Oxygen	Glutamate antagonists	Calcium	
L	–	–	N
L	–	H	I
L	+	–	N
L	+	H	N
H	–	–	N
H	–	H	N
H	+	–	N
H	+	H	N

Key: L = low concentration, H = high concentration
+ = present, – = absent
N = normal, I = increase

Experiment 2:

Several cultured neurons were bathed in a solution containing high concentrations of calcium, sodium, and chloride ions, but not oxygen. The cells experienced marked swelling and eventually an action potential was evoked. After the action potential, internal ion levels were measured every 30 seconds. Intracellular levels of both calcium and sodium were elevated.

Based on these two experiments, researchers have proposed that the initial effects of activation of the NMDA receptor can be modeled as follows:

Figure 1

Further experiments suggested that the NMDA receptor also allowed K^+ to exit the cell.

1. Flow of calcium into cells is essential to which of the following processes?

A) Opening of voltage-gated sodium channels
B) Propagation of action potentials in motor neuron axons
C) Cardiac muscle contraction
D) ATP hydrolysis

2. In the increased biosynthesis of neurotransmitter receptors, activity of the rough endoplasmic reticulum increases because:

A) the cell is undergoing the process of exocytosis.
B) it is the primary site of complex lipid synthesis.
C) it is the primary site of plasma membrane protein synthesis.
D) more vesicles arrive at the rough ER from the Golgi apparatus.

3. Regarding Experiment 2, which of the following is the most likely reason that the cells experienced marked swelling?

A) Activation of the NMDA receptor due to ischemia blocked aquaporins, preventing the efflux of water from the cell.

B) The failure of the Na^+/K^+ ATPase led to osmotic influx of water.

C) The high intracellular concentrations of sodium and calcium led to the osmotic influx of water.

D) The influx of sodium due to the action potential led to the osmotic influx of water.

4. Which of the following amino acids would most likely be found in the transmembrane portion of the NMDA receptor?

A) Leu
B) Pro
C) Arg
D) Asn

5. Regarding Experiment 1, if glutamate is the only neurotransmitter that can bind to the NMDA receptor to increase the inward flow of calcium, which of the following would account for the lack of calcium flow in the presence of oxygen, extracellular calcium, and no glutamate antagonists?

A) No glutamate was supplied to the cells in the extracellular medium.

B) Other glutamate receptor subtypes inhibit the flow of calcium into the cell.

C) In the presence of oxygen, the cell does not depolarize.

D) Ischemic conditions prevent the normal functioning of the Na^+/K^+ ATPases.

SOLUTIONS TO CHAPTER 8 FREESTANDING PRACTICE QUESTIONS

1. **B**   The macula contains both rods and cones; the fovea centralis is a region of the macula that contains only cones. In macular degeneration, both rods and cones would be affected (choice A is wrong). Rods and cones are electromagnetic receptors, not mechanoreceptors, at the back of the eye (choice C is wrong, and choice B is correct). Bipolar cells and ganglion cells would be affected, but they are not nociceptors (choice D is wrong).

2. **D**   The correct order of events is: 1) an action potential reaches the end of an axon at the synaptic knob, 2) depolarization of presynaptic membrane, 3) voltage-gated calcium channels open, 4) neurotransmitter is released from the presynaptic cell, 5) neurotransmitter crosses the synaptic cleft, 6) neurotransmitter binds to ligand-gated ion channels on the postsynaptic membrane, 7) membrane depolarization of postsynaptic cell, 8) voltage-gated sodium channels open, 9) an action potential is initiated, and 10) neurotransmitter in the synaptic cleft is degraded and/or removed (choices A, B, and C are wrong).

3. **A**   The corpus callosum is a bundle of axons that connects the left and right hemispheres of the brain and is responsible for the vast majority of the communication between the two hemispheres. Cutting this structure in half prevents the rapid cross-hemispheric communication that is observed during seizures in patients with severe epilepsy. The medulla and pons are part of the hindbrain and play roles in basic autonomic processes (choices B and D are wrong), and the thalamus is a relay station for somatic sensory stimuli located in the diencephalon (choice C is wrong).

4. **D**   Acetylcholine is a neurotransmitter in several areas in the body including the neuromuscular junction, pre- and postganglionic parasympathetic neurons, and preganglionic sympathetic neurons (choice D is the false statement and the correct answer choice). As acetylcholine receptors become nonfunctional with the binding of antibody, patients have difficulty with muscle contraction, and opening of the eyes may be one possible symptom of this (choice A is a true statement and can be eliminated). Repeated injection of an acetylcholine receptor into an animal model will result in an immune response and subsequent attack of the endogenous acetylcholine receptors, producing myasthenia gravis symptoms (choice B is a true statement and can be eliminated). The antibodies attack the postsynaptic neuron receptors and do not result in a direct change in neurotransmitter release (choice C is a true statement and can be eliminated).

5. **C** Cortisol is a steroid hormone. Steroids are synthesized in the smooth ER (choices B and D can be eliminated). It is hydrophobic, so it needs to be bound to a carrier protein (usually albumin) to travel in the bloodstream (choice A can be eliminated). Steroid hormones are synthesized only when needed, and released immediately (choice C is correct).

6. **D** Hyperparathyroidism means having an abnormally high level of parathyroid hormone. The functions of parathyroid hormone include 1) enhancing the breakdown of bone by osteoclasts and the release of calcium into the bloodstream, 2) enhancing the reabsorption of calcium in the nephrons of the kidneys, and 3) enhancing the absorption of calcium in the small intestine. Item I is true: high PTH levels cause calcium to leave the bone and enter the bloodstream, resulting in weak bones that can fracture easily (choice B can be eliminated). Item II is false: PTH leads to increased reabsorption of calcium to increase serum calcium levels (choice C can be eliminated). Item III is true: high PTH levels cause serum calcium levels to rise since it is being removed from the bone, reabsorbed by the kidneys, and absorbed by the small intestines (choice A can be eliminated). The correct answer is choice D.

7. **D** Make sure to highlight the word "EXCEPT" and write "A B C D" on your noteboard. Evaluate each answer choice, writing "Y" if it would activate a second messenger system or "N" if it would not. Insulin is a peptide hormone. Peptide hormones are generally unable to cross the cell membrane, so they bind to receptors on the cell surface and trigger second messenger systems (write "Y" next to "A" on the noteboard). Glucagon and epinephrine are also peptide hormones and activate second messenger systems (write "Y" next to "B" and "C" on the noteboard). Progesterone, however, is a steroid hormone, and exerts its effects on the target cell by binding to intracellular receptors that ultimately regulate DNA transcription (write "N" next to "D" on the noteboard). Since choice D stands out with an "N" instead of a "Y," it is the correct answer choice.

8. **A** Since this is a Roman numeral question, start by analyzing the Roman numeral item that appears in exactly two of the answer choices, in this case, Item I or III. Whether it is true or false, you can eliminate half the answer choices. Item I is true: the patient is probably dehydrated if they are experiencing elevated levels of blood creatinine and urea nitrogen in the absence of kidney disease. In response to dehydration, the posterior pituitary will secrete ADH, leading to increased water retention to help counteract the dehydration (choices B and C can be eliminated). You can evaluate either Item II or III to get to the correct answer. Item II is false: the patient has low blood pressure, which stimulates the release of renin from the kidney (choice D can be eliminated, and choice A is correct). Note that Item III is also false: a downstream effect of renin release is increased release of aldosterone.

SOLUTIONS TO CHAPTER 8 PRACTICE PASSAGE

1. **C** The action potential in cardiac muscle includes the opening of slow voltage-gated calcium channels. The opening of these channels allows calcium into cardiac muscle cells, which plays a role in the release of the troponin/tropomyosin complex from actin filaments, allowing myosin heads to bind and initiate contraction. Voltage-gated sodium channels open in response to changes in membrane potential, not calcium influx, and the changes in potential are typically due to sodium influx through ligand-gated channels (choice A is wrong). Propagation of action potentials in motor neurons relies on sodium and potassium flux, not calcium (choice B is wrong), and ATP hydrolysis is not calcium-dependent (choice D is wrong).

2. **C** Neurotransmitter receptors are integral plasma membrane proteins, all of which are translated on the rough ER. Increased plasma membrane protein translation requires more activity in the rough ER. The receptors are not released via exocytosis, they are embedded in the plasma membrane (choice A is wrong), lipid synthesis occurs in the smooth ER, not the rough ER (choice B is wrong), and vesicles travel from the ER to the Golgi apparatus, not the other way around (choice D is wrong).

3. **B** The cells were kept in ischemic (low oxygen) conditions. Oxygen is required for ATP synthesis, and ATP is required to operate the Na^+/K^+ ATPase. In the absence of oxygen, the lack of ATP would cause the Na^+/K^+ ATPases to fail. One of the functions of the ATPases is to maintain osmotic equilibrium for the cell; as it pumps ions out, water doesn't want to come in. The failure of the pump would lead to osmotic influx of water (choice B is correct). There is nothing in the passage to support the idea that NMDA receptors block aquaporins, and even if they did, the movement of water through the aquaporins is not restricted to just efflux (choice A is wrong). While the increase in intracellular concentrations of sodium and calcium could lead to osmotic influx of water, this would happen after the action potential was induced, and the swelling occurred prior to the induction of the action potential (choices C and D are wrong).

4. **A** Proteins that span the plasma membrane must contain hydrophobic (nonpolar) amino acid residues in the transmembrane region. Of the amino acids listed, only leucine and proline are nonpolar; arginine and asparagine are both polar (choices C and D can be eliminated). Proline, while nonpolar, does not fit well into the alpha helical shape of most transmembrane regions, making leucine the more likely of the two to be found there (choice B can be eliminated, and choice A is correct).

5. **C** In the presence of oxygen, the Na^+/K^+ ATPases would not fail, and the cell would not depolarize. If the cell doesn't depolarize, then glutamate would not be released to stimulate the NMDA receptor and open the calcium channels (choice C is correct). It is true that no glutamate was supplied to the cells, but this was by design; the experiment was designed to test what happens with glutamate release and NMDA receptor stimulation in the absence of oxygen. Supplying glutamate in the extracellular medium would prevent any effect of ischemia from being seen since the cell would automatically be stimulated (choice A is wrong). It is also true that ischemic conditions prevent the normal activity of the ATPases, but these cells are not exposed to ischemic conditions (choice D is wrong), There is no reason to assume any other glutamate receptor subtypes (choice B can be eliminated).

Chapter 9
The Circulatory, Lymphatic, and Immune Systems

9.1 OVERVIEW OF THE CIRCULATORY SYSTEM

The cells of a multicellular organism have the same basic requirements as unicellular organisms. Living so close to billions of other cells has many advantages, but there are drawbacks too. Each cell must compete with its neighbors for nutrients and oxygen and must also cope with the waste products that are inevitable in so dense a civilization. Other requirements of community living are efficient communication and homeostasis. The circulatory system addresses these problems by accomplishing the following goals:

1) Distribute nutrients from the digestive tract, liver, and adipose (fat) tissue.
2) Transport oxygen from the lungs to the entire body and carbon dioxide from the tissues to the lungs.
3) Transport metabolic waste products from tissues to the excretory system (i.e., the kidneys).
4) Transport hormones from endocrine glands to targets and provide feedback.
5) Maintain homeostasis of body temperature.
6) *Hemostasis* (blood clotting). This does not address a need of a multicellular organism *per se*, but rather is necessitated by the presence of the circulatory system itself.

The flow of blood through a tissue is known as **perfusion**. Inadequate blood flow, known as **ischemia**, results in tissue damage due to shortages of O_2 and nutrients, and buildup of metabolic wastes. When adequate circulation is present but the supply of oxygen is reduced, a tissue is said to suffer from **hypoxia**. [What's the difference between ischemia and hypoxia?[1]]

In the following sections we will study the components of the circulatory system. We will not delve into its thermoregulatory role, which will be covered in Chapter 12 (The Respiratory System and the Skin).

Components of the Circulatory System

The functions of the circulatory system involve transport of blood throughout the body and exchange of material between the blood and tissues. The **heart** is a muscular pump that forces blood through a branching series of vessels to the lungs and the rest of the body. Vessels that carry blood away from the heart at high pressure are **arteries**, and vessels that carry blood back toward the heart at low pressure are **veins**. As arteries pass farther from the heart, the pressure of blood decreases, and they branch into increasingly smaller arteries called **arterioles**. The arterioles then pass into the **capillaries**, very small vessels, often just wide enough for a single blood cell to pass. Arterioles have smooth muscle in their walls that can act as a control valve to restrict or increase the flow of blood into the capillaries of tissues. The capillaries have thin walls made of a single layer of cells and are designed to allow the exchange of material between the blood and tissues. After passing through capillaries, blood collects in small veins called **venules**, and then into the veins leading back to the heart. Except for the largest vessels near the heart, veins lack a muscular wall. From the heart, the blood can be pumped out once again through the arteries to the capillaries in the tissues.

- If the arterioles constrict in a tissue, will material diffuse through the wall of the arterioles into the tissue?[2]

---

[1] In hypoxia, wastes are adequately removed, but in ischemia they build up. Ischemia is worse.

[2] No. All exchange of material between the blood and tissues must occur in capillaries. The walls of arterioles are too thick and muscular for exchange to occur.

The inner lining of all blood vessels is formed by a thin layer of **endothelial cells**; the walls of capillaries are formed from a single layer of such cells. These cells have important roles in a number of vascular functions such as:

- Vasodilation and vasoconstriction: The secretion of substances like nitric oxide and endothelin can regulate vessel diameter. This is important in maintaining blood pressure, tissue oxygenation, and thermoregulation.
- Inflammation: The release of inflammatory chemicals from injured tissues stimulate endothelial cells to increase their expression of adhesion molecules. These molecules allow white blood cells to adhere to the endothelial cells and ultimately enter the injured tissue.
- Angiogenesis (the formation of new blood vessels): Angiogenic growth factors stimulate endothelial cells to break free from an existing vessel and proliferate in surrounding tissues, ultimately forming new vessels altogether. This property has important implications for cancer treatments, as many tumors secrete angiogenic growth factors. The resulting vascular increase supplies oxygen and nutrients to a developing tumor to help sustain its extraordinary cell division and growth. Angiogenesis inhibitors are drugs that can be used to restrict blood flow to tumors and help reduce or halt their growth.
- Thrombosis (blood clotting): Undamaged endothelial cells secrete substances that inhibit the coagulation cascade, thus preventing the formation of potentially life-threatening clots inside undamaged or unbroken vessels.

Endothelial cell dysfunction can lead to a number of pathogenic conditions, such as hypercholesterolemia, hypertension, inappropriate clot formation, and coronary artery disease and atherosclerosis; in fact, endothelial cell dysfunction is key to the development of atherosclerosis, and predates any clinical vascular signs by several years.

To achieve both efficient oxygenation of blood in the lungs and transport of oxygenated blood to the tissues, the heart has evolved in humans to have two sides separated by a thick wall to pump blood in two separate circuits. The right side of the heart pumps blood to the lungs, and the left side of the heart pumps blood to the rest of the body. The flow of blood from the heart to the lungs and back to the heart is the **pulmonary circulation**, and the flow of blood from the heart to the rest of the body and back again is the **systemic circulation** (Figure 1, next page).

- In fish, blood passes from the heart to the gills and then to the rest of the body. Why have mammals evolved a separate circulation for the lungs?[3]

By having two separate circulations, most blood passes through only one set of capillaries before returning to the heart. There are exceptions to this, however: **portal systems**. In the hepatic portal system, blood passes first through capillaries in the intestine, then collects in veins to travel to the liver, where the vessels branch and the blood passes again through capillaries. Another example is the hypothalamic-hypophysial portal system, in which blood passes through capillaries in the hypothalamus to the portal veins, then to capillaries in the pituitary (Chapter 8). The portal systems evolved as direct transport systems, to transport nutrients directly from the intestine to the liver or hormones from the hypothalamus to the pituitary, without passing through the whole body.

---

[3] Blood is pumped away from the heart at high pressure in arteries to pass through the capillaries. If the blood is to pass through one bed of capillaries, and then through another bed of capillaries, the pressure must be very high in the first set of capillaries or blood will not have enough pressure to pass through the second set of capillaries. Having two separate circulations solves this problem.

- If the hypothalamic-hypophysial portal circulation is severed, how does this affect the function of the pituitary?[4]

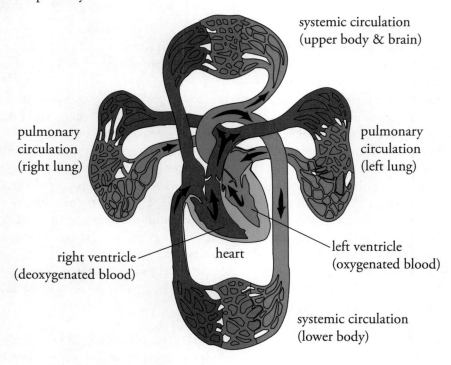

Figure 1 Pulmonary and Systemic Circuits

9.2 THE HEART

The heart has two kinds of chambers involved in pumping blood, the **atria** and the **ventricles** (Figure 2). The atria are reservoirs or "waiting rooms" where blood can collect from the veins before getting pumped into the ventricles. The muscular ventricles pump blood out of the heart at high pressures into the arteries. The systemic circulation and the pulmonary circulation are separated within the heart, so the right and left sides of the heart each have one atrium and one ventricle. The right atrium receives deoxygenated blood from the systemic circulation (from the large veins: the **inferior vena cava** and the **superior vena cava**) and pumps it into the right ventricle. From the right ventricle, blood passes through the pulmonary artery to the lungs. Oxygenated blood from the lungs returns through the pulmonary veins to the left atrium and is pumped into the left ventricle before being pumped out of the heart in a single large artery, the **aorta**, to the systemic circulation.

- Do all of the arteries of the body carry oxygenated blood?[5]

---

[4] Normally, the pituitary receives hormones directly from the hypothalamus. If the portal system is severed, hormones must take a longer route and will be diluted and degraded before they reach the pituitary. As a result, secretion by the pituitary will not be effectively regulated by the hypothalamus.

[5] No. The pulmonary artery carries deoxygenated blood from the heart to the lungs.

- Based on the above, you can conclude that blood flows:[6]
  A) from the lungs into the right atrium, since the right side of the heart deals with deoxygenated blood.
  B) from the right ventricle to the right atrium, since the atrium is a low-pressure chamber.
  C) from the right atrium to the left ventricle, since the right side of the heart deals with deoxygenated blood and the left side must pump blood to the body.
  D) from the lungs into the left atrium and from there to the left ventricle, since the left side of the heart deals with oxygenated blood.

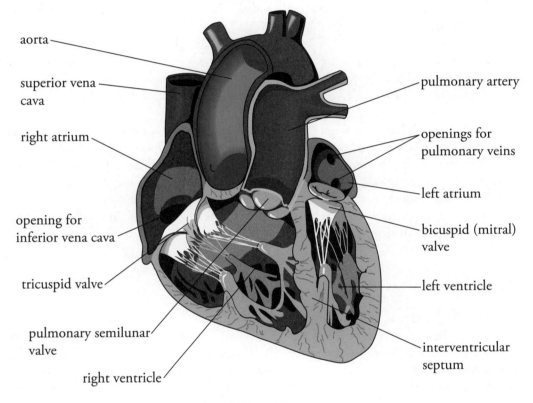

Figure 2 The Heart

The heart is a large muscular organ which requires a blood supply of its own. The very first branches from the aorta are **coronary arteries,** which branch to supply blood to the wall of the heart. They are called "coronary" because they encircle the heart, forming a crown shape. Deoxygenated blood from the heart collects in **coronary veins**, which merge to form the **coronary sinus**, located beneath a layer of fat on the outer wall of the heart. (A sinus is an open space; in the case of the cardiovascular system, it is a pool of low-pressure blood.) Blood in the coronary sinus is the only deoxygenated blood that does not end up in the inferior vena cava or superior vena cava. Instead, the coronary sinus drains directly into the right atrium.

---

[6] Oxygenated blood flows from the lungs to the left atrium (choice A is wrong), then to the left ventricle (choice **D** is right, and choice C is wrong). The atrium is a low pressure chamber, however, blood flow from the ventricles to the atria is prevented by the atrioventricular valves (choice B is wrong).

Valves

Valves are necessary to ensure one-way flow through the circulatory system. Valves in the heart are especially important, since the pressure differentials there are so extreme. In particular, ventricular pressure is very high and atrial pressure is lower. Hence, an **atrioventricular valve** (**AV valve**) between each ventricle and its atrium is necessary to prevent backflow.

The AV valve between the left atrium and the left ventricle is the **bicuspid** (or **mitral**) **valve**. [The mitral valve must withstand enormous pressures. What would happen if it ruptured?[7]] The AV valve between the right atrium and the right ventricle is the **tricuspid valve**. [What valve prevents blood flow between the left ventricle and the right ventricle?[8]]

Another set of valves is needed between the large arteries and the ventricles; these are the **pulmonary** and **aortic semilunar valves**. [Since the ventricles are ultra-high pressure chambers, why is it necessary to put valves between them and the arteries?[9]] Together these two valves are known simply as the *semilunar valves*.

There are also valves throughout the venous system. This is necessary because in passing through capillaries, blood loses its pressure. Thus, there is not much of a driving force pushing it toward the heart. Contraction of skeletal muscle becomes important, because normal body movements push and squeeze the veins, pressurizing venous blood and pushing it along. Venous valves prevent backflow; as long as the valves hold up, the blood moves toward the heart. When the valves fail, **varicose veins** result. Pregnant women often suffer from varicose veins because the growing fetus presses against the inferior vena cava, causing venous pressure in the legs to rise.

The Cardiac Cycle

The heart contracts, then relaxes, in a cycle which ends only in death. The left and right sides of the heart proceed through the same cycle at the same time. The cardiac cycle is divided into two periods, **diastole** and **systole** (pronounced dy-AS-toe-lee and SIS-toe-lee). During diastole, the ventricles are relaxed, and blood is able to flow into them from the atria. In fact, the atria contract during diastole, to propel blood into the ventricles more rapidly. [How strong is atrial compared to ventricular contraction?[10]] At the end of diastole, the ventricles contract, initiating systole. The ensuing buildup of pressure causes the AV valves to slam shut. Over the next few milliseconds, the pressure in the ventricles increases rapidly, until the semilunar valves fly open and blood rushes into the aorta and pulmonary artery. Systole is the period of time during which the ventricles are contracting, beginning at the "lub" sound and ending at the "dup." At the end of systole, the ventricles are nearly empty[11] and stop contracting. As a result, the pressure inside falls rapidly, and blood begins to flow backward, from the pulmonary artery into the right ventricle,

---

[7] The left ventricle would pump blood in both directions; out the aorta and back into the left atrium. The result will be elevated pulmonary blood pressure and pulmonary edema.

[8] None! The two ventricles are separated by a thick muscular wall. Remember: the left and right halves are separate.

[9] The ventricles are only pressurized while contracting. When they are not contracting, they must have a very low pressure so that blood can flow into them from the atria.

[10] Much weaker. The atria really only contract to ensure that most of the blood they contain passes into the ventricles. In contrast, the ventricles must propel blood through arteries, capillary beds, and veins. Therefore, the muscular walls of the atria are much thinner than those of the ventricles.

[11] Actually, only about 2/3 of the blood is normally ejected from the ventricle; this is the **ejection fraction**.

and from the aorta into the left ventricle. But very little backflow actually occurs, because the semilunar valves slam shut when the pressure in the ventricles becomes lower than the pressure in the great arteries. At this point, the heart has completed a full cardiac cycle and is back in diastole.

- Which one of the following is true during systole?[12]
  A) The bicuspid valve is open.
  B) Blood does not flow through the aortic valve.
  C) Both semilunar valves are closed.
  D) Pressure in the atria is low, and thus the atria fill with blood from the vena cava and pulmonary veins.

Heart Sounds, Heart Rate, and Cardiac Output

The "lub-dup" of the heartbeat is produced by valves slamming shut. The "lub" results from the closure of the AV valves at the beginning of systole, and the "dup" is the sound of the semilunar valves closing at the end of systole. [Based on this, which is longer: systole or diastole?[13]]

The **heart rate** (HR) or **pulse** is the number of times the "lub-dup" cardiac cycle is repeated per minute. The normal pulse rate is about one beat per second, ranging from 45 beats per minute (b.p.m.) in athletes to 80 or more beats per minute in the elderly and in children. The explanation for this variation is that a stronger heart pumps more blood each time it contracts, and thus may beat fewer times per minute and still provide adequate circulation. Athletes have strong hearts, while children and the elderly have weaker hearts. The amount of blood pumped with each systole is known as the **stroke volume** (SV). The total amount of blood pumped per minute is termed the **cardiac output** (CO), defined by the equation

$$\text{cardiac output (L/min)} = \text{stroke volume (L/beat)} \times \text{heart rate (beats/min)}$$
$$\text{CO} = \text{SV} \times \text{HR}$$

- An overweight child weighing 110 pounds, a female athlete weighing 110 pounds, and an elderly man weighing 110 pounds all require a cardiac output of about 5 L/min. But the child and the old man have a stroke volume of 1/16 L, while the athlete's stroke volume is 1/9 L. How can the child and the old man supply enough blood to their bodies?[14]
- Which is larger: the cardiac output of the right ventricle or of the left ventricle?[15]

---

[12] During systole the ventricles are contracting. The bicuspid valve separates the left atrium from the left ventricle, and must be closed to prevent backflow into the left atrium (choice A is wrong). The high pressures generated during systole force blood out of the ventricles through the aortic and pulmonary semilunar valves (choices B and C are wrong). While the ventricles are contracting, the atria are resting, and blood can flow into them from the vena cava and pulmonary veins. This flow would be prevented if there were any pressure in the atria (choice **D** is correct). Note that closure of the AV valves ensures that the super-high ventricular pressure does not spread to the atria.

[13] Diastole is longer, since it occupies the space between *lub-dup* and *lub-dup*. Systole is shorter, since it occupies the space between *lub* and *dup*.

[14] The athlete's heart can provide the necessary cardiac output by pumping at a leisurely rate of 45 beats per minute. But the hearts of the child and old man will have to work hard to pump enough blood; their pulses will be 80 beats per minute.

[15] Neither; they are equal. The same amount of blood must pass through both sides of the heart or blood would back up in either the pulmonary or systemic circulatory system.

The Frank-Starling Mechanism and Venous Return

There are several ways to increase cardiac output. One is increasing heart rate, as we saw above. Also, a stronger heart has a larger stroke volume and is capable of a greater cardiac output. Another mechanism of increased stroke volume is termed the **Frank-Starling mechanism**. If the heart muscle is stretched, it will contract more forcefully. How can the heart muscle be stretched? By filling it with more blood, of course. The return of blood to the heart by the vena cava is termed **venous return**. If venous return is increased, the heart fills more. As a result, its muscle fibers are stretched, and they respond by contracting more force-fully. The result is that a larger volume of blood enters the heart *and* the heart contracts better. The stroke volume can be increased significantly in this manner. The control of cardiac output in this manner is largely automatic: the more blood the heart receives from the tissues, the more it pumps out to the tissues.

There are two principal ways to increase venous return: 1) Increase the total volume of blood in the circulatory system. The body does this by retaining water (by urinating less). 2) Contraction of large veins can propel blood toward the heart. The presence of valves throughout the venous system is essential here; without valves, contraction of the veins would cause blood to flow backward, through the venules to the capillaries. [If the arterioles in a large part of the systemic circulation dilate, how will this affect cardiac output?[16]]

Cardiac Muscle

The force of contraction in the ventricles and atria is generated by the cardiac muscle cells that form the muscular walls of the chambers of the heart. The nature of the force generation in contractile cells and the differences between skeletal muscle, cardiac muscle, and smooth muscle will be presented in Chapter 11, but it is necessary to present some aspects of cardiac muscle to understand the heart. All muscle cells, including those of cardiac muscle, share with neurons the ability to propagate an action potential across their surface. The action potential in all muscle cells, as in neurons, is a wave of depolarization of the plasma membrane. [Do ligand-gated ion channels propagate action potentials in cardiac muscle?[17]]

A difference between neurons and cardiac muscle cells is that cardiac muscle is a **functional syncytium**. A syncytium is a tissue in which the cytoplasm of different cells can communicate via gap junctions. In cardiac muscle, the gap junctions are found in the **intercalated disks**, the connections between cardiac muscle cells. The depolarization of a cardiac muscle cell can be communicated directly through the cytoplasm to neighboring cardiac muscle cells through these gap junctions. (Recall that this is an example of an electrical synapse; there are no chemical synapses between cardiac muscle cells.) As a result, once an action potential starts, it spreads in a wave of depolarization throughout the cardiac muscle tissue in the atria or the ventricles. The atria and the ventricles are separate syncytia. The action potential in the heart is transmitted from the atrial syncytium to the ventricles by the **cardiac conduction system**. Transmission of the action potential is delayed slightly as it passes through the part of the conduction system known as the A-V node (Figure 5). [Why?[18] What would happen if gap junctions in the heart were blocked, but voltage-gated ion channels remained functional?[19]]

---

[16] If the arterioles open, more blood will flow through the tissues. The more blood that flows through the tissues, the greater the venous return and the greater the cardiac output.

[17] No. Ligand-gated ion channels may help to create the threshold depolarization required to trigger an action potential but do not play a role in propagating an action potential. Propagation of action potentials requires *voltage*-gated ion channels.

[18] In order for the heart to function normally, the atria must contract first (during diastole) to completely fill the ventricles with blood before they begin contracting during systole. Thus, the action potential must be propagated through the atrial syncytium before being propagated through the ventricular syncytium.

[19] The gap junctions between cells are necessary for the propagation of action potentials in cardiac muscle. A cell with blocked gap junctions could have an action potential on its own membrane in this circumstance if it reached threshold depolarization, but it would be unable to transmit the action potential to neighboring cells.

Voltage-gated sodium channels, also called **fast sodium channels**, play an important role in cardiac muscle, as in neurons, but, in addition, another type of voltage-gated channel, the **slow calcium channel**, is involved in the cardiac muscle action potential. Like all voltage-gated channels, these channels open in response to a change in membrane potential to a specific voltage (the threshold voltage) and, when open, allow the passage of calcium down its gradient. These channels also stay open longer than the fast sodium channels do, causing the membrane depolarization to last longer in cardiac muscle than in neurons, producing a plateau phase (Figure 4, on page 339).

The nature of the action potential in cardiac muscle affects the function of this tissue. Cardiac cells, like all cells with an excitable membrane, have a period during and just after the action potential during which they are refractory to new action potentials. Another result of the long depolarization in cardiac muscle is that the contraction of muscle lasts a long time, strengthening the force with which blood is expelled. To maximize the entry of calcium in the cell, cardiac muscle has involutions of the membrane called **T tubules**. The action potentials travel down along T tubules, allow the entry of calcium from the extracellular environment, and also induce the sarcoplasmic reticulum to release calcium. The combination of intracellular and extracellular calcium causes the contraction of actin-myosin fibers. [Will the absolute refractory period, during which a cell will not fire an action potential, be longer in cardiac or neuronal cells?[20] Will the strength of contraction by cardiac muscle be affected by the extracellular concentration of calcium ions?[21]]

Rhythmic Excitation of the Heart

Once an action potential is initiated, it will spread throughout the cardiac muscle of the heart. Interestingly, the heart is *not* stimulated to contract by neuronal or hormonal influences, although these can change the rate and strength of contraction (the **contractility** of the heart). Isolated cardiac muscle cells will in some circumstances continue contracting on their own, free of any external influences. So, what initiates the action potential in heart tissue? The initiation of each action potential that starts each cardiac cycle occurs automatically from within the heart itself, in a special region of the right atrium called the **sinoatrial (SA) node**. Under normal circumstances, the cells of the SA node act as the **pacemaker of the heart**. The SA node exhibits automaticity and its action potential is commonly divided into 3 separate phases; Phase 0, Phase 3, and Phase 4. (*Note*: Other cardiac myocytes (muscle cells) additionally have Phases 1 and 2, but the SA node does *not*; see Figure 3 on the next page).

The SA node is unique in that it has an *unstable resting potential* (not really resting, huh?). This is **Phase 4** (automatic slow depolarization) and is caused by special **sodium leak channels** that are responsible for its rhythmic, automatic excitation. This inward sodium leak brings the cell potential to the threshold for voltage-gated calcium channels; when they open they cause **Phase 0**, the upstroke of the pacemaker potential. It is caused mainly by an inward flow of Ca^{2+}. (*Note*: Skeletal muscle cells and other myocytes depolarize because of a *Na*$^+$ influx, not *Ca*$^{2+}$ like the SA node.) This Ca^{2+} drives the membrane potential of the SA nodal cells toward the positive Ca^{2+} equilibrium potential. Note also that the Ca^{2+} channels operate more slowly than the Na^+ channels, leading to a more gradual upsweep in the action potential.

---

[20] The absolute refractory period is the period during the action potential in which a new action potential cannot be induced. If the membrane is still depolarized as part of an action potential, it will be refractory to new action potentials. Cardiac muscle action potentials last much longer than neuronal (or skeletal muscle) action potentials, and will therefore have a longer absolute refractory period.

[21] Yes. A significant portion of the calcium that stimulates contraction comes from the extracellular pool, entering the cell as part of the action potential.

Phase 3 is repolarization. It is caused by closure of the Ca^{2+} channels and opening of the K^+ channels, leading to an outward flow of K^+ from the cell. This loss of positively charged K^+ ions drives the membrane potential back down toward the negative K^+ equilibrium potential.

The SA node cells transmit their action potential through intercalated discs to the rest of the conduction cells in the heart (as well as to the atrial myocytes), repolarize, then start the process over again, repeated once per heartbeat for the life of the individual (Figure 3).

- Why don't potassium leak channels cause spontaneous action potentials in neurons or muscle cells?[22]

Note that while several regions of the heart can spontaneously depolarize (e.g., the AV node, Purkinje fibers), the SA node has the most Na^+ leak channels of all of the conduction system. Thus, it reaches threshold before any other region of the heart does, and sets the rate of heart contraction (that's why it's called the "**pacemaker**" of the heart). When the SA nodal cells are injured or the pathway of atrial depolarization is blocked, these other regions of the heart will take over the pacemaking responsibility, but pace the heart at a slower rate.

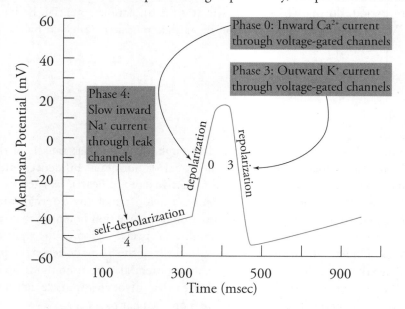

Figure 3 The Pacemaker Potential of the SA Node

The cardiac muscle cells of the heart have an action potential that differs from the SA node and the other conduction system cells. These muscle cells have a resting membrane potential of about –90 mV (very close to the K^+ equilibrium potential). The action potentials here have a long duration, up to 300 milliseconds normally. The phases of the action potential in these cells are Phases 0–4 (see Figure 4).

---

[22] Potassium leak channels allow potassium to leave the cell, down a gradient, polarizing the membrane; the *opposite* effect of sodium leak channels. Sodium is at a higher concentration outside of the cell, so sodium leak channels allow sodium to enter the cell and depolarize the membrane.

Phase 0 (depolarization) is again the upstroke of the action potential and is caused by the transient increase in Na⁺ conductance (just like in neurons). Action potentials propagating through the intercalated discs stimulate myocytes to reach threshold for voltage-gated Na⁺ channels. Once threshold is reached, the Na⁺ channels open and Na⁺ rushes into the cell.

In **Phase 1** (initial repolarization) the Na⁺ channels inactivate and K⁺ channels open. This leads to an efflux of K⁺ and a slight drop in cell potential. Furthermore, the increased potential due to the initial Na⁺ influx causes the opening of voltage-gated Ca²⁺ channels; this leads to **Phase 2**, the **plateau** phase. During the plateau, the influx of Ca²⁺ ions balance the K⁺ efflux from phase one, leading to a transient equilibrium in cell potential.

Phase 3 (repolarization) occurs when the Ca²⁺ channels close and the K⁺ channels continue to allow K⁺ to leave the cell (again, this is just like in neurons). **Phase 4** (the resting membrane potential) is the period during which inward and outward current are equal. Remember, this is dictated by action of the Na⁺/K⁺ ATPase and slow K⁺ leak channels.

Figure 4 Phases of the Membrane Potential in a Cardiac Muscle Cell

Thus, each heartbeat begins as an action potential in the **sinoatrial (SA) node** then spreads throughout the atria, causing them to contract and fill the ventricles with blood. The action potential also spreads down the special conduction pathway which transmits action potentials very rapidly without contracting. The pathway connects the SA node to the **atrioventricular (AV) node.** Since this pathway connects the two nodes, it is referred to as the **internodal tract**. Note that while the impulse travels to the AV node almost instantaneously, it spreads through the atria more slowly, because contracting heart muscle cells pass the impulse more slowly than specialized conduction fibers. At the AV node, the impulse is delayed slightly, then passes from the node to the ventricles via the conduction pathway again. This part of the conduction pathway is known as the **AV bundle** (**bundle of His**). The AV bundle divides into the **right** and **left bundle branches**, and then into the **Purkinje fibers**, which allow the impulse to spread rapidly and evenly over both ventricles. Note that the Purkinje fibers spread over the inferior portion of the ventricles (paradoxically called the "apex" of the heart). The result is that this region of the ventricles contracts first, and blood is pushed toward the superior region of the heart (paradoxically called the "base"), where the valves and arteries are (Figure 5).

Figure 5 The Cardiac Conduction System

Regulation of the Heart by the Autonomic Nervous System

The autonomic nervous system does not initiate action potentials in the heart, but it does regulate the rate of contraction. The intrinsic firing rate of the SA node is about 120 beats per minute. The reason the normal heart rate is only about 60–80 beats/minute is that the parasympathetic nervous system continually inhibits depolarization of the SA node. In particular, the **vagus nerve** (a cranial nerve) contains preganglionic axons which synapse in ganglia near the SA node. The postganglionic neurons innervate the SA node, releasing acetylcholine (ACh). The ACh inhibits depolarization by binding to receptors on the cells of the SA node. The constant level of inhibition provided by the vagus nerve is known as **vagal tone**. [Does ACh always inhibit postsynaptic cells? If not, how can different responses be elicited by the same neurotransmitter?[23]] In summary, the role of the *parasympathetic* system in controlling the heart is to modulate the rate by *inhibiting rapid automaticity*.

---

[23] ACh is the neurotransmitter released by all autonomic preganglionic neurons, all parasympathetic postganglionic neurons, and all somatic motor neurons. In most cases it is stimulatory, i.e., causes an action potential to occur, causes an effect in an organ. Whether a neurotransmitter is stimulatory or inhibitory depends only on the nature of its receptor on the postsynaptic cell.

The sympathetic system can also influence the heart. At rest, however, most nervous input is from the vagus. The sympathetic system kicks in when increased cardiac output is needed during a "fight or flight" response. The sympathetic system affects the heart in two ways: first, sympathetic postganglionic neurons directly innervate the heart, releasing norepinephrine. Second, epinephrine secreted by the adrenal medulla binds to receptors on cardiac muscle cells. The effect of sympathetic activation is stimulatory. The heart rate increases, and so does the force of contraction.

The heart rate and blood pressure are tightly regulated. In any regulatory system, three components are required: input (afferent information), integration (the function of the central nervous system), and output (efferent information, discussed in the above two paragraphs). The input in this regulatory system is complex, but we can highlight one key element: in the aortic arch and in the carotid arteries there are special receptors known as **baroreceptors**, which monitor pressure (like a *baro*meter). When they notify the central nervous system that the pressure is too high, the CNS sends out information to correct the problem: increased vagal tone and decreased sympathetic input. When the pressure is too low, the opposite happens. People with high blood pressure have a poorly functioning regulatory system and must take medications designed to keep things under control.

9.3 HEMODYNAMICS

Resistance

Hemodynamics is the study of blood flow. The driving force for blood flow is a difference in pressure from arteries to veins. The force opposing flow is friction, which results when blood squeezes through many tiny branching vessels. The technical term for this opposing force is **resistance**. Ohm's law summarizes the relationship between these variables: $\Delta P = Q \times R$. Here, ΔP is the pressure gradient (in mm Hg) from the arterial system to the venous system, Q stands for blood flow (or cardiac output in L/min), and R denotes resistance. The usefulness of this simple equation is twofold: first, it shows us that blood pressure is directly proportional to both cardiac output and peripheral resistance. If either of these change, blood pressure changes similarly. [How would an increase in stroke volume change blood pressure?[24]] Second, it shows us that if we want to change blood flow, we can only change it by changing either the pressure or the resistance; those are the only independent variables in the equation.

We know that pressure can be varied by increasing the *force* (thus changing the stroke volume) or *rate* (beats per minute) of cardiac contraction. What about resistance? The principal determinant of resistance is the degree of constriction of arteriolar smooth muscle, also known as **precapillary sphincters**. If arteriolar smooth muscles contract, it becomes more difficult for blood to flow from arteries into capillaries; that is, the resistance goes up. The resistance of the entire systemic circuit is easily calculated using the above equation in the form $R = \Delta P/Q$. We can measure ΔP and Q, then solve for R. This quantity is known as the **peripheral resistance**.

---

[24] Recall that CO = SV × HR, therefore, an increase in stroke volume would increase cardiac output. Since blood pressure and cardiac output are directly proportional, an increase in cardiac output would increase blood pressure as well.

The sympathetic nervous system controls the peripheral resistance. A certain amount of pressure in the arterial system is always desirable; otherwise not all tissues would be perfused. This basal level of pressure is provided by a constant level of norepinephrine released by millions of sympathetic postganglionic axons innervating precapillary sphincters. This constant nervous input is known as **adrenergic tone**. (Adrenergic means sympathetic; the word comes from adrenaline, which is another name for epinephrine.) [Why might tense, stressed out people tend to have high blood pressure?[25]]

The sympathetic system can increase the overall peripheral resistance, thus increasing blood pressure. It can also specifically divert blood away from one tissue so that another is preferentially perfused. In particular, sympathetic activation causes precapillary sphincters in the gut to contract, while arterioles supplying skeletal muscle are allowed to relax. The result is that blood flow is diverted from the gut to skeletal muscle, which facilitates the fight or flight response.

Blood Pressure

When physicians measure blood pressure, what they are actually measuring is **systemic arterial pressure**. This is the force per unit area exerted by blood upon the walls of arteries. You may recall that a typical blood pressure reading looks like this: 120/80, pronounced "120 over 80." What do the two numbers mean? 120 mm Hg is the **systolic pressure**, and 80 mm Hg is the **diastolic pressure**. In other words, 120 mm Hg is the highest pressure that ever occurs in the circulatory system of this particular patient during the time the blood pressure is being measured. This level is attained as the ventricles contract (that is, during systole). 80 mm Hg is as low as the pressure gets between heartbeats (that is, during diastole) during the measurement. The **pulse pressure** is the difference between systolic and diastolic pressures.

The measurement is taken using a **sphygmomanometer**, or "blood pressure cuff." This is an inflatable bag attached to a manometer (pressure-measuring device). The physician wraps the cuff around the upper arm and places a stethoscope at a point below the cuff where the pulse can be heard. Then she inflates the cuff until no blood flows into the arm (silence is heard in the stethoscope). Then she gradually reduces the cuff pressure, until a pulse first becomes audible. The significance of this point is that systolic arterial pressure is just greater than the pressure of the cuff. Thus, this pressure level is written down as the systolic pressure (120 in our example above). The pulse is very loud; this sound comes from blood slamming into arteries (which are constricted by the cuff) each time the heart beats. Then the physician continues to release pressure from the cuff. At a certain level, the pulse becomes much more quiet (usually inaudible). The significance of this is that now the cuff is loose enough so that blood flows smoothly through arteries and does not create the pounding noise described above. The point at which the pulse becomes inaudible is written down as the diastolic pressure. This is the lowest arterial pressure occurring at any time during the cardiac cycle.

It is important to emphasize the last sentence: this is the lowest *arterial* pressure occurring at any time during the cardiac cycle. You must realize that throughout the cardiac cycle, the pressure in the vena cava is about *zero* mm Hg. The highest pressures in the circulatory system are achieved in the left ventricle, aorta, and other large arteries. (That's what we measured with the cuff.) But every large artery branches, giving rise to many arterioles, and every arteriole gives rise to many capillaries. The result of all this branching is that the pressure generated by the heart is dissipated (Figure 6). By the time blood reaches the vena cava, it depends on valves to prevent backflow because the driving pressure is negligible.

---

[25] Tension and stress are similar to fear. Both involve activation of the sympathetic nervous system.

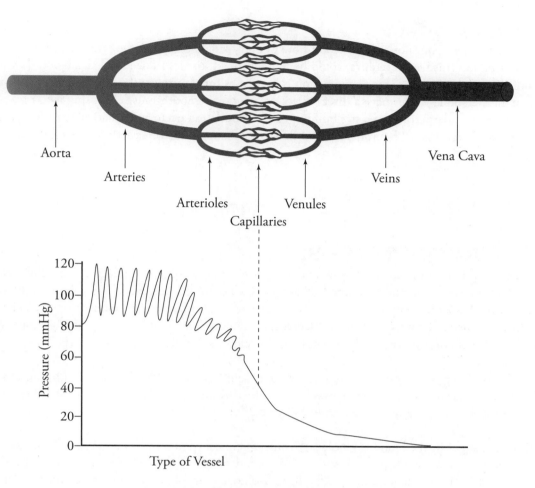

Figure 6   Pressures Throughout the Circulatory System

Why is the diastolic arterial pressure as high as it is? In other words, between heartbeats, why does the arterial pressure remain elevated? Without the heart contracting, wouldn't you expect the pressure to fall rapidly? This is the reason arteries are highly elastic and muscular. When the heart contracts, the arteries distend like balloons. During diastole, the arteries exert pressure on the blood, just as an inflated balloon exerts pressure on the air it contains. This maintains diastolic pressure, which is important because it provides a continued driving force for blood.

- Which one of the following will increase cardiac output?[26]
    A) Blocking sodium leak channels in the sinoatrial node
    B) Stimulation of the heart by the parasympathetic nervous system
    C) Significant dehydration due to prolonged exercise in the heat
    D) Contraction of smooth muscle in the walls of the large veins

---

[26] Blocking the sodium leak channels will slow the spontaneous firing of action potentials by the sinoatrial node and slow the heart rate. Slowing the heart rate will decrease, not increase the cardiac output (choice A is wrong). The parasympathetic nervous system slows the heart rate and therefore decreases the cardiac output (choice B is wrong). Dehydration will reduce venous return and reduce the stroke volume of the heart, leading to a reduction in cardiac output (choice C is wrong). However, the large veins do have smooth muscle, although less than arteries, and can constrict in response to sympathetic stimulation. This would increase the filling pressure (the pressure gradient), driving blood into the right atrium, thus increasing venous return, stroke volume, and cardiac output (choice **D** is correct). Note that this is a difficult and complex question because we do not normally think of the veins as having smooth muscle, and furthermore, we tend to think of blood flow *reduction* when a vessel constricts. The MCAT also has difficult and complex questions. The key to answering this question correctly is to have confidence in the elimination of choices A, B, and C. Thus, choice D, however improbable it may seem, must be the correct answer.

Local Autoregulation

The nervous system does not control blood flow to every single region of the body. The amount of feedback information this would require would be huge. Instead, tissues in need of extra blood flow are able to requisition it themselves. This phenomenon is known as **local autoregulation**. The mechanism is simple: certain metabolic wastes have a direct effect on arteriolar smooth muscle, causing it to relax. Hence, when a tissue is underperfused, wastes build up, and vasodilation occurs automatically. Autoregulation is the principal determinant of coronary blood flow (blood supply to the heart); it generally overrides nervous input.

9.4 COMPONENTS OF BLOOD

Blood has a liquid portion called **plasma**, and a portion which is composed of cells. The cellular elements of blood are known as **formed elements**. Plasma accounts for 55 percent of the volume of blood, and consists of the following items dissolved in water: electrolytes, buffers, sugars, blood proteins, lipoproteins, CO_2, O_2, and metabolic waste products. **Electrolytes** refer to Na^+, K^+, Cl^-, Ca^{2+}, and Mg^{2+} ions. **Buffers** in the blood maintain a constant pH of 7.4; the principal blood buffer is bicarbonate (HCO_3^-).

- During exercise, a significant amount of lactic acid is produced by fermentation in muscles that are not receiving adequate oxygen. Despite this increase in lactic acid, the pH of the blood does not change dramatically. Why not?[27]

The principal sugar in the blood is glucose. A constant concentration must be maintained so that all the cells of the body receive adequate nutrition. The blood proteins, most of which are made by the liver, include albumin, immunoglobulins (antibodies), fibrinogen, and lipoproteins. **Albumin** is essential for maintenance of **oncotic pressure** (osmotic pressure in the capillaries due only to plasma proteins). The **immunoglobulins** are a key part of the immune system (Section 9.7). **Fibrinogen** is essential for blood clotting (hemostasis). **Lipoproteins** are large particles consisting of fats, cholesterol, and carrier proteins. Their role is to transport lipids in the bloodstream. CO_2 and O_2 are involved in respiration, of course. However, CO_2 is also important for its role in buffering the blood (see the reaction in footnote 27). The principal *metabolic waste product* is **urea**, a breakdown product of amino acids. Urea is basically a carrier of excess nitrogen. There are other important waste products too, such as **bilirubin**, a breakdown product of heme (the oxygen-binding moiety of hemoglobin, discussed below).

By centrifuging whole blood, one can separate the plasma from the formed elements, as shown below. The volume of blood occupied by the red blood cells (**erythrocytes**) is known as the **hematocrit** (Figure 7). The normal hematocrit in adult males is 40–45 percent; in females it is lower, approximately 35–40 percent. White blood cells (**leukocytes**) and platelets account for a small volume (about 1 percent). All the formed elements of the blood develop from special cells in the bone marrow, known as **bone marrow stem cells**.

If whole blood is allowed to clot, one is left with a solid clot plus a clear fluid known as **serum**. Thus, serum is similar to plasma except that it lacks all the proteins involved in clotting.

---

[27] The HCO_3^- buffer system prevents pH changes via the reaction $CO_2 + H_2O \rightleftharpoons H_2CO_3 \rightleftharpoons HCO_3^- + H^+$.

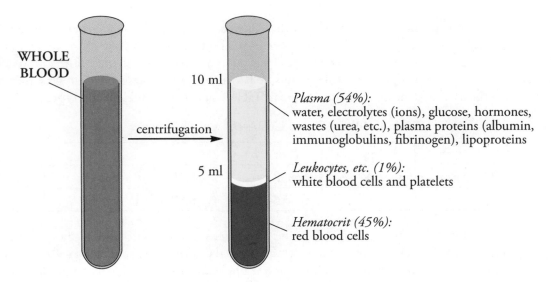

WHOLE BLOOD

10 ml

centrifugation

5 ml

Plasma (54%):
water, electrolytes (ions), glucose, hormones, wastes (urea, etc.), plasma proteins (albumin, immunoglobulins, fibrinogen), lipoproteins

Leukocytes, etc. (1%):
white blood cells and platelets

Hematocrit (45%):
red blood cells

Figure 7   The Hematocrit and the Components of Blood

Erythrocytes (Red Blood Cells—RBCs)

The hormone **erythropoietin** (made in the kidney) stimulates RBC production in the bone marrow. Aged RBCs are eaten by phagocytes in the spleen and liver.

The erythrocyte is a cell, but it has no nucleus or other organelles such as mitochondria. However, it does require the energy of ATP for processes such as ion pumping and basic maintenance of cell structure during its 120-day lifetime in the bloodstream. Lacking mitochondria, the RBC relies on glycolysis for ATP synthesis. The purpose of the RBC is to transport O_2 to the tissues from the lungs and CO_2 from the tissues to the lungs. Thus, it requires a large surface area for gas exchange. A high surface-to-volume ratio is achieved by the RBC's flat, biconcave shape (like a deflated basketball or a throat lozenge, see Figure 8). The RBC is able to carry oxygen because it contains millions of molecules of **hemoglobin** (more on hemoglobin below).

Figure 8   Red Blood Cells (Erythrocytes)

Blood Typing

Blood typing is the classification of a person's blood based on the presence or absence of certain surface antigens on their red blood cells. The two most important blood group antigens are the **ABO blood group** and the **Rh blood group**. The ABO blood group consists of glycoproteins that are coded for by three different alleles: I^A, I^B, and i. These alleles and their genotypes and phenotypes were discussed in more detail in Chapter 7 (Genetics and Evolution).

The other main antigen used in blood typing is the Rh (rhesus) factor. The expression of this antigen follows a classically dominant pattern: *RR* and *Rr* genotypes lead to the expression of the protein on the surface of the red blood cell (Rh positive), and the *rr* genotype leads to the absence of the protein (Rh negative). The combinations of the ABO alleles and the Rh alleles (and the respective antigens they code for) determine the overall blood type of an individual. Table 1 summarizes these blood types.

Table 1   Blood Group Genotypes and Phenotypes

	$I^A I^A$ or $I^A i$	$I^B I^B$ or $I^B i$	$I^A I^B$	ii
RR or *Rr*	type A+	type B+	type AB+	type O+
rr	type A-	type B-	type AB-	type O-

Determining blood type is critical when performing blood transfusions. Antibodies to the A and B antigens are produced early in infancy and can cause clumping and destruction of red blood cells bearing the incorrect antigen (called a **transfusion reaction**). For example, a person with A+ blood produces anti-B antibodies; if transfused with type B blood, these antibodies will clump and destroy the donated type B cells, possibly leading to the death of the recipient. Note that this early production of antibodies without prior exposure to the antigen is unusual; typically the immune system must be exposed to a foreign protein before it produces antibodies against it.

Antibodies to the Rh antigen do not develop unless a person with Rh– blood is exposed to Rh+ blood, an event called "sensitization"; note that this is the typical response of the immune system to a foreign protein (antigen). Subsequent exposure to Rh+ blood can then result in a transfusion reaction. This is particularly dangerous in the case of an Rh– mother carrying an Rh+ baby. Typically, if it is the first baby there are no complications (unless the mother had been previously sensitized); the mother's blood and the baby's blood do not mix during pregnancy. However, on delivery, some Rh+ cells from the child can mix with the mother's Rh– blood and lead to her sensitization. Future Rh+ babies are then at risk, since the anti-Rh antibodies can cross the placental barrier to clump and/or destroy the Rh+ baby's red blood cells. This is known as **hemolytic disease of the newborn** or *erythroblastosis fetalis*, and can be fatal. Injection of the mother at the time of birth with anti-Rh antibodies can clump and lead to the destruction of any stray Rh+ cells from the baby; this can prevent sensitization of the mother and protect any future unborn Rh+ children.

Two special blood types are AB+ and O–. Type AB+ individuals do not make antibodies to any of the blood group antigens, since their red blood cells possess all three of the antigens. Thus, type AB+ individuals are known as "**universal recipients**" because they can receive any of the other blood types without complication. Type O– individuals do not possess any of the surface antigens that could trigger a reaction in an individual with a different blood type. Thus, O– individuals are known as "universal donors" because they can donate blood to any of the other blood types, typically without complication. (Note that type O– individuals do make anti-A and anti-B antibodies, and these can sometimes cause issues in recipients. It is always best to match blood types between donors and recipients when possible.)

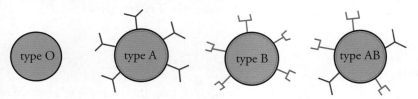

Figure 9   RBC Surface Antigens

Leukocytes

The white blood cell's role is to fight infection and dispose of debris. All white blood cells are large complex cells with all the normal eukaryotic cell structures (nucleus, mitochondria, etc.). Some white blood cells (**macrophages** and **neutrophils**) move by amoeboid motility (crawling). This is important because they are able to squeeze out of capillary intercellular junctions (spaces between capillary endothelial cells) and can therefore roam free in the tissues, hunting for foreign particles and pathogens. Some white blood cells exhibit **chemotaxis**, which means movement directed by chemical stimuli. The chemical stimuli can be toxins and waste products released by pathogens, or can be chemical signals released from other white blood cells. There are six types of white blood cells (Table 2).

Table 2 Roles of the Six Types of Leukocytes

Cell	Role
monocytes:	
macrophage	phagocytose debris and microorganisms; amoeboid motility; chemotaxis
lymphocytes:	
B cell	mature into *plasma cell* and produce antibodies
T cell	kill virus-infected cells, tumor cells, and reject tissue grafts; also control immune response
granulocytes:	
neutrophil	phagocytose bacteria resulting in pus; amoeboid motility; chemotaxis
eosinophil	destroy parasites; allergic reactions
basophil	store and release histamine; allergic reactions

Platelets and Hemostasis

Like red blood cells, platelets have no nuclei and a limited lifespan. They are derived from the fragmentation of large bone marrow cells called **megakaryocytes**, which are derived from the same stem cells that give rise to red blood cells and white blood cells. The function of platelets is to aggregate at the site of damage to a blood vessel wall, forming a **platelet plug**. This immediately helps stop bleeding. **Hemostasis** is a term for the body's mechanism of preventing bleeding.

The other component of the hemostatic response is **fibrin**. This is a threadlike protein which forms a mesh that holds the platelet plug together. When the fibrin mesh dries, it becomes a scab, which seals and protects the wound. The plasma protein **fibrinogen** is converted into fibrin by a protein called **thrombin** when bleeding occurs. A blood clot, or **thrombus**, is a scab circulating in the bloodstream. Calcium as well as many accessory proteins are necessary for the activation of thrombin and fibrinogen. Several of the proteins depend on vitamin K for their function. Defects in these proteins result in **hemophilia** ("loving to bleed"), an X-linked recessive group of diseases involving excessive bleeding.

9.5 TRANSPORT OF GASES

Oxygen

Oxygen is too hydrophobic to dissolve in the plasma in significant quantities. Therefore, RBCs are used to bind and carry O_2. RBCs are able to carry oxygen because they contain millions of molecules of **hemoglobin** (Hb). This is a complex protein composed of four polypeptide subunits. Each subunit contains one molecule of **heme**, which is a large multi-ring structure that has a single iron atom bound at its center. The role of heme with its iron atom is to bind O_2. Since each hemoglobin has four subunits and each subunit has one heme, each molecule of hemoglobin can carry four molecules of oxygen. Hemoglobin has some important properties which make it an excellent oxygen carrier.

The four subunits of hemoglobin do not bind oxygen independently of one another. When none of the subunits have oxygen bound, all four subunits assume a **tense** conformation that has a relatively low affinity for oxygen. (A *conformation* is a specific three-dimensional structure of a protein.) When one of the subunits binds oxygen, its conformation changes from a tense to a **relaxed** state that has a higher affinity for oxygen. The change in the three-dimensional structure of the subunit with oxygen bound is then communicated to the other subunits through contacts between the polypeptides to alter their conformation and increase their affinity for oxygen as well. Thus, hemoglobin is said to bind oxygen **cooperatively**.

- Myoglobin is a molecule with a structure very similar to hemoglobin, but with a single subunit that has one binding site. Does myoglobin display cooperativity in oxygen binding?[28]
- If binding of oxygen is cooperative, is it saturable?[29]
- Does hemoglobin have higher affinity for oxygen in the tissues or in the lungs?[30]

This has monumental significance for the ability of the blood to transport oxygen efficiently. The level of O_2 in active tissues is very low, because they use it in oxidative phosphorylation. Thus, in the tissues, hemoglobin has low affinity for oxygen and tends to release any oxygen which it carries. The level of O_2 in the lungs is of course very high. Hence, when a red blood cell is passing through a capillary in the lungs, the hemoglobin it contains will have higher affinity due to cooperative binding and will tend to bind oxygen very strongly. The result is that a lot of oxygen is picked up by RBCs in the lungs, and most of it is released as they pass through active tissues that need oxygen. This is an amazing example of how structural biochemistry determines physiology (or vice versa).

There is even more complexity to the hemoglobin story. It turns out that certain factors stabilize the tense configuration (which has a low O_2 affinity). These factors are:

1) decreased pH,
2) increased P_{CO_2} (level of CO_2 in the blood), and
3) increased temperature.

---

[28] Cooperativity requires more than one binding site in a protein so that one binding site can alter the affinity of another. Myoglobin cannot be cooperative in oxygen binding since it has only one binding site.

[29] There are a limited number of binding sites, even if they are cooperative, so binding will be saturated at a high concentration (partial pressure) of oxygen. There is a limit to the oxygen carrying capacity of the blood.

[30] At higher partial pressure of oxygen, more of the hemoglobin protein will have at least one of the subunits occupied with oxygen. Since binding is cooperative, the more oxygen that is bound, the higher the affinity for oxygen. The partial pressure of oxygen is higher in the lungs than in the tissues, so hemoglobin will have higher affinity for oxygen in the lungs.

The fact that these factors stabilize tense hemoglobin and thus reduce its oxygen affinity is known as the **Bohr effect**. This system is truly incredible when you realize that these three factors perfectly characterize the environment within active tissues. [What is the significance of this?[31]]

The affinity of hemoglobin for oxygen can be quantified by measurement of the fraction of O_2-binding sites which have bound O_2. If hemoglobin is in the relaxed configuration, then as more oxygen becomes available, much more of it will be bound up. But if it is in the tense configuration, the tendency to bind oxygen is reduced, and less will be bound. This can be described mathematically using the notion of **percent saturation (% sat.)**:

$$\text{\% sat.} = (\text{\# of } O_2 \text{ molecules bound}) \div (\text{\# of } O_2 \text{ binding sites}) \times 100\%$$

• At a given P_{O_2}, which has a higher % sat.: tense or relaxed hemoglobin?[32]

This information can be depicted graphically, using an **O_2-Hemoglobin Dissociation Curve**, which plots % sat. vs. P_{O_2} (Figure 10). The sigmoidal shape of the curve resembles the behavior of cooperative enzymes.

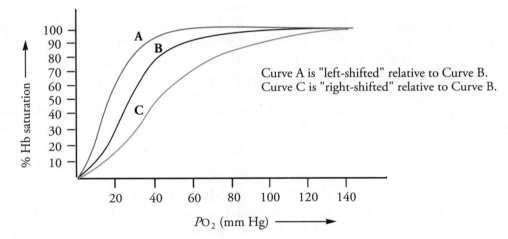

Curve A is "left-shifted" relative to Curve B.
Curve C is "right-shifted" relative to Curve B.

Figure 10 O_2-Hemoglobin Dissociation Curves

---

[31] When a tissue is active, its cells metabolize a lot of glucose and this results in an elevated P_{CO_2}. Soon the cells run low on oxygen and begin to perform lactic acid fermentation. The result is a drop in pH. Finally, whenever there is a lot of metabolic activity, the temperature increases. So, due to the Bohr effect, hemoglobin is most ready to release its load of oxygen in regions of the body where oxygen is most needed!

[32] Relaxed, since it has a higher affinity. This just means that at any O_2 level, relaxed hemoglobin will bind more O_2 than tense hemoglobin will.

Answer all of the following questions about Figure 10 before looking at the footnote.[33]

- Curve _____ represents Hb with the highest affinity of all.
- Curve C could be the result of _____.
- Curve A would most likely be seen in what region of the body?
- Why do all the curves level off?
- It is interesting to note that fetal hemoglobin is a bit different from adult hemoglobin. The fetus must be able to "steal" oxygen away from the mother's blood. Hence, the O_2 dissociation curve for fetal hemoglobin is _____-shifted relative to the curve for adult hemoglobin.

Carbon Dioxide

Carbon dioxide is transported in the blood in three ways:

1) 73% of CO_2 transport is accomplished by the conversion of CO_2 to **carbonic acid**, which can dissociate into **bicarbonate** and a **proton** according to this reaction: $CO_2 + H_2O \rightleftharpoons H_2CO_3 \rightleftharpoons HCO_3^- + H^+$. These compounds are extremely water-soluble and are thus easily carried in the blood. The conversion of CO_2 into carbonic acid is catalyzed by an RBC enzyme called **carbonic anhydrase**. Remember that this reaction is also important as the principal plasma pH buffer.

2) Some CO_2 (~ 20%) is transported by simply being stuck onto hemoglobin. It does *not* bind to the oxygen-binding sites, but rather to other sites on the protein. Binding of CO_2 to hemoglobin is important in the Bohr effect because it stabilizes tense Hb.

3) CO_2 is somewhat more water-soluble than O_2, so a fair amount (~ 7%) can be dissolved in the blood and carried from the tissues to the lungs. Virtually no oxygen can be dissolved in the blood.

Exchange of Substances Across the Capillary Wall

The capillaries are the site of exchange between the blood and tissues. To facilitate exchange, capillaries have walls of only a single layer of flattened endothelial cells, and there are spaces (**intercellular clefts**) between the endothelial cells that make up the capillary wall. Three types of substances must be able to pass through the clefts: nutrients, wastes, and white blood cells. We will discuss each of these in turn. [Is it necessary for O_2 and CO_2 to pass through the clefts?[34]]

There are three main types of nutrients: amino acids, glucose, and lipids. Amino acids and glucose are absorbed from the digestive tract and carried by a special vein called the **hepatic portal vein** to the liver. It is called a *portal vein* because it connects two capillary beds: the one in the intestinal wall and the one inside the liver. The liver stores amino acids and glucose and releases them into the bloodstream as needed. From the bloodstream they can pass through capillary clefts into the tissues. The journey of lipids through the bloodstream is different. Fats are absorbed from the intestine and packaged into **chylomicrons**, which are a type of lipoprotein. The chylomicrons enter tiny lymphatic vessels in the intestinal wall called **lacteals**. The lacteals empty into larger lymphatics, which eventually drain into a large vein near the neck. Hence, dietary fats bypass the hepatic vein. The result is that after eating a fatty meal, a person's

---

[33] Curve A is farthest to the left and thus represents the highest affinity. Curve C could be the result of the Bohr effect. At a given O_2 level, the hemoglobin studied in Curve C has less of a tendency to bind oxygen (a lower affinity). Curve A would most likely be seen in the lungs, where there is plenty of oxygen and relaxed hemoglobin predominates. All the curves level off because 100% is the maximum degree of saturation; all the hemoglobin molecules become completely saturated. Fetal Hb has a left-shifted curve (higher affinity).

[34] No, they can pass straight through any cell by simple diffusion.

blood will appear milky. (The term for this is **lipemia**, which means "lipids flowing in the blood.") The chylomicrons are taken up by the liver and converted into another type of lipoprotein, which is released into the bloodstream. This lipoprotein carries fats to **adipocytes** (fat cells) for storage. When fats are to be used for energy, adipocyte triglycerides are hydrolyzed, and free fatty acids are released into the bloodstream. They pass easily through capillary pores and thus can be picked up by cells of various tissues.

Many wastes are produced during cellular metabolism. They diffuse through the capillary walls into the bloodstream. The liver removes many wastes and converts them into forms which can be excreted in the feces. Such compounds are passed into the gut as **bile**. Other wastes are excreted directly by the kidneys.

White blood cells must be able to pass out of capillaries in order to patrol the tissues for invading microorganisms. Two of the six types of white blood cell can squeeze through the clefts: the _____ and the _____. These are large cells which depend on _____ in order to fit through the clefts, which are too small to allow RBCs to pass.[35]

It is also important to realize that water has a great tendency to flow out of capillaries through the clefts. There are two reasons: 1) The hydrostatic pressure (fluid pressure) created by the heart simply tends to squeeze water out of the capillaries, and 2) the high osmolarity of the tissues tends to draw water out of the bloodstream. The circulatory system deals with this problem by giving the plasma a high osmolarity. [Would dissolving NaCl in the plasma accomplish this?[36]] Plasma osmolarity is provided by high concentrations of large plasma proteins, mainly albumin. Albumin is too large and rigid to pass through the clefts, so it remains in the capillaries and keeps water there too. The osmotic pressure provided by plasma proteins is given a special name: **oncotic pressure**. However, some water does leak out, resulting in an interesting cycle.

1) At the beginning of the capillary, the hydrostatic pressure is high. The result is that water squeezes out into the tissues.
2) As water continues to leave the capillary, the relative concentration of plasma proteins increases.
3) At the end of the capillary the hydrostatic pressure is quite low, but since the blood is now very concentrated, the oncotic pressure is very high. As a result, water flows back into the capillary from the tissues.

Thus, some water is lost into the tissues, but due to the oncotic pressure of the plasma proteins, the net loss is normally low. Occasionally the system breaks down and a significant amount of water is lost into the tissues. For example, during **inflammation**, capillaries dilate, increasing the size of the intercellular clefts. This allows more space for white blood cells to migrate into the tissues. The unfortunate side-effect is that plasma proteins and a lot of water are lost into the tissues. The result is water in the tissues, or swelling, termed **edema**. Small amounts of fluid loss into the tissues are normal; even some protein is normally lost. Fluid, proteins, and white blood cells in the tissues are returned to the bloodstream via the lymphatic system.

- What would occur if capillaries throughout the circulatory system were made more permeable?[37]
- Albumin is made in the liver. Alcoholics with diseased livers make insufficient amounts of albumin, and thus have insufficient plasma oncotic pressure. What result would you predict?[38]

---

[35] Macrophages and neutrophils can squeeze through the clefts, even though they are larger than RBCs, because they are capable of *amoeboid motility*, as noted in Table 2. RBCs are not capable of independent motility.

[36] No, because salts can freely pass out of the capillaries.

[37] A significant volume of fluid will be lost from the plasma into tissues, decreasing the blood volume and cardiac output. Circulatory shock can result.

[38] The result is edema of the entire body, including the limbs, abdomen, and lungs.

9.6 THE LYMPHATIC SYSTEM

The lymphatic system (Figure 11) is a one-way flow system which begins with tiny lymphatic capillaries in all the tissues of the body that merge to form larger lymphatic vessels. These merge to form large lymphatic ducts. Lymphatic vessels have valves, and the larger lymphatic ducts have smooth muscles in their walls. As a result, the lymphatic system acts like a suction pump to retrieve water, proteins, and white blood cells from the tissues. The fluid in lymphatic vessels is called **lymph**. The lymph is filtered by numerous **lymph nodes**. The lymph nodes are an important part of the immune system because they contain millions of white blood cells that can initiate an immune response against anything foreign that may have been picked up in the lymph. The large lymphatic ducts merge to form the **thoracic duct**, which is the largest lymphatic vessel, located in the chest. The thoracic duct empties into a large vein near the neck. Also, lymphatic vessels from the intestines dump dietary fats in the form of chylomicrons into the thoracic duct.

Figure 11 The Lymphatic System: Vessels and Lymph Nodes

9.7 THE IMMUNE SYSTEM

The interior of the body provides a warm, protective, nourishing environment where microorganisms can flourish. We could not survive without a versatile and efficient immune system to destroy invaders without destroying the body itself. There are three types of immunity: innate, humoral, and cell-mediated.

Innate Immunity

Innate immunity refers to the general, nonspecific protection the body provides against various invaders. The simplest example of innate immunity is the barrier to the outside world known as **skin**. The skin prevents many types of pathogens from infecting us. Here is a list of the principal components of innate immunity:

1) The skin is an excellent barrier against the entry of microorganisms.
2) Tears, saliva, and blood contain **lysozyme**, an enzyme that kills some bacteria by destroying their cell walls.
3) The extreme acidity of the stomach destroys many pathogens which are ingested with food or swallowed after being passed out of the respiratory tract.
4) Macrophages and neutrophils indiscriminately phagocytize microorganisms.[39]
5) The **complement system** is a group of about 20 blood proteins that can nonspecifically bind to the surface of foreign cells, leading to their destruction.

---

[39] Do not confuse this portion of innate immunity with cell-mediated immunity. You are correct to notice that cells are involved, but this activity is placed in the "innate" category because we are referring to nonspecific phagocytosis. Humoral and cell-mediated immunity are highly specific. There is one other subtlety: when a macrophage eats an antigen which has been coated with specific antibodies, we are dealing with humoral immunity; this is different from the indiscriminate, nonspecific pathogen phagocytosis discussed above.

Humoral Immunity, Antibodies, and B Cells

Humoral immunity refers to specific protection by proteins in the plasma called **antibodies** (**Ab**) or **immunoglobulins** (**Ig**). Antibodies specifically recognize and bind to microorganisms (or other foreign particles), leading to their destruction and removal from the body. Each antibody molecule is composed of two copies of two different polypeptides, the **light chains** and the **heavy chains**, joined by disulfide bonds (Figure 12). In addition, each antibody molecule has two regions, the **constant region** and the **variable (antigen binding) region**. There are several different classes of immunoglobulins, differentiated by their constant regions: IgG, IgA, IgM, IgD, and IgE. The classes of immunoglobulins have slightly different functions (see Table 3), with most of the antibody circulating in plasma in the IgG class. The variable regions are responsible for the specificity of antibodies in recognizing foreign particles.

Figure 12   Antibody Structure

Constant Region Class	Location in Body	Function
IgM	blood and B cell surface	Involved in initial immune response; pentameric structure in blood, monomeric structure on B cell as antigen receptor
IgG	blood	Involved in ongoing immune response; the majority of antibody in the blood is IgG; can also cross the placental barrier
IgD	B cell surface	Serves with IgM as antigen receptor on B cells
IgA	secretions (saliva, mucus, tears, breast milk, etc.)	Secreted in breast milk; helps protect newborns, dimeric structure
IgE	blood	Involved in allergic reactions

Table 3   Classes of Antibodies

Each antibody forms a unique variable region that has a different binding specificity. The molecule that an antibody binds to is known as the **antigen** (**Ag**). Examples of antigens are viral capsid proteins, bacterial surface proteins, and toxins in the bloodstream (such as tetanus toxin). [Would an antibody against a cytoplasmic bacterial protein help the immune system to remove the bacteria?[40]] The specificity of antigen binding is determined by the fit of antigen in a small three-dimensional cleft formed by the variable region of the antibody molecule (Figure 12). [If the antigen binding site is small, can antibodies recognize

---

[40] No. Antibodies are soluble in the plasma, so they can only recognize antigens on surfaces that are accessible to them. A protein in the cytoplasm of a bacteria would never be accessible to antibodies in the plasma and therefore could not be recognized.

9.7

large proteins as antigens?[41] Why might an antibody that binds tightly to a small region of a protein, five amino acids out of 200, have very low affinity for the same five amino acids of the protein when presented as an isolated peptide?[42]] Antigens are often large molecules which have many different recognition sites for different antibodies. The small site that an antibody recognizes within a larger molecule is called an **epitope**. Very small molecules often do not elicit the production of antibodies on their own but will when bound to an antigenic large molecule like a protein. The protein in this case is called a **carrier**, and the small molecule that becomes antigenic is known as a **hapten**. When antibody binds to an antigen, the following can contribute to removal of the antigen from the body:

1) Binding of antibody may directly inactivate the antigen. For example, binding of antibody to a viral coat protein may prevent the virus from binding to cells.
2) Binding of antibody can induce phagocytosis of a particle by macrophages and neutrophils.
3) The presence of antibodies on the surface of a cell can activate the complement system to form holes in the cell membrane and lyse the cell.

Antibodies are produced by a type of lymphocyte called **B cells**. Antibodies produced by an individual B cell can recognize only one specific antigen, but B cells in general produce antibodies that recognize an immense array of antigens. How do B cells produce such a broad array of antibodies? Does the genome encode a gene for every possible antibody molecule, a million genes for a million different potential antibodies? No. Immature B cells are derived from precursor stem cells in the bone marrow. The genes that encode antibody proteins are assembled by recombination from many small segments during B cell development. Thus, there are many different B cell clones, each with a different variable region. The immature B cells express antibody molecules on their surface. When antigen binds to the antibody on the surface of a specific immature B cell, that cell is stimulated to proliferate and differentiate into two kinds of cells: **plasma cells** and **memory cells**. Plasma cells actively produce and secrete antibody protein into the plasma. Memory cells are produced from the same clone and have the same variable regions, but do not secrete antibody; they are like pre-activated, dormant B cells. The memory cells remain dormant, sometimes for years, waiting for the same antigen to reappear. If it does, the memory cells *then* become activated, and start producing antibody very quickly; so quickly that no symptoms of illness appear. This method of selecting B cells with specific antigen binding is called **clonal selection**. [In general, every cell of the body is said to possess the same copy of the genome. Is this true in the immune system?[43]]

---

[41] Yes. Antibodies often recognize proteins as antigens, but they do not recognize the whole protein. Usually antibodies recognize a small part of a protein as an antigen.

[42] In the intact protein the five amino acids assume a specific three-dimensional conformation that is recognized well by the antibody. The five amino acids as a small peptide, however, will not fold the same way and probably would not be as well recognized by the antibody.

[43] No. Recombination during development of B cells and T cells makes these an exception to the generalization that every cell contains the whole genome.

- Which one of the following best describes the mechanism by which production of specific antibody is achieved in response to antigen exposure?[44]
  - A) Immature B cell clones expressing several different antibody genes select for one gene and turn off expression of the others.
  - B) Antigen stimulates proliferation of a specific B cell clone expressing a single antibody protein that recognizes that antigen.
  - C) The variable regions of antibody proteins on an immature B cell clone form a pocket around the antigen, and the antibody genes are recombined to fit the bound antigen.
  - D) Antibody light and heavy chains are mixed on each B cell's surface in different combinations to produce different antigen recognition.

The first time a person encounters an antigen during an infection, it can take a week or more for B cells to proliferate and secrete significant levels of antibody. This is known as the **primary immune response** and is too slow to prevent symptoms of the infection from occurring. The immune response to the same antigen the second time a person is exposed, the **secondary immune response**, is much swifter and stronger, so much so that symptoms never develop, and the person is said to "be immune." This immunity can last for years and is due to the presence of the memory cells produced during the first infection. **Vaccination** is used to improve the response to infection by exposing the immune system to an antigen associated with a virus or bacterium, thus building up the secondary immune response if the live pathogen is encountered in the future. [Vaccination against some viruses is ineffective in preventing future infection, while it is highly effective against other viruses. Does the failure of vaccination to protect against some viruses indicate a failure in the ability to produce memory cells?[45]]

Cell-Mediated Immunity and the T Cell

There are two types of **T cells**: **T helpers** ("CD4 cells") and **T killers** (cytotoxic T cells, "CD8 cells").[46] The role of the T helper is to activate B cells, T killer cells, and other cells of the immune system. Hence, the T helper is the central controller of the whole immune response. It communicates with other cells by releasing special hormones called **lymphokines** and **interleukins**.[47] The T helper cell is the host of HIV, the virus that causes AIDS.

The role of the T killer cell is to *destroy abnormal host cells*, namely:

1) Virus-infected host cells
2) Cancer cells
3) Foreign cells such as the cells of a skin graft given by an incompatible donor

---

[44] Choice **B** is correct. The two key features of clonal selection in B cells are 1) recombination during development to produce many clones, each with a single antigen recognition specificity, and 2) selection of a clone out of the many clones based on specific recognition of antigen by preexisting antibody genes.

[45] No. It is probably the result of mutation by the virus. Vaccination against one form of virus and production of memory cells will not protect against a virus if the viral antigen mutates so that it is no longer recognized by the immune system.

[46] "CD" stands for "Cell Differentiation marker."

[47] *Lympho-* is short for lymphocytes, and *-kine* means move or activate. *Inter-* means between, and *-leukin* is for leukocytes or white blood cells.

The "T" in "T cell" stands for **thymus**. T cells are named after this gland because this is where they develop during childhood. Trillions of different T cells are produced in the bone marrow during childhood. Each of these is specific for a particular antigen, just as with B cells. [If a T cell is specific for an antigen, does that mean it releases antibodies that bind to the antigen?[48]] The protein on the T cell surface that can bind antigen is the **T cell receptor**.

The function of T cells is exceedingly complex. As a brief introduction, the way a T cell recognizes a bad cell is by "examining" (binding to) proteins on its surface. One important group of cell-surface proteins is known as the **major histocompatibility complex** (**MHC**). Our cells are all programmed to have MHC proteins on their surfaces so that the immune system can keep an eye on what is going on inside every cell. There are two kinds of MHCs, known as MHC class I and MHC class II, or simply **MHC I** and **MHC II**. MHC I proteins are found on the surface of every nucleated cell in the body. Their role is to randomly pick up peptides from the inside of the cell and display them on the cell surface. This allows T cells to monitor cellular contents. For example, if a cell is infected with a virus, one of its class I MHC complexes will display a piece of a virus-specific protein. When a T killer cell detects the viral protein (by binding to it) displayed on the cell's MHC I, it becomes activated and will proliferate.

The role of MHC II is more complex. Only certain special cells have MHC II. These cells are known as **antigen-presenting cells** (**APCs**). The antigen-presenting cells include macrophages and B cells. Their role is to phagocytize particles or cells, chop them up, and display fragments using the MHC II display system, which T helpers then recognize (bind to). After a T helper is activated by antigen displayed in MHC II, it will activate B cells (and stimulate proliferation of T killer cells) that are specific for that antigen. The activated B cells mature into plasma cells and secrete antibodies specific for the antigen. The complexity of this process helps explain why the primary immune response takes a week or more.

- Can a T helper cell become activated after encountering a foreign particle floating in the blood? If so, how? If not, why not, and what else is required?[49]

Note that full activation of T cells only occurs when the T cell binds to both antigen (displayed on MHC I or II) and the MHC molecule itself.

Other Tissues Involved in the Immune Response

The **bone marrow** is the site of synthesis of all the cells of the blood from a common progenitor. The cell that gives rise to all the various blood cells is called the bone marrow stem cell. **Lymph nodes** were discussed earlier in this chapter. The **spleen** filters the blood and is a site of immune cell interactions, just like lymph nodes. The spleen also destroys aged RBCs. The **thymus** is the site of T cell maturation. The thymus shrinks in size in adults since the maturation of the immune system and T cells is most active in children. The **tonsils** are masses of lymphatic tissue in the back of the throat that help "catch" pathogens which enter the body through respiration or ingestion. The **appendix** is very similar to the tonsils, both in structure and function, and is found near the beginning of the large intestine. Neither the appendix nor the tonsils are required for survival and are often removed if they become infected.

---

[48] No, only B cells make antibodies. If a T helper is specific for an antigen, it will activate B cells or T killers to destroy it.

[49] No, T helpers are only activated by antigen presented on MHC II. For a foreign particle to activate a helper T cell, the particle must first be displayed by an antigen-presenting cell (macrophage or B cell). The antigen-presenting cell must phagocytize the particle, hydrolyze it into fragments in a lysosome, and allow it to bind to an MHC II which will be displayed on the cell surface.

9.8 AUTOIMMUNITY

Ideally, the immune system will only recognize and destroy foreign antigen; it should ignore (not become activated against) all normal proteins and cell structures; this is called **tolerance**. However, the production of these trillions of different B cells and T cells with different receptors is random, and as a result, many of them will be specific for normal molecules found in the human body, or *self* antigens. Thus, B cells and T cells must go through a selection process in order to eliminate any self-reactive cells.

For B cells, this generally occurs in the bone marrow, but can also occur in lymph nodes. An immature B cell whose surface receptor binds to normal cell surface proteins (for example, MHCs or other proteins on a macrophage or other bone marrow cell) is induced to die through apoptosis. Those whose surface receptors bind to normal soluble proteins (for example, hemoglobin or lipoproteins) do not go through apoptosis, but become unresponsive or **anergic**. Only those B cells whose surface receptors bind to no normal proteins during maturation are released into the circulation. For T cells, the process is similar, but occurs in the thymus or in the lymph nodes. Immature T cells whose antigen receptors bind normal proteins in the thymus undergo apoptosis, and (because not all proteins are expressed in the thymus), some T cells are released that may bind surface proteins in the periphery; these cells become anergic. The result of this is that billions of B and T cells survive, but billions of others do not. The ones that survive go on to proliferate if stimulated by antigen in the proper context, each producing a group of identical B or T cells, all specific for a particular antigen. Such a group is known as a **B cell or T cell clone**. Clonal selection in response to antigen recognition is similar in B and T cells.

It is very important to get rid of all cells specific for self-antigen, because such cells can cause an **auto-immune reaction**, in which the immune system attacks normal body cells or proteins. Obviously, this would cause problems as normal body structures become inflamed or destroyed. Some autoimmune diseases include type I diabetes mellitus, rheumatoid arthritis, Graves' disease, myasthenia gravis, and celiac disease. Autoimmune diseases are often treated with immunosuppressant drugs or with steroids to reduce the inflammatory response.

9.8

Chapter 9 Summary

- The circulatory and lymphatic systems transport materials (O_2, CO_2, nutrients, wastes, hormones, etc.) around the body. The lymphatic system helps to filter and return tissue fluid (lymph) to the circulatory system.

- Deoxygenated blood returning from the body enters the heart at the right atrium, and is pumped to the lungs by the right ventricle. The oxygenated blood returns to the heart at the left atrium, and is pumped to the body by the left ventricle.

- AV valves (tricuspid on the right and bicuspid, or mitral, on the left) separate the atria and ventricles. Semilunar valves (pulmonary on the right and aortic on the left) separate the ventricles and the arteries.

- Veins always return blood to the heart. Most veins carry deoxygenated blood; an exception are the pulmonary veins, which return blood from the lungs to the heart.

- Arteries always carry blood away from the heart. Most arteries carry oxygenated blood; an exception are the pulmonary arteries, which carry blood from the heart to the lungs.

- Endothelial cells line the insides of blood vessels and form the walls of capillaries. They are important mediators of vasoconstriction, vasodilation, the inflammatory response, blood clotting, and angiogenesis.

- The cardiac muscle cell action potential is prolonged by the opening of voltage-gated calcium channels. The influx of calcium causes a long plateau in the action potential.

- Cardiac muscle is a functional syncytium; cells are connected by intercalated disks, which contain gap junctions. The gap junctions are electrical synapses that easily allow the transmission of the action potential, and thus contraction, to spread from cell to cell.

- The SA node is the "pacemaker" of the heart. It has an unstable resting potential that rises until threshold is reached and an action potential is fired. This action potential (and subsequent contraction) is then transmitted throughout the heart.

- Systemic blood pressure is directly proportional to cardiac output (the volume of blood pumped per minute) and to peripheral resistance (the force opposing blood flow through the vessels).

- Cardiac output is directly proportional to stroke volume and heart rate, while peripheral resistance is inversely related to vessel diameter.

- Blood is approximately 55 percent plasma, 40 to 45 percent erythrocytes (red blood cells), and 1 percent leukocytes (white blood cells) and platelets.

- ABO and Rh antigens on the surface of erythrocytes determine blood type; type AB+ is the universal recipient and type O− is the universal donor.

- Oxygen is transported in the blood bound to hemoglobin, a protein in red blood cells. Carbon dioxide is transported in the blood primarily as bicarbonate ion; some also binds to hemoglobin.

- Innate immunity is nonspecific and includes things like the skin, lysozyme, stomach acid, phagocytes, and the complement system.

- Humoral immunity is the production of antibodies by B cells that are highly specific for particular antigens (foreign molecules).

- There are five classes of antibodies: IgM (pentameric, primary immune response), IgG (secondary immune response and main blood antibody), IgA (dimeric, found in secretions like saliva and breast milk), IgD (B cell antigen receptor), and IgE (allergic reactions).

- Cell-mediated immunity is handled by T cells. Killer (cytotoxic) T cells destroy "self" cells that are displaying abnormal antigen on MHC I. Helper T cells are activated by antigen displayed on MHC II, and secrete chemicals to help activate and stimulate the proliferation of killer T cells and B cells.

- Autoimmunity occurs when the immune system targets normal body cells or tissues and destroys them. It is the result of a failure to eliminate self-reactive B cells and T cells during their development and maturation. Elimination of self-reactive lymphocytes is referred to as "developing tolerance."

CHAPTER 9 FREESTANDING PRACTICE QUESTIONS

1. The cardiac cycle is divided into systole and diastole, during which the ventricles contract and relax, respectively. During systole, blood is ejected from the ventricles and is pumped into either the aorta or pulmonary artery. The pressure in the ventricles rapidly increases; however, the volume of blood in the ventricles initially remains unchanged. This is referred to as *isovolumetric contraction*. Which of the following is the most likely reason for isovolumetric contraction?

A) Decreased ventricular contractility due to over-stretching of cardiac sarcomeres.
B) The pressure in the aorta is initially greater that of the left ventricle.
C) The pressure within the pulmonary vein is initially lower than that of the right ventricle.
D) The action potential that propagates through the bundle of His and Purkinje fibers has not yet depolarized all of the ventricles.

2. The ductus arteriosus is a shunt in the fetal circulation that diverts a portion of the blood from the pulmonary circulation into the aorta. Failure of the ductus arteriosus to close shortly after birth results in a condition referred to as a *patent ductus arteriosus* and, in severe cases, the generation of a left-to-right shunt. A left-to-right shunt would result in all of the following EXCEPT:

A) increased mixing of oxygenated blood with deoxygenated blood.
B) decreased blood flow into the systemic circulation.
C) increased blood flow into the pulmonary circulation.
D) decreased vascular pressure in the pulmonary circulation.

3. Blood pressure is directly proportional to cardiac output and peripheral resistance. Which of the following will raise blood pressure?

A) Consumption of a large meal, because it increases the heart rate
B) Exercise, because it increases cardiac output
C) Sizable blood loss, because it increases epinephrine levels due to the fear response
D) A localized allergic reaction, because it causes fluid loss to the tissue at the site

4. What are the names of the two portal systems in the body?

A) The pancreatic and the hypothalamic-hypophyseal
B) The pancreatic and the renal-urinary
C) The hepatic and the hypothalamic-hypophyseal
D) The hepatic and the renal-urinary

5. T cell antigen receptors are different from antibodies because:

A) T cell receptors must interact with antigen uniquely presented by other cells but not with free antigen.
B) T cell receptors bind various cytokines.
C) T cell receptors bind complement proteins to lyse cells.
D) T cell receptors are mediators of allergic reactions.

6. Hepatitis B is an inflammatory disease of the liver. While the virus itself is relatively benign, the body's attempt to eradicate it causes unwanted liver inflammation. Which of the following blood test results could be from an individual who has been vaccinated against Hepatitis B and does not have an active infection?

A) Negative for anti-Hepatitis B antibodies and negative for Hepatitis B antigen
B) Negative for anti-Hepatitis B antibodies and positive for Hepatitis B antigen
C) Positive for anti-Hepatitis B antibodies and positive for Hepatitis B antigen
D) Positive for anti-Hepatitis B antibodies and negative for Hepatitis B antigen

7. Individuals affected with DiGeorge syndrome have a T cell deficiency due to congenital lack, or incomplete development, of the thymus. Based on this statement, individuals affected with this syndrome will:

A) have normal humoral immunity.
B) have normal cell-mediated immunity.
C) be susceptible to infection.
D) be resistant to infection.

8. Which of the following statements about antibodies is true?

   I.   Antibodies are produced by B cells.
  II.   Antibodies only recognize peptide antigens.
 III.   Antibodies can mark an antigen for destruction by killer T cells.

A) I only
B) II only
C) I and II
D) I and III

Drill

MCAT BIOLOGY REVIEW

CHAPTER 9 PRACTICE PASSAGE

Endurance training, also known as aerobic exercise, causes adaptations in the cardiovascular system. The principal parameters involved in this adaptation are *maximum oxygen consumption*, *blood pressure*, and *blood flow*.

Maximum oxygen consumption is the product of cardiac output (CO) and the maximum difference in oxygen concentration between the arteries and the veins, known as the arterio-venous oxygen difference ($\Delta A-V_{O_2}$). Figure 1 shows the $\Delta A-V_{O_2}$ before and after endurance training in a 40-year-old man.

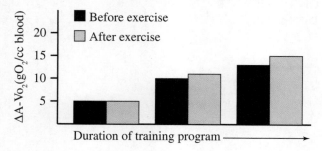

Figure 1

Blood pressure is a measure of the force per unit area with which blood pushes against the walls of the blood vessels. The pressure is determined by the pumping of the heart and by vascular *tone*. Tone refers to the level of muscular tension and is determined by sympathetic nervous input and by *autoregulation*. Autoregulation refers to changes in vascular tone determined by local factors, i.e., the buildup of metabolic end-products. It causes vessels to dilate when end products build up, indicating a need for more blood flow. The blood pressure readings of a 40-year-old man before and after an endurance training program are shown in Figure 2.

Figure 2

Blood flow is directly proportional to blood pressure, except when autoregulation is present, in which case dilation of vessels allows increased flow without increased pressure. Figure 3 shows the coronary and brain blood flow values of a 40-year-old man before and after endurance training.

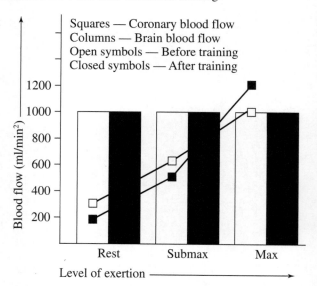

Figure 3

Adapted from *Exercise Physiology*, by George Brooks and Thomas Fahey, © 1985 by Macmillan Publishing Co.

1. Each of the following could account for the changes induced by endurance training in $\Delta A–V_{O_2}$ seen in Figure 1 EXCEPT increased:

A) numbers of mitochondria in muscle.
B) O_2 affinity of hemoglobin.
C) lactate buildup due to increased muscle mass.
D) muscle capillary density.

2. In Figure 2, the after-training blood pressure of the 40-year-old man at submaximal work rate is approximately:

A) 120/60.
B) 120/80.
C) 160/80.
D) 160/60.

3. Figure 3 supports which of the following conclusions?

A) The brain's oxygen requirements increase with increase in work rate.
B) The heart is more active at submax work rate after training.
C) After training, coronary metabolic requirements are greatest at maximal exercise.
D) Vasoconstriction increases in the heart during exercise.

4. Cardiac output is influenced by which of the following?

   I.   Nervous input
   II. Hormones
   III. Blood pressure

A) I only
B) II only
C) I and II only
D) I, II, and III

5. It can be inferred from Figures 2 and 3 that:

A) increasing blood pressure increases brain blood flow.
B) blood pressure and blood flow are inversely proportional.
C) the brain vasculature responds to exercise differently than does cardiac muscle.
D) autoregulation leads to vasoconstriction in the heart during exercise.

6. It can be inferred from the passage that:

A) during exertion and during rest, blood pressure between heartbeats changes less than the pressure during heartbeats.
B) the maximum blood pressure measured in an individual during exercise changes more with training than the level measured during rest.
C) blood flow to the brain decreases during sleep.
D) athletes use oxygen less efficiently than people who are in poor physical shape.

SOLUTIONS TO CHAPTER 9 FREESTANDING PRACTICE QUESTIONS

1. **B** At the start of systole the semilunar valves are closed, and although the ventricles are contracting, no blood is ejected. The semilunar valves will remain closed until the pressure within the ventricle exceeds that of the aorta or pulmonary artery (choice B is correct), at which point the semilunar valves open and blood is ejected from the ventricles. While overstretching of the cardiac sarcomeres could lead to decreased contractility (because of less overlap between actin and myosin filaments), this would not explain why the contraction is isovolumetric (choice A is wrong). It is true that the pulmonary vein has very low pressure and would be at a lower pressure than the right ventricle, but this does not explain why contraction (which pumps blood into the pulmonary artery rather than into the pulmonary *vein*) would be isovolumetric (choice C is wrong). Ventricular depolarization, initiated by the atrioventricular node, propagates through the bundle of His and Purkinje fibers and depolarizes all of the ventricles in about 120 to 200 ms. The approximate duration of ventricular contraction is 300 to 450 ms; in other words, depolarization of the ventricles is very rapid, and all of the myocytes of the ventricles have been depolarized well before the pressure within the ventricles begins to change (choice D is wrong).

2. **D** Since the left side of the heart deals with oxygenated blood and the right side of the heart deals with deoxygenated blood, a left-to-right shunt would cause increased mixing of oxygenated and deoxygenated blood (choice A would occur and can be eliminated). A left-to-right shunt, particularly one connecting the aorta and pulmonary artery, would result in blood flow from the high-pressure aorta into the lower-pressure pulmonary artery (both choices B and C would occur and can be eliminated). This additional flow into the pulmonary artery would result in an increased blood volume in the pulmonary circulation and a subsequent increase (not decrease) in pulmonary vascular pressure (choice D would not occur and is the correct answer choice).

3. **B** Exercise will cause muscle contraction, which pushes blood along the veins, increasing venous return to the heart. According to the Frank-Starling mechanism, the increase in venous return will increase stroke volume, increasing cardiac output and therefore blood pressure. Further, the increased heart rate due to exercise will also increase cardiac output and blood pressure. Consumption of a large meal will activate the parasympathetic nervous system (rest and digest), so the vagus nerve will be stimulated and the heart rate will decrease. This will decrease the cardiac output and decrease blood pressure (choice A is wrong). Blood loss will decrease blood volume and thus blood pressure. If the blood loss is sizable, the decrease in pressure will be larger than the increase in heart rate from the epinephrine produced by the fear response (choice C is wrong). The loss of fluid to the tissues will decrease blood volume, and thus also blood pressure (choice D is wrong).

4. **C** A portal system consists of two capillary beds connected by a vein. The hepatic portal system connects the small intestine's nutrient absorption to the detoxification systems of the liver, and the hypothalamic-hypophyseal portal system provides a short connection for the hormones of the hypothalamus to control the hormones of the anterior pituitary. The renal system (kidney) and the urinary system (bladder) are connected by the ureter (which carries urine, not blood). Also, do not get confused by the connection of the glomerular capillaries

to the peritubular capillaries (the vasa recta); these are connected by an artery (the efferent arteriole), not a vein (choices B and D can be eliminated). The pancreas has an exocrine duct system and a single capillary bed (choice A can be eliminated).

5.   **A**   T cell receptors must bind antigen that is presented by MHC proteins on the surface of other cells. They are unable to bind free antigen. Cytokines have their own family of receptors and are not bound by T cell receptors or antibodies (choice B is wrong). T cell receptors do not bind complement proteins; the complement system is a set of proteins that can be activated, sometimes by antibodies, to cause nonspecific cell lysis (choice C is wrong). IgE and some other antibodies are involved with allergic reactions, but T cell receptors are not (choice D is wrong).

6.   **D**   Vaccination involves the introduction of non-pathogenic antigen into the body in order to trigger the production of antibodies and memory lymphocytes. Individuals who have been vaccinated against Hepatitis B would test positive for anti-Hepatitis B antibodies (choices A and B can be eliminated). Individuals who do not have an active Hepatitis B infection would test negative for Hepatitis B antigens (choice C can be eliminated, and choice D is correct).

7.   **C**   DiGeorge syndrome is also known as *thymic aplasia*. The T cells (or cell-mediated arm) of the immune system are affected and there is an increased susceptibility to infection (choice D is wrong), both from the lack of killer T cells (choice B is wrong), and from the lack of helper T cells and the subsequent effect on the humoral branch of the immune system (choice A is wrong).

8.   **A**   Item I is true: antibodies are produced by the B cells of the immune system (choice B can be eliminated). Item II is false: antibodies can recognize a great diversity of antigens which include, but are not limited to, peptides (choice C can be eliminated). Item III is false: antibodies can mark an antigen for destruction by macrophages and other phagocytes. Killer T cells do not directly destroy antigens; rather, they kill cells that are producing antigens (such as cells infected by a virus). Further, the mechanism of cell destruction by killer T cells does not involve antibodies (choice D can be eliminated, and choice A is correct).

SOLUTIONS TO CHAPTER 9 PRACTICE PASSAGE

1.   **B**   Figure 1 shows that as the training program progresses, the arterio-venous oxygen difference increases; in other words, after undergoing training, oxygen is extracted more efficiently from the blood. Increased numbers of mitochondria would lead to more efficient oxygen extraction (choice A could account for the changes and can be eliminated). Lactate buildup would reduce blood pH, reducing hemoglobin's affinity for oxygen and allowing oxygen to be taken from the blood more easily (choice C could account for the changes and can be eliminated). Muscle capillary density does increase during training; this would bring more blood to the muscle and make it easier for oxygen to diffuse out of the blood (choice D could account for the changes and can be eliminated). However, if hemoglobin had an increased affinity for oxygen, it would hold on to the oxygen and not release it to the muscle. This would decrease the arterio-venous oxygen difference (choice B cannot account for the changes and is the correct answer choice).

2.   **A**   Blood pressure is defined as systolic pressure over diastolic pressure, and the after-training values are indicated by closed symbols. The systolic value after training at submax work rate is 120 (choices C and D are wrong), and the diastolic value is 60 (choice B is wrong, and choice A is correct).

3.   **C**   Figure 3 shows that as the level of exertion increases, the blood flow to the brain remains constant while the blood flow to the heart increases (note that this is due to vasodilation, not vasoconstriction; choice D is wrong). This is true both before and after training. Since the brain blood flow is constant regardless of the level of exertion, its oxygen requirements must not be increasing (choice A is wrong). Coronary blood flow is higher at submax work rate before training, indicating that the heart is working harder than it is after training (choice B is wrong). Coronary blood flow is highest at maximal exercise, indicating that the metabolic requirements of the heart must be very high (need for oxygen, need to eliminate carbon dioxide, etc.; choice C is correct).

4.   **D**   Item I: True. Parasympathetic nerves to the SA node keep the heart rate slow when one is resting, and sympathetic stimulation increases the heart rate (choice B can be eliminated). Item II: True. Circulating hormones affect cardiac performance. The key example is epinephrine from the adrenal gland, which increases cardiac output (choice A can be eliminated). Item III: True. Increased blood pressure makes it more difficult for the heart to eject its load of blood, and decreased blood pressure impairs cardiac function when not enough blood is returned to the pumping heart (choice C can be eliminated, and choice D is correct).

5.   **C**   Combining Figures 2 and 3, you can see that both blood pressure and cardiac blood flow increase as exertion increases, but brain blood flow stays the same (choice C is correct, and choice A is wrong). Since both pressure and flow are increasing, they must be directly proportional, not inversely proportional (choice B is wrong). Since cardiac flow is increasing, it must be due to vasodilation, not vasoconstriction (choice D is wrong).

6.   **A**   Figure 2 shows that the diastolic pressure (the pressure between heartbeats) changes much less during exertion and rest than the systolic pressure (the pressure during heartbeats; choice A is correct). It also shows that the highest blood pressure reached during exercise does not change as much after training as does the resting systolic pressure (in other words, the "Max" squares are closer together than the "Rest" squares; choice B is wrong). There is no information given on brain blood flow during sleep, and if anything, you might assume it stays constant based on Figure 3 (choice C is wrong). Based on Figure 1, you can assume that athletes use oxygen more efficiently, since the arterio-venous difference is greater after training (choice D is wrong).

Chapter 10
The Excretory and Digestive Systems

10.1   OVERVIEW OF THE EXCRETORY SYSTEM

Excretion is the disposal of waste products. "The excretory system" generally refers to the kidneys, even though the liver, large intestine, and skin are involved in excretion too. Let's begin by summarizing the excretory roles of these organs to see where the kidneys fit into the picture.

Liver

The **liver** is responsible for excreting many wastes by chemically modifying them and releasing them into bile (discussed later in this chapter). In particular, the liver deals with hydrophobic or large waste products, which cannot be filtered out by the kidney. (The kidney can only eliminate small hydrophiles dissolved in plasma.) For example: in the liver, old heme units are broken down into bilirubin, which is then tagged with a molecule called glucuronate; the resulting bilirubin glucuronate is excreted with bile.

The liver is also very important in excretion because it synthesizes **urea** (Figure 1) and releases it into the bloodstream. Urea is a carrier of excess nitrogen resulting from protein breakdown. Excess nitrogen must be converted to urea because free ammonia is toxic. Urea derives its name from the fact that it is excreted in urine.

Figure 1   Urea

Colon

The **large intestine** reabsorbs water and ions (sodium, calcium, etc.) from feces. In this sense it doesn't really excrete anything, but merely processes wastes already destined for excretion. However, the colon is also capable of excreting excess ions (e.g., sodium, chloride, calcium) into the feces using active transport.

Skin

The skin produces sweat, which contains water, ions, and urea. In other words, sweat is similar to urine. In this sense, the skin is an excretory organ. However, sweating is not primarily controlled by the amount of waste that needs to be excreted, but rather by temperature and level of sympathetic nervous system activity. Therefore, the excretory role of the skin is secondary.

Kidneys

The final responsibility for excretion of hydrophilic wastes lies with the kidneys. Substances which must be excreted in the urine include urea, sodium, bicarbonate, and water. "But wait," you say, "sodium, bicarbonate, and water aren't waste products!" Actually, they sometimes are wastes, when they are present at abnormally high concentrations. You begin to see that the kidney is not like the colon, a passive container for wastes waiting to be excreted. It is a sensitive regulator that must keep concentrations at *optimum levels*, as opposed to simply dumping things.

This is the homeostatic role of the kidneys. **Homeostasis** refers to the constancy of physiological variables. For example, the normal serum Na^+ concentration is 142 mEq/L. Variations in this level greater than 15 percent are fatal due to dysfunction of neurons, cardiac muscle cells, and other cell types. There are other components to homeostasis which the kidney does not control (e.g., temperature maintenance).

Excretory and Homeostatic Roles of the Kidney
1) Excretion of hydrophilic wastes
2) Maintenance of constant solute concentration and constant pH
3) Maintenance of constant fluid volume (important for blood pressure and cardiac output)

As a simplification, we can say that these goals are accomplished via three processes:

- The first process is **filtration**. This entails the passage of pressurized blood over a filter (like a coffee filter). Cells and proteins remain in the blood (like coffee grinds), while water and small molecules are squeezed out into the **renal tubule** (like java). During filtration, water, waste products, and useful small molecules such as glucose are filtered into the renal tubule. The fluid in the tubule is called **filtrate**, and it will eventually be made into urine.
- The second process is **selective reabsorption**. Here we take back useful items (glucose, water, amino acids), while leaving wastes and some water in the tubule.
- The third process is **secretion**. This involves the addition of substances to the filtrate. Secretion can increase the rate at which substances are eliminated from the blood; because not only are the substance filtered out, more of them are added to the filtrate *after* filtration.

The last step in urine formation is **concentration and dilution**. This involves the selective reabsorption of water, and is where we decide whether to make concentrated urine or dilute urine. After this step, whatever remains in the renal tubule gets excreted as urine.

10.2 ANATOMY AND FUNCTION OF THE URINARY SYSTEM

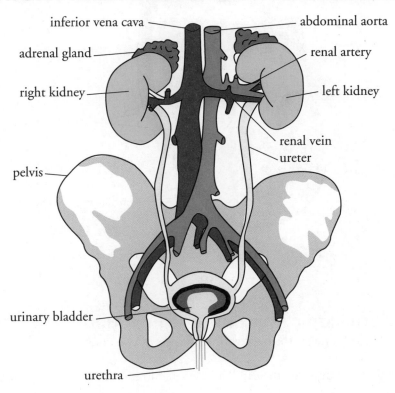

Figure 2 Gross Anatomy of the Urinary System

Each kidney is a filtration system that removes unwanted materials from the blood and passes them to the bladder for storage and eventual elimination. Blood enters the kidney from a large **renal artery**, which is a direct branch of the lower portion of the aorta (the abdominal aorta). Purified blood is returned to the circulatory system by the large **renal vein**, which empties into the inferior vena cava. Urine leaves each kidney in a **ureter**, which empties into the **urinary bladder**. The bladder is a muscular organ that stretches as it fills with urine. When it becomes full, signals of urgency are sent to the brain. There are two sphincters controlling release of urine from the bladder: an **internal sphincter** made of smooth (involuntary) muscle and an **external sphincter** made of skeletal (voluntary) muscle. The internal sphincter relaxes reflexively (and the bladder contracts) when the bladder wall is stretched. If a person decides the time is appropriate, they can relax the external sphincter, allowing urine to flow from the bladder into the urethra and out of the body.

A frontal section (separating front from back) through the kidney demonstrates its internal anatomy (Figure 3). The outer region is known as the **cortex**, and the inner region is the **medulla**. The **medullary pyramids** are pyramid-shaped striations within the medulla. This appearance is due to the presence of many **collecting ducts**. Urine empties from the collecting ducts and leaves the medulla at the tip of a pyramid, known as a **papilla** (plural: **papillae**). Each papilla empties into a space called a **calyx** (plural: **calyces**). The calyces converge to form the **renal pelvis**, which is a large space where urine collects. The renal pelvis empties into the ureter.

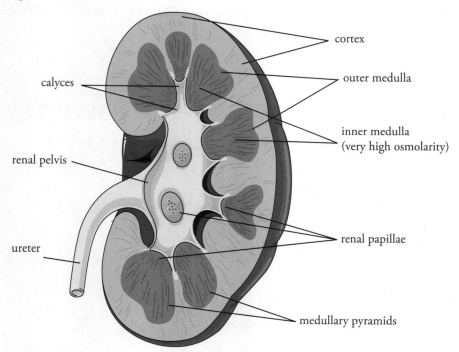

Figure 3   Internal Anatomy of the Kidney

Simplified Microscopic Anatomy and Function

The functional unit of the kidney is the **nephron**. It consists of two components:

1)   a rounded region surrounding the capillaries where filtration takes place, known as the **capsule**, and

2) a coiled tube known as the **renal tubule** (Figure 4). The tubule receives filtrate from the capillaries in the capsule at one end and empties into a **collecting duct** at the other end. The collecting duct dumps urine into the renal pelvis.

Figure 4   Simplified View of the Renal Tubule

Many blood vessels surround the nephron. They carry arterial blood toward the capillaries of the capsule for filtration, then surround the tubule to carry filtered blood and reabsorbed substances away from the tubule (Figure 5).

Figure 5   Simplified View of the Renal Tubule Plus Blood Vessels

Figures 4 and 5 depict most of the structures responsible for the three processes involved in urine formation. Let's go through the steps again, but this time in more detail.

Filtration

Blood from the renal artery flows into an **afferent arteriole**, which branches into a ball of capillaries known as the **glomerulus**. From there the blood flows into an **efferent arteriole**. Constriction of the efferent arteriole results in high pressure in the glomerulus, which causes fluid (essentially blood plasma) to leak out of the glomerular capillaries. The fluid passes through a filter known as the **glomerular basement membrane** and enters **Bowman's capsule**. As you can see from the figures, the lumen of Bowman's capsule is continuous with the lumen of the rest of the tubule. Substances which are too large to pass through the glomerular basement membrane are not filtered; they remain in the blood in the glomerular capillaries and drain into the efferent arteriole.[1] Examples are blood cells and plasma proteins.

- Which of the following are present in the filtrate in Bowman's capsule in concentrations similar to those seen in blood?[2]
    - I. Albumin (a plasma protein)
    - II. Glucose
    - III. Sodium

    - A) I and II only
    - B) II only
    - C) I and III only
    - D) II and III only

Selective Reabsorption

The filtrate in the tubule consists of water and small hydrophilic molecules such as sugars, amino acids, and urea. Some of these substances must be returned to the bloodstream. They are extracted from the tubule, often via active transport, and picked up by **peritubular capillaries**, which drain into venules that lead to the renal vein. For example, glucose is actively transported out of the filtrate and returned to the bloodstream by a cotransporter identical to the one involved in glucose absorption in the small intestine. A lot (most) of the reabsorption occurs in the part of the tubule nearest to Bowman's capsule, called the **proximal convoluted tubule** (PCT). All solute movement in the PCT is accompanied by water movement. As a result, a lot of water reabsorption occurs in this region also; roughly 70 percent of the volume of the filtrate is reabsorbed here. The amount (final volume) of urine we make is determined by much smaller fluxes taking place in the distal nephron. This makes sense if you think about it: about 5 percent of our circulating blood is continuously being filtered out of the glomerulus; most of this must be taken

---

[1] The glomerular basement membrane is actually a layer lining *each capillary* of the glomerulus.

[2] Item I: False. Plasma proteins are too large to pass through the filter. **Item II: True.** Glucose passes through into the filtrate and must be reclaimed during selective reabsorption. **Item III: True.** Sodium also passes into the filtrate. It will be reclaimed or left in the filtrate to be urinated out, depending on physiological needs. The answer is choice **D**.

back. Note that reabsorption in the PCT is selective in that it chooses what to reabsorb, but it is not overly regulated, since it reabsorbs "as much as possible," not a certain amount.

Selective reabsorption takes place further along the nephron as well, in the **distal convoluted tubule** (**DCT**). Reabsorption in this location is more regulated than in the PCT, usually via hormones (see Concentration and Dilution).

- Which one of the following best describes selective reabsorption?[3]
  - A) In normal individuals, only a small portion of the serum glucose is filtered into the tubule. Of this amount, about 50% is reabsorbed by the epithelial cells of the tubule.
  - B) In normal individuals, the concentration of glucose which is filtered into the tubule is identical to the serum [glucose]. Of the filtered glucose, 100% is reabsorbed by the epithelial cells of the tubule.
  - C) Epithelial cells of the renal tubule actively transport glucose into the filtrate.
  - D) Glucose is kept in the bloodstream by the filtering action of the glomerular basement membrane.

Secretion

Secretion is the movement of substances into the filtrate (usually via active transport) thus increasing the rate at which they are removed from the plasma. Not everything that needs to be removed from the blood gets filtered out at the glomerulus; secretion is a "back-up" method that ensures what needs to be eliminated, gets eliminated. As with reabsorption, secretion occurs all along the tubule; however unlike reabsorption, most secretion takes place in the DCT and the collecting duct. Note also that this is the primary way that many drugs and toxins are deposited in the urine.

Concentration and Dilution

Before filtrate is discarded into the ureter as urine, adjustments are made so that the urine volume and osmolarity are appropriate. This occurs in the last part of the tubule, known as the **distal nephron** (meaning the most distant part of the tubule), which includes the **DCT** and the **collecting duct**. It is controlled by two hormones: **ADH** and **aldosterone**.

1) *ADH:* When you are dehydrated, the *volume of fluid* in the bloodstream is low and the *solute concentration* in the blood is high. Therefore, you need to make small amounts of highly concentrated urine. Under these conditions (low blood volume and high blood osmolarity) **antidiuretic hormone** (**ADH** or **vasopressin**) is released by the posterior pituitary. This prevents **diuresis** (water loss in the urine) by increasing water reabsorption in the distal nephron.

---

[3] As stated in the section on filtration, glucose is small enough that all of it freely passes through the glomerular basement membrane (choice D is wrong), as are ions, amino acids, and water. However, even though glucose is filtered into the tubule, it must be reclaimed into the bloodstream or we would constantly lose glucose into the urine. 100 percent of filtered glucose is normally reclaimed (choice **B** is correct, and choice A is wrong), and in no instance is glucose ever transported *into* the filtrate (choice C is wrong). Note that in diabetes, the blood glucose level is so high that the cotransporters responsible for glucose reabsorption become saturated, and large amounts of glucose are left in the urine.

This is accomplished by making the distal nephron (primarily the collecting duct) permeable to water. (Without ADH, this region is impermeable to water. Note that this is the first time we have encountered a layer in the body which is impermeable to water.) As a result, water flows out of the filtrate into the tissue of the kidney, where it is picked up by the peritubular capillaries, and thus returned to the blood. [Why would water tend to flow out of the tubule into the tissue of the kidney?[4]] A drop in blood pressure can also trigger ADH release (renal regulation of blood pressure will be discussed later).

After drinking a lot of water, the plasma volume is too high, and a large volume of dilute urine is necessary. In this case, no ADH is secreted. The result is that the collecting duct is not permeable to water. This means that any water in the filtrate remains in the tubule and is lost in the urine, or *diuresed*. The reason alcohol causes people to diurese is that it inhibits ADH secretion by the posterior pituitary.

2) *Aldosterone:* When the blood *pressure* is low, **aldosterone** is released by the adrenal cortex. It causes increased reabsorption of Na^+ by the distal nephron (distal convoluted tubule and the cortical region of the collecting duct). The result is increased plasma osmolarity, which leads to increased thirst and water retention, which raises the blood pressure. (The fact that increased serum $[Na^+]$ increases blood pressure is the reason people with high blood pressure have to avoid salty foods.) When the blood pressure is high, aldosterone is not released. As a result, sodium is lost in the urine. Plasma osmolarity (and eventually blood pressure) falls. Other triggers for the release of aldosterone are low blood osmolarity, low blood volume, and **angiotensin II** (discussed below).

ADH and aldosterone work together to increase blood pressure. First, aldosterone causes sodium reabsorption, which results in increased plasma osmolarity. This causes ADH to be secreted, which results in increased water reabsorption and thus increased plasma volume.

Actual Microscopic Anatomy and Function

Up to this point we have presented a conceptual outline of kidney function, and we have referred to a simplified nephron, depicted as a straight tube. But the nephron is more complex than that (Figure 6). Bowman's capsule empties into the first part of the tubule, known as the proximal convoluted tubule (PCT). Again, *proximal* means "near" (near the glomerulus), and *convoluted* just means "twisting and turning." Both Bowman's capsule and the PCT are located in the **renal cortex**, the outer layer of the kidney. The PCT empties into the next region of the nephron, known as the **loop of Henle**. This is a long loop that dips down into the **renal medulla**, the inner part of the kidney. The part that heads into the medulla is called the **descending limb of the loop of Henle**, and the part that heads back out toward the cortex is the **ascending limb**. The descending limb is thin walled, but part of the ascending limb is thin and the other part is thick. These are referred to simply as the *thin ascending limb* and the *thick ascending limb* of the loop of Henle. [What might be the structural difference between a thick portion of the tubule and a thin portion?[5]] As we continue down the tubule, the loop of Henle becomes the distal

---

[4]   Because the renal medulla has a very high osmolarity, which causes water to exit the tubule by osmosis. This will be discussed later in more detail.

[5]   The two portions are composed of different types of epithelial cells. Thin portions of the tubule are composed of *squamous* (flat) epithelial cells, which are not very metabolically active. Thick portions are composed of *cuboidal* epithelial cells, which are large thick cells busily performing active transport.

convoluted tubule (DCT). The DCT dumps into a **collecting duct**. Many collecting ducts merge to form larger tributaries which empty into renal calyces. Figure 6 shows the actual anatomy and function of the nephron. You should familiarize yourself with the information in the figure, but this level of detail is too advanced to warrant extensive discussion. The conceptual material presented above is more typical of MCAT questions.

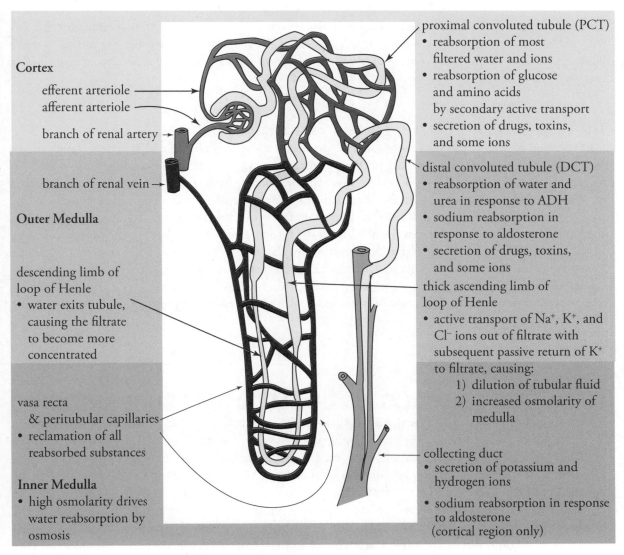

Cortex

efferent arteriole
afferent arteriole

branch of renal artery

branch of renal vein →

Outer Medulla

descending limb of loop of Henle
• water exits tubule, causing the filtrate to become more concentrated

vasa recta
  & peritubular capillaries
• reclamation of all reabsorbed substances

Inner Medulla
• high osmolarity drives water reabsorption by osmosis

proximal convoluted tubule (PCT)
• reabsorption of most filtered water and ions
• reabsorption of glucose and amino acids by secondary active transport
• secretion of drugs, toxins, and some ions

distal convoluted tubule (DCT)
• reabsorption of water and urea in response to ADH
• sodium reabsorption in response to aldosterone
• secretion of drugs, toxins, and some ions

thick ascending limb of loop of Henle
• active transport of Na^+, K^+, and Cl^- ions out of filtrate with subsequent passive return of K^+ to filtrate, causing:
  1) dilution of tubular fluid
  2) increased osmolarity of medulla

collecting duct
• secretion of potassium and hydrogen ions

• sodium reabsorption in response to aldosterone (cortical region only)

Figure 6   Regions and Functions of the Nephron

The Loop of Henle Is a Countercurrent Multiplier

Although we do not intend to go into too much detail on renal physiology, one concept is important to mention: the notion of a **countercurrent multiplier**. The significance of the loop of Henle is that the ascending and descending limbs go in opposite directions and have different permeabilities. The descending limb is permeable to water, but not to ions. Hence, water exits the descending limb, flowing into the high-osmolarity medullary interstitium.[6] Thus, the filtrate becomes concentrated. The thin ascending

---

6   *Interstitium* is a generic word for "tissue." It literally means "an in-between region"; in this case it means tissue in-between renal tubules.

limb is *not* permeable to water, but passively loses ions from the high-osmolarity filtrate into the renal medullary interstitium. Additionally, the thick ascending limb actively transports salt out of the filtrate into the medullary interstitium, and the medullary interstitium becomes *very* salty. This is important because the medulla will suck water out of the collecting duct by osmosis whenever the collecting duct is permeable to water (e.g., in the presence of ADH).

Don't spend too much time pondering over this now (you will in medical school). Just remember that *the loop of Henle is a countercurrent multiplier that makes the medulla very salty, and that this facilitates water reabsorption from the collecting duct. This is how the kidney is capable of making urine with a much higher osmolarity than plasma.*

The Vasa Recta Are Countercurrent Exchangers

Like the loop of Henle, the **vasa recta** form a loop that helps to maintain the high concentration of salt in the medulla. In short, the ascending portions of the vasa recta are near the descending limb of the loop of Henle and thus carry off the water that leaves the descending limb. Also, the vasa recta are branches of efferent arterioles. The vasa recta are "eager" to reabsorb water because the blood they contain is like coffee grinds which have been drained. The important thing to remember is that the vasa recta return to the bloodstream any water that is reabsorbed from the filtrate. Because the blood in the vasa recta moves in the opposite direction of the filtrate in the nephron, the vasa recta perform countercurrent exchange. Other biological systems use countercurrent exchange because it is very efficient. For example, oxygen and blood flow in opposite directions in fish gills. This mechanism increases the efficiency of the respiration process by maintaining the concentration gradient and preventing the oxygen levels from reaching an equilibrium.

10.3 RENAL REGULATION OF BLOOD PRESSURE AND pH

Since the **glomerular filtration rate** (**GFR**) depends directly on pressure, the kidney has built-in mechanisms to help regulate systemic and local (glomerular) blood pressure. The **juxtaglomerular apparatus** (**JGA**) is a specialized contact point between the afferent arteriole and the distal tubule. At this contact point, the cells in the afferent arteriole are called **juxtaglomerular** (**JG**) **cells**, and those in the distal tubule are known as the **macula densa**. The JG cells are baroreceptors that monitor systemic blood pressure. When there is a decrease in blood pressure, the JG cells secrete an enzyme called **renin** into the bloodstream. Renin catalyzes the conversion of **angiotensinogen** (a plasma protein made by the liver) into **angiotensin I,** which is further converted to **angiotensin II** by **angiotensin-converting enzyme** (**ACE**) in the lungs. Angiotensin II is a powerful vasoconstrictor that immediately raises the blood pressure. It also stimulates the release of aldosterone, which (as discussed previously) helps raise the blood pressure by increasing sodium (and, indirectly, water) retention.

The cells of the macula densa are chemoreceptors, and monitor filtrate osmolarity in the distal tubule. When filtrate osmolarity decreases (indicating a reduced filtration rate), the cells of the macula densa stimulate the JG cells to release renin. The macula densa also causes a direct dilation of the afferent arteriole, increasing blood flow to (and thus blood pressure and filtration rate in) the glomerulus.

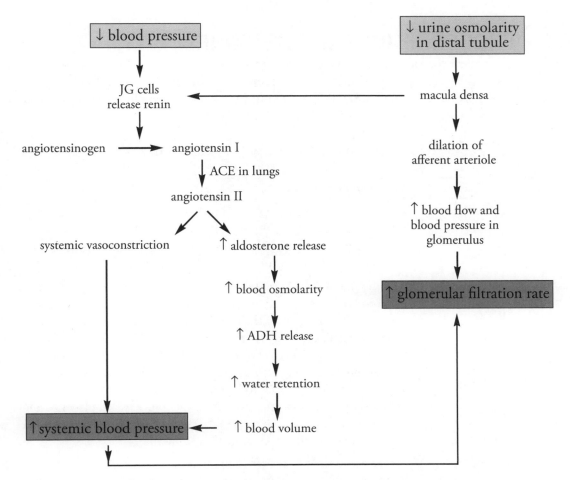

Figure 7   Regulation of Blood Pressure and GFR by the Kidney

Renal Regulation of pH

The kidney is essential for maintenance of constant blood pH. It accomplishes this by a very simple and direct mechanism: when the plasma pH is too high, HCO_3^- is excreted in the urine; when the plasma pH is too low, H^+ is excreted. We will not go into the details. Just be aware that the enzyme **carbonic anhydrase** is involved. It is found in epithelial cells throughout the nephron, except the flat (squamous) cells of the thin parts of the loop of Henle. Carbonic anhydrase catalyzes the conversion of CO_2 into carbonic acid (H_2CO_3), which dissociates into bicarbonate plus a proton. Once this reaction has taken place, the kidney can reabsorb or secrete bicarbonate or protons as needed. (Recall that carbonic anhydrase was discussed in Chapter 9, as it is found in RBCs.) Generally speaking, protons are secreted and bicarbonate is reabsorbed; the amounts are adjusted to adjust pH.

Renal pH adjustments are slow, requiring several days to return plasma pH to normal after a disturbance. The other organ important for pH regulation is the lung. By exhaling excess CO_2, the lung removes an acid (H_2CO_3) from the blood, thus raising the pH. Thus, *hyperventilation* (deep, rapid breathing) raises plasma pH. Respiratory adjustments to the plasma pH are rapid, taking effect in just minutes.

10.4 ENDOCRINE ROLE OF THE KIDNEY

Several hormones affect the kidney, and the kidney makes one as well. All are peptides except aldosterone, which is a steroid. The one made by the kidney is **erythropoietin** (**EPO**). You should know the basic role and source of each of the following hormones. You're unlikely to see very detailed memory-oriented questions on the MCAT, but as a doctor you will know this stuff like the back of your hand.

Table 1   Hormones Affecting or Secreted by Kidney

Hormone	Source	Target and effect
aldosterone	adrenal cortex	Causes sodium reabsorption and potassium secretion by increasing the synthesis of basolateral Na^+/K^+ ATPases in the distal nephron. End result: increased serum $[Na^+]$, increased blood volume (through the action of ADH), and thus increased blood pressure.
ADH	posterior pituitary	ADH is secreted when plasma volume is too low, blood pressure is too low, or plasma osmolarity is too high. It causes water reabsorption by causing epithelial cells of the distal nephron to become permeable to water, which allows water to flow out of the filtrate into the medullary interstitium. Vasa recta return this water to the bloodstream. The result is more concentrated urine, and more diluted blood. ADH and aldosterone work together to increase blood pressure: first, aldosterone causes sodium reabsorption, which results in increased plasma osmolarity; this causes ADH to be secreted, which results in increased water reabsorption and thus increased plasma volume.
calcitonin	C cells	C cells are located in the thyroid gland but do not secrete thyroid hormone. They secrete calcitonin when the serum $[Ca^{2+}]$ is too high. Calcitonin causes $[Ca^{2+}]$ to be removed from the blood by 1) deposition in bone, 2) reduced absorption by the gut, and 3) excretion in urine.
parathyroid hormone	parathyroid	There are four parathyroid glands, found embedded in the thyroid gland. The function of parathormone (PTH) is opposite that of calcitonin.
EPO	kidney	Erythropoietin (EPO) causes increased synthesis of red blood cells in the bone marrow. It is released when blood oxygen content falls.

10.5   OVERVIEW OF THE DIGESTIVE SYSTEM

Food contains molecules that are substrates in **catabolic reactions** (reactions that break down molecules to supply energy) and **anabolic reactions** (synthesis of macromolecules). Digestion is the breakdown of polymers (polypeptides, fats, starch) into their building blocks. This breakdown is accomplished by **enzymatic hydrolysis** (Figure 8). Food also contains vitamins, which are not substrates, but rather serve a catalytic role as enzyme cofactors or prosthetic groups. Digestion and absorption of foodstuffs is the primary function of the digestive system. A secondary function, which we will touch on only briefly, is protection from disease.

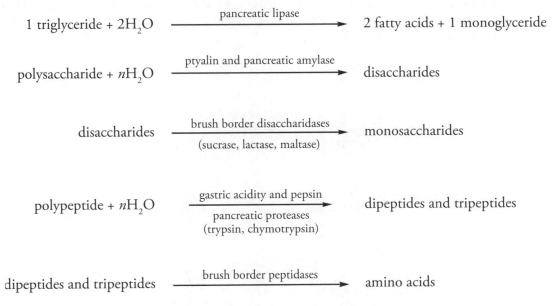

Figure 8   Enzymatic Hydrolysis of Biological Macromolecules

Digestion is accomplished along the **gastrointestinal (GI) tract**, also known as the **digestive tract**, the **alimentary canal**, or simply the **gut**. The GI tract is a long, muscular tube extending from the mouth to the anus. This tube is derived from the cavity produced by **gastrulation** during embryogenesis; the anus is derived from the **blastopore** (discussed in Chapter 13). The inside of the gut is the **GI lumen**. The lumen is continuous with the space outside the body. (Food could go from the plate into the lumen and from there into the toilet bowl without ever contacting the bloodstream, the muscles, the bones, etc.) The GI lumen is a compartment where the usable components of foodstuffs are extracted, while wastes are left to be excreted as feces. The entire GI tract is composed of specific tissue layers which surround the lumen (Figure 9).

Figure 9   Layers of the GI Tract

GI Epithelium

Because it is exposed to substances from the outside world, the innermost lining of the lumen is composed of the same type of cells that line the outer surface of the body and the inner surface of the respiratory tract: epithelial cells. By definition, epithelial cells are attached to a **basement membrane**.[7] The surface of the epithelial cell which faces into the lumen is the **apical surface** (*apex* means "top"; *apical* is the adjective). In the small intestine, the apical surfaces of these cells have outward folds of their plasma membrane called **microvilli** to increase their surface area. The apical surface is separated from the remainder of the cell surface by **tight junctions**, which are bands running all the way around the sides of epithelial cells, creating a barrier that separates body fluids from the extracellular environment (see Chapter 6). The sides and bottom of an epithelial cell form the surface opposite the lumen, known as the **basolateral** surface (Figure 10). As discussed below, specialized epithelial cells are responsible for most of the secretory activity of the GI tract.

Figure 10   Epithelial Cells

GI Smooth Muscle

GI muscle is known as **smooth muscle** because of its smooth microscopic appearance. This contrasts with **striated muscle**, which appears striped under magnification. Skeletal (voluntary) muscle and cardiac (heart) muscle are striated. (The differences between smooth, skeletal, and cardiac muscle cells will be covered in Chapter 11.) Note in Figure 9 that there are two layers of smooth muscle lining the gut. The **longitudinal layer** runs along the gut lengthwise, while the **circular layer** encircles it.

GI motility refers to the rhythmic contraction of GI smooth muscle. It is determined by a complex interplay between five factors:

1) Like cardiac muscle, GI smooth muscle exhibits *automaticity*. In other words, it contracts periodically without external stimulation, due to spontaneous depolarization.

---

[7] *Epi-* means "upon," and *-thelial* refers to the bumpy microscopic appearance of the basement membrane (it means "nippley").

2) Like cardiac muscle, GI smooth muscle is a **functional syncytium**, meaning that when one cell has an action potential and contracts, the impulse spreads to neighboring cells.

3) The GI tract contains its own massive nervous system, known as the **enteric nervous system**. The enteric nervous system plays a major role in controlling GI motility.

4) GI motility may be increased or decreased by hormonal input.

5) The parasympathetic nervous system stimulates motility and causes sphincters to relax (allowing the passage of food through the gut), while sympathetic stimulation does the opposite.

GI motility serves two purposes: mixing of food and movement of food down the gut. Mixing is accomplished by disordered contractions of GI smooth muscle, which result in churning motions. Movement of food down the GI tract is accomplished by an orderly form of contraction known as **peristalsis** (Figure 11). During peristalsis, contraction of circular smooth muscle at point A prevents food located at point B from moving backward. Then longitudinal muscles at point B contract, with the result being shortening of the gut so that it is pulled up over the food like a sock. As a result, the food moves toward point C. Then circular smooth muscles at point B contract to prevent the food from moving backward, and longitudinal muscles at point C contract, with the result being movement of food past point C, and so on. A ball of food moving through the GI tract is called a **bolus**.

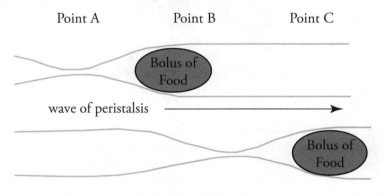

Figure 11   Peristalsis

Enteric Nervous System

The enteric nervous system is the branch of the **autonomic nervous system** that helps to control digestion via innervation of the gastrointestinal tract, pancreas, and gall bladder. Specifically, it helps to regulate local blood flow, gut movements, and the exchange of fluid from the gut to and from its lumen. This branch can operate independently of the other two branches of the autonomic nervous system, but both of those branches can modulate the activity of the enteric nervous system. [What are the two main branches of the autonomic nervous system? What effects would they have on the enteric branch?[8]]

The enteric nervous system is made up of two networks of neurons: the **myenteric plexus** and the **submucosal plexus**. The myenteric plexus is found between the circular and longitudinal muscle layers and helps primarily to regulate gut motility. The submucosal plexus is found in the submucosa and helps to regulate enzyme secretion, gut blood flow, and ion/water balance in the lumen. In areas where these functions are minimal (e.g., the esophagus or anus), the submucosal plexus is sparse.

---

[8]   The two main branches of the autonomic nervous system are the sympathetic nervous system (fight or flight) and parasympathetic nervous system (rest and digest). The sympathetic nervous system generally inhibits digestive processes and so would inhibit the enteric branch, whereas the parasympathetic nervous system stimulates the enteric branch and thus stimulates digestion.

GI Secretions

Generally speaking, GI secretion (release of enzymes, acid, bile, etc.) is stimulated by food in the gut and by the parasympathetic nervous system and is inhibited by sympathetic stimulation. There are two types of secretion: **endocrine** and **exocrine**. [What's the difference?[9]] Exocrine glands are composed of specialized epithelial cells, organized into sacs called **acini** (singular: **acinus**). Acinar cells secrete products which pass into ducts. It is important to keep the contrast between endocrine and exocrine in mind. Figure 12 shows the microscopic structure of an exocrine gland.

Figure 12 Exocrine Gland Structure

Most exocrine secretion in the GI tract is performed by exocrine glands within special digestive organs. These glands release enzymes into ducts (see Figure 12) that ultimately empty into the GI lumen. The digestive organs primarily involved in exocrine secretion include the liver, gallbladder, and pancreas. However, some exocrine secretion is performed by specialized individual epithelial cells in the wall of the gut itself. These cells are miniature exocrine glands, releasing secretions directly into the gut lumen. Important examples are the cells of the **gastric glands** in the stomach and specialized mucus-secreting cells called **goblet cells**. The gastric glands secrete acid and pepsinogen (a protease zymogen discussed below). Goblet cells are found along the entire GI tract. Mucus is a slimy liquid which protects and lubricates the gut; any body surface covered with mucus is known as a **mucus membrane**. One last secretion must be mentioned: water. Whenever a meal is to be digested it must be dissolved in water. Hence, each day, gallons of water are secreted into the GI lumen. Most of it is reabsorbed in the small intestine, and the colon is responsible for reclaiming whatever water is left.

Endocrine secretion is also accomplished by both specialized organs (the pancreas) and by cells in the wall of the gut. Remember that endocrine secretions (hormones) do not empty into ducts but instead are picked up by nearby capillaries. In other words, you should realize that when the same organ has both endocrine and exocrine activities, these functions are accomplished by separate cells, which are usually grouped in such a way as to be microscopically distinguishable. For example, the two principal cell types in the pancreas are: 1) exocrine cells, referred to simply as **pancreatic acinar cells**, which are organized into acini that drain into ducts, and 2) endocrine cells clumped together in groups known as **islets of Langerhans**, which are supplied with capillaries.

---

[9] *Exocrine* glands secrete their products (digestive enzymes, etc.) into *ducts* that drain into the GI lumen. *Endocrine* glands are ductless glands; their secretions (hormones) are picked up by capillaries and thus enter the bloodstream.

10.6 THE GASTROINTESTINAL TRACT

Although the GI tract is a continuous tube, each portion is seen as a separate organ: mouth, pharynx, esophagus, etc. Here we will summarize the major structures and functions of each GI organ. The liver, gallbladder, and pancreas, known as **accessory organs**, are covered in Section 10.7. Section 10.8 details the absorptive process.

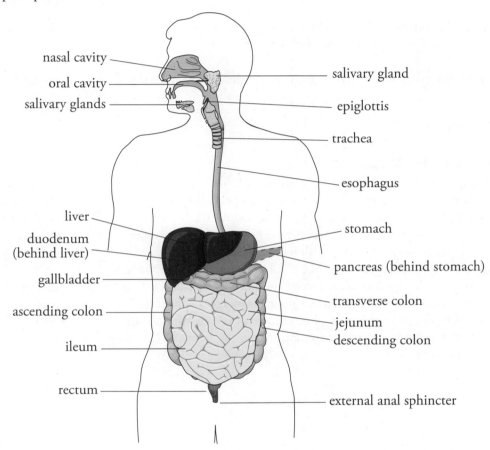

Figure 13 Organs of the Digestive System

Mouth

The mouth has three roles in the digestion of foodstuffs:

1) Fragmentation
2) Lubrication
3) Some enzymatic digestion

Fragmentation is accomplished by **mastication** (**chewing**). The **incisors** (front teeth) are for cutting, the **cuspids** (canine teeth) are for tearing, and the **molars** are for grinding.

Lubrication and some digestion are accomplished by **saliva**, a viscous fluid secreted by salivary glands. Saliva contains **salivary amylase** (**ptyalin**), which hydrolyzes starch, breaking it into fragments. The smallest fragment yielded by salivary amylase is the disaccharide; digestion to monosaccharides occurs only at the intestinal brush border (discussed below). Saliva also contains a small amount of **lingual lipase** for fat digestion. No digestion of proteins occurs in the mouth. Lastly, saliva also contains **lysozyme**, which attacks _____.[10] Therefore, the mouth also participates in innate immunity.

The muscles of the mouth and the muscular tongue are important for compacting chewed food into a smooth lump which can be swallowed, a **bolus**.

10.6

- When carbohydrates are broken down by ptyalin, can they be absorbed in the mouth?[11]

Pharynx and Esophagus

The **pharynx** is what we commonly call the throat. [Key trivia: The floppy thing that hangs down at the back of the throat is called the _____.[12]] The pharynx contains the openings to two tubes: the **trachea** and the **esophagus**. The trachea is a cartilage-lined tube at the front of the neck which conveys air to and from the lungs. The esophagus is a muscular tube behind the trachea which conveys food and drink from the pharynx to the stomach. During swallowing, solids and liquids are excluded from the trachea by a flat cartilaginous flap, the **epiglottis**. A bolus of food passes through the pharynx, over the epiglottis, and into the esophagus, where it is conveyed to the stomach by peristalsis. Two muscular rings regulate movement of food through the esophagus. The **upper esophageal sphincter** is near the top of the esophagus, and the **lower esophageal sphincter** (also known as the **cardiac sphincter** since it is found near the heart) is at the end of the esophagus, at the entrance to the stomach. [Does the lower esophageal sphincter regulate movement of substances into or out of the esophagus?[13]]

Stomach

The stomach is a large hollow muscular organ which serves three purposes: partial digestion of food, regulated release of food into the small intestine, and destruction of microorganisms. The following list highlights some of the attributes and secretions that allow the stomach to accomplish these goals. **Gastric** is an adjective meaning "related to the stomach."

---

[10]   bacterial cell walls. Remember, lytic phages make lysozyme too.

[11]   No. Sugars are not broken down into monosaccharides until they reach the intestinal brush border. Only monosaccharides can be absorbed into the body. Absorption requires special transmembrane transporters located on the intestinal brush border; each transporter is specific for a particular monosaccharide.

[12]   uvula

[13]   It is there to prevent reflux from the stomach into the esophagus. There is no reason to regulate movement of substances out of the esophagus into the stomach, since nothing is stored in the esophagus; it's just a conduit.

Acidity

Gastric pH is about 2, due to the secretion of HCl by parietal cells, located in the gastric mucosa. Effects of low gastric pH include: 1) destruction of microorganisms, 2) acid-catalyzed hydrolysis of many dietary proteins, and 3) conversion of pepsinogen to pepsin.

Pepsin

This is an enzyme secreted by **chief cells** in the stomach wall. It catalyzes proteolysis (protein breakdown). Pepsin is secreted as **pepsinogen**, which is an inactive precursor that must be converted to the active form (pepsin). As noted above, this conversion is catalyzed by gastric acidity. The secretion of an inactive precursor is a common theme in the GI tract; the inactive form is known as a **zymogen**. Most zymogens are activated by proteolysis (cleavage of the protein at a specific site that activates it). Pepsinogen is unique because it is activated by _____ instead of _____.[14]

10.6

Motility

The stomach constantly churns food. Like chewing, this breaks up food particles so that they are exposed to gastric acidity and enzymes. Food mixed with gastric secretions is known as **chyme**.

Sphincters

The lower esophageal sphincter prevents reflux of chyme into the esophagus. The **pyloric sphincter** prevents the passage of food from the stomach into the duodenum. Opening of the pyloric sphincter (stomach emptying) is inhibited when the small intestine already has a large load of chyme. More specifically, stretching or excess acidity in the duodenum inhibits further stomach emptying, by causing the pyloric sphincter to contract. This effect is mediated both by nerves connecting the duodenum and stomach, and by hormones. The main hormone responsible is **cholecystokinin**, secreted by epithelial cells in the wall of the duodenum. [Is this hormone secreted into the lumen of the duodenum or into the lumen of the stomach?[15]]

Gastrin

This is a hormone secreted by cells in the stomach wall known as **G cells**. It stimulates acid and pepsin secretion and gastric motility. Gastrin secretion is stimulated by food in the stomach and by parasympathetic stimulation. The small molecule **histamine** (which is secreted in response both to stomach stretching and to gastrin) binds to parietal cells to stimulate acid release. The ulcer-healing drugs cimetidine (Tagamet) and ranitidine (Zantac) function by blocking the binding of histamine to its receptor (the "H_2 receptor") on parietal cells. This results in less gastric acidity, which allows ulcers to heal.

Small Intestine

Food leaving the stomach enters the small intestine, a tube which is about an inch wide and 10 feet long. (After death, it measures about 25 feet due to relaxation of longitudinal muscles.) The small intestine is divided into three segments: the **duodenum**, **jejunum**, and **ileum**. Digestion begins in the mouth

---

[14] Pepsinogen is unusual in that it is activated to pepsin by acidic proteolysis (autocleavage) instead of proteolytic cleavage by another enzyme.

[15] Neither! It's a hormone; by definition, it is secreted into the bloodstream.

(ptyalin), continues in the stomach, and is completed in the duodenum and jejunum. Absorption begins in the duodenum and continues throughout the small intestine. The anatomy and function of the small intestine are described below. In Section 10.8 we will detail the specific mechanisms of digestion and absorption of carbohydrates, proteins, and fats.

Surface Area

The key feature that allows the small intestine to accomplish absorption is its large surface area; this results from 1) length, 2) villi, and 3) microvilli. **Villi** (singular: **villus**) are macroscopic (multicellular) projections in the wall of the small intestine. **Microvilli** are microscopic foldings of the cell membranes of individual intestinal epithelial cells. The lumenal surface of the small intestine is known as the **brush border** due to the brush-like appearance of microvilli.

The Intestinal Villus

The villus is a finger-like projection of the wall of the gut into the lumen. It has three very important structures:

1) The villus contains capillaries, which absorb dietary monosaccharides and amino acids. The capillaries merge to form veins, which merge to form the large **hepatic portal vein**, which transports blood containing amino acid and carbohydrate nutrients from the gut to the liver.

2) The villus also contains small lymphatic vessels called **lacteals**, which absorb dietary fats. The lacteals merge to form large lymphatic vessels, which transport dietary fats to the thoracic duct, which empties into the bloodstream.

3) **Peyer's patches** are part of the immune system. They are collections of lymphocytes dotting the villi that monitor GI contents and thus confer immunity to gut pathogens and toxins.

Figure 14 An Intestinal Villus

Bile and Pancreatic Secretions in the Duodenum

A key anatomical feature of the duodenum is that two ducts empty into it (Figure 15). One is the **pancreatic duct**, which delivers the exocrine secretions of the pancreas (digestive enzymes and bicarbonate). The other is the **common bile duct**, which delivers **bile**. This is a green fluid containing **bile acids**, which are made from cholesterol in the liver and are normally absorbed and recycled. Bile is stored in the **gallbladder** until it is needed. Bile has two functions: it is a vehicle for the disposal (excretion) of waste products by the liver, and it is essential for the digestion of fats, as discussed below. The bile duct and the pancreatic duct empty into the duodenum via the same orifice, known as the **sphincter of Oddi** (Figure 15).

- If a gallstone became lodged in the sphincter of Oddi, what would happen?[16]
- Bile acids secreted into the duodenum are normally reabsorbed in the ileum. Bile acid sequestrants are drugs which bind bile acids in the small intestine, causing them to remain in the GI lumen and eventually be excreted as feces. Each of the following is most likely true about such drugs EXCEPT that:[17]
  - A) they are stable at low pH levels.
  - B) they result in a decrease in the level of cholesterol in the bloodstream.
  - C) it would be reasonable to be concerned that they might disrupt fat absorption.
  - D) they would be administered intravenously (injected into a vein).

10.6

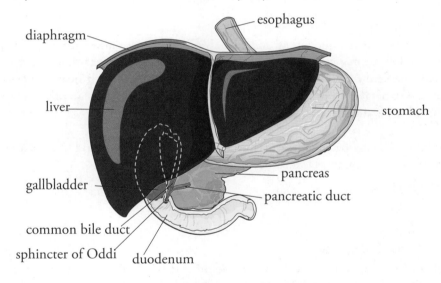

Figure 15   Anatomy around the Duodenum

---

[16]   Both the bile and the pancreatic ducts would be blocked, and digestion would be severely impaired (especially fat digestion, but also protein and carbohydrate digestion due to failure of pancreatic zymogens and amylase to reach the intestinal lumen).

[17]   Since the drugs must pass through the stomach, they should be stable at low pH levels (choice A is true and can be eliminated). The text states that bile acids are made from cholesterol and normally recycled. It is reasonable to assume that blocking this recycling would require the conversion of more cholesterol into bile acids, which would lower the serum cholesterol level. This is, in fact, what bile acid sequestrants are used for (choice B is true and can be eliminated). It would be reasonable to be concerned about fat absorption, based on the fact that bile acids are necessary for this absorption, as stated in the text (choice C is true and can be eliminated). However, the drugs would have to be *swallowed* to end up within the GI lumen, not injected (choice **D** is false and is the correct answer choice).

Duodenal Enzymes

Some duodenal epithelial cells secrete enzymes. Duodenal **enterokinase** (also known as **enteropeptidase**) activates the pancreatic zymogen **trypsinogen** to trypsin (Section 10.7). Other duodenal enzymes are peculiar in that they are not truly secreted, but rather do their work inside or on the surface of the brush border epithelial cell. These duodenal enzymes are called **brush border enzymes**. Their role is to hydrolyze the smallest carbohydrates and proteins (like disaccharides and dipeptides) into monosaccharides and amino acids (Section 10.8).

Duodenal Hormones

Other duodenal epithelial cells secrete hormones. The three main duodenal hormones are **cholecystokinin (CCK)**, **secretin**, and **enterogastrone**. CCK is secreted in response to fats in the duodenum. It causes the pancreas to secrete digestive enzymes, stimulates gallbladder contraction (bile release), and decreases gastric motility. Note that all these processes cooperate to deal with fats in the duodenum, by digesting them and preventing further stomach emptying. Secretin is released in response to acid in the duodenum. It causes the pancreas to release large amounts of a high-pH aqueous buffer, namely HCO_3^- in water. This neutralizes HCl released by the stomach. Duodenal pH must be kept neutral or even slightly basic for pancreatic digestive enzymes to function. Enterogastrone decreases stomach emptying.

Jejunum and Ileum

Substances not absorbed in the duodenum must be absorbed in these lower segments of the small intestine. The lower small intestine performs special absorptive processes. For example, absorption of vitamin B_{12} occurs only in the ileum (and only when vitamin B_{12} is complexed with **intrinsic factor**, a glycoprotein secreted by the parietal cells of the stomach). A valve called the **ileocecal valve** separates the ileum from the cecum, which is the first part of the large intestine.

- True or false? When a pancreatic exocrine cell secretes an alkaline fluid into the duodenum, a corresponding decrease in pH must occur in that cell's cytoplasm.[18]

Colon (Large Intestine)

Like the rest of the intestine, the colon is a muscular tube. It is 3 or 4 feet long and several inches wide. Its role is to absorb water and minerals, and to form and store feces until the time of defecation. Abnormalities of colon function result in poor fluid absorption and diarrhea, which can cause dehydration and death. The first part of the colon is the **cecum**. Entrance of chyme into the cecum is controlled by the ileocecal valve. The **appendix** is a finger-like appendage of the cecum. It is composed primarily of lymphatic tissue and was mentioned in the preceding chapter. The last portion of the colon is called the **rectum**. Exit of feces (**defecation**) from the rectum occurs through the **anus**. Defecation is controlled by the **anal sphincter**, which has an internal portion and an external portion. The internal anal sphincter consists of smooth muscle, which is under autonomic control. The external anal sphincter consists of skeletal muscle and is under voluntary control. (Note that this is the same arrangement as seen in the

---

[18] True. In the pancreas, CO_2 is converted to carbonic acid by carbonic anhydrase. Carbonic acid dissociates into bicarbonate (HCO_3^-) plus a proton. If the bicarbonate is secreted into the gut, the proton is left behind, thus the pH falls. Severe diarrhea may involve the loss of large amounts of bicarbonate from the gut, and this may cause a significant decrease in the plasma pH level.

urinary sphincters.) Most of the wastes from a meal are defecated about a day after it is eaten. However, the wastes from a meal are first present in stool after just a few hours and some residue of a meal is typically still present in the colon after several days.

The colon contains billions of bacteria of various species. Many are facultative or obligate anaerobes. Undigested materials are metabolized by colonic bacteria. This often results in gas, which is given off as a waste product of bacterial metabolism. **Colonic bacteria** are important for two reasons: 1) the presence of large numbers of normal bacteria helps keep dangerous bacteria from proliferating, due to competition for space and nutrients, and 2) colonic bacteria supply us with **vitamin K,** which is essential for blood clotting.

10.7 THE GI ACCESSORY ORGANS

The GI accessory organs are those that play a role in digestion, but are not actually part of the alimentary canal. They include the **pancreas**, **liver**, **gallbladder**, and the large **salivary glands** found outside the mouth. We have already discussed saliva, so the salivary glands will not be discussed further here. The pancreas and liver are essential for GI function. The gallbladder is not essential, but can become infected, obstructed, or cancerous, and is thus medically important.

Exocrine Pancreas

Pancreatic enzymes released into the duodenum are essential for digestion. **Pancreatic amylase** hydrolyzes polysaccharides to disaccharides. **Pancreatic lipase** hydrolyzes triglycerides at the surface of a micelle (see Liver and Gallbladder). **Nucleases** hydrolyze dietary DNA and RNA. Several different **pancreatic proteases** are responsible for hydrolyzing polypeptides to di- and tripeptides. Pancreatic proteases are secreted in their inactive **zymogen** forms. [Why do you suppose digestive enzymes are stored and released in an inactive form?[19]] Zymogens must be activated by removal of a portion of the polypeptide chain. **Trypsinogen** is a zymogen which is converted to the active form, **trypsin**, by **enterokinase**, an intestinal enzyme. Other pancreatic enzymes are then activated by trypsin. These include **chymotrypsinogen** (active form: **chymotrypsin**), **procarboxypeptidase** (active form: **carboxypeptidase**), and **procollagenase** (active form: **collagenase**).

Control of the Exocrine Pancreas

Two hormones discussed previously help to control pancreatic secretion. **Cholecystokinin** (CCK) secreted into the bloodstream by the duodenum causes the pancreas to secrete enzymes. **Secretin**, also released by the duodenum, causes the pancreas to secrete water and bicarbonate (high pH). Parasympathetic nervous system activation increases pancreatic secretion; sympathetic activation reduces it.

---

[19] It is a safety mechanism. Active digestive enzymes could be dangerous to the pancreatic cells themselves.

Endocrine Pancreas

The endocrine pancreas consists of small regions within the pancreas known as **islets of Langerhans**. There are three types of cells in the islets, and each secretes a particular hormone into the bloodstream.

1) α cells secrete **glucagon** in response to low blood sugar. Glucagon functions to mobilize stored fuels by stimulating the liver to hydrolyze glycogen and release glucose into the bloodstream, and by stimulating adipocytes (fat cells) to release fats into the bloodstream.
2) β cells secrete **insulin** in response to elevated blood sugar (e.g., after a meal). Its effects are opposite those of glucagon: insulin stimulates the removal of glucose from the blood for storage as glycogen and fat.
3) δ cells secrete **somatostatin**. It inhibits many digestive processes.

Focus on Blood Glucose

1) **Lowering blood glucose:** Insulin is essential for life because it causes sugar to be removed from the bloodstream and stored. Diabetics lack insulin or have dysfunctional insulin receptors. Their blood sugar levels are extraordinarily high. The excess glucose directly destroys many physiological systems at the cellular level, including neurons, blood vessels, and the kidneys.

2) **Raising blood glucose:** Three hormones can raise the blood glucose level: glucagon (a polypeptide hormone from the pancreas), epinephrine (an amino acid derivative from the adrenal medulla), and cortisol (a steroid or glucocorticoid from the adrenal cortex). Note that of these three hormones, one is a steroid, one is a polypeptide, and one is an amino acid derivative. Also note that there is only one hormone that can lower blood glucose, while three different hormones can raise blood glucose. It makes sense to have many ways to raise blood glucose, and for it to be less easy to lower blood glucose, since low blood glucose levels are immediately fatal, while elevated blood glucose is harmless in the short term. (Over several years, however, it is harmful.)

- Which one of the following statements is true?[20]
  A) Insulin stimulates the release of glucose into the blood and also stimulates peristalsis in the small intestine.
  B) Gastrin stimulates stomach emptying and inhibits secretion of gastric acid.
  C) Cholecystokinin stimulates peristalsis in the intestine and inhibits stomach emptying.
  D) Glucagon stimulates the storage of glucose and stimulates small intestinal peristalsis.

Liver and Gallbladder

The exocrine secretory activity of the liver is simple: it secretes bile. The liver actually produces about 1 liter of bile a day. The principal ingredients of bile include bile acids (known as **bile salts** in the deprotonated—anionic—form), cholesterol, and bilirubin (from RBC breakdown). Bile emulsifies large fat particles in the duodenum, creating smaller clusters of fat particles called **micelles**. The smaller particles have a greater collective surface area than the large particles, and thus are more easily digested by hydrophilic lipases (from the pancreas). Also, bile helps fatty particles to diffuse across the intestinal mucosal membrane.

---

[20] Insulin stimulates the *removal* of glucose from the blood (choice A is false), gastrin *causes* acid secretion (choice B is false), and glucagon functions to *raise* blood glucose (choice D is false). Choice **C** is a true statement.

Bile made in the liver can go to one of two places: it is either directly secreted into the duodenum or it is stored for later use in the **gallbladder**. Bile stored in the gallbladder is concentrated, and released when a fatty meal is eaten. A **gallstone** is a large crystal formed from bile made with ingredients in incorrect proportions.

The gallbladder itself has no secretory activity. Bile release from this organ is dictated by both the endocrine system and the nervous system. Both CCK (released by the duodenal cells) and the parasympathetic nervous system stimulate contraction of the gallbladder wall.

The liver plays a more complicated role in the *processing* of absorbed nutrients than it does in digestion (breakdown). In order to understand this process, it helps to consider the **hepatic portal system**. The liver receives blood from two places. First, it receives oxygenated blood from the hepatic arteries. Second, it receives venous blood draining the stomach and intestines through the **hepatic portal vein**. (*Hepatic* means "relating to the liver.") As this blood percolates through the liver, nutrients are extracted by hepatocytes (liver cells). The hepatocytes monitor the blood and make changes to the body's physiology based on what is and is not present (much as the hypothalamus does in the hypothalamic-pituitary portal system). For example, if blood glucose is low, the liver will initiate a cascade that leads to glycogen breakdown as well as new glucose production (gluconeogenesis). The free glucose can be released to raise blood glucose levels.

Both the liver and the skeletal muscles are capable of storing glucose as glycogen and subsequently breaking glycogen down when glucose is needed. However only the liver is able to release free glucose to the bloodstream. The product of glycogen breakdown is glucose-6-phosphate; in order to move into the bloodstream, this product must be dephosphorylated, and only the liver contains the enzyme needed to accomplish this (glucose-6-phosphatase).

The waste products from protein catabolism (breakdown) are also regulated through the liver. When proteins are broken down into amino acids, and amino acids are broken down even further (e.g., to enter the Krebs cycle to generate ATP during starvation), nitrogenous by-products are released in the form of NH_3 (ammonia). Ammonia in high levels is toxic to the body, so it is transported to the liver where it is converted into urea. Urea is then absorbed into the bloodstream and excreted by the kidney in urine.

Lipid metabolism is assisted by the liver as well. Lipids exit the intestine and enter the lymphatic system in molecules called **chylomicrons**. Chylomicrons are degraded by lipases into triglycerides, glycerol, and cholesterol-rich **chylomicron remnants**. These remnants are taken up by hepatocytes and combined with proteins to make lipoproteins (HDL, LDL, VLDL, etc.). These lipoproteins then re-enter the blood and are the source of cholesterol and triglycerides for the other tissues of the body.

Many important plasma proteins (such as albumin, globulins, fibrinogens, and other clotting factors necessary to stop bleeding) are made in the liver and secreted into the plasma. People with liver disease often have problems with sealing wounds due to a lack of clotting factors. They also have a tendency to swell up; the lack of albumin allows fluid to leave the bloodstream and enter the tissues.

Finally, the liver is the major center for drug and toxin detoxification in the body. The smooth ER in hepatocytes contains enzyme pathways that break down drugs and toxins into forms that are less toxic and more readily excreted by the renal and gastrointestinal systems. Interestingly, sometimes these same enzyme pathways in hepatocytes are used to convert some drugs into their active forms. Therefore, people with liver disease must have drug levels in their blood monitored closely when they are on medications that are affected by the detoxification system of the liver.

10.7

Hormonal Control of Appetite

The desire to eat between meals is subject to hormonal control. When the stomach is empty, gastric cells produce the hormone **ghrelin** to stimulate appetite. When the colon is full, the jejunum (lower intestine) produces **peptide YY** to reduce appetite. The hormone **leptin**, produced by white adipose tissue (fat), is an appetite suppressant that acts as an "adipostat"—maintaining stable lipid content in adipose tissue. Leptin is secreted in response to increased triglyceride levels, and it works to suppress appetite until appropriate levels are restored. All three of these hormones can affect multiple target tissues, but their effects on appetite are primarily mediated by the arcuate nucleus of the hypothalamus.

Leptin has been a focus of obesity research, particularly because disruption of leptin signaling in animal models causes the animals to become obese. Disruptions include the inability to synthesize leptin or a malfunction of the leptin receptor. In humans, obesity is often associated with high levels of leptin but a lack of appetite suppression. This suggests that the hypothalamus may become resistant to leptin, possibly due to down-regulation of the receptors.

10.8

10.8   A DAY IN THE LIFE OF FOOD

In order to draw the above information together, let's trace the path of each of the three main types of dietary nutrients: carbohydrates, proteins, and fats.

Carbohydrates

You purchase a sourdough baguette and tear off a hunk. Chewing increases the bread's surface area, allowing it to soak up more saliva. Ptyalin hydrolyzes starch into fragments, while the tongue and cheeks form a bolus. As you swallow, the upper esophageal sphincter relaxes. Peristalsis carries the bolus to the stomach; the lower esophageal sphincter relaxes to let it pass. In the stomach, strong acid destroys most of the microorganisms which were present in the bread, while further hydrolyzing some polysaccharides. The stomach thoroughly churns the bread, forming acidic chyme, which is gradually released into the duodenum. In the duodenum, pancreatic amylase chops the polysaccharides into disaccharides, which diffuse to the intestinal brush border. Here the disaccharides are hydrolyzed to monosaccharides. Digestion is complete. Up to this point, none of the sugar composing the bread has entered your body; it remains on the lumenal side of GI epithelial tight junctions.

Since they are bulky and hydrophilic, monosaccharides must be taken up into the intestinal epithelial cell by active transport. An apical symport transports one sugar into the cell while allowing sodium to flow in, down its large concentration gradient (Figure 16). [Is this primary or secondary active transport?[21]] The large sodium concentration gradient is created by constant activity of Na+/K+ ATPases on the basolateral surface of the cell, pumping Na+ out. As secondary active transport continues to pack the epithelial cell with monosaccharides, their concentration gets quite high. Thus, there is now a concentration gradient driving them out of the cell into nearby capillaries. This movement occurs by facilitated diffusion (uniports) at the basolateral surface of the cell. In the bloodstream, sugars dissolve into the plasma as it flows into the hepatic portal vein toward the liver.

---

[21] Secondary, since transport is powered by a pre-existing gradient, not directly by ATP hydrolysis.

Figure 16   Absorption of Hydrophilic Food Monomers

The liver takes up some of the sugars and begins to store them or use their energy. Nonetheless, the blood sugar level increases rather suddenly. When the pancreas is exposed to elevated blood glucose levels, the β cells of the islets of Langerhans secrete insulin. The insulin causes many different cells (liver, muscle, nerve, and fat cells) to take up, utilize, and store glucose. Soon the blood sugar level returns to normal, and you're ready for dessert.

Proteins

The next day, you're well rested from an iron-pumping session and are ready for a nice can of albacore in spring water. You buy generic because it's the same quality but cheaper (and check to make sure it's dolphin-safe).

In your mouth, the tuna is ground and mixed with saliva. No digestion of protein occurs in the mouth. A bolus is formed, and you swallow. Churning of the stomach mixes the tuna with acid, mucus, and enzymes. The low pH kills microorganisms and causes many peptide bonds to hydrolyze. Activated pepsin attacks polypeptides, breaking them into fragments. Chyme is gradually released into the duodenum.

Chyme in the duodenum causes duodenal epithelial cells to secrete CCK and secretin. As a result, the gallbladder releases concentrated bile and the pancreas secretes a basic (high pH) solution of bicarbonate plus digestive zymogens. In the gut, trypsinogen is activated to trypsin by enterokinase. Trypsin then activates other zymogens. The activated proteases go to work on polypeptides from the tuna until all that's left are dipeptides and tripeptides. These are hydrolyzed by brush border peptidases.

Amino acid absorption is similar to monosaccharide absorption: a secondary active transporter (symport) specific to each amino acid couples the uptake of an amino acid to the entrance of sodium into the cell, and a uniporter facilitates movement out of the intestinal epithelial cell into the interstitium. Just as with carbohydrates, the amino acid ends up in the liver, where it is catabolized for energy or used in synthesis (anabolism).

Fats

"Enough of sourdough and tuna fish!" you declare, as you enter an ice cream shop. The almost-pure triglycerides melt in your mouth and are swallowed. The stomach's churning mixes the triglycerides with acid and mucus to some extent, but because they are extremely hydrophobic, they end up just floating in a layer above the aqueous contents of the stomach. Eventually they are emptied into the duodenum where they stimulate CCK release into the bloodstream. Then the pancreas sends enzymes into the gut, via the sphincter of Oddi. But there is a problem: pancreatic lipase cannot digest the fats if they are organized into huge hydrophobic droplets.

Fortunately, CCK in the bloodstream also stimulates gallbladder contraction. This sends bile down the bile duct into the duodenum. Bile acids emulsify the lipids from the ice cream, forming tiny micelles. Then pancreatic lipase can go to work. It hydrolyzes triglycerides to monoglycerides plus free fatty acids, as shown below. These move into intestinal epithelial cells by simple diffusion, which they are able to do thanks to their greasy hydrophobicity and small size. Once inside, they are converted back to triglycerides, which are packaged into **chylomicrons**. These are large particles composed of fats and proteins which are designed to transport fats in the bloodstream (Figure 17).

Figure 17   Fat Absorption

The chylomicrons do not enter intestinal blood capillaries. Instead, they enter tiny lymphatic capillaries known as **lacteals**. These merge to form larger lymphatic vessels, which eventually empty into the thoracic duct. This empties into a large vein near the heart. A few minutes after your sundae, huge amounts of fat are released from the thoracic duct directly into the bloodstream. Your plasma attains a milky yellow color which is easily noticeable when a blood sample is taken. The term for milky plasma is **lipemia**, meaning "fat in the blood."

The chylomicrons circulate throughout the body and are gradually whittled away by removal of fat. In particular, adipose and liver tissues contain the enzyme **lipoprotein lipase**, which hydrolyzes chylomicron triglycerides into monoglycerides and free fatty acids. These diffuse into adipocytes and liver cells, are remade into triglycerides, and then stored.

10.9   VITAMINS

Vitamins are nutrients which must be included in the diet because they cannot be synthesized in the body. They are divided into **fat-soluble** and **water-soluble** categories. Fat-soluble vitamins require bile acids for solubilization and absorption. Excess fat-soluble vitamins are stored in adipose tissue. Excess water-soluble vitamins are excreted in urine by the kidneys.

10.9

Table 2   Vitamins

Vitamin	Function
fat-soluble	
A (retinol)	A visual pigment that changes conformation in response to light
D	Stimulates Ca^{2+} absorption from the gut; helps control Ca^{2+} deposition in bones
E	Prevents oxidation of unsaturated fats
K	Necessary for formation of blood coagulation factors
water-soluble	
B_1 (thiamine)	Needed for enzymatic decarboxylations
B_2 (riboflavin)	Made into FAD, an electron transporter
B_3 (niacin)	Made into NAD^+, an electron transporter
B_6 (pyridoxine)	A coenzyme involved in protein and amino acid metabolism
B_{12} (cobalamin)	A coenzyme involved in the reduction of nucleotides to deoxynucleotides
C (ascorbic acid)	Necessary for collagen formation; deficiency results in scurvy
Biotin	Prosthetic group essential for transport of CO_2 groups
Folate	Enzyme cofactor used in the transport of methylene groups; synthesis of purines and thymine; required for normal fetal nervous system development

Chapter 10 Summary

- The kidneys filter the blood to remove hydrophilic wastes. They also play a major role in homeostasis by regulating blood pressure, pH, ion balance, and water balance.

- Urine is produced by first filtering the blood, and then by modifying the filtrate via reabsorption (moving substances from the filtrate to the blood) and secretion (moving substances from the blood to the filtrate), and finally by concentrating the filtrate to conserve body water.

- Filtration occurs at the glomerulus, most reabsorption and secretion occurs in the PCT, selective reabsorption and secretion occur in the DCT, and concentration occurs in the collecting duct.

- The loop of Henle establishes a concentration gradient in the medulla; this gradient is critical to the reabsorption of water and the creation of a concentrated urine.

- ADH increases the water permeability of the collecting duct to allow reabsorption of water, and aldosterone increases Na^+ reabsorption at the distal tubule. Both hormones work together to help regulate blood pressure.

- When systemic blood pressure falls, the kidneys release renin. Renin is an enzyme that converts the blood protein angiotensinogen into angiotensin I, which is further converted to angiotensin II. Angiotensin II is a potent vasoconstrictor, and it increases the release of aldosterone; the ultimate goal is to increase blood pressure.

- The digestive system organs are divided into two categories: the alimentary canal and the accessory organs. The alimentary canal is the long muscular tube consisting of the mouth, esophagus, stomach, small intestine, and large intestine. The accessory organs have a digestive role, but are not part of the tube. They include the salivary glands, the liver, the gallbladder, and the pancreas.

- The mouth breaks down food mechanically by chewing, and it begins starch digestion via salivary amylase.

- The stomach is primarily a storage tank for food. Mechanical digestion occurs through churning of the food, acid hydrolysis begins chemical digestion, and protein digestion is begun via pepsin.

- Almost all chemical digestion and nutrient absorption takes place in the small intestine. The large intestine primarily reabsorbs water and stores feces; no digestion takes place in the large intestine.

- The liver produces bile (secreted into the small intestine), which emulsifies fat to increase the efficiency of fat digestion. The gallbladder stores and concentrates bile.

- The pancreas secretes the majority of the digestive enzymes used in the small intestine, along with bicarbonate to help neutralize the acid entering the small intestine from the stomach. The pancreas is also a major endocrine organ, secreting insulin and glucagon to regulate blood glucose.

- The enteric nervous system consists of the myenteric plexus and the submucosal plexus. It helps to regulate gut movement, local blood flow, and ion/water exchange.

- Ghrelin is a hormone produced by gastric cells when the stomach is empty to stimulate appetite, while peptide YY is a hormone released by the jejunum when the colon is full to reduce appetite.

- Leptin is produced by fat cells and suppresses appetite when lipid levels in the blood are high.

CHAPTER 10 FREESTANDING PRACTICE QUESTIONS

1. The loop of Henle uses a countercurrent multiplier system to create an area of high ion concentration in the renal medulla. Which of the following statements about the loop of Henle is true?

A) The descending limb is permeable to ions and water.
B) The descending limb is permeable to water but not to ions.
C) The ascending limb is permeable to ions and water.
D) The ascending limb is permeable to water but not to ions.

2. All of the following would increase glomerular filtration rate EXCEPT:

A) constriction of efferent arterioles in the kidney.
B) increased circulatory volume.
C) dilation of afferent arterioles in the kidney.
D) increased filtrate osmolarity.

3. The kidneys play a role in all of the following processes EXCEPT:

A) erythropoiesis.
B) increased absorption of calcium in the intestine.
C) vasoconstriction.
D) stimulation of the sympathetic nervous system.

4. Which of the following statements about angiotensin II is true?

I. Angiotensin II is a vasodilator.
II. Angiotensin II is a substrate for ACE.
III. Angiotensin II stimulates aldosterone release from the adrenal cortex.

A) I only
B) II only
C) III only
D) II and III

5. Which of the following is *not* an effect of gastrin?

A) Promote parietal cell atrophy
B) Decrease stomach pH
C) Activate chief cells
D) Indirectly stimulate protein degradation

6. A defect in pancreatic amylase would prevent digestion of which of the following nutrients?

A) Starch
B) Maltose
C) Fructose
D) Proteins

7. Hydrochloric acid is present in the stomach, resulting in an approximate pH of 2. Which of the following is NOT a correct statement about HCl?

A) It destroys microorganisms in the stomach.
B) It is secreted by G cells.
C) It converts pepsinogen to pepsin.
D) It participates in the acid hydrolysis of proteins.

8. The hepatic portal vein carries deoxygenated blood from the alimentary canal into the liver, where it is filtered before continuing to the heart via the hepatic vein and inferior vena cava. Blood from which of the following organs does NOT drain into the hepatic portal vein?

A) Stomach
B) Small intestine
C) Colon
D) Kidneys

CHAPTER 10 PRACTICE PASSAGE

The kidneys are critical in regulating and maintaining fluid balance and blood pressure. The functional unit of the kidney is the nephron, a tubule that starts at the glomerulus, enters the cortex, descends into the medulla, loops around, and returns to the cortex. These tubules empty into collecting ducts, which empty into the renal calyces and then into the ureter. Aldosterone and vasopressin are two main hormones that affect renal function.

Aldosterone is the primary effector hormone in the *renin-angiotensin-aldosterone system* (RAAS). It is secreted in response to low blood pressure, low plasma sodium levels, and high plasma potassium levels. Renin is an enzyme secreted by the JG cells of the kidney; it converts angiotensinogen into angiotensin I, which is then converted into angiotensin II by angiotensin converting enzyme (ACE). Angiotensin II is a powerful vasoconstrictor and stimulator of aldosterone release. Aldosterone acts to increase sodium reabsorption, thereby increasing water retention.

Vasopressin is a peptide hormone and is secreted by the posterior pituitary. The main effect of vasopressin is to increase permeability of the collecting ducts to water by stimulating the insertion of *aquaporins* into the epithelial cells of these ducts. Vasopressin can also stimulate increased reabsorption of sodium in the thick ascending loop of Henle. Vasopressin release is stimulated by a decreased plasma volume (via pressure receptors), and by an increased plasma osmotic pressure (via osmoreceptors) in the hypothalamus.

Other hormones acting on or produced by the kidneys include atrial natriuretic peptide (ANP) and erythropoietin (EPO). Although EPO does not act on the kidneys, it is released by the kidneys and stimulates red blood cell production. ANP, on the other hand, is released by atrial myocytes in response to excess atrial stretch. ANP acts as a vasodilator, and increases glomerular filtration rate; this hormone also inhibits renin secretion and reduces aldosterone secretion.

Kidney function can be assessed by analyzing glomerular filtration rate (GFR). GFR is defined as the sum of the filtration rates of all functioning nephrons. An approximate value for normal GFR can be obtained by using the equation: GFR = 140 – [patient age]. Various conditions can affect GFR, as evidenced by Figure 1, which shows the prevalence of various GFR rates by function of age for patients with hyperphosphatemia and patients with hypertension.

Figure 1 Prevalence of GFR rates as a function of age

Figure adapted from Bowling, Inker, Gutiérrez, Allman, Warnock, McClellan, et. al. (2011). Age-Specific Associations of Reduced Estimated Glomerular Filtration Rate with Concurrent Chronic Kidney Disease Complications. *Clinical Journal of the American Society of Nephrology*, 6 (12) 2822-2828

1. Which of the following could be the result of a hormone-secreting tumor of the kidneys?

A) Increased sodium retention
B) Elevated hemoglobin
C) Concentrated urine
D) Increased thirst

2. According to Figure 1, which of the following is true?

A) In those with hypertension, it is more common for people to have a GFR of more than 60 mL/min versus less than 45 mL/min across all ages groups.

B) The prevalence of a GFR of 50 mL/min in hypertensive 50-year-old adults is approximately 85%.

C) In those with hypertension, GFR directly increases with age.

D) In those with hyperphosphatemia, the prevalence of a GFR of 60 mL/min and above is roughly similar for ages 60–69 and 70–79.

3. Which of the following statements is correct?

A) Glomeruli are circular in shape, and contain a capillary system, which separates two arterioles.

B) Vasa recta can be found accompanying the loop of Henle in the adrenal cortex.

C) The distal tubules empty into the minor calyx via the renal papilla.

D) Aldosterone acts to increase potassium reabsorption.

4. Alcohol acts as a diuretic; consumption of alcohol produces large quantities of dilute urine. Which of the following statements is NOT a possible explanation for this observation?

A) Alcohol decreases the action of ACE, thereby inhibiting the release of aldosterone from the adrenal gland and decreasing water reabsorption by the collecting duct.

B) Alcohol acts to stimulate renin release.

C) Alcohol inhibits the secretion of vasopressin, therefore diminishing the kidneys' ability to concentrate urine.

D) Alcohol stimulates the release of ANP from the atria.

5. Hyperphosphatemia refers to an elevated amount of phosphate in the blood. A 45-year-old patient with hyperphosphatemia is tested for kidney function. His GFR value is 55 mL/min. Which of the following is/are true?

   I.   The patient would have high levels of aldosterone in his blood.

   II.   The patient's GFR would be considered normal.

   III.   The prevalence of a GFR of 55 mL/min for his age range and condition is 13%.

A) I only

B) II only

C) I and III only

D) I, II, and III

6. Which of the following statements comparing ANP and angiotensin is correct?

A) ANP increases blood pressure and urine volume, whereas angiotensin II decreases blood pressure and urine volume.

B) ANP decreases blood pressure and increases urine volume, whereas angiotensin II increases blood pressure and decreases urine volume.

C) ANP decreases blood pressure and urine volume, whereas angiotensin II increases blood pressure and urine volume.

D) ANP increases blood pressure and decreases urine volume, whereas angiotensin II decreases blood pressure and increases urine volume.

SOLUTIONS TO CHAPTER 10 FREESTANDING PRACTICE QUESTIONS

1. **B** The descending limb of the loop of Henle is permeable to water but not to ions (choice B is correct, and choice A is wrong); water leaves the filtrate, thereby concentrating it. The ascending limb is permeable to ions but not to water (choices C and D can be eliminated). Na^+, K^+, and Cl^- are actively transported out of the filtrate, and K^+ is passively transported, concentrating the renal medulla.

2. **D** Constricting efferent arterioles would restrict flow out of the glomerulus, and dilating afferent arterioles would increase flow into the glomerulus; in either case, pressure at the glomerulus would rise and filtration rate would increase (choices A and C can be eliminated). An increase in circulatory volume will increase blood pressure and further enhance this effect on a systemic level (choice B can be eliminated). However, if the filtrate osmolarity is high, the macula densa will not send signals to stimulate the juxtaglomerular cells and the GFR will not be increased (choice D would not increase GFR and is the correct answer choice).

3. **D** Erythropoietin is released by the kidneys and stimulates red blood cell production in bone marrow (the kidneys play a role in choice A, so it can be eliminated). Calcitriol (vitamin D) is activated in the kidneys and promotes the uptake of calcium in the intestines (the kidneys play a role in choice B, so it can be eliminated). Renin is released by the kidneys and triggers the production of angiotensin II, which causes vasoconstriction (the kidneys play a role in choice C, so it can be eliminated). However, sympathetic nervous system stimulation comes from the products of the adrenal glands, not the kidneys (the kidneys do not play a role in choice D, so it is the best answer choice).

4. **C** Item I is false: angiotensin II acts as a vasoconstrictor to increase blood pressure (choice A can be eliminated). Item II is false: angiotensin I is the substrate for ACE, which converts angiotensin I into angiotensin II (choices B and D can be eliminated, and choice C is correct). Item III is true: angiotensin II stimulates the release of ADH from the posterior pituitary gland and aldosterone from the adrenal cortex, thereby increasing blood pressure.

5. **A** Gastrin acts on parietal cells in a stimulatory manner, causing them to release HCl (choice B is an effect and can be eliminated). Parietal cell atrophy occurs in the *absence* of gastrin (choice A is not an effect of gastrin and is the correct answer choice). Additionally, gastrin activates chief cells to release pepsinogen (choice C is an effect and can be eliminated). The combination of pepsinogen from the chief cells and acid from the parietal cells stimulates the cleavage and activation of pepsinogen to pepsin, with subsequent degradation of proteins (choice D is an effect and can be eliminated).

6. **A** Amylase hydrolyzes starch into maltose, which is further broken down into individual glucose molecules by brush border enzymes in the small intestine (choice A is correct, and choice B is wrong). Fructose is already a monosaccharide and can be absorbed without further digestion (choice C is wrong), and proteins are digested by proteases like trypsin or pepsin (choice D is wrong).

7. **B** Choices A, C, and D are all consistent with the function of HCl in the stomach. The statement in choice B is incorrect (and, therefore, the correct answer) because HCl is secreted by parietal cells, not G cells. G cells secrete gastrin, a hormone.

8. **D** The stomach, small intestine, and colon (large intestine) are part of the alimentary canal, and their blood supplies drain into the hepatic portal vein to be filtered by the liver (choices A, B, and C can be eliminated). Blood that passes through the kidneys drains directly into the inferior vena cava via the renal veins (choice D is correct).

SOLUTIONS TO CHAPTER 10 PRACTICE PASSAGE

1. **B** EPO is the only hormone secreted by the kidneys. It will act to increase red blood cell production, thus increasing hemoglobin. Don't confuse renin with a hormone! Renin is an enzyme that acts on an existing blood protein (angiotensinogen) to convert it to an active form (angiotensin). It does not bind to receptors anywhere and does not have a direct role on cellular function (as do hormones). Certainly, if the secretion of renin were increased, then all other answer choices would also occur. There would be an increase in aldosterone and a subsequent increase in sodium reabsorption. The increased sodium reabsorption would increase vasopressin release and the urine would be concentrated. Both the increased sodium and vasopressin would act to increase thirst, but since renin is not a hormone and this question specifically asks about a "hormone-secreting tumor of the kidney," choices A, C, and D are wrong.

2. **D** In people ages 20–59 with hypertension, there is approximately an 85% prevalence of a GFR of less than 45 mL/min versus approximately 15% prevalence of a GFR of more than 60 mL/min. Since the answer choice says "across all age groups," the finding of even one age group for which this is not the case makes the answer false (choice A can be eliminated). The prevalence values are calculated for age ranges, so you cannot infer from the graph what the prevalence of the GFR for a 50-year-old specifically would be (choice B can be eliminated). The graph shows the prevalence of certain GFR values as a function of age, not the exact correlation between age and GFR (choice C can be eliminated). As shown on the graph, the prevalence of a GFR of 60 mL/min or higher in those with hyperphosphatemia is approximately 6% for both ages 60–69 and 70–79 (choice D is correct).

3. **A** The glomeruli are small knots of capillaries, supplied with blood by the afferent arterioles and drained of blood by the efferent arterioles. Although the vasa recta do surround the loop of Henle, they are found in the medulla, not the cortex (choice B is wrong). The distal tubules empty into the collecting ducts (which then empty into the minor calyces; choice C is wrong). Aldosterone acts to increase sodium reabsorption (not potassium), and in any case, the passage states that the release of aldosterone can be triggered by high plasma potassium. If its release is triggered by high plasma potassium, aldosterone is unlikely to stimulate the reabsorption of potassium, driving the levels up even higher (choice D is wrong).

4. **B** Decreased water reabsorption means increased water elimination; in other words, the production of large quantities of dilute urine (choice A could explain the observation and can be eliminated). Similarly, since the passage describes the action of vasopressin in reclaiming water from the nephron, an inhibition of vasopressin secretion would lead to decreased water reclamation (reabsorption) and the production of dilute urine (choice C could explain the observation and can be eliminated). The passage states that ANP acts to increase glomerular filtration rate (increase urine production) and to decrease renin and aldosterone secretion; both of these would decrease water reabsorption and lead to the production of dilute urine (choice D could explain the observation and can be eliminated). However, if alcohol were to stimulate renin release, more aldosterone would be secreted, leading to the reabsorption of more water and the production of a concentrated urine (choice B does not explain the observation and is the correct answer choice). Note that the actual action of alcohol is to inhibit vasopressin, but the question only asks which of the answer choices was a *possible* explanation.

5. **C** Since this is a Roman numeral question, start by analyzing the Roman numeral item that appears in exactly two of the answer choices, in this case Item II or III. Item II is shorter, so start with that one; whether it is true or false, you can eliminate half the answers. Item II is false: the passage states that normal GFR can be approximated by subtracting a patient's age from 140; this would give an approximate GFR of 95 ml/min, which is much higher than the patient's actual GFR (choices B and D can be eliminated). Since both remaining choices include Item I, it must be true and you can evaluate Item III. Item III is true: in Figure 1, the prevalence of a GFR of 45–59 ml/min for the age range of 20–59 for those with hyperphosphatemia is approximately 13% (choice A can be eliminated, and choice C is correct). Note that Item I is in fact true: the passage states that aldosterone is secreted in response to high blood potassium levels.

6. **B** Both ANP and angiotensin II act on arteries but in opposite ways. The passage states that ANP acts as a vasodilator and thus would decrease blood pressure, but angiotensin II is a vasoconstrictor and would increase blood pressure (choices A and D can be eliminated). Angiotensin II would decrease urine volume by stimulating aldosterone (and indirectly vasopressin); the passage states that ANP reduces aldosterone secretion, and thus it would increase urine volume (choice C can be eliminated, and choice B is correct).

SEQUENTIAL NEPHRON BLOCKADE WITH COMBINED DIURETICS IMPROVES DIASTOLIC FUNCTION IN PATIENTS WITH RESISTANT HYPERTENSION

David Fouassier, Anne Blanchard, Antoine Fayol, Guillaume Bobrie, Pierre Boutouyrie, Michel Azizi, Jean-Sébastien Hulot

ESC Heart Failure 2020; 7:2561–2571 Published online 29 June 2020 in Wiley Online Library

INTRODUCTION

Heart failure with preserved ejection fraction (HFpEF) has been reported to account for almost half of all heart failure (HF) patients. HFpEF typically occurs in association with advanced age, cardiovascular, metabolic, and proinflammatory comorbidities. One of the most common comorbidities associated with HFpEF is arterial hypertension, which is thought to favour the development of left ventricular (LV) stiffening, hypertrophy, and consequent diastolic dysfunction. Patients with resistant hypertension (RHTN), defined as a failure to reach seated office systolic blood pressure < 140 mmHg or diastolic blood pressure < 90 mmHg while treated with an appropriate three drug regimen that includes a diuretic have a higher risk to develop HF, notably HFpEF.

Consequently, current European and U.S. guidelines recommend treating hypertension in HFpEF patients with diuretics, angiotensin-converting enzyme inhibitors (ACEIs)/angiotensin-II-receptor blockers (ARBs), mineralocorticoid receptor antagonists (MRAs), or beta-blockers. These anti-hypertensive drugs have different pharmacological targets with potential impact on myocardial remodelling or on the further development of cardiac dysfunction. For instance, one of the major contributors to RHTN is fluid retention, which also contributes to increase LV filling pressures. Aldosterone blockade with mineralocorticoid receptor antagonist has been shown to reduce myocardial fibrosis, an important component observed in HFpEF. Reciprocally, the use of beta-blockers in HFpEF patients is debated as potentially associated with increased risk of cardiovascular outcomes. The optimal antihypertensive strategy in patients with RHTN to both treat hypertension and improve cardiac diastolic dysfunction is thus currently undetermined.

The 'Management of Resistant Hypertension: Comparison of Two Treatment Strategies: Increase Sodium Depletion or Combined Blockage of Renin-angiotensin System (RAS)' ('PHARES trial,' NCT00224549) compared the efficacy of two different anti-hypertensive pharmacological strategies in RHTN patients. The primary results showed that sequential nephron blockade (NBD) with different diuretics (i.e., furosemide, spironolactone, and amiloride) acting on three segments of renal tubule of the nephron induced a large and well-tolerated reduction in BP compared with a strategy with combined renin-angiotensin system blockade (RASB) with irbesartan, ramipril, and bisoprolol.

In this pre-specified substudy of the PHARES trial, we aimed to evaluate and compare the changes in cardiac biomarkers (BNP) [B-type natriuretic peptide] and echocardiographic parameters of diastolic dysfunction according to the two anti-hypertensive strategies in RHTN patients.

METHODS

Study design

The design of this 12-week, single-centre, prospective, randomized, open, blinded endpoint trial with optional drug titration has been described elsewhere and will be summarized briefly here.

Briefly, eligible men or women were aged 18 to 75 years, with essential hypertension resistant to three or more antihypertensive drugs including a diuretic (supine office blood pressure BP at least 140 and or 90 mmHg). The main exclusion criteria were secondary hypertension, history of severe cardiovascular disease (cardiac surgery or percutaneous coronary angioplasty), or stroke in the past 3 months, atrial fibrillation, uncontrolled diabetes (HbA1c > 8%), and estimated glomerular filtration rates less than 40 mL/min (modification of diet in renal disease formula). The patients entered a 4-week standardized triple-therapy regimen comprising hydrochlorothiazide (12.5 mg/day), irbesartan (300 mg/day), and amlodipine (5 mg/day) (Figure 1A). After 4 weeks of the standardized triple-therapy regimen, patients with a mean daytime ambulatory systolic blood pressure ≥ 135 mmHg and/or mean daytime ambulatory diastolic blood pressure ≥ 85 mmHg were randomized 1:1 to the NBD regimen or to the RASB regimen at week 0 (W0, baseline). Treatment intensity was increased at week 4, 8, or 10 if home BP was ≥135/85 mmHg, by sequentially adding 25 mg spironolactone, 20–40 mg furosemide, and 5 mg amiloride (NBD group) or 5–10 mg ramipril and 5–10 mg bisoprolol (RASB group). No other antihypertensive drug was allowed during the study.

At W4, W8, W10, and W12, patients reported to the centre at approximately 0830 h, without having taken their morning dose, to undergo safety, office BP, and laboratory assessments.

Evaluation of cardiac biomarkers and diastolic function

BNP levels were measured at baseline and at the 12-week follow-up visit. The cut-offs BNP levels were defined in line with current guidelines in non-acute settings: BNP levels above 100 pg/mL were considered as likely indicating the presence of HF while BNP levels below 35 pg/mL were considered as invalidating the presence of HF. The grey zone was comprised between these two limits.

Trans-thoracic echocardiography was also performed at baseline (W0) and at the last follow-up visit (W12) by the same experienced operator blind to the randomization group. Cardiac dimensions including wall thickness, ventricular diameters, and left atrial area were measured. Pulse wave Doppler recordings of the LV inflow were obtained.

Haemodynamic and vascular measurements

Supine office BP was measured. Twenty four-hour ambulatory, daytime and nighttime BP and heart rate (HR) monitoring was performed.

Systemic vascular resistance (SVR) was calculated using the formula: SVR = (daytime mean arterial BP blood pressure − central venous pressure) × 79.92/cardiac output.

Mean arterial blood pressure was calculated with the formula: (daytime mean arterial systolic blood pressure + 2 × daytime mean arterial diastolic blood pressure). Cardiac output was estimated with the formula: [π/2 × (LV outflow tract diameter)^2 × LV outflow tract sub-valvular velocity time integral)] × heart rate.

Laboratory parameters

Blood was sampled at baseline and at the last follow-up visit in fasting conditions to measure plasma renin, aldosterone, BNP, creatinine, sodium, potassium, and protein concentrations.

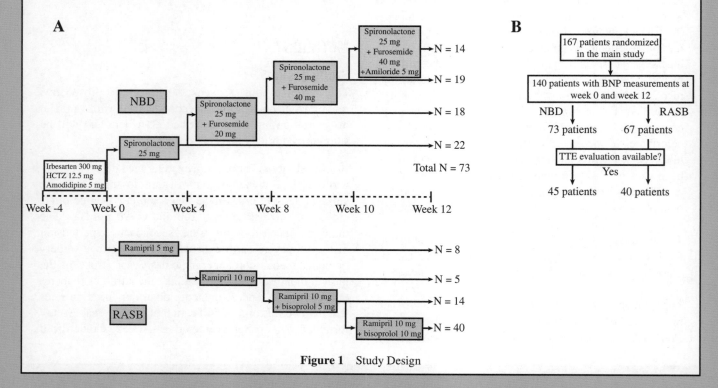

Figure 1   Study Design

Statistical analysis

Continuous variables are expressed as means ± standard deviations. Categorical variables are expressed as numbers and percentages. A Student's t-test was used for continuous variable and a χ^2 square test or Fisher's exact test for categorical variable was performed for comparison between groups and between baseline and week 12. Statistical results are presented as mean differences, with two-tailed 95% confidence intervals. To adjust for multiple testing, a P value < 0.01 was considered statistically significant.

RESULTS

Patients characteristics at randomization

Among the 167 patients randomized for the main study, the baseline characteristics, laboratory parameters, and plasma hormones (BNP, renin, and aldosterone) did not significantly differ between the NBD and the RASB groups (Tables 1 and 2). None of these patients had previous history of HF or current symptoms of congestive HF.

The proportion of patients with baseline plasma BNP concentrations < 35 pg/mL, between 35 and 100 pg/mL, and >100 pg/mL did not significantly differ between the two groups (Figure 2A and 2B). Only three (4.1%) patients of the NBD group and one (1.5%) of the RASB group had baseline plasma BNP concentrations > 100 pg/mL.

Table 1   Baseline characteristics of patients with resistant hypertension randomized to nephron blockade or renin-angiotensin system blockade group and complete BNP evaluation

n = 140	NBD group n = 73	RASB group n = 67	P
Age (years)	55.8 ± 10	53.7 ± 10.3	0.233
Men, n (%)	54 (74)	53(79)	0.475
BMI (kg/m²)	30.0 ± 4.9	28.3 ± 3.8	0.031
Obesity (BMI > 30 kg/m²), n (%)	32 (44)	24 (36)	0.334
Diabetes mellitus, n (%)	12 (15)	15 (22)	0.609
Dyslipidemia, n (%)	46 (63)	40 (60)	0.326
Duration of hypertension (years)	14.3 ± 10.3	12.7 ± 10.6	0.352
Daytime ambulatory SBP (mmHg)	148.7 ± 12.4	149.9 ± 12.1	0.569
Daytime ambulatory DBP (mmHg)	91.4 ± 10.1	93.3 ± 9.3	0.245
Daytime ambulatory HR (bpm)	79.6 ± 9.9	81.7 ± 10.2	0.375
Night-time ambulatory SBP (mmHg)	137.2 ± 13.1	135.4 ± 13.5	0.419
Night-time ambulatory DBP (mmHg)	81.0 ± 9.9	80.9 ± 9.5	0.941
Night-time ambulatory HR (bpm)	70.3 ± 8.8	69 ± 9.9	0.446

BMI, body mass index; DBP, diastolic blood pressure; PP, pulse pressure; SBP, systolic blood pressure.
Results are mean ± SD or mediane (IQR)

Table 2   Comparison between the two arms of treatment of haemodynamic and biological parameters at weeks 0 and 12

	Week 0			Week 12		
	NBD (n = 73)	RASB (n = 67)	P value	NBD (n = 73)	RASB (n = 67)	P value
Plasma BNP (pg/mL)	21 (11–33)	17 (10–27)	0.216	12 (8–22)	40 (17–64)	<0.0001
Daytime ambulatory SBP (mmHg)	148.7 ± 12.4	149.9 ± 12.1	0.569	128.0 ± 11.7	142.1 ± 17.7	<0.0001
Daytime ambulatory DBP (mmHg)	91.4 ± 10.1	93.3 ± 9.3	0.245	79.5 ± 9.9	86.1 ± 9.9	<0.0001
Systemic vascular resistance (Wood)	3064.9 ± 856.3	3131.5 ± 786.8	0.687	1396.5 ± 382.6	16423 ± 383.4	0.0024
Daytime ambulatory HR (bpm)	79.6 ± 9.9	81.7 ± 10.2	0.375	80.9 ± 9.8	68.4 ± 11.8	<0.0001
Plasma potassium (mmol/L)	3.8 ± 0.4	3.9 ± 0.4	0.199	4.3 ± 0.5	4.0 ± 0.4	<0.0001
Plasma sodium (mmol/L)	140.6 ± 2.2	140.8 ± 2.4	0.682	138 ± 3	140 ± 2	<0.0001
eGFR (ml/min per 1.73m²)	83.5 ± 18.6	89.7 ± 18.9	0.055	73 ± 20	86 ± 18	<0.0001
Plasma proteins (g/L)	69.5 ± 4.9	68.2 ± 4.2	0.122	70 ± 5	68 ± 4	0.0018
Plasma renin (mUI/M)	19 (10–39)	20.5 (9–37.8)	0.922	122 (52–327)	8 (5–29)	<0.0001
Plasma aldosterone (pmol/L)	104 (69–152)	95 (63.3–132)	0.362	270 (177–344)	91 (58–137)	<0.0001

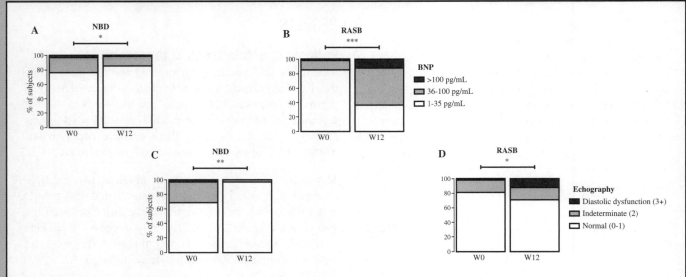

Figure 2 Evolution from randomization (W0) to week 12 (W12) of BNP and echocardiographic parameters of diastolic dysfunction in nephron blockade and renin-angiotensin system blockade arms of treatment.

Among the 140 patients with BNP measurements, 45 patients in NBD group and 40 in RASB group had TTE recordings available for analysis (Figure 1B). At baseline, there was no significant difference in echocardiographic parameters between the two groups (Table 3). A total of 21 patients (11 women and 10 men) had LV hypertrophy. The echocardiographic parameters required to score diastolic dysfunction were available in 32 patients of the NBD and 31 patients of the RASB arm. Nine patients in NBD group and five patients in RASB group had undetermined level of diastolic function, and one patient in each group had echocardiographic diastolic dysfunction ($p = 0.676$, Table 3, Figure 2C and 2D).

After 12 weeks, nephron blockade and renin-angiotensin system blockade had different effects on BNP levels

At 12 weeks, plasma BNP concentrations decreased significantly from baseline in the NBD group but increased in the RASB group (Figure 3 and Table 2). Consequently, the number of patients with plasma BNP concentrations between 35 and 100 pg/mL and >100 pg/ml decreased from baseline to W0 to nine (12%) and one (1.4%) patients in the NBD group, respectively, whereas it increased to 37 (55%) and 7 (10.4%) patients in the RASB group, respectively ($p < 0.001$; Figure 2A and 2B).

Table 3 Echocardiographic parameters at randomization (week 0) and after 12 weeks of nephron blockade or renin-angiotensin system blockade treatment

	Week 0			Week 12		
	NBD $N = 45$	RAS $N = 40$	p value	NBD $n = 45$	RAS $n = 40$	p value
LVED diameter (mm)	48.3 ± 5.2	50.7 ± 4.2	0.0244	48.4 ± 4.6	51.6 ± 5.8	0.0059
LVEF (%)	68.0 ± 8.2	66.1 ± 8.5	0.299	66.9 ± 8.1	67.0 ± 7.5	0.968
Cardiac output (l/min)	6.1 ± 1.7	5.8 ± 1.4	0.529	5.8 ± 1.5	5.3 ± 1.2	0.083
LVED volume (mL/m²)	65.9 ± 18.7	63.6 ± 11.9	0.532	66.6 ± 17.2	66.7 ± 16.6	0.977
LVES volume (mL/m²)	20.9 ± 8.3	21.9 ± 7.8	0.589	22.4 ± 9.6	22.2 ± 8.6	0.922
Left atrial area (cm²)	17.7 ± 4.2	18.5 ± 4.0	0.401	16.5 ± 3.6	19.2 ± 3.9	0.0021
	Assessment of diastolic function					
	NBD $n = 32$	RAS $n = 31$	p value	NBD $n = 32$	RAS $n = 31$	p value
Normal, n (%)	22	25	0.676	31	21	0.0048
Undetermined, n (%)	9	5		1	6	
Diastolic dysfunction, n (%)	1	1		0	4	

Full data of echographic parameters for assessment of diastolic function were available in 43% and 46% of subjects in NBD arm and RASB arm, respectively.

Figure 3 Evolution of BNP levels at baseline and after 12 weeks according to the nephron blockade or renin-angiotensin system blockade.

In the univariate analysis, NBD treatment was significantly associated with decrease in BNP levels over the 12 weeks of the study (Table 4). The influence of NBD treatment was also significant after adjustment on classical factors influencing BNP levels including age, sex, renal function, and BMI.

Table 4 Factors influencing difference in BNP levels between week 12 and week 0 in univariable linear regression

	B	p value
Age (years)	0.17 ± 0.36	0.636
Women	−1.02 ± 8.76	0.907
NBD versus RASB treatment	−42.51 ± 6.50	<0.0001
Difference in daytime SBP (mmHg)	1.12 ± 0.24	<0.0001
Difference in daytime PP (mmHg)	2.67 ± 0.44	<0.0001
Difference in aortic SBP (mmHg)	0.73 ± 0.22	0.0013
Difference in aortic PP (mmHg)	0.86 ± 0.34	0.0122
Difference in pulse Wave velocity (m/s)	4.55 ± 2.55	0.077
Difference in HR (bpm)	−1.68 ± 0.28	<0.0001
Difference in systemic vascular resistance (Wood)	−0.01 ± 0.01	0.924
eGFR (mL/min per 1.73m²)	0.28 ± 0.18	0.134
BMI (kg/m²)	0.63 ± 0.84	0.455

Nephron blockade has an independent effect on changes in BNP levels

We further looked at haemodynamics differences between the two groups that could explain the observed difference in BNP changes (Table 2). At the end of the study (week 12), the mean decrease from baseline in daytime systolic BP, diastolic BP, aortic systolic BP, and pulse pressure (PP) was significantly higher in the NBD group as compared with the RASB group (Table 2), in line with previous results in the main study. PWV tended to decrease in both groups, a trend that however did not reach significance. SVR were significantly lower after 12 weeks in the NBD arm compared with the RASB arm (Table 2). HR was significantly lower in the RASB group than the NBD group due to bisoprolol's effect.

At week 12, patients in the NBD group had lower plasma sodium, higher potassium, and higher plasma creatinine resulting in lower estimated glomerular filtration rate than RASB group (Table 2). Similarly, renin and aldosterone plasma concentrations increased more in NBD than in RASB (Table 2). However, none of these factors has significant influence on changes in BNP levels.

Nephron blockade improved diastolic function assessed by echocardiography

After 12 weeks, we observed that LV diastolic diameter, LV mass index, and left atrial area decreased in NBD group, while these parameters slightly increased in the RASB group (Table 3). In both NBD and RASB, cardiac index did not change significantly between W0 and W12.

In line with our results on changes in BNP levels, we observed an improvement of diastolic parameters in NBD group: at week 12, 97% of patients had a normal diastolic function compared with 69% at baseline ($p = 0.001$). Only one patient in NBD group remained with undetermined diastolic function, none with diastolic dysfunction (Table 3, Figure 2C). Reciprocally, echography indicated worsening of diastolic function at week 12 in patients of the RASB group (Figure 2D). At week 12, only 68% of patients in RASB group presented normal diastolic function (Table 3, Figure 2).

DISCUSSION

We report that in patients without symptomatic HF but with RHTN as a major risk factor for HF, a 12-week treatment based on sequential NBD with combined diuretics significantly and rapidly improves biological and echocardiographic markers of diastolic function while a strategy of triple RASB (with ARB, ACEI, and beta-blocker) did not improve these markers. This study was a pre-specified substudy of the PHARES trial, a prospective, randomized, open-blinded endpoint study, where 167 patients with mean baseline daytime ambulatory blood pressure of 135 mmHg or more and/or 85 mmHg or more despite 4-week treatment with irbesartan 300 mg/day, were randomized to NBD vs. RASB. The PHARES study showed a significantly higher reduction in blood pressure and in LV mass in patients receiving NBD. In this sub-study focusing on the biological and echographic markers of cardiac function, we further show a positive and significant impact of the NBD strategy on the changes in BNP levels and cardiac parameters of diastolic dysfunction after 12 weeks of treatment. Importantly, in the multivariable analysis, the effect of NBD remained significant after adjustment for multiple factors, notably BP reduction and changes in renal function. In addition, while the RASB therapeutic strategy was also associated with BP reduction, we observed opposite effects on changes in BNP levels and echocardiographic parameters of diastolic function. This result suggests that an aggressive strategy to reduce sodium balance in patients with RHTN is preferable to rapidly reduce cardiac wall stress and improve cardiac relaxation.

RHTN combines several pathophysiological mechanisms including increased peripheral resistance, fluid retention, and salt sensitivity. RHTN is considered as major risk factor for diastolic dysfunction, a setting in which impaired relaxation is associated with an increase in telediastolic pressure, indirectly reflected by higher levels of BNP. As compared with RASB, NDB was associated with a greater reduction in blood volume as indicated by larger reduction in systemic vascular resistance and in GFR and higher increase in renin levels as compared with RASB. However, our results indicate that the improvement in cardiac function with NBD is likely explained by additional effects beyond the plasma volume reduction. A link between salt overload and increased arterial thickness has been well established experimentally and is independent of BP. Arteries play an important role in adapting to an acute sodium load by endothelium-dependent and endothelium-independent mechanisms. In a mouse model of chronic sodium loading, it was shown that the consequent increase in arterial stiffness could be partially prevented by spironolactone or amiloride. In our study, it is possible that modamide and spironolactone have induced a decrease in arterial stiffness (thus increasing compliance) leading to a greater decrease in the PP in the NBD group.

On the other hand, the achievement of a complete RASB with ARB, ACEI, and beta-blocker resulted in a significant increase of BNP levels and echographic markers of diastolic function. In the multivariable analysis, the changes in HR were significantly associated with the changes in BNP levels with lower HRs being associated with higher BNP levels. This suggests that an important part of our observation could be explained by a direct detrimental effect of beta-blockers. Beta-blockers and bisoprolol have, however, been reported to exert a positive lusitropic effect in different animal models, an observation that potentially does not translate into humans. In line with our results, it was shown in a substudy of the ASCOT clinical trial that hypertensive patients treated with atenolol displayed higher LV filling pressure and BNP levels as compared with patients receiving amlodipine while the on-treatment BP was similar in both groups. In another study, bisoprolol improved echographic parameters of diastolic function after 3 months of treatment, but these patients did not have RHTN as in our study.

As RHTN is a major risk factor for HF, notably with HFpEF, our results can also be interpreted in the context of the different clinical studies that evaluated therapeutic strategies in patients with HFpEF. Indeed, there is currently no evidence to support a therapeutic benefit for the use of beta-blockers, ACEi, and ARB in patients with HFpEF. Furthermore, these results are in line with the ONTARGET study, which did not show any benefit of a double RAS blockade in terms of cardiovascular events or hospitalization for HF but on the contrary an increased risk of hypotension and renal failure. Reciprocally, the use of spironolactone is likely associated with a reduction in HF rehospitalization in HFpEF patients, but the effects on mortality and quality of life remain unclear. Our results further suggest that spironolactone, in combination with other diuretics, might be beneficial to prevent further development of HF, notably with preserved ejection fraction. This observation would however deserve further long-term studies.

Study limitations

The studied population has a major risk factor of HF, but none had a history of HF, so the results cannot be extrapolated to HFpEF patients. BNP and echocardiography were only available at week 0 and week 12 and in a fraction of the patients, so we could not analyse the effect of each titration of the treatment on these parameters. Moreover, some more recent echocardiographic parameters such as left atrial volume and LV longitudinal strain were not measured in our study. The scores to estimate cardiac diastolic dysfunction were derived using left atrial areas rather than volumes as lastly recommended. However, similar trends with improvement in the NBD group were also observed after deriving the scores without considering LA areas (data not shown), thus suggesting that using LA areas instead of LA volumes was not changing our overall results.

In conclusion, our data suggest that combined diuretic treatment (NBD strategy) that targets fluid retention improves diastolic dysfunction and decreases arterial stiffness. Reciprocally, our results suggest that a more complete inhibition of the renin-angiotensin system does not improve diastolic function. These differences involve mechanisms associated with BP reduction and improved ventriculararterial coupling. An intensive strategy with a combination of diuretics should be preferably considered in patients presenting RHTN.

JOURNAL ARTICLE EXERCISE 2

Remember that the science sections on the MCAT include a significant number of passages with experiments. You'll need to be able to extract information efficiently and analyze data effectively in order to do well on these passages.

This is the second of three "Journal Article Exercises" in this book. In the first exercise, we showed you the type of information you should be able to extract from the article and the sorts of things to pay attention to in the data. In this exercise, you'll do more of that on your own, and in the final exercise we'll show you how that article might get turned into an MCAT-style passage.

As a reminder, when analyzing an experiment, you should be able to:

- identify the control group(s)
- extract information from graphs and data tables
- determine how the experimental group(s) change relative to the control
- determine if the results are statistically significant
- come to a reasonable conclusion about WHY the results were observed
- consider potential weaknesses in the study
- determine how to increase the power of the study
- decide what the next most logical experiment or study should be

Again, the goal of these exercises is NOT to learn content from the articles, just to get a little more comfortable reading and extracting information from them.

For the (abridged) article on pages 403–408, try to summarize the purpose of the experiment and the methods in 4–5 sentences. Consider the following mnemonic: Oh ouR Car Won't Start (ORCWS).

- O = Organism and Organization: is the research being conducted on humans or on animals or on bacteria in a petri dish, or something else? What is being done to these organisms? Are there any unique qualities to these organisms? Are there multiple groups? Is the study conducted over a long period of time with multiple data points, or is it a short-term study? Does it have a large or small n?
- R = Results: where and how are the results presented? Is it a graph? A data table? Figures and images? What is/are the independent variable(s)? What is/are the dependent variable(s)? What are the results? Do the results show correlation or cause and effect, or both? Describe.
- C = Control and Comparison: is there a control group? How does it differ from the experimental group? Is it given a placebo or nothing at all? Is it held under different conditions? If there are multiple experimental groups, how do they differ from one another? Is it a blinded study? If so, double blind or single blind?
- W = Weirdness: does anything or do any of the results stand out as unexpected?
- S = Statistics: was any sort of statistical analysis done? How is it presented? Are there error bars on a graph? Standard errors around a mean? Are there p-values? Is there an asterisk indicating statistical significance? Is there any data that is not statistically significant?

Try interpreting the data on your own before reading the results/discussion section. When you do read the discussion, consider:

- What are the conclusions of the study?
- How are the conclusions supported by the data?
- What potential weaknesses or flaws do you see in the experimental design? Are these addressed in the discussion section?
- How might this study be potentially biased?
- How might this study be improved?
- What would be the next most logical experiment?

Let's answer the above questions for the article on pages 403–408.

1. **O = Organism and Organization:**
   - Is the research being conducted on humans or on animals or on bacteria in a petri dish, or something else?

     _____

     _____

   - What is being done to these organisms?

     _____

     _____

   - Are there any unique qualities to these organisms?

     _____

     _____

   - Are there multiple groups?

     _____

     _____

   - Is the study conducted over a long period of time with multiple data points, or is it a short-term study?

     _____

     _____

   - Does it have a large or small n?

     _____

     _____

2. **R = Results:**
   - Where and how are the results presented? Is it a graph? A data table? Figures and images?

     _____

     _____

- What is/are the independent variable(s)?

_____

_____

- What is/are the dependent variable(s)?

_____

_____

- What are the results of the study?

_____

_____

- Do the results show correlation or cause and effect, or both? Describe.

_____

_____

3. **C = Control and Comparison:**
   - Is there a control group?

   _____

   _____

   - How does it differ from the experimental group? Is it given a placebo or nothing at all? Is it held under different conditions?

   _____

   _____

   - If there are multiple experimental groups, how do they differ from one another?

   _____

   _____

   - Is it a blinded study? If so, double blind or single blind?

   _____

   _____

4. **W = Weirdness:**
   - Does anything or do any of the results stand out as unexpected?

   _____

   _____

5. **S = Statistics:**
   - Was any sort of statistical analysis done?

   _____

   _____

- How is it presented? Are there error bars on a graph? Standard errors around a mean? Are there *p*-values? Is there an asterisk indicating statistical significance?

   _____

   _____

- Is there any data that is not statistically significant?

   _____

   _____

6. **Interpreting the data:**
   - What are the conclusions of the study?

      _____

      _____

   - How are the conclusions supported by the data?

      _____

      _____

   - What potential weaknesses or flaws do you see in the experimental design? Are these addressed in the discussion section?

      _____

      _____

   - How might this study be potentially biased?

      _____

      _____

   - How might this study be improved?

      _____

      _____

   - What would be the next most logical experiment?

      _____

      _____

7. **Final Summary of Experiment and Results:**

   _____

   _____

   _____

   _____

   _____

   _____

SOLUTIONS TO JOURNAL ARTICLE EXERCISE 2

1. **O = Organism and Organization:**
   - Is the research being conducted on humans or on animals or on bacteria in a petri dish, or something else? *Humans (33 women, 107 men).*
   - What is being done to these organisms? *A baseline drug treatment for hypertension was given to 167 people. Of those, 140 demonstrated hypertension resistant to the treatment so they were randomized to two additional drug treatment profiles with additional medication being added depending on how their blood pressure did or did not change during the trial.*
   - Are there any unique qualities to these organisms? *No unique qualities, though the study population included those with obesity, elevated levels of lipids, and/or diabetes so comorbid conditions were not excluded.*
   - Are there multiple groups? *Yes, the treatment is split into those receiving spironolactone (plus possibly furosemide and amiloride) and those receiving ramipril (plus possibly bisoprolol).*
   - Is the study conducted over a long period of time with multiple data points, or is it a short-term study? *The initial treatment ran for four weeks and the two split treatment groups ran for 12 weeks with multiple measurements taken through the duration.*
   - Does it have a large or small n? *The n for the study is relatively small, but it is still reasonable given the challenges in recruiting human subjects.*

2. **R = Results:**
   - Where and how are the results presented? Is it a graph? A data table? Figures and images? *The results are presented in tables and graphs as well as a figure that combines study design with part of the results.*
   - What is/are the independent variable(s)? *Time, particular drug protocol.*
   - What is/are the dependent variable(s)? *Measurement of blood pressure, B-type natriuretic peptide (BNP), diastolic dysfunction.*
   - What are the results of the study? *The treatment with sequential nephron blockage (NBD) improved resistant hypertension, while treatment with sequential renin-angiotensin system blockade (RASB) did not.*
   - Do the results show correlation or cause and effect, or both? Describe. *The results appear to be causative as both groups were subject to the same drug treatment prior to starting either of the protocols in the study and had similar demographics and conditions. Other anti-hypertension drugs were not permitted so the cause of the improvement would have been the particular drug protocol.*

3. **C = Control and Comparison:**
   - Is there a control group? *No.*
   - How does it differ from the experimental group? Is it given a placebo or nothing at all? Is it held under different conditions? *Both groups received a drug protocol. There was not a group that was not receiving treatment or simply stayed on their current treatment.*
   - If there are multiple experimental groups, how do they differ from one another? *The difference between the two groups is the administration of the NSD protocol versus the RASB protocol.*

- Is it a blinded study? If so, double blind or single blind? *Yes, double-blinded.*

4. **W = Weirdness:**
   - Does anything or do any of the results stand out as unexpected? *The lack of effectiveness of the RASB protocol was unexpected, but it does explain why more people in that group received escalating levels of treatment.*

5. **S = Statistics:**
   - Was any sort of statistical analysis done? *Yes.*
   - How is it presented? Are there error bars on a graph? Standard errors around a mean? Are there *p*-values? Is there an asterisk indicating statistical significance? *P-values, asterisk, standard errors reported on means, error bars on graphs.*
   - Is there any data that is not statistically significant? *The RASB results were not found to make a statistically significant improvement in resistant hypertension.*

6. **Interpreting the data:**
   - What are the conclusions of the study? *For those with resistant hypertension, an NBD treatment protocol would be more effective in treatment than a RASB protocol.*
   - How are the conclusions supported by the data? *The conclusions are supported based on the improvement in diastolic function, BNP, and blood pressure measurements as seen in the NBD group in comparison to the RASB group.*
   - What potential weaknesses or flaws do you see in the experimental design? Are these addressed in the discussion section? *The protocol worked to recruit across a broad range of ages (18 to 75 years), but the study population was mostly male and the paper does not report on race, ethnicity, or descriptors of the diversity of the population. The number of subjects would need to be larger and would need to be reported to match the overall impacted patient population to make further treatment recommendations.*
   - How might this study be potentially biased? *This study may be biased based on the composition of its patient population.*
   - How might this study be improved? *A larger n with reporting done on other patient demographics.*
   - What would be the next most logical experiment? *An additional trial with a larger pool of subjects run at multiple centers.*

7. **Final Summary of Experiment and Results:**
   - *In this journal article, the effect of an NBD treatment protocol for resistant hypertension was measured in comparison to a RASB treatment protocol. The study was blinded and included male and female subjects across a range of ages and conditions. Treatments were run over the course of 12 weeks with measurements including B-type natriuretic peptide, diastolic function, and blood pressure being taken. The NBD protocol was found to make a statistically significant improvement, while the RASB protocol did not.*

Chapter 11
The Muscular and Skeletal Systems

11.1 OVERVIEW OF MUSCLE TISSUE

There are three types of muscle which differ in cellular physiology, anatomy, and function. The type we are all familiar with is **skeletal muscle** (Section 11.2), which is also known as *voluntary* muscle, because its role is to contract in response to conscious intent. The next muscle type is called **cardiac muscle** because it is found only in the wall of the heart. Skeletal and cardiac muscle are said to be **striated** because of their microscopic appearance. The third type of muscle is **smooth muscle**, which is found in the walls of all hollow organs such as the GI tract, the urinary system, the uterus, etc. It is responsible for GI motility, constriction of blood vessels, uterine contractions, and so on. We have no conscious control over cardiac or smooth muscle because they are innervated only by the autonomic nervous system. The three types of muscle share some characteristics and differ in others. In Sections 11.3 and 11.4, we characterize cardiac and smooth muscle by comparison with skeletal muscle.

11.2 SKELETAL MUSCLE

Movement of Joints

Skeletal muscle provides voluntary movement of the body in response to stimulation by somatic motor neurons, but skeletal muscle alone cannot move the body. Skeletal muscle requires the framework of the bones of the skeleton for movement to occur. Skeletal muscles are attached at each end to two different bones. Muscles are often attached to bones by **tendons**, strong connective tissue formed primarily of collagen. By contracting, skeletal muscle can draw the points of attachment on the two bones closer together. [What effect does expansion of skeletal muscle have on the two bones the muscle is connected to?[1]] Skeletal muscles can move a joint by **flexing** (reducing the angle of the joint), **extending** (increasing the angle of the joint), by **abducting** (moving away from the body's midline) or **adducting** (moving toward the body's midline), as well as many other types of movement. [Which of these movements involve contraction of skeletal muscle?[2] Does flexing the elbow bring the hand closer to or farther from the shoulder?[3]] One of the two bones joined by a skeletal muscle is generally closer to the center of the body and tends to stay in place when the muscle contracts. The point on this bone where the muscle attaches is called the **origin** of that skeletal muscle, and the point where the muscle attaches on the bone more distant from the center of the body is referred to as the muscle's **insertion**. When a muscle contracts, its insertion point is brought closer to its origin.

An example of a skeletal muscle and its action is the flexion of the elbow joint by the biceps brachii (Figure 1). The origin of this muscle lies in the shoulder joint, and the insertion lies in the bones of the forearm. Contraction of the biceps brachii brings its insertion (the forearm) closer to its origin (the shoulder). Since muscles can only *contract* to move a joint, different muscles are necessary for flexion and extension (opposite movements) of a joint. For the elbow, the *triceps* brachii (the muscle on the back of the upper

---

[1] None. Muscle cannot expand with force. Muscle can only contract (get shorter) to cause force on bones and movement.

[2] All of them. It is the only way to move bones and joints: by contracting skeletal muscles.

[3] Flexing decreases the angle of a joint. If the elbow is flexed, the hand will be closer to the shoulder.

arm) is responsible for extension. [Where is the origin of the triceps brachii?[4]] The origin and the insertion for the triceps brachii are on the opposite side of the arm as for the biceps brachii, so that contraction of the triceps has the opposite effect on the lower arm as contraction of the biceps. [Do both the biceps brachii and the triceps brachii contract vigorously simultaneously to cause movement?[5]] Muscles that are responsible for movement in opposite directions are termed **antagonistic**, while muscles that move a joint in the same direction are **synergistic**. Usually, the contraction of antagonistic muscles is coordinated by the nervous system so that one muscle relaxes while the other contracts. [Do antagonistic muscles receive stimulation by neurons that release different neurotransmitters?[6]]

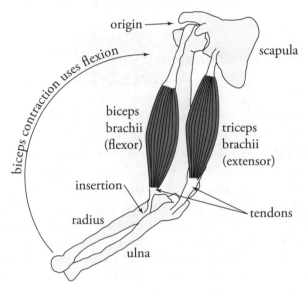

Figure 1   Skeletal Muscle

Structure of Skeletal Muscle

Each skeletal muscle is composed not only of muscle tissue, but also of connective tissue that holds the contractile tissue together in bundles called **fascicles** to allow flexibility within the muscle (Figure 2). Looking within each bundle, it is possible to see many fine **muscle fibers** (also called **myofibers**). Each muscle fiber is a single skeletal muscle cell. Skeletal muscle cells are **multinucleate syncytia** formed by the fusion of individual cells during development. They are innervated by a single nerve ending, and stretch the entire length of the muscle. The myofiber has a cell membrane, called the **sarcolemma**, that is made of the plasma membrane and an additional layer of polysaccharide and collagen. This additional layer helps the cell to fuse with tendon fibers. Within each skeletal muscle cell (myofiber) there are many smaller units called **myofibrils**. The myofibril in the muscle cell is like a specialized organelle; it is responsible for the striated appearance of skeletal muscle and generates the contractile force of skeletal muscle.

---

[4]   The origin of the triceps is the point of attachment nearer the center of the body, or the shoulder, on the opposite side of the biceps attachment.

[5]   Usually, no. Muscles that oppose each other's action are usually regulated by the nervous system in the opposite manner, so that one relaxes while the other contracts.

[6]   No. All skeletal muscle is innervated by somatic motor neurons which release acetylcholine at the neuromuscular junction. The difference in regulation is not the *form* of the signal (i.e., the *type* of neurotransmitter) that is sent to the muscle, but the *timing* of the signal (i.e., the *frequency* of stimulation, and thus the *amount* of neurotransmitter released).

Figure 2   Levels of Skeletal Muscle Organization

The proteins in the myofibril that generate contraction are polymerized **actin** and **myosin**. Actin polymerizes to form **thin filaments** visible under the microscope, and myosin forms **thick filaments** (Figure 3). The striated appearance of skeletal muscle is due to the overlapping arrangement of bands of thick and thin filaments in **sarcomeres**. A myofibril is composed of many sarcomeres aligned end-to-end. Each sarcomere is bound by two **Z lines**. Thin filaments (actin) attach to each Z line and overlap with thick filaments (myosin) in the middle of each sarcomere; the thick filaments are not attached to the Z lines. The regions of the sarcomere composed only of thin filaments are referred to as the **I bands**. The full length of the thick filament represents the **A band** within each sarcomere; this includes both the overlapping regions of thick and thin filaments (where contraction is generated), as well as the region composed of only thick filaments (this is seen in resting sarcomeres only and is referred to as the **H zone**). See Figure 3.

Figure 3   The Sarcomere and a Cross-Section of a Myofiber

The Sliding Filament Model of Muscle Contraction

Within each sarcomere, actin and myosin filaments overlap with each other (Figures 3 and 4). Contraction occurs when the thin and thick filaments slide across each other, drawing the Z lines of each sarcomere closer together and shortening the length of the muscle cell. [During muscle contraction, do the thin and thick filaments shorten?[7]] Filament sliding is powered by ATP hydrolysis. Myosin is an enzyme that uses the energy of ATP to create movement. (You will hear the term "myosin ATPase.") Each myosin monomer contains a **head** and a **tail**. The head attaches to a specific site on an actin molecule (the **myosin binding site**). When it is attached, myosin and actin are said to be connected by a **cross bridge**. Contraction occurs when the angle between the head and tail decreases. Filament sliding occurs in four steps. It is important to remember which step requires a new ATP molecule.

Steps of the contractile cycle:
1) Binding of the myosin head to a myosin binding site on actin, also known as **cross bridge formation**. At this stage, myosin has ADP and P_i bound.
2) The **power stroke**, in which the myosin head moves to a low-energy conformation, and pulls the actin chain toward the center of the sarcomere. ADP is released.
3) Binding of a new ATP molecule is necessary for *release* of actin by the myosin head (key!).
4) ATP hydrolysis occurs immediately and the myosin head is *cocked* (set in a high-energy conformation, like the hammer of a gun). Another cycle begins when the myosin head binds to a new binding site on the thin filament.

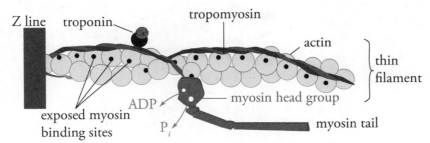

a) original position of filaments and Z line
prior to cocking of myosin head group

b) new position of filaments and Z line
after cocking of myosin head group

Figure 4 Filament Sliding

---

[7] No. The thin and thick filaments slide across each other to shorten the sarcomere without themselves changing in length.

Excitation-Contraction Coupling in Skeletal Muscle

The above four steps in the contractile cycle occur spontaneously. In other words, if you put actin and myosin into a beaker and add ATP and Mg^{2+} (necessary for all reactions involving ATP), ATP will be hydrolyzed and the filaments will slide past one another. But in the myofiber, contraction occurs only when the cytoplasmic $[Ca^{2+}]$ increases. This is because in addition to polymerized actin, the thin filament contains the **troponin-tropomyosin complex** (Figure 5) that prevents contraction when Ca^{2+} is not present. **Tropomyosin** is a long fibrous protein that winds around the actin polymer, blocking all the myosin-binding sites. **Troponin** is a globular protein bound to the tropomyosin that can bind Ca^{2+}. When troponin binds Ca^{2+}, troponin undergoes a conformational change that moves tropomyosin out of the way, so that myosin heads can attach to actin and filament sliding can occur.

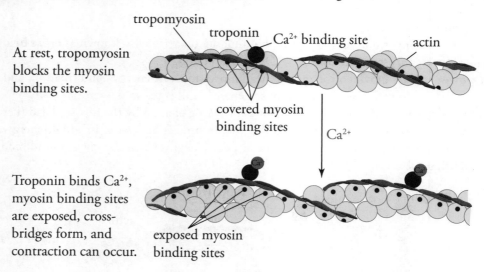

At rest, tropomyosin blocks the myosin binding sites.

Troponin binds Ca^{2+}, myosin binding sites are exposed, cross-bridges form, and contraction can occur.

Figure 5 The Troponin/Tropomyosin Complex

- What protein is responsible for ATP hydrolysis during muscle contraction?[8]
- In the absence of actin, which step in ATP hydrolysis by myosin is prevented, the hydrolysis of ATP or the release of ADP?[9]
- If troponin-tropomyosin is added to myosin and actin filaments in a test tube along with ATP, which one of the following will be true?[10]
  - A) The hydrolysis of ATP will become insensitive to the concentration of calcium.
  - B) The hydrolysis of ATP will become sensitive to the concentration of calcium.
  - C) ATP will be hydrolyzed when actin binds myosin.
  - D) ATP will be hydrolyzed during the power stroke.

---

[8] Myosin is the protein with the ATPase activity.

[9] In the absence of actin, myosin can still hydrolyze ATP, but it cannot release ADP after hydrolysis.

[10] Choice **B** is correct. Without troponin-tropomyosin, ATP hydrolysis will begin as soon as ATP, actin, and myosin are mixed. In the presence of troponin-tropomyosin, myosin cannot bind actin, but if calcium is added, the troponin-tropomyosin complex allows binding and ATP hydrolysis can occur once again.

The Neuromuscular Junction and Impulse Transmission

The **neuromuscular junction** (**NMJ**) is the synapse between an axon terminus (synaptic knob) and a myofiber. The NMJ is not a single point, but rather a long trough or invagination (infolding) of the cell membrane; the axon terminus is elongated to fill the long synaptic cleft. The purpose of this arrangement is to allow the neuron to depolarize a large region of the postsynaptic membrane at once. The postsynaptic membrane (the myofiber cell membrane) is known as the **motor end plate**. ACh is the neurotransmitter at the NMJ.

Impulse transmission at the NMJ is typical of chemical synaptic transmission: an action potential arrives at the axon terminus, triggering the opening of _____ channels; the resulting increase in _____ triggers the _____ of acetylcholine.[11] The postsynaptic membrane contains ACh receptors, which are ligand-gated Na^+ channels. The ACh must reach its receptor by diffusing across the synaptic cleft. Binding of ACh to its receptor results in a postsynaptic sodium influx, which depolarizes the postsynaptic membrane. This depolarization is known as an **end plate potential** (**EPP**). The smallest measurable EPP, caused by exocytosis of a single ACh vesicle, is known as a **miniature EPP** (**MEPP**).

ACh will continue to stimulate postsynaptic receptors until it is destroyed. This is accomplished by the enzyme **acetylcholinesterase**, which hydrolyzes ACh to choline plus an acetyl unit.

As in neurons, summation is required to initiate an AP in the postsynaptic cell. In other words, a single MEPP is insufficient to cause the myofiber to contract. When a sufficient EPP occurs, threshold is reached, and _____ channels open in the postsynaptic membrane.[12] This initiates an AP in the myofiber. The AP is propagated as in neurons, by a continuing wave of voltage-gated sodium channel opening. The shape of this AP on a graph is similar to the shape of the neuronal AP (see Chapter 8).

This AP must depolarize the entire myofiber if contraction is to occur. But there is a problem: action potentials occur only at the cell surface, because they are by nature a depolarization of the cell membrane. The myofiber is so thick that an AP on its surface will not depolarize its interior. The solution is to have deep invaginations of the cell membrane, which allow the AP to travel into the thick cell. These deep infoldings are called **transverse tubules** (**T-tubules;** see Figure 3).

Another specialized membrane in the myofiber is the **sarcoplasmic reticulum** (**SR**). This is a huge, specialized smooth endoplasmic reticulum, which enfolds each myofibril in the cell (Figure 3). The SR is specialized to sequester and release Ca^{2+}. Active transporters in the SR rapidly remove calcium from the *sarcoplasm* (myofiber cytoplasm). Then, when an AP travels down the T-tubular network, it depolarizes the cell, and with it, the SR. The SR contains voltage-gated Ca^{2+} channels, which allow Ca^{2+} to rush out of the SR into the sarcoplasm upon depolarization. The increase in sarcoplasmic $[Ca^{2+}]$ causes troponin-tropomyosin to change conformation, allowing myosin to bind actin. Actin and myosin fibers slide across each other, and the muscle fiber contracts. When the cell repolarizes, calcium is actively sequestered by the SR, and contraction is ended.

---

[11] An action potential arrives at the axon terminus, triggering the opening of **voltage-gated Ca^{2+}** channels; the resulting increase in **intracellular Ca^{2+}** triggers the **release of vesicles** of acetylcholine.

[12] voltage-gated sodium channels

Mechanics of Contraction

The smallest measurable muscle contraction is known as a muscle **twitch**. The nervous system can increase the force of contraction in two ways.

1) **Motor unit recruitment**. A motor unit is a group of myofibers innervated by the branches of a single motor neuron's axon. A muscle twitch results from the activation of one motor neuron, and a larger twitch can be obtained by activating ("recruiting") more motor neurons (and thus more myofibers).

2) **Frequency summation**. Each contraction ends when the SR returns the [Ca^{2+}] to low resting levels. If a second contraction occurs rapidly enough, however, there is insufficient time for the Ca^{2+} to be sequestered by the SR, and the second contraction builds on the first. The force of contraction increases. A rapidly repeating series of stimulations results in the strongest possible contraction, known as tetanus. This is a normal occurrence which the nervous system uses to obtain strong contractions.[13]

A note of clarification: the skeletal muscle action potential has a refractory period as does the neural AP. For frequency summation to occur, the amount of time between successive stimulations must be greater than the duration of the refractory period, but brief enough so that the cytoplasmic [Ca^{2+}] has not been returned to its low resting level.

One topic of muscle physiology which is less likely to appear on the MCAT, but worth mentioning, is the **length-tension relationship**. A muscle contracts most forcefully at an optimum length. This corresponds to a sarcomere length of 2.2 microns. The explanation is that at this length, a maximum degree of overlap between thick and thin filaments occurs. A greater sarcomere length makes the overlap smaller with fewer myosin heads able to bind to actin. A shorter length causes filaments to obstruct each other's movement by bumping together.

- The central nervous system can increase the strength of skeletal muscle contraction by:[14]
    A) increasing the size of action potentials in somatic motor neurons that innervate the muscle.
    B) increasing the number of neurons that innervate each skeletal muscle cell.
    C) increasing the number of motor neurons leading to a muscle that are firing action potentials.
    D) decreasing firing by inhibitory neurons that innervate the skeletal muscle.

Energy Storage in the Myofiber

ATP provides the energy for contraction, and supplies must be regenerated by glucose catabolism. However, glycolysis and the TCA cycle are not fast enough to keep pace with the rapid ATP utilization during

---

[13] Do not confuse this with the disease tetanus, caused by *tetanospasmin*, a bacterial toxin. The disease is an exaggerated, uncontrolled example of the normal process.

[14] Each muscle cell is innervated by a single neuron (choice B is wrong), and the more neurons that fire, the more muscle cells that will contract; the more muscle cells that contract, the greater the total force of contraction (choice **C** is correct). Action potentials are all-or-none events; the depolarization is the same size in a given neuron (choice A is wrong), and there are no inhibitory neurons that innervate the neuromuscular junction. Only acetylcholine, which is excitatory to muscle cells, is released at these synapses (choice D is wrong). (All motor neurons release a constant, small, baseline amount of ACh onto the muscle cell; this provides a baseline level of contraction that we commonly call "muscle tone." To inhibit a muscle, the amount of baseline ACh is reduced.)

extended contraction. There is a need for an *intermediate-term* energy storage molecule. **Creatine phosphate** is that molecule. During contraction, its hydrolysis drives the regeneration of ATP from ADP + P$_i$.

Muscle is highly aerobic tissue, with abundant mitochondria. **Myoglobin** is a globular protein and is similar to one of the four subunits of hemoglobin. The role of myoglobin is to provide an oxygen reserve by taking O$_2$ from hemoglobin and then releasing it as needed.

Nonetheless, during prolonged contraction, the supply of oxygen runs low, and metabolism becomes anaerobic. Lactic acid is produced and moves into the bloodstream, causing a drop in pH. The liver picks up this lactate and converts it into pyruvate, which can be used in various pathways.

Cramps may result from exhaustion of energy supplies (temporary lack of ATP) in muscle cells. **Rigor mortis** is rigidity of skeletal muscles which occurs soon after death. It results from complete ATP exhaustion; without ATP, myosin heads cannot release actin, and the muscle can neither contract nor relax.

Muscle Fiber Types

Skeletal muscle fibers generally fall into one of two categories, slow twitch fibers and fast twitch fibers. "Slow" and "fast" refer to their contractile speeds; slow twitch fibers take around three times as long as fast twitch fibers to reach their maximum tension after stimulation.

Type I Slow Twitch Fibers

These fibers are also known as **red slow twitch** or **red oxidative** fibers because of their high myoglobin content. They also have a much better blood supply than fast twitch fibers due to an extensive surrounding capillary network. The combination of good oxygen delivery from the blood stream and the ability to store oxygen on their myoglobin allows these fibers to maintain contraction for extended periods of time without fatigue. These are the fibers that allow marathoners and long distance cyclists to run or bike for hours at a time.

Type II Fast Twitch Fibers

These fibers actually fall into two subcategories according to their ability to resist fatigue. Both fiber types contract quickly, but Type IIA fast twitch fibers have more mitochondria than Type IIB fast twitch and are thus more fatigue resistant.

- *Type IIA:* also known as fast twitch oxidative fibers, these are somewhat resistant to fatigue. They cannot maintain activity for as long as slow twitch fibers can (only around 30 minutes or so), but far exceed the duration of use of the Type IIB fibers.
- *Type IIB:* also known as white fast twitch fibers due to their lack of mitochondria, these fibers contract very quickly with great force. However, they fatigue just as quickly, maxing out at around one minute of use. These are the fibers that provide the explosive force needed for jump shots and pole vaults.

Table 1 compares the three fiber types.

Table 1   Comparison of Muscle Fiber Types

Fiber type	Slow Twitch	Type IIA	Type IIB
Other names	Red slow twitch, red oxidative	Intermediate, fast twitch oxidative	White fast twitch
Speed of contraction	Slow	Intermediate	Very fast
Force generated	Low	Medium	High
Mitochondria	Many	Some	Very few
Capillaries	Very dense	Medium	Very few
Fatigue resistance	High Hours of use	Medium 30 minutes of use	Low 1 minute of use

11.3   CARDIAC MUSCLE COMPARED TO SKELETAL MUSCLE

Cardiac muscle is similar to skeletal muscle in the following ways:

1) Thick and thin filaments are organized into sarcomeres. Therefore, both cardiac and skeletal muscle are microscopically striated (striped).
2) T-tubules are present and serve the same function (transmission of APs into the interior of the large, thick cell).
3) Troponin-tropomyosin regulates contraction in the same way.
4) The length-tension relationship works the same way and is more significant in cardiac muscle. Skeletal muscle is fixed at a certain maximum length due to its attachments to bones, but cardiac muscle has no such limitations. Increasing the amount of blood that returns to the heart (e.g., through vigorous skeletal muscle contraction during exercise) can stretch cardiac muscle to optimize the length-tension relationship and maximize cardiac output, however *excess* stretch on cardiac muscle (e.g., dilation and enlargement of the heart, which can occur in heart failure) can lead to a *decrease* in contraction strength and a *decrease* in the ejection fraction (the fraction of blood the left ventricle ejects with each contraction). If the ejection fraction drops too low, death results.

Cardiac muscle is *different* from skeletal muscle in some important ways:

1) Cardiac muscle cells are not structurally syncytial (they each have only one nucleus), while skeletal muscle cells are syncytial. But all the muscle cells of the heart are interconnected by gap junctions known as **intercalated disks**, which allow action potentials to propagate throughout the entire heart without allowing nuclei and cytoplasmic contents to be shared; only small items like ions can pass. Heart muscle is thus called a ***functional* syncytium** because it acts like a syncytium (but isn't really).
2) Cardiac muscle cells are each connected to several neighbors by intercalated disks.

3) Some of the calcium required for cardiac muscle-cell contraction comes from the extracellular environment, through the voltage-gated calcium channels. In skeletal muscle, all the calcium for contraction comes from the sarcoplasmic reticulum, an intracellular structure.

4) Cardiac muscle contraction does *not* depend on stimulation by motor neurons. In fact, the most important nerve releasing ACh at chemical synapses with the heart is inhibitory! This is the vagus nerve, a parasympathetic nerve. It synapses with the sinoatrial node, where it releases ACh to inhibit spontaneous depolarization (discussed below), with the result being a slower heart rate. Contrast this with skeletal muscle innervation, in which neurons release ACh to stimulate contraction. [If neurons don't trigger cardiac contraction, what does?[15]]

5) The AP in cardiac muscle depends not only on voltage-gated sodium channels (**fast sodium channels**, as in skeletal muscle), but also on voltage-gated calcium channels. These are called **slow channels** because they respond more slowly to threshold depolarization, opening later than the fast channels and taking longer to close. The voltage-gated calcium channels cause the cardiac AP to have the distinctive plateau shown in Figure 6.

Note: All ion movement is through voltage-gated channels; all channels open and close at the beginning of the phase.

Phase 0: Fast Na⁺ channels open
 Na⁺ influx

Phase 1: Na⁺ channels inactivate
 K⁺ channels open
 K⁺ efflux

Phase 2: Ca²⁺ channels open
 Ca²⁺ influx
 K⁺ channels still open
 K⁺ efflux

Phase 3: Ca²⁺ channels close
 K⁺ channels still open
 K⁺ efflux

Phase 4: K⁺ channels close

Figure 6 The Cardiac Muscle Cell Action Potential

The significance of the plateau phase is twofold: 1) a longer duration of contraction facilitates ventricular emptying (better ejection fraction), and 2) a longer refractory period helps prevent disorganized transmission of impulses throughout the heart, and makes summation and tetanus impossible. This is

---

[15] Pacing by the sinoatrial node, as discussed in Chapter 9.

advantageous because the heart must relax after each contraction. So remember: skeletal muscle cells and neurons have the same steeply spiking AP, while cardiac muscle cells have a spike and a plateau. Figure 6 shows the phases of the cardiac action potential. This was discussed in more detail in Chapter 9.

11.4 SMOOTH MUSCLE COMPARED TO SKELETAL MUSCLE

Smooth muscle is like skeletal muscle in that contraction is accomplished by sliding of actin and myosin filaments; the four-step contractile cycle is the same. Another similarity is that contraction is triggered by an increase in cytoplasmic [Ca^{2+}]. Like skeletal muscle cells, smooth muscle cells do not branch. However, smooth muscle is different from skeletal muscle in many ways:

1) Smooth muscle cells are much narrower and shorter than skeletal muscle cells.
2) T-tubules are *not* present. The smooth muscle cell is so small that they are unnecessary; a depolarization on the surface can depolarize the entire cell.
3) Each smooth muscle cell has only one nucleus and is connected to its neighbors by gap junctions (like cardiac muscle cells) which allow impulses to spread from cell to cell. Thus, both smooth and cardiac muscle are functional syncytia.
4) Thick and thin filaments are not organized into sarcomeres in smooth muscle. Instead they are dispersed in the cytoplasm. This is why the cell appears smooth instead of striated (no regular A band, H zone, etc.).
5) The troponin–tropomyosin complex is not present. Instead, contraction is regulated by **calmodulin** and **myosin light-chain kinase** (**MLCK**). In brief, calmodulin binds Ca^{2+} and then activates MLCK. MLCK phosphorylates a portion of the myosin molecule, thus activating its enzymatic/mechanical activity.
6) While skeletal muscles rely heavily on Ca^{2+} from sarcoplasmic reticulum, the SR in smooth muscles is poorly developed. It stores some Ca^{2+} that can be released upon depolarization, but the cell also relies heavily on extracellular stores of Ca^{2+} for contraction.
7) The smooth muscle cell action potential varies depending on the location of the smooth muscle cell. Most smooth muscle cells can elicit action potentials (also called **spike potentials**) similar to skeletal muscle action potentials, but since smooth muscle cells have almost no sodium fast channels and their action potential is determined by slow channels only, it takes ten to twenty times as long as a skeletal muscle action potential (Figure 7).
8) Some smooth muscle that must sustain prolonged contractions (such as the uterus or vascular smooth muscle) has action potentials similar to those of cardiac muscle, although with a less-sharp spike.
9) Smooth muscles have a constantly fluctuating resting potential. Ions pass through the gap junctions between neighboring cells, causing the changes in resting potential to propagate like waves through the connected smooth muscle cells. These fluctuations in resting potential are called "slow waves." Slow waves are NOT spike potentials and do NOT elicit muscle contractions, but they are necessary to help *coordinate* the action potentials. In response to local stimuli (e.g., stretching of smooth muscle in the gut wall due to a food bolus), neurotransmitter from parasympathetic neurons is released. The neurotransmitter binds to receptors on smooth muscle cells and primes them for an action potential by pushing their electrical potential closer to threshold. Slow waves then pass through these "primed" smooth muscle cells, they reach threshold and undergo an action (spike) potential (Figure 7). The amplitude of these slow waves is increased by ACh and decreased by NE (e.g., stimulating the gut during a parasympathetic response, and slowing it down during a sympathetic one).

10) Like skeletal muscle, smooth muscles are innervated by motor neurons, but in the case of smooth muscle, they are *autonomic* motor neurons instead of somatic motor neurons. Individual neurons do activate smooth muscle cells (as in skeletal muscle), but, as mentioned previously, the action potential then spreads from cell to cell. (Recall that in skeletal muscle, each action potential is limited to one large myofiber, while the heart is one large functional syncytium in which each action potential spreads to every cell. Therefore, regarding innervation and the spread of impulses, smooth muscle shares features of both skeletal and cardiac muscle.)

Acetylcholine increases amplitude of slow wave.
Norepinephrine decreases amplitude of slow wave.

Figure 7   The Smooth Muscle Cell Spike Potential and Slow Waves

Table 2 Comparison of Skeletal, Cardiac, and Smooth Muscle

Feature	Skeletal Muscle	Cardiac Muscle	Smooth Muscle
Appearance	Striated	Striated	No striations
Upstroke of action potential	Inward Na^+ current	Inward Ca^{2+} (SA node) Inward Na^+ (atria, ventricles, Purkinje)	Inward Na^+
Plateau	No	Yes (except for SA node)	No
Duration of AP	2–3 msec	150 msec (SA node) 300 msec (other cells)	20 msec
Calcium from	AP opens voltage-gated Ca^{2+} channels in SR, Ca^{2+} released from SR	AP opens voltage-gated Ca^{2+} channels, inward Ca^{2+} current during plateau Ca^{2+}-induced-Ca^{2+} release from SR	AP opens Ca^{2+} channels in cell membrane, inward Ca^{2+} current
Molecular basis for contraction	Ca^{2+} troponin binding	Ca^{2+} troponin binding	Ca^{2+} calmodulin binding, myosin light-chain kinase activation
Functional syncytium	No	Yes	Yes
Contraction dependent on extracellular Ca^{2+}	No	Partially	Yes

Figure 8 Three Types of Muscle Tissue

11.5   OVERVIEW OF THE SKELETAL SYSTEM

As vertebrates, we have an **endoskeleton** made of bone. This contrasts with the chitinous exoskeleton of arthropods. The vertebrate skeletal system serves five roles:

1) support the body
2) provide the framework for movement
3) protect vital organs (brain, heart, etc.)
4) store calcium
5) synthesize the formed elements of the blood (red blood cells, white blood cells, platelets). This occurs in the marrow of flat bones and is called **hematopoiesis**.

The vertebrate endoskeleton is divided into **axial** and **appendicular** components. The axial skeleton consists of the skull, the vertebral column, and the rib cage. All other bones are part of the appendicular skeleton (see Figure 9).

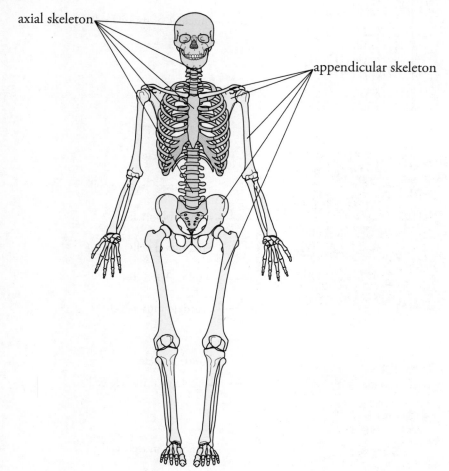

axial skeleton

appendicular skeleton

Figure 9 Axial and Appendicular Skeletons

11.6 CONNECTIVE TISSUE

Bone is an example of **connective tissue**. Connective tissue consists of cells and the materials they secrete. All connective tissue cells are derived from a single progenitor, the **fibroblast**. This name derives from its ability to secrete fibrous material such as **collagen**, a strong fibrous protein. Another important fibrous extracellular protein is **elastin**, which gives tissue the ability to stretch and regain its shape. Fibroblast-derived cells include **adipocytes** (fat cells), **chondrocytes** (cartilage cells), and **osteocytes** (bone cells).

Connective tissue differs from the other tissue types in the body (epithelial, muscle, and nervous tissue) because it is primarily extracellular material with a few cells scattered in it (the other three tissue types are the opposite; mostly cellular, with little extracellular material). The extracellular material is known as the **matrix** and consists of the fibers described above and **ground substance**, a thick, viscous material. The main ingredients of the ground substance are proteoglycans; these are large macropolymers consisting of a protein core with many attached carbohydrate chains. The carbohydrate chains are called glycosaminoglycans (GAGs) and like all carbohydrates, they are very hydrophilic. Hence, in the body, they are always surrounded by a large amount of water ("water of solvation"). This gives tissues their characteristic thickness and firmness. For example, dehydration results in saggy skin because of decreased hydration of the ground substance in the extracellular matrix.

There are two types of connective tissue: loose and dense. **Loose connective tissues** are basically packing tissues, and include areolar tissue (the soft material located between most cells throughout the body) and adipose tissue (fat). **Dense connective tissue** refers to tissues that contain large amounts of fibers (especially collagen), such as tendons, ligaments, cartilage, and bone. Cartilage and bone are sometime classified as supportive connective tissues, because of the role they play in physical support of body structures.

11.7   BONE STRUCTURE

Macroscopic

There are two primary bone shapes: **flat** and **long**. Flat bones, such as the scapula, the ribs, and the bones of the skull, are the location of hematopoiesis and are important for protection of organs. The bones of the limbs are long bones, important for support and movement. The main shaft of a long bone is called the **diaphysis**. The flared end is called the **epiphysis**.

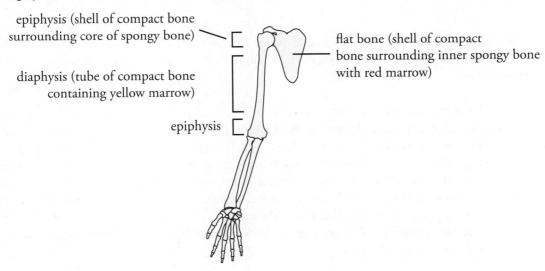

epiphysis (shell of compact bone surrounding core of spongy bone)

diaphysis (tube of compact bone containing yellow marrow)

epiphysis

flat bone (shell of compact bone surrounding inner spongy bone with red marrow)

Figure 10   Gross Anatomy of Bone

The general structure of bone may be either **compact** or **spongy**. As the names imply, compact bone is hard and dense while spongy bone is porous. Spongy bone is always surrounded by a layer of compact bone. The diaphysis of long bones is a tube composed only of compact bone.

Figure 11 Compact and Spongy Bone

Bone marrow is non-bony material found in the shafts of long bones and in the pores of spongy bones. **Red marrow**, found in spongy bone within flat bones, is the site of hematopoiesis. Its activity increases in response to erythropoietin, a hormone made by the kidney. **Yellow marrow**, found in the shafts of long bones, is filled with fat and is inactive.

Microscopic

Bone is composed of two principal ingredients: collagen and **hydroxyapatite**, which is a solid material consisting of calcium phosphate crystals. During bone synthesis, collagen is laid down in a highly ordered structure. Then, hydroxyapatite crystals form around the collagen framework, giving bone its characteristic strength and inflexibility.

Spongy bone under the microscope looks like a sponge. It has a disorganized structure in which many spikes of bone surround marrow-containing cavities. The spikes of bone in spongy bone are called **spicules** or **trabeculae**.

Compact bone has a specific organization (Figure 12). The basic unit of compact bone structure is the **osteon** (sometimes referred to as a **Haversian system**). In the center of the osteon is a hole called the **central** (or **Haversian**) **canal**, which contains blood, lymph vessels, and nerves. Surrounding the canal are concentric rings of bone termed **lamellae** (which just means "sheets" or "layers"). Tiny channels, or **canaliculi**, branch out from the central canal to spaces called **lacunae** ("lakes"). In each lacuna is an **osteocyte**, or mature bone cell. Osteocytes have long processes which extend down the canaliculi to contact other osteocytes through gap junctions. This allows the cells to exchange nutrients and waste through an otherwise impermeable membrane. **Perforating** (or **Volkmann's**) **canals** are channels that run perpendicular to central canals to connect osteons.

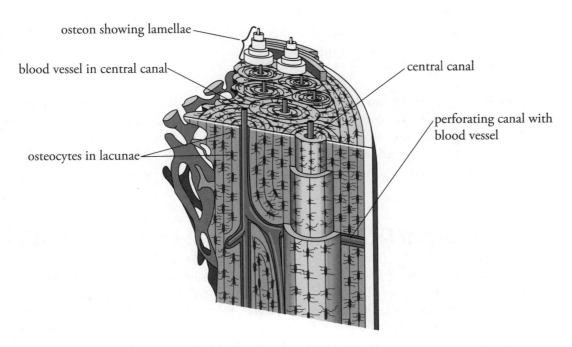

osteon showing lamellae

blood vessel in central canal

central canal

perforating canal with blood vessel

osteocytes in lacunae

Figure 12 Microscopic Structure of Compact Bone

11.8 TISSUES FOUND AT JOINTS

Cartilage

Cartilage is a strong but very flexible extracellular tissue secreted by cells called **chondrocytes**. There are three types of cartilage: hyaline, elastic, and fibrous. **Hyaline cartilage** is strong and somewhat flexible. The larynx and trachea are reinforced by hyaline cartilage, and joints are lined by hyaline cartilage known as **articular cartilage**, as shown in Figure 11. **Elastic cartilage** is found in structures (such as the outer ear and the epiglottis) that require support and more flexibility than hyaline cartilage can provide; it contains elastin. **Fibrous cartilage** is very rigid and is found in places where very strong support is needed, such as the pubic symphysis (the anterior connection of the pelvis) and the intervertebral disks of the spinal column. Cartilage is not innervated and does not contain blood vessels (it is **avascular**). It receives nutrition and immune protection from the surrounding fluid. [Why do cartilage injuries take a long time to heal?[16]]

Ligaments, Tendons, and Joints

Ligaments and tendons are strong tissues composed of dense connective tissue. **Ligaments** connect bones to other bones, and **tendons** connect bones to muscles. The point where one bone meets another is called a **joint**. Immovable joints, called **synarthroses**, are basically points where two bones are fused together. For example, the skull is formed from many fused bones. Slightly movable joints, called **amphiarthroses**, provide both movability and a great deal of support (*amphi-* means "both"). The vertebral joints are

---

[16] Cells in cartilage are not directly supplied by blood and have a low rate of metabolism. Thus, they are slow to repair damage. Often the damaged cartilage is simply removed or repaired surgically.

an example. Freely movable joints (i.e., most of the joints in the body) are called **diarthroses**. There are several types, for example, ball and socket (hip, shoulder) and hinge (elbow). All movable joints are supported by ligaments.

Movable joints are lubricated by **synovial fluid**, which is kept within the joint by the **synovial capsule**. The surfaces of the two bones that contact each other are perfectly smooth because they are lined by special **articular cartilage** (composed of hyaline cartilage). Like all cartilage, articular cartilage lacks blood vessels. Hence, it is easily damaged by overuse or infection. Inflammation of joints (**arthritis**) leads to destruction of the articular cartilage, which causes pain and stiffness.

11.9 BONE GROWTH AND REMODELING; THE CELLS OF BONE

Growth of long bones proceeds as follows: during childhood, a structure called the **epiphyseal plate** is seen between the diaphysis and the epiphysis. The epiphyseal plate is a disk of hyaline cartilage that is actively being produced by chondrocytes. As the chondrocytes divide, the epiphysis and diaphysis are forced apart. Then the cartilage is replaced by bone (ossified). This process is stimulated by growth hormone, and the rate of ossification is slightly faster than the rate of chondrocyte cell division (cartilage growth). Thus, at about the age of 18, the diaphysis and epiphyses meet and fuse together, and lengthening can no longer occur. This "fusion of the epiphyses" is easily observed in X-rays and can be used to notify adolescents when they have stopped growing taller. In adults, the fusion point is referred to as the **epiphyseal line**.

During adulthood, bones do not elongate. However, bone is continually degraded and remade in a process termed **remodeling**. The cells which make bone by laying down collagen and hydroxyapatite are called **osteoblasts**. The osteoblast synthesizes bone until it is surrounded by bone. The space it is left in is now called a lacuna, and the osteoblast is now called an **osteocyte**. Cells called **osteoclasts** continually destroy bone by dissolving the hydroxyapatite crystals. The osteoclast is a large phagocytic cousin of the macrophage. Bone destroyed by osteoclasts must be replaced by osteoblasts.

An increased ratio of osteoclast to osteoblast activity results in the liberation of calcium and phosphate into the bloodstream (and a decreased ratio has the opposite effect). Thus, activity of these cells is important not only for bone structure, but also for maintenance of proper blood levels of calcium and phosphate. The hormones **PTH (parathyroid hormone)**, **calcitonin**, and **calcitriol** (derived by the kidney from vitamin D) regulate their activity and thus blood calcium levels. PTH and calcitriol increase blood calcium, and calcitonin reduces it. The specific effects of these hormones are listed in Table 3.

Table 3 Hormonal Control of Calcium Homeostasis

Hormone	Effect on bones	Effect on kidneys	Effect on intestines
PTH	stimulates osteoclast activity	increases reabsorption of calcium, stimulates conversion of vitamin D into calcitriol	indirectly (via calcitriol) increases intestinal calcium absorption
calcitriol	may stimulate osteoclast activity, but minor effect	increases reabsorption of phosphorus	increases intestinal absorption of calcium
calcitonin	inhibits osteoclast activity	decreases reabsorption of calcium	n/a

Chapter 11 Summary

- There are three types of muscle tissue: skeletal, cardiac, and smooth.

- Skeletal muscles are voluntary, striated, multinucleate, and attached to the bones. They are individually innervated.

- The group of skeletal muscle cells controlled by a single neuron is called a motor unit, and each muscle is made of several motor units. All the cells in a motor unit contract together; to increase the strength of a contraction, additional motor units are recruited.

- Skeletal muscles are bundled into fascicles of many myofibers (cells), which are composed of myofibrils (strings of sarcomeres).

- Actin and myosin are organized into sarcomeres, which are the contractile units of the skeletal muscle cell. The arrangement of actin and myosin produces a characteristic banding pattern (striations): A band, I band, A band, I band, etc. Overlap of actin and myosin during the sliding filament theory produces sarcomere shortening.

- The four steps of the sliding filament theory involve the binding of myosin to actin (crossbridge formation), the pulling of actin toward the center of the sarcomere (power stroke), the release of actin (ATP binding), and resetting myosin to a high-energy conformation (ATP hydrolysis).

- Depolarization of the muscle cell triggers the release of calcium into the cytosol from the sarcoplasmic reticulum. Calcium binds to troponin, changing its shape, and subsequently changing the position of the tropomyosin to which the troponin is bound. This exposes the myosin binding sites on actin and allows contraction to occur. This is known as excitation-contraction coupling.

- Slow twitch fibers contract slowly, but have many mitochondria and a good blood supply, so are fatigue resistant.

- Fast twitch fibers contract quickly. Type IIA fibers have some mitochondria and are somewhat fatigue resistant, while Type IIB fibers lack mitochondria and fatigue quickly.

- Cardiac muscle is also striated, meaning that it, too, is organized into sarcomeres. Sliding filaments and excitation-contraction occur as in skeletal muscle. However, cardiac muscle is involuntary and autorhythmic. The cells are uninuclear and connected by gap junctions to form a functional syncytium.

- Cardiac muscle cells have an action potential that includes a long plateau phase. The plateau is the result of the opening of voltage-gated Ca^{2+} channels.

- Smooth muscle lacks striations and sarcomeres; however, calcium is still needed for smooth muscle cells to contract. They are involuntary.

- Bone is a dense connective tissue that functions primarily in body support and protection. Bones also play a role in mineral storage; resorption and deposition of bone is regulated by parathyroid hormone and calcitonin, respectively, to regulate blood calcium levels.

- Compact bone is organized into osteons, long cylinders of hard, dense bone. Compact bone forms the outer shell of all bones and the shaft (diaphysis) of long bones.

- Spongy bone contains much more space than compact bone and is filled with red bone marrow; this is where blood cell formation takes place. Spongy bone forms the core of flat bones and is found at the ends (epiphyses) of long bones.

CHAPTER 11 FREESTANDING PRACTICE QUESTIONS

1. Which of the following is NOT true regarding smooth muscle cells?

A) They are uninucleate and relatively small in size compared to skeletal muscle.
B) Gap junctions may exist between adjacent smooth muscle cells.
C) Ca^{2+} influx and binding to troponin results in actin and myosin binding and contraction.
D) They lack striations due to nonlinear alignment of the sarcomeres.

2. Rigor mortis, the stiffening of body limbs after death, is due to:

A) the inability of the myosin head to detach from actin due to loss of ATP.
B) the inability of the myosin head to attach to actin due to the loss of ATP.
C) the inability of the myosin head to detach from actin due to loss of ADP.
D) the inability of the myosin head to attach to actin due to the loss of ADP.

3. The neurotransmitter released at somatic axon synapses is:

A) dopamine.
B) norepinephrine.
C) acetylcholine.
D) epinephrine.

4. Lambert-Eaton syndrome is characterized by the formation of antibodies to voltage-gated calcium channels, rendering them inactive. Which of the following processes involved in generating a muscle contraction would be directly affected?

A) Saltatory conduction
B) Release of neurotransmitter at the synaptic cleft
C) Binding of neurotransmitter at the muscle end plate
D) Release of calcium from the sarcoplasmic reticulum

5. Which of the following is a possible way to distinguish between muscle types?

A) Skeletal muscle can contract via peristalsis, while smooth muscle cannot.
B) Skeletal muscle contraction depends on motor neuron stimulation, while cardiac muscle does not.
C) Cardiac muscle cells are syncytial, while smooth muscle cells are not.
D) Cardiac muscle contractions are regulated by influxes of calcium, while smooth muscle is not.

6. A young patient is found to have signs and symptoms of osteoporosis, or decreased bone density. The patient undergoes a variety of studies and is found to have a tumor secreting excessive levels of a particular hormone. What hormone could this tumor be secreting?

A) Parathyroid hormone
B) Calcitonin
C) Vitamin D
D) Thyroxine

7. Bisphosphonates are drugs that prevent the loss of bone mass and are used to treat osteoporosis and similar diseases. Which of the following is the most likely mechanism of action for this drug class?

A) Osteoblast inhibition
B) Osteoclast inhibition
C) Stimulation of PTH
D) Calcitonin inhibition

8. Synovial fluid is an essential lubricant for highly movable joints. Which of the following joints does not have synovial fluid?

A) Shoulder
B) Hip
C) Finger
D) Cranium (frontal-parietal)

CHAPTER 11 PRACTICE PASSAGE

Peristaltic smooth muscle contractions of the small intestine are essential to digestion and are under the control of two competing neural pathways, noradrenergic and cholinergic. Stimulation of noradrenergic fibers causes the release of norepinephrine and epinephrine, which inhibit smooth muscle contractions. Stimulation of cholinergic fibers causes the release of acetylcholine (ACh), which stimulates smooth muscle contractions. These two systems work together to regulate smooth muscle contraction and digestion.

The regulatory effects of these two competing nervous pathways have been demonstrated in the laboratory. To study the effects of cholinergic and noradrenergic neural stimulation on smooth muscle contraction in the rabbit, various concentrations of ACh, norepinephrine, and epinephrine were applied to the ileum of a rabbit.

Experiment:

Step 1: A 2- to 3-cm strip of mature rabbit ileum was removed from an animal and was attached to a kymograph, a device designed especially for the study of muscle contractions. Preparation temperature was maintained between 35°C and 36°C, and the sample was kept well-aerated. Acetylcholine was applied to stimulate contractions and then epinephrine was added to the preparation in concentrations ranging from 0.4 to 0.8 µg per l00 mL of bath solution. This was done in order to determine the minimum dose required to inhibit contractions.

Step 2: The same procedure was repeated using norepinephrine in similar concentrations.

Step 3: ACh was added to restimulate muscle contractions. After a one-minute waiting period, epinephrine was added in order to determine its depressive effect. One minute later, ACh was reapplied to the preparation in order to determine its excitatory effect.

Results: When norepinephrine and epinephrine concentrations were increased relative to constant ACh levels, muscle contractions were predictably and significantly inhibited. The degree of inhibition was directly proportional to the relative amounts of noradrenergic and cholinergic neurotransmitters present.

1. Which of the following activities will NOT cause the release of epinephrine in large quantities?

A) Digesting food one hour after a large meal
B) Watching a frightening movie
C) Running in the second half of a marathon
D) Performing a difficult task under pressure

2. After a meal, when will the greatest amount of acetylcholine be released?

A) Within the first two hours
B) After 6 hours
C) After 10 hours
D) After an all-night fast

3. In the experiment, muscle contractions were significantly decreased because epinephrine causes:

A) an immediate increase in levels of ACh.
B) an increase in smooth muscle fiber nervous stimulation.
C) a decrease in the number of cholinergic fibers.
D) a decrease in the effect of acetylcholine on smooth muscle activity.

4. To conclude that both epinephrine and acetylcholine are supplied to stomach smooth muscle by nerve fibers, what information would be necessary?

A) Denervation of rabbit stomach muscle decreases food absorption.
B) Denervation of rabbit stomach muscle decreases both contractions and inhibition of contractions.
C) Epinephrine has an antagonistic effect to acetylcholine.
D) Acetylcholine and epinephrine have similar functional groups.

5. In stimulating peristaltic activity, acetylcholine is an organic molecule that has the effect of causing:

A) a decrease in actin–myosin contractions due to increased intracellular Ca^{2+} concentration.
B) a decrease in actin–myosin contractions due to decreased ATP concentration.
C) an increase in actin–myosin contractions due to increased intracellular Ca^{2+} concentration.
D) an increase in actin–myosin contractions due to decreased ATP concentration.

6. Why was the degree of inhibition in the experiment directly proportional to the relative amounts of neurotransmitters?

A) Acetylcholine and epinephrine bind to each other in the synapse in a one-to-one ratio.
B) Inhibition and excitation cause opposing ion fluxes.
C) After a certain point, acetylcholine's effects dominate over epinephrine's.
D) After a certain point, only excitatory effects are registered by the cell.

SOLUTIONS TO CHAPTER 11 FREESTANDING PRACTICE QUESTIONS

1. **C** It is important to remember that smooth muscle is activated very differently from cardiac or skeletal muscle. Smooth muscle lacks troponin and tropomyosin and utilizes other regulatory enzymes including MLCK, or myosin light-chain kinase. All the other statements are true regarding smooth muscle (choices A, B, and D can be eliminated).

2. **A** During muscle contraction, the binding of ATP to the myosin head group is required to detach myosin from the actin filament. If there is no detachment (myosin and actin remain connected), the muscles remain stiff and immovable (choices B and D are wrong). Because ATP formation is an active process that requires living cells, levels of ATP decline rapidly after death, and ADP levels rise correspondingly. Thus, it is the lack of ATP after death that leads to rigor mortis (choice A is correct, and choice C is wrong). Note that this is a two-by-two question: a single piece of information can be used to eliminate two answer choices.

3. **C** Somatic axons stimulate skeletal muscle, so the synapse under discussion is the motor end plate, and acetylcholine is always released at the motor end plate. Dopamine is a neurotransmitter used in the brain (choice A is wrong), norepinephrine is the neurotransmitter secreted by sympathetic neurons (choice B is wrong), and epinephrine is a hormone (choice D is wrong).

4. **B** Release of neurotransmitter from the axon terminal is dependent upon calcium influx from voltage-gated channels, and is greatly impaired in Lambert-Eaton syndrome (choice B is correct). Saltatory conduction is primarily dependent on sodium channels, not calcium (choice A is wrong), binding of neurotransmitter at the motor end plate does not depend on calcium (choice C is wrong), and although the calcium channels of the sarcoplasmic reticulum are voltage-gated, they are intracellular and are not likely to encounter antibodies (choice D is wrong).

5. **B** It is true that skeletal muscle contraction depends on motor neuron stimulation; remember that skeletal muscles are voluntary. However, cardiac muscle is not voluntary; contraction is controlled by the sinoatrial node. This is a possible way to distinguish between these muscle types (choice B is correct). Smooth muscle, not skeletal muscle, contracts using peristalsis, such as in the digestive tract (choice A is wrong). Cardiac muscle cells form a functional syncytium; the cells are connected by gap junctions and function as unit. Smooth muscle also functions in this manner (choice C is wrong). All muscle contractions are regulated by influxes of calcium (choice D is wrong).

6. **A** The patient is described as having signs and symptoms of decreased bone density. This could be the result of either excessive bone resorption or poor bone formation. Of the hormones listed, parathyroid is known to cause bone resorption by stimulating osteoclasts. Calcitonin functions to inhibit osteoclasts, preventing bone resorption (choice B is wrong). Excessive levels of vitamin D would result in increased calcium absorption in the small intestine and, more likely, subsequent bone formation (choice C is wrong). Thyroxine is not involved in calcium regulation (choice D is wrong).

7. **B**   Osteoporosis is a disease where bone mineral density is reduced due to increased bone resorption. The cells that are responsible for resorbing bone matrix are osteoclasts; these are stimulated by PTH and inhibited by calcitonin. In contrast, osteoblasts build bone and are stimulated by calcitonin. If bisphosphonates help prevent bone loss, they must either inhibit bone resorption or stimulate bone building. Inhibiting osteoclasts would reduce bone resorption and could be a mechanism of action of bisphosphonates (choice B is correct). Inhibiting osteoblasts is the opposite effect and would not help build bone (choice A is wrong); an increase of PTH stimulates osteoclasts and would increase bone resorption (choice C is wrong). Calcitonin reduces osteoclast activity and stimulates osteoblasts, so inhibiting calcitonin would not help bone loss (choice D is wrong).

8. **D**   Synovial fluid lubricates movable joints. Of the joints listed, the only stationary one is the frontal-parietal joint or the frontal-parietal suture (choices A, B, and C are wrong).

SOLUTIONS TO CHAPTER 11 PRACTICE PASSAGE

1. **A**   In general, the sympathetic nervous system, which releases epinephrine at post-ganglionic synapses, is stimulated by the "fight or flight" response. Choices B, C, and D will all stimulate the sympathetic nervous system and cause the release of epinephrine. However, digestion (choice A) stimulates the parasympathetic nervous system, which releases acetylcholine at the post-ganglionic synapse; choice A is correct.

2. **A**   Digestion quickly causes stimulation of the parasympathetic nervous system, which in turn stimulates secretion and motility in the GI tract. The response should be strongest while digestion is occurring (choice A is the best response).

3. **D**   Acetylcholine and epinephrine bind to cell-surface receptors with ligand-gated ion channels which either hyperpolarize or depolarize the membrane. Acetylcholine depolarizes the membrane, while epinephrine hyperpolarizes the membrane, causing the neurotransmitters to oppose each other (choice D is correct). Increased ACh would cause increased, not decreased contraction (choice A is wrong), and since the strip of ileum was removed from the animal, it had no neural stimulation (choices B and C are wrong).

4. **B**   If both are supplied by nerves, then it should be possible to eliminate the effect of both by denervation.

5. **C**   Acetylcholine increases peristalsis, not decreases (choices A and B are wrong). Calcium release plays a role in smooth muscle contraction (as it does in cardiac and skeletal muscle as well; choice C is correct). A decrease in ATP would lead to a decrease in contraction (choice D is wrong).

6. **B**   Neurotransmitters exert their effects on cells through opening ion channels which either depolarize or hyperpolarize the membrane. Acetylcholine and epinephrine bind to their receptors, not to each other (choice A is wrong). Neither choice C nor choice D answers the question.

Chapter 12
The Respiratory
System and the Skin

12.1 FUNCTIONS OF THE RESPIRATORY SYSTEM

Single-cell eukaryotes that require oxygen to perform oxidative phosphorylation can acquire it by simple diffusion of oxygen from the surrounding medium. Even simple multicellular organisms such as coelenterates (jellyfish and hydra) can still receive sufficient oxygen by diffusion between cells and the environment. Larger organisms, such as the vertebrates, evolved a respiratory system to exchange O_2 and CO_2 between the atmosphere and the blood and a circulatory system to transport those gases between the respiratory system and the rest of the tissues of the body. Note that at the cellular level, all organisms exchange respiratory gases via simple diffusion across the plasma membrane. However, the respiratory system ensures the efficient delivery of O_2 and removal of CO_2 for all cells in a complex, multicellular animal. [What parts of glucose metabolism produce CO_2, and what point in glucose metabolism utilizes oxygen?[1]]

The simple movement of air into and out of the lungs is properly called **ventilation**, whereas the actual exchange of gases (between either the lungs and the blood or the blood and the other tissues of the body) is called **respiration**.[2] The parts of the respiratory system that participate *only* in ventilation are referred to as the **conduction zone**, and the parts that participate in actual gas exchange are referred to as the **respiratory zone**. Additional tasks performed by the respiratory system include the following:

1) *pH regulation.* In the blood, CO_2 is converted to carbonic acid by the RBC enzyme carbonic anhydrase (Chapter 9). When CO_2 is exhaled by the lungs, the amount of carbonic acid in the blood is decreased, and as a result the pH of the blood increases (becomes more alkaline). Hence, minute-to-minute variations in respiration affect blood pH. **Hyper**ventilation (too much breathing) causes alkalinization of the blood, known as **respiratory alkalosis**. **Hypoventilation** (too little breathing) causes acidification of the blood, or **respiratory acidosis**. [Which organ regulates pH over a period of hours to days?[3]]

2) *Thermoregulation.* Breathing can result in significant heat loss. Heat loss from the respiratory system occurs through **evaporative water loss**, which functions under the same principles as sweating. The respiratory structures are necessarily moist. Liquid water absorbs heat as it changes into water vapor, and this heat is removed from the body during the process. Dogs, for example, depend on panting for the dissipation of excess heat, because they cannot sweat. Some animals manage to conserve both water and heat by utilizing **countercurrent exchange** within the nasal passages. The nasal passages warm and humidify the air entering the respiratory system, and the exiting air is cooled and de-humidified. Breathing through the mouth (as with panting, or during exercise) will bypass this mechanism and increase rates of heat loss.

3) *Protection from disease and particulate matter.* The lungs provide a large moist surface where chemicals and pathogens can do harm. The **mucociliary escalator** and alveolar macrophages, discussed below, protect us from harmful inhaled particles.

---

[1] Pyruvate dehydrogenase and the Krebs cycle produce CO_2 during oxidative respiration, and oxygen is reduced to water by the last electron carrier in electron transport, cytochrome *c* oxidase.

[2] Sometimes these terms are used interchangeably. For example, we refer to "respiratory rate" when we really mean "ventilation rate."

[3] The kidney

12.2 ANATOMY OF THE RESPIRATORY SYSTEM

The Conduction Zone

As mentioned earlier, the part of the respiratory system designed only to allow gases to enter and exit the system is called the conduction zone (Figure 1). Inhaled air follows this pathway: **nose → nasal cavity → pharynx → larynx → trachea → bronchi → terminal bronchioles → respiratory bronchioles → alveolar ducts → alveoli** (the respiratory bronchioles, alveolar ducts, and alveoli are parts of the respiratory zone and will be discussed later). The nose is important for warming, humidifying, and filtering inhaled air; nasal hairs and sticky mucus act as filters. The nasal cavity is an open space within the nose. The pharynx is the throat (a common pathway for air and food) at the bottom of which is the larynx. The larynx has three functions: 1) it is made entirely of cartilage and thus keeps the airway open, 2) it contains the **epiglottis**, which seals the trachea during swallowing to prevent the entry of food, and 3) it contains the **vocal cords**, which are folds of tissue positioned to partially block the flow of air and vibrate, thereby producing sound. The **trachea** is a passageway which must remain open to permit air flow. Rings of cartilage prevent its collapse. The trachea branches into two **primary bronchi**, each of which supplies one lung. Each bronchus branches repeatedly to supply the entire lung. Collapse of bronchi is prevented by small plates of cartilage. Very small bronchi are called **bronchioles**. They are about 1 mm wide and contain no cartilage. Their walls are made of smooth muscle, which allows their diameters to be regulated to adjust airflow into the system. The smallest (and final) branches of the conduction zone are aptly called the **terminal bronchioles**.

The smooth muscle of the walls of the terminal bronchioles is too thick to allow adequate diffusion of gases; this is why no gas exchange occurs in this region. The conduction zone is strictly for ventilation.

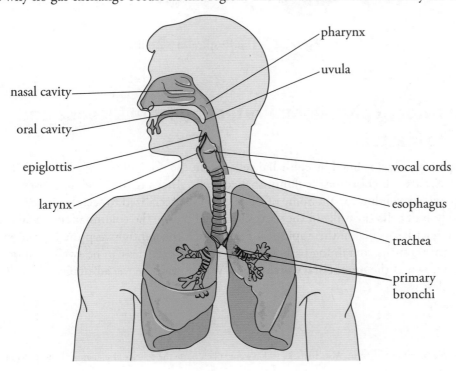

Figure 1 The Conduction Zone

The Respiratory Zone

The region of the system where gas exchange occurs is the respiratory zone (Figure 2). The actual structure across which gases diffuse is called the **alveolus** (plural: **alveoli**). Alveoli are tiny sacs with very thin walls (they're so thin that they're transparent!). The wall of the alveolus is only one cell thick, except where capillaries pass across its outer surface. The duct leading to the alveoli is called an **alveolar duct**, and its walls are entirely made of alveoli. The alveolar duct branches off a **respiratory bronchiole**. This is a tube made of smooth muscle, just like the terminal bronchioles, but with one important difference: the respiratory bronchiole has a few alveoli scattered in its walls. This allows it to perform gas exchange, so it is part of the respiratory zone.

respiratory bronchioles

alveoli

smooth muscle

capillaries

Figure 2   The Respiratory Zone

The Respiratory Epithelium: Protection from Disease and Particulate Matter

The entire respiratory tract is lined by epithelial cells. From the nose all the way down to the bronchioles, the epithelial cells are tall **columnar** (column-shaped) cells. They are too thick to assist in gas exchange; they merely provide a conduit for air. Some of these cells are specialized to secrete a layer of sticky mucus and are called **goblet cells** (just like in the gastrointestinal tract). The columnar epithelial cells of the upper respiratory tract have cilia on their apical surfaces which constantly sweep the layer of mucus toward the pharynx, where mucus containing pathogens and inhaled particles can be swallowed or coughed out. This system is known as the **mucociliary escalator**. [What would be the advantage of swallowing pathogens and particles?[4]]

---

[4]   Gastric acidity destroys many pathogens. Also, particles which would likely harm the delicate alveoli are unlikely to harm the tough lining of the GI tract.

The alveoli, alveolar ducts, and the smallest bronchioles (respiratory bronchioles) are involved in gas exchange. Oxygen and CO_2 must be able to diffuse across the layer of epithelial cells in order to pass freely between the bloodstream and the air in the lungs. Tall columnar cells with cilia would be too large to permit rapid diffusion. Thus, gas-exchanging surfaces are lined with a single layer of thin, delicate squamous epithelial cells. (Squamous means flat.) A single layer of squamous epithelial cells is called *simple squamous epithelium*. It would also be unacceptable to have a layer of mucus covering the gas exchange surface, so another method of protection from disease and inhaled particles is necessary. Alveolar macrophages fill this role by patrolling the alveoli, engulfing foreign particles.

Surfactant

Imagine a beehive made of tissue paper. If you put it in a steamy bathroom, what would happen? Would all the small air spaces remain filled with air? No, the hive would collapse into a wet ball, because the mutual attraction of water molecules would overcome the flimsy support structure provided by the fine paper fibers. The tendency of water molecules to clump together creates **surface tension**, which is the force that causes wet hydrophilic surfaces (e.g., the tissue paper) to stick together in the presence of air. Think of it this way: air is hydrophobic, so hydrophilic substances in the presence of air tend to clump together. Now imagine a beehive made of thin wax paper. If you put it into a steamy room, does it collapse? No, because the wax on the surface of the paper prevents adjacent pieces of paper from being strongly attracted. In other words, the wax destroys the surface tension.

The alveoli are as fine and delicate as tissue paper, and they too tend to collapse due to surface tension (Figure 3). This problem is solved by a soapy substance called **surfactant** (*surf*ace *acti*ve substance), which coats the alveoli. Just like the wax in our example above, surfactant reduces surface tension. Surfactant is a complex mixture of phospholipids, proteins, and ions secreted by cells in the alveolar wall. [Is it likely that these are the principal lining cells of the alveolar wall?[5]]

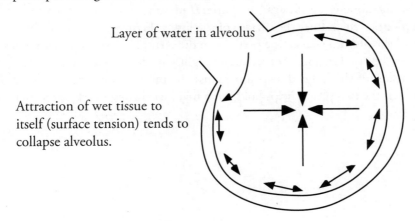

Layer of water in alveolus

Attraction of wet tissue to itself (surface tension) tends to collapse alveolus.

Figure 3   Surface Tension in an Alveolus

---

[5] No, the principal cells of the alveolar wall are thin squamous cells designed to allow diffusion of gases. Cells which actively secrete substances (i.e., surfactant) are large, metabolically active cells with many mitochondria. The basic alveolar lining cells (simple squamous epithelium) are called Type 1 alveolar cells. The fat (cuboidal) epithelial cells that secrete surfactant are called Type 2 alveolar cells.

- There is not sufficient surfactant within a fetus's lungs until about the eighth month of gestation, so some premature infants lack the protective effects of surfactant when they are born. Which of the following statements best describes resulting effects upon respiration in "preemies" (babies born prematurely)?[6]
  - A) Surface tension would be abnormally low.
  - B) The alveoli would collapse.
  - C) Oxygen would be unable to diffuse through water.
  - D) Respiration is unnecessary, since the infant is dependent on the mother.

12.3 PULMONARY VENTILATION

Pulmonary ventilation is the circulation of air into and out of the lungs to continually replace the gases in the alveoli with those in the atmosphere. The drawing of air into the lungs is termed **inspiration**, and the movement of air out of the lungs is termed **expiration**. Inspiration is an active process driven by the contraction of the diaphragm, which enlarges the chest cavity (and the lungs along with the chest cavity) drawing air in. Passive expiration is driven by the elastic recoil of the lungs and does not require active muscle contraction. These processes will be described in more detail below.

The Pleural Space and Lung Elasticity

The lungs are large elastic bags that tend to collapse in upon themselves if removed from the chest cavity. However, the structures of the chest prevent this collapse and allow the lungs to remain inflated during inspiration and expiration. The lungs are not directly connected to the chest wall, however. Each lung is surrounded by two membranes, or **pleura**: the **parietal pleura**, which lines the inside of the chest cavity, and the **visceral pleura**, which lines the surface of the lungs (Figure 4). Between the two pleura is a very narrow space called the **pleural space**. The pressure in the pleural space (the **pleural pressure**) is negative, meaning that the two pleural membranes are drawn tightly together by a vacuum. This negative pressure keeps the outer surface of the lungs drawn up against the inside of the chest wall. Additionally, a thin layer of fluid between the two pleura helps hold them together through surface tension.

---

[6] In the absence of surfactant, surface tension would be high (choice A is wrong), and the alveoli would collapse on every exhalation like tissue-paper beehives (choice **B** is correct). It would take an enormous exertion to reopen the collapsed alveoli to get any air (oxygen) into them; the result is poor oxygen delivery to the alveoli and thus to the blood (for this reason, preemies are typically kept on ventilators until their surfactant levels are higher and they are stronger in general). Note that oxygen has some ability to diffuse through water, but choice C is wrong mostly due to irrelevance. It's not as though in the absence of surfactant the lungs suddenly fill with water. Respiration is always necessary once a baby is born; this question specifically refers to infants born prematurely (choice D is wrong).

Figure 4 The Lungs and Pleura

- If the pleural space is punctured, opening it to the external atmosphere, which one of the following will occur?[7]

  A) Fluid will leak out of the pleural space.

  B) Air will leak out of the pleural space.

  C) Air will leak into the pleural space.

  D) Since the pressure within the pleural space is equal to atmospheric pressure during expiration, nothing will happen.

Inspiration is caused by muscular expansion of the chest wall, which draws the lungs outward (expands them), and causes air to enter the system. The lungs expand along with the chest due to the negative pressure in the pleural space. The expansion of the chest during inspiration is driven primarily by contraction of the **diaphragm**, a large skeletal muscle that is stretched below the ribs between the abdomen and the chest cavity. When resting, the diaphragm is shaped like a dome, bulging upward into the chest cavity. When it contracts, the diaphragm flattens and draws the chest cavity downward, forcing it and the lungs (which are stuck to the inside wall of the chest cavity) to expand. The external **intercostal muscles** between the ribs also contract during inspiration, pulling the ribs upward and further expanding the chest cavity. Inspiration is an *active* process, requiring contraction of muscles to occur.

Resting expiration, by contrast, is a *passive* process (no muscle contraction required). When the diaphragm and rib muscles relax, the elastic recoil of the lungs draws the chest cavity inward, reducing the volume of the lungs and pushing air out of the system into the atmosphere. During exertion (or at other times when a more forcible exhalation is required), contraction of abdominal muscles helps the expiration process by pressing upward on the diaphragm, further shrinking the size of the lungs and forcing more air out. This is called a **forced expiration** and is an active process.

---

[7] The pleural space is always at negative pressure, or the lung would collapse. If the pleural pressure is negative, and an opening to the atmosphere is made, then air will rush into the pleural space and the lungs will collapse. The correct answer is choice **C**. (Note that choice A will probably also occur, but the amount of fluid is so minimal as to be insignificant. Choice C is the better answer.)

12.3

The pressure of air in the alveoli and the pleural pressure vary during inspiration and expiration. During inspiration, the following steps occur:

1) The diaphragm contracts and flattens (moves downward).
2) The volume of the chest cavity expands.
3) The pleural pressure decreases, becoming more negative.
4) The lungs expand outward.
5) The pressure in the alveoli becomes negative.
6) Air enters the lungs and the alveoli.

The opposite steps occur during expiration. Typically inspiration and expiration are not consciously controlled although they are mediated by voluntary muscle (which means we *can* control the processes if we want to!).

- At the beginning of inspiration, does the pleural pressure increase, decrease, or remain the same?[8]
- When is the alveolar pressure exactly zero (equal to atmospheric)?[9]
- What would be the result of a hole in the lung that allowed inhaled air to flow into the pleural cavity?[10]

Pulmonary Ventilation: Volumes and Capacities

Spirometry is the measurement of the volume of air entering or exiting the lungs at the various stages of ventilation.[11] A **spirometer** is a device used for these measurements. Data can be plotted on a **spirometric graph** (Figure 5). The volumes and capacities defined below should be familiar to you but do *not* need to be memorized.

Figure 5 Lung Volumes and Capacities

---

[8] At the beginning of inspiration, pleural pressure decreases (becomes more negative), sucking the lungs open.

[9] At the end of a resting expiration, air tends to neither enter nor leave the lungs, until another inspiration begins. This is when alveolar pressure is zero. Also, just after inspiration, before expiration begins, there is an instant of zero pressure.

[10] A hole in the lung would allow air to flow into the pleural cavity, just like a hole from the pleural space to the exterior. This would cause the lung to collapse, because negative pleural pressure is the only significant force opposing lung collapse. Inspiration would be impossible.

[11] *Spir-* is from re*spir*ation.

The **tidal volume** (**TV**) is the amount of air that moves in and out of the lungs with normal light breathing and is equal to about 10 percent of the total volume of the lungs (0.5 liters out of 5–6 liters). The **expiratory reserve volume** (**ERV**) is the volume of air that can be expired after a passive resting expiration. The **inspiratory reserve volume** (**IRV**) is the volume of air that can be inspired after a relaxed inspiration. The **functional residual capacity** (**FRC**) is the volume of air left in the lungs after a resting expiration. The **inspiratory capacity** (**IC**) is the maximal volume of air which can be inhaled after a resting expiration. The **residual volume** (**RV**) is the amount of air that remains in the lungs after the strongest possible expiration. The **vital capacity** (**VC**) is the maximum amount of air that can be forced out of the lungs after first taking the deepest possible breath. The **total lung capacity** (**TLC**) is the vital capacity plus the residual volume (TLC = VC + RV).

- Is the total volume of the lungs exchanged with each breath?[12]

- In emphysema, lung elasticity is greatly reduced. Each of the following occurs EXCEPT:[13]
  A) residual volume increases.
  B) total lung capacity increases.
  C) resting expiration becomes active instead of passive.
  D) pleural pressure becomes more negative.

12.4 GAS EXCHANGE

The Pulmonary Circulation

Deoxygenated blood is carried toward the lungs by the pulmonary artery, which has left and right branches. These large arteries branch many times, eventually giving rise to a huge network of **pulmonary capillaries**, also called **alveolar capillaries**. Each alveolus is surrounded by a few tiny capillaries, which are just wide enough to permit the passage of RBCs, and have extremely thin walls to permit diffusion of gases between blood and alveolus. The capillaries drain into venules, which drain into the pulmonary veins. The lungs are supplied with lymphatic vessels as well.

Small increases in left atrial pressure have very little effect on the pulmonary circulation because pulmonary veins can dilate, accommodating excess blood. However, if the pressure in the left atrium increases above a certain level, the pressure will increase in pulmonary capillaries, and fluid (essentially blood plasma) will be forced out of the capillaries and into the surrounding lung tissue. Fluid in the lungs resulting from increased blood pressure is known as **pulmonary edema**. Normally, the lymphatic system prevents pulmonary edema from developing by carrying interstitial fluid out of the lungs.

---

[12] No, some air always remains in the lungs; the FRC during relaxed breathing or the RV during deep breathing.

[13] Typically, when the lungs are stretched on inspiration, elastic recoil draws them inward and leads to expiration. The loss of elasticity means that the lungs do not want to recoil as strongly (or at all) and remain in their stretched position (choice B would occur and can be eliminated). Thus, expiration is not as efficient and more air remains in the lungs after expiration than normal (choice A would occur and can be eliminated). In order to make expiration more efficient, contraction of internal intercostal and abdominal muscles must be used to compress the chest cavity and push air out (choice C would occur and can be eliminated). Even at rest, alveoli are typically stretched somewhat and elastic recoil tends to draw them inward; this helps create the negative pleural pressure. However, if lung elasticity is reduced, there is less of a force drawing them inward, and the pleural pressure would be less negative, not more (choice **D** would not occur and is the correct answer choice).

- Which of the following may result from increased pulmonary capillary hydrostatic pressure?[14]
    - I. Accumulation of interstitial fluid in the lungs
    - II. Fluid accumulation in the alveoli
    - III. Decreased oxygenation of the blood due to excess fluid slowing O_2 diffusion

    A) I and II only
    B) I and III only
    C) II and III only
    D) I, II, and III

The lungs are "designed" to expose a large amount of blood to a large amount of air. Thus the primary property of the lung is its enormous surface area, close to that of a tennis court. The goal is to allow O_2 from the atmosphere to diffuse into pulmonary capillaries, where it is bound by hemoglobin in RBCs. Simultaneously, CO_2 diffuses from the blood to the alveolar gas. [To review, how is CO_2 carried in the blood?[15]]

Air is a complex mixture of many gases, with nitrogen and oxygen as its primary components and other gases such as water vapor and carbon dioxide forming small percentages of the total (Table 1). In cities, poisons such as carbon monoxide may attain significant concentrations (partial pressures).

Table 1 Approximate Atmospheric Gas Compositions

Gas	% of atmosphere
N_2	80%
O_2	20%
H_2O	0.5%
CO_2	0.04%

Each gas that is part of a mixture contributes to the total pressure of the mixture in proportion to its abundance. The contribution of each individual gas to the total pressure is termed the **partial pressure**. The partial pressure of Gas X is abbreviated PX. For example, P_{O_2} designates the partial pressure of oxygen. [If the total atmospheric pressure is 760 torr, what is the partial pressure of oxygen (P_{O_2}) in the atmosphere?[16]] The total pressure is the sum of all partial pressures.

Henry's Law

Gases in the air equilibrate with gases in liquids. If you place a beaker of water in a room, after a time the gases in the room will diffuse into the water. Therefore, partial pressures are also used to describe the amount of gases carried in the bloodstream.

---

[14] If the hydrostatic pressure is high enough, all of these will result (choice **D**).

[15] Most is transported as $HCO_3^- + H^+$ (carbonic anhydrase is the key enzyme); some is bound nonspecifically to Hb; a little can dissolve in plasma.

[16] Oxygen forms 20% of the atmosphere (Table 1). The partial pressure of oxygen in the atmosphere is 20% of 760 torr, or about 150 torr.

In order to diffuse into a cell, gas molecules from the air must dissolve into a liquid (e.g., extracellular fluid). According to **Henry's Law**, the amount of gas that will dissolve into liquid is dependent on the partial pressure of that gas as well as the solubility of that gas in the liquid. If we use oxygen as an example, Henry's Law states:

$$[O_2] = P_{O_2} \times S_{O_2}$$

where $[O_2]$ is the concentration of dissolved oxygen, P_{O_2} is the partial pressure of oxygen in the air above the fluid, and S_{O_2} is the solubility of oxygen in that liquid. Thus, an increase in pressure increases the amount of gas dissolved in a liquid.

Note that gases become less soluble in liquids as temperatures increase; this is why a soda goes flat faster on a hot day, and it is why a goldfish will gulp for air when the water is too warm. [Scuba divers breathe pressurized air. Why do they have to worry about nitrogen bubbles forming in the extracellular fluid if they ascend too quickly?[17]]

In the lungs, oxygen and carbon dioxide diffuse between the alveolar air and blood in the alveolar capillaries (Figure 6). The driving force for the exchange of gases in the lungs is the difference in partial pressures between the alveolar air and the blood. For diffusion to occur (from the air to the blood) gases must first pass across the alveolar epithelium, and then through the interstitial liquid, and finally across the capillary endothelium. These three barriers to diffusion together form the **respiratory membrane** (the pathway is obviously reversed for diffusion from the blood to the air). [Do the lipid membranes of the alveolar and capillary cells act as barriers to the diffusion of oxygen and carbon dioxide?[18]]

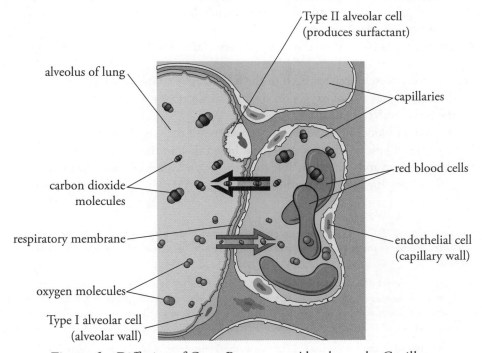

Figure 6   Diffusion of Gases Between an Alveolus and a Capillary

---

[17]   Gases are more soluble in liquids at high pressures. At depth, gases dissolve into the blood and extracellular fluids more readily because of the high pressure of the surrounding water. If a diver ascends too quickly, the gases come out of solution before they can be transported to the respiratory system. This results in air bubbles that primarily contain nitrogen, the most abundant gas in the air we breathe. These bubbles tend to form most abundantly at the joints, and cause decompression sickness, a painful condition commonly known as "the bends." To treat decompression sickness, afflicted divers are put into a hyperbaric (high pressure) chamber to redissolve the gases before slowly restoring the tissues to atmospheric pressure.

[18]   No, lipid bilayers do not act as barriers to the diffusion of such small hydrophobic molecules.

As blood passes through the alveolar capillaries, the oxygen pressure gradient between the alveolar air and the blood drives the net diffusion of oxygen into the blood. The arterial Po_2 is denoted P_aO_2.

- Is the Po_2 at the arterial end of pulmonary capillaries greater than, less than, or equal to the Po_2 in the venous end?[19]

- Although the partial pressures of oxygen and nitrogen in the atmosphere are relatively constant, the partial pressure of water vapor can vary considerably. If water vapor in the atmosphere increases, which one of the following will occur?[20]
  - A) The total atmospheric pressure will increase.
  - B) The partial pressures of oxygen and nitrogen will decrease.
  - C) The partial pressure of oxygen will decrease, and the partial pressure of nitrogen will increase.
  - D) The partial pressure of oxygen will increase, and the partial pressure of nitrogen will decrease.

- Atmospheric Po_2 is 150 torr, while the arterial Po_2 is 100 torr. Which one of the following is the best explanation for this discrepancy?[21]
  - A) Due to the short amount of time blood spends in the lungs, atmospheric gases do not fully equilibrate with arterial gases.
  - B) The barrier to diffusion formed by the alveolar epithelium plus the capillary endothelium prevents full equilibration of atmospheric and arterial gases.
  - C) The P_{H_2O} and Pco_2 in the alveolus are much higher than in the atmosphere; as a result, the Po_2 is lower.
  - D) The hydrophobic nature of oxygen prevents large amounts from dissolving in blood.

- During vigorous muscle activity, each of the following is true EXCEPT:[22]
  - A) the partial pressure of oxygen in the muscle decreases; as a result, oxygen diffuses from the blood into the muscle.
  - B) the flow of blood in the venous system through the muscle is reduced.
  - C) arteriolar dilation increases the rate of blood flow to the muscle.
  - D) myoglobin in muscle cells is able to take oxygen from RBC hemoglobin because myoglobin has a higher oxygen affinity.

---

[19] Less than. Deoxygenated blood (Po_2 = 40 torr) enters the pulmonary system in the pulmonary artery. As the deoxygenated blood passes through the capillaries, it becomes increasingly oxygenated until it emerges at the venous end equilibrated with the alveolar oxygen pressure (Po_2 = 100 torr).

[20] Total atmospheric pressure is defined as the force exerted against a surface due to the weight of the air above that surface; thus, it is determined primarily by gravitational forces and changes very little (choice A is wrong). Partial pressure, however, is defined as the portion of total pressure due to a particular gas; thus, if the partial pressure of water increases (and since the total pressure remains the same), the relative partial pressures of oxygen and nitrogen would have to decrease (choice **B** is correct, and choices C and D are wrong).

[21] The alveolar Po_2 is only 100 torr because water and CO_2 take up a greater proportion of gases in the alveolus than in the atmosphere. The gases in the alveolus do not have the same composition as the atmosphere since they are not fully exchanged with each breath (choice **C** is correct). While it is true that blood spends only a short amount of time in the lungs, the barrier (respiratory membrane) is extremely thin, allowing for rapid and complete equilibration of gases under normal circumstances (choices A and B are wrong). Choice D is true but irrelevant; most oxygen in the blood is carried on hemoglobin.

[22] During vigorous exertion, blood flow to the muscle through arterioles is increased (choice C is true and can be eliminated); thus, flow from the muscles through veins and venules must also increase; blood does not pool in the muscles during activity (choice **B** is false and the correct answer choice). As O_2 is used to make ATP, Po_2 in the muscle decreases and the resulting increased O_2 gradient from blood to muscle tissue allows oxygen to diffuse into the muscle cells (choice A is true and can be eliminated). This effect is enhanced by the fact that myoglobin has a higher affinity for oxygen than hemoglobin (choice D is true and can be eliminated).

12.5 REGULATION OF VENTILATION RATE

Proper regulation of the rate and depth of breathing is essential. Although breathing can be voluntarily controlled for short periods of time, it is normally an involuntary process directed by the **respiratory control center** in the medulla of the brain stem. The stimuli that affect ventilation rate are both mechanical and chemical (Table 2, next page).

The principal chemical stimuli that affect ventilation rate are increased P_{CO_2}, decreased pH, and decreased P_{O_2} (with CO_2 and pH being the primary regulators and O_2 secondary). These variables are monitored by special autonomic sensory receptors. **Peripheral chemoreceptors** are located in the aorta and the carotid arteries and monitor the P_{CO_2}, pH, and P_{O_2} of the blood, while **central chemoreceptors** are found in the medullary respiratory control center and monitor P_{CO_2} and pH of the cerebrospinal fluid (CSF). Recall that pH and P_{CO_2} are connected through the carbonic acid buffer system of the blood (discussed briefly in Chapters 9 and 10).

$$CO_2 + H_2O \rightleftharpoons H_2CO_3 \rightleftharpoons H^+ + HCO_3^-$$

Respiration eliminates CO_2 from the body. Thus, changes in ventilation rate can have rapid effects on pH due to the decrease or increase in P_{CO_2} and the resulting shift to maintain the above equilibrium. For example, a person hyperventilating during an anxiety attack can have an elevated pH. [Why do we give these folks a paper bag to breathe into?[23]] A person whose ventilation rate has been reduced due to extreme alcohol intoxication can become acidotic. Similarly, changes in pH can be compensated for by increasing or decreasing ventilation rate. For example, diabetics who are acidotic due to the metabolism of proteins and fats instead of glucose will have an increased ventilation rate to remove CO_2 and increase pH.

Mechanical stimuli that affect ventilation rate include physical stretching of the lungs and irritants. The mechanical stretching of lung tissue stimulates stretch receptors that inhibit further excitatory signals from the respiratory center to the muscles involved in inspiration. The walls of bronchi and larger bronchioles contain smooth muscle. Contraction of this smooth muscle is known as **bronchoconstriction**. Irritation of the inner lining of the lung stimulates irritant receptors, and reflexive contraction of bronchial smooth muscle prevents irritants from continuing to enter the passageways. This contractile response is determined by parasympathetic nerves that release ACh. During an allergy attack, mast cells release histamine, which also causes bronchoconstriction. Epinephrine opposes this; it increases ventilation by causing airway smooth muscles to relax (this is **bronchodilation**). [Asthma is caused by spasm of airway smooth muscles. Patients with asthma carry "inhalers," which are small aerosol cans whose contents they spray into their lungs during an asthma attack. Based on this discussion, what might inhalers contain?[24]]

There are also **irritant receptors** in the lung that trigger coughing and/or bronchoconstriction when an irritating chemical (such as smoke) is detected.

---

[23] Breathing into a paper bag forces them to rebreathe their exhaled CO_2. This pushes the equilibrium of the equation to the right and brings pH back down to normal.

[24] They contain epinephrine, antihistamines (drugs that block histamine receptors on smooth muscle cells), and anticholinergics (drugs that block acetylcholine receptors on smooth muscle cells).

Table 2 Factors that Regulate Ventilation Rate

Stimulus	Receptor	Effect
stretch of lung	stretch receptor in lung	inhibits inspiration
$\uparrow P_{CO_2}$	peripheral chemoreceptors and medullary respiratory center	increased P_{CO_2} causes $\downarrow$pH via carbonic anhydrase; the $\downarrow$pH is what is actually sensed (see below)
$\downarrow$pH	as above	increases respiratory rate
$\downarrow P_{O_2}$	peripheral chemoreceptors	increases respiratory rate
chemical irritation	irritant receptor in lung	coughing and/or bronchoconstriction

12.6 STRUCTURE AND LAYERS OF THE SKIN

The skin is the largest organ in the body, by size and by weight (Figure 7). Its role is to protect us from pathogens, to prevent excessive evaporation of water, and to regulate body temperature (Section 12.7). The outermost layer of the skin is called the **epidermis**; it lies upon the deeper **dermis**, which rests on **subcutaneous tissue** or **hypodermis**. The hypodermis is a protective, insulating layer of fat (adipose tissue).

The epidermis is composed of stratified (many layers of) squamous epithelial cells. These cells are constantly sloughed off and then replenished by mitosis of cells at the deepest part of the epidermis, the **stratum basale**. A cell in this layer divides, and one of the resulting daughter cells moves outward. Soon this cell will die and be pushed farther and farther outward by continued mitosis below, until it flakes away from the surface of the body. The significance of many layers of epithelial cells is that they provide a strong protective structure.

Another important facet of the stratified squamous cells of the epidermis is that they are **keratinized**. This means that as they die, they become filled with a thick coating of the tough, hydrophobic protein **keratin**. Keratin helps make the skin waterproof.

Epidermal epithelial cells also contain **melanin**. This is a brown pigment, produced by specialized cells in the epidermis termed *melanocytes*, that helps absorb the ultraviolet light of the Sun to prevent damage to underlying tissues.

Beneath the epidermis lies the **dermis**. The dermis consists of various cell-types embedded in a connective tissue matrix. It contains blood vessels that nourish both the dermis and the epidermis (the epidermis has no blood vessels of its own). The dermis also contains **sensory receptors**, which convey information about touch, pressure, pain, and temperature to the central nervous system. Also found in the dermis are **sudoriferous** (sweat) glands, **sebaceous** (oil) glands, and **hair follicles**. Hairs consist of dead epithelial cells bound tightly together. Some specialized regions of skin contain **ceruminous** (wax) glands (e.g., the external ear canal).

The sudoriferous gland is composed of a tube-like structure that originates in the dermis and leads through the epidermis to a pore on the surface of the skin. The purpose of sweat is to allow loss of excess heat by evaporation. Sweat contains water, electrolytes, and urea. Sweat glands are responsive to aldosterone. People living in hot climates must sweat a lot. In order to conserve sodium, they have a high level of aldosterone, and thus their sweat does not waste salt.

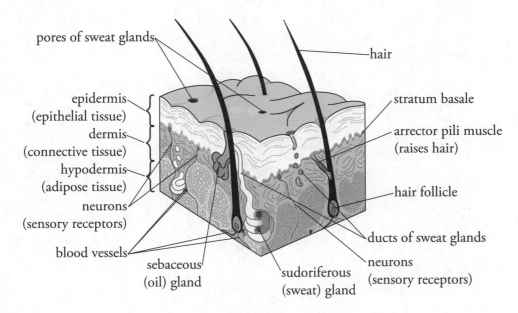

pores of sweat glands
hair

epidermis
(epithelial tissue)
stratum basale

dermis
(connective tissue)
arrector pili muscle
(raises hair)

hypodermis
(adipose tissue)
hair follicle

neurons
(sensory receptors)

blood vessels
ducts of sweat glands

neurons
(sensory receptors)

sebaceous
(oil) gland

sudoriferous
(sweat) gland

Figure 7   Skin Layers

12.7   TEMPERATURE REGULATION BY THE SKIN

Humans are **homeotherms**, meaning their body temperature is relatively constant. Heat is generated by metabolic processes and muscle contraction. Some homeotherms (e.g., bears) can maintain their temperature by burning special fat called **brown adipose tissue**; this process is called **chemical thermogenesis** or **nonshivering thermogenesis**. But this is *not* an important mechanism of temperature regulation in adult humans. Also, while it is true that an increased level of thyroid hormone can increase the metabolic rate and thus increase body temperature, this mechanism takes several weeks to kick in and is not thought to be important in day-to-day temperature regulation. So, practically, only four strategies are available to cope with cold weather:

1) Contraction of skeletal muscles produces heat, whether it is involuntary (shivering) or voluntary (jumping up and down).
2) The skin insulates us so that we conserve heat generated by metabolism. Subcutaneous (beneath the skin) tissue contains a layer of insulating fat, which helps.
3) Heat loss by conduction is minimized by constriction of blood vessels in the dermis (**cutaneous vasoconstriction**). Cutaneous vasoconstriction occurs in response to cold weather or upon activation of the sympathetic nervous system. This is why the skin becomes cold and pale when one is frightened.
4) Obviously, contrivances such as clothing and blankets help us conserve heat.

A mechanism for dissipation of excess heat is also necessary. This is accomplished by two mechanisms in the skin:

1) Sweating, which allows heat loss by evaporation
2) Dilation of blood vessels in the dermis (**cutaneous vasodilation**), which results in heat loss by conduction or convection, when air blows past the skin (as with a fan or a breeze)

Chapter 12 Summary

- The primary functions of the respiratory system are gas exchange and pH regulation. pH regulation by the respiratory system is very fast.

- The organs of the respiratory system are divided into the conduction zone and the respiratory zone.

- The conduction zone is for ventilation only and includes the nose and nasal cavity, the pharynx, the larynx, the trachea, and the respiratory tree from the primary bronchi to the terminal bronchioles.

- The larynx is made entirely of cartilage and includes the epiglottis (which separates food and air) and the vocal cords (for sound production).

- The respiratory zone is for gas exchange and includes the respiratory bronchioles, the alveolar ducts, and the alveoli.

- Surfactant reduces surface tension inside alveoli, making them easier to inflate.

- Inspiration is an active process and requires the contraction of the diaphragm to expand the chest cavity. An increase in the size of the chest cavity (and lungs) reduces their pressure, and air flows in.

- Expiration is primarily a passive process; the diaphragm relaxes and lung elastic recoil helps return them to their resting state. Forced expiration requires the contraction of the abdominal muscles to forcibly reduce the size of the chest cavity. In either case, the reduction in the size of the chest cavity increases their pressure and pushes the air out.

- Ventilation rate is determined primarily by P_{CO_2} and the need to regulate pH, according to the following equilibrium: $CO_2 + H_2O \rightleftharpoons H_2CO_3 \rightleftharpoons H^+ \rightleftharpoons + HCO_3^-$. As CO_2 levels increase, pH falls, and ventilation rate increases (the reverse is also true).

- The skin is made of three main layers: the epidermis (epithelial tissue), the dermis (connective tissue), and the hypodermis (adipose tissue).

- The epidermis provides a barrier to infection and water loss, the dermis is where sweat glands, nerves, blood vessels, and sensory receptors are found, and the hypodermis is a layer of fat for insulation and protection.

- Thermoregulation is primarily a function of the dermis. When temperatures rise, blood vessels in the dermis dilate to release heat, and sweat glands are activated. When temperature falls, blood vessels constrict to retain heat. Also, involuntary skeletal muscle contractions occur (shivering) to produce heat.

CHAPTER 12 FREESTANDING PRACTICE QUESTIONS

1. Patients injected with agents that paralyze muscles during surgeries must be artificially ventilated until they recover. These drugs interfere with which neurotransmitter?

    A) Acetylcholine
    B) Norepinephrine
    C) Dopamine
    D) GABA

2. A patient presents to the emergency room in diabetic ketoacidosis (DKA), a life-threatening complication of diabetes, which results in metabolic acidosis, as well as very high serum glucose levels. Which of the following vital signs would be expected in this patient, as compared to baseline?

    A) Increased blood pressure
    B) Increased respiratory rate
    C) Decreased heart rate
    D) Decreased respiratory rate

3. Patients can often alleviate symptoms of an asthma attack by using drugs called sympathomimetics that mimic the effects of norepinephrine. Based on this information, which is the most likely explanation for why patients with asthma have difficulty breathing?

    A) Constriction of bronchial smooth muscle leads to diminished air flow.
    B) Dilation of bronchial smooth muscle leads to diminished air flow.
    C) Constriction of smooth muscle surrounding blood vessels leads to decreased blood flow to the lungs.
    D) Interference with skeletal muscle neurons leads to decreased force of contraction of the diaphragm.

4. A middle-aged man is in a coma after a motor vehicle accident. His respiratory rate has significantly decreased due to trauma to the medulla. All of the following are true EXCEPT:

    A) there will be a decrease in the $[H^+]$ of his blood.
    B) normal regulation of ventilation rate has been disrupted.
    C) there will be an increase in P_{CO_2} of his blood.
    D) there will be a decrease in P_{O_2} of his blood.

5. All of the following are functions of the respiratory system EXCEPT:

    A) regulation of pH.
    B) protection from particulate matter.
    C) removal of nitrogenous waste.
    D) regulation of body temperature.

6. Which of the following homeostatic responses maximizes the dissipation of excess heat through the skin?

    A) Increased release and evaporation of sudoriferous gland secretions and constriction of dermal blood vessels
    B) Increased release and evaporation of sudoriferous gland secretions and dilation of dermal blood vessels
    C) Decreased release and evaporation of sudoriferous gland secretions and constriction of dermal blood vessels
    D) Decreased release and evaporation of sudoriferous gland secretions and dilation of dermal blood vessels

7. A cancer of the skin is more likely to involve which population of cells?

    A) Cells in the outer (most superficial) layer of the epidermis that have uncontrolled mitosis
    B) Cells in the outer (most superficial) layer of the epidermis that have uncontrolled meiosis
    C) Cells in the deepest layer of the epidermis that have uncontrolled mitosis
    D) Cells in the deepest layer of the epidermis that have uncontrolled meiosis

CHAPTER 12 PRACTICE PASSAGE

Occupational and environmental lung diseases are estimated to affect more than 20 million individuals in the United States alone. These diseases are generally caused by inhalation of toxic dusts and fumes and include silicosis, asbestosis, coal worker's pneumoconiosis (black lung disease), and berryliosis, as well as several diseases caused by the inhalation of dust and spores associated with agricultural businesses. Exposure to mineral dusts often leads to restrictive lung diseases (where the total lung capacity is reduced), whereas exposure to chemical agents leads to occupational asthma and other obstructive diseases (where air flow through the bronchial tubes is restricted).

Coal worker's pneumoconiosis (CWP) is a restrictive lung disease caused by long-term exposure to and inhalation of coal dust. Once inhaled, coal dust cannot be destroyed or removed, and consequently is simply engulfed by resident alveolar macrophages. These macrophages tend to aggregate and can be visualized microscopically as granular black areas that give the disease its common name. The aggregations lead to inflammation, damage to the lung tissue, fibrosis, and the formation of nodules throughout the lungs.

CWP is generally divided into simple and complicated classes. Simple CWP can develop early on from chronic exposure to coal dust; chest X-ray reveals nodules between 5 mm and 1 cm in diameter. Symptoms are similar to those experienced with cigarette smoking (cough, excess mucus, etc.). Upon continued, long-term exposure to coal dust (>10-15 years), simple CWP can progress to complicated CWP, which is characterized by lung nodules anywhere from 1 cm in diameter to the size of an entire lung lobe, significant reduction in lung volume and gas diffusion capacity, and premature mortality. Alveolar hypoxia can lead to pulmonary vasoconstriction; thus, complicated CWP can also be associated with right-side heart failure (*cor pulmonare*).

Lung function can be assessed by measurement of flow volumes during inspiration and expiration. Obstructive diseases tend to have increased total lung capacity and residual volume along with reduced flow. Restrictive diseases caused by damage to lung tissue tend to have reduced lung capacity and residual volumes, but normal flow. Restrictive diseases caused by damage to the inspiratory muscles or chest wall have reduced lung capacity, increased residual volume, and reduced flow. Figure 1 shows the expiratory flow-volume curves for four different patients.

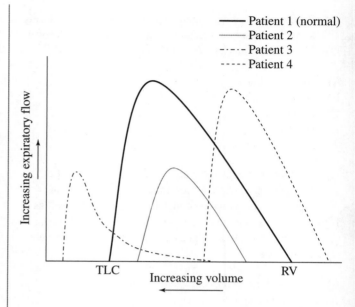

Figure 1 Expiratory flow-volume curves. Total lung capacity (TLC) and residual volume (RV) are indicated on the normal curve.

1. Agonistic drugs increase a particular response, while antagonistic drugs reduce a response. Which of the following drugs would be the best choice to treat occupational asthma?

A) Parasympathetic agonist
B) Parasympathetic antagonist
C) Sympathetic agonist
D) Sympathetic antagonist

2. The FEV_1 is a measurement of the total amount of air that can be forcibly expired in 1 second after a complete inhalation. In which of the following conditions would a reduced FEV_1 be expected?

I. CWP
II. Occupational asthma
III. Chronic obstructive pulmonary disease (COPD)

A) I only
B) II only
C) II and III only
D) I, II, and III

3. Which of the following would NOT be associated with complicated CWP?

A) Lung nodules 2–3 cm in diameter
B) Decreased pressure in the pulmonary vasculature
C) Right ventricular hypertrophy
D) Granular blackened areas in the lungs

4. Botulism is a type of food poisoning in which a toxin released by the bacteria *Clostridium botulinum* inhibits the release of acetylcholine from motor neurons. In severe cases, this can lead to paralysis of the diaphragm. Which of the following would be expected in an individual suffering from severe botulism?

A) Decreased total lung capacity, decreased residual volume, and normal flow
B) Decreased total lung capacity, increased residual volume, and decreased flow
C) Increased total lung capacity, decreased residual volume, and normal flow
D) Increased total lung capacity, increased residual volume, and decreased flow

5. Which of the following statements about the respiratory system is true?

A) The ratio of cartilage to smooth muscle decreases as the bronchial tubes branch smaller and smaller.
B) The respiratory zone participates in gas exchange only, while the conduction zone participates in both ventilation and gas exchange.
C) Contraction of the diaphragm is mediated entirely by the autonomic nervous system.
D) An increase in carbon dioxide leads to an accumulation of carbonic acid, a decrease in blood pH, and a decrease in ventilation rate.

6. Which of the patients in Figure 1 is most likely suffering from CWP?

A) Patient 1
B) Patient 2
C) Patient 3
D) Patient 4

SOLUTIONS TO CHAPTER 12 FREESTANDING PRACTICE QUESTIONS

1. **A** The diaphragm is the primary ventilatory muscle; it is a skeletal muscle, and acetylcholine is the neurotransmitter that mediates nerve transmission to skeletal muscle (choice A is correct). Norepinephrine is the neurotransmitter used at postsynaptic synapses in the sympathetic nervous system; although interference with this neurotransmitter could affect the smooth muscle surrounding the bronchi, it would not affect the diaphragm and ventilation (choice B is incorrect). Dopamine and GABA are neurotransmitters that are found only in the central nervous system; paralysis in these patients is produced at the level of the muscle itself, not the central nervous system (choices C and D are incorrect).

2. **B** The metabolic acidosis (decreased blood pH) would lead to hyperventilation (increased respiratory rate) in an attempt to compensate for the low pH by reducing the amount of CO_2 (thus raising the pH; choice B is correct, and choice D is wrong). It is important to remember the equation: $CO_2 + H_2O \rightleftharpoons H_2CO_3 \rightleftharpoons H^+ + HCO_3^-$. This is enough to answer the question; however, it is also true that patients in DKA have very high levels of serum glucose, which overwhelm the glucose reabsorption mechanisms of the kidney, leading to glucose in the urine. This glucose has an osmotic pressure effect and leads to severe water loss in the urine (diuresis). This in turn leads to potentially severe dehydration, which would ultimately result in lower blood pressure (choice A is incorrect), and elevated heart rates (choice C is incorrect).

3. **A** In asthma, constriction of bronchial smooth muscle decreases the diameter of the bronchi, leading to diminished air flow. Sympathomimetics stimulate the adrenergic receptors on smooth muscle, causing the muscle to dilate and improving air flow through the bronchi (choice A is correct). Dilation of bronchial smooth muscle would improve air flow, rather than diminish it, as flow is proportional to diameter (choice B is incorrect). Norepinephrine causes constriction of smooth muscle around blood vessels, not dilation, which would lead to less blood flow to the lungs. In any case, asthma is primarily a problem of ventilation (moving air in and out), not perfusion (the flow of blood to the lungs; choice C is incorrect). Acetylcholine, not norepinephrine, is the neurotransmitter that mediates contraction of skeletal muscle (choice D is incorrect).

4. **A** The centers that regulate respiratory rate are found in the medulla. Since the question text states his respiratory rate has significantly decreased due to trauma in this region, the normal feedback mechanisms (such as pH and P) will not be effective in restoring normal ventilatory patterns (choice B is true and can be eliminated). The reduced rate of respiration will lead to an accumulation of CO_2 and a drop in O_2 in his blood (choices C and D are true and can be eliminated). The excess CO_2 will shift the equilibrium of $CO_2 + H_2O \rightleftharpoons H_2CO_3 \rightleftharpoons H^+ + HCO_3^-$ to the right, leading to an increase in $[H^+]$ and a drop in pH (choice A is false and is the correct answer choice).

5. **C** The respiratory system participates in pH regulation via changes in the ventilation rate. An increase in ventilation (hyperventilation) will lead to rapid removal of CO_2 and, due to the carbonic anhydrase buffer system, an increase in the pH ($CO_2 + H_2O \rightleftharpoons H_2CO_3 \rightleftharpoons H^+ + HCO_3^-$). A decrease in ventilation (hypoventilation) will lead to a decrease in pH (choice A is a function of the respiratory system and can be eliminated). The mucociliary escalator protects the body from particulate matter by either swallowing or coughing out the mucus-coated particle (choice B is a function of the respiratory system and can be eliminated). Hyperventilation also leads to heat loss; in order to dissipate excess heat, dogs depend on panting (choice D is a function of the respiratory system and can be eliminated). However, the respiratory system is not involved in the removal of nitrogenous waste; that is a function of the renal excretory system (choice C is not a function of the respiratory system and is the correct answer choice).

6. **B** Sudoriferous (sweat) glands are exocrine glands found within the skin that secrete water and electrolytes. As water evaporates from the skin surface, heat is dissipated. Thus, the hotter you are, the more you sweat (choices C and D are wrong). Dilating dermal blood vessels will increase blood flow to the skin and increase conductive heat loss (choice B is correct, and choice A is wrong).

7. **C** Meiosis only occurs in sperm and ova (choices B and D are wrong). Stem cells (basal cells) located in the deepest layer of the epidermis undergo mitosis throughout an individual's life. With each mitotic event, daughter cells arise, move outward (superficially), and differentiate as they do so; eventually, they die and are sloughed off. The daughter cells that differentiate lose their ability to divide; thus, it is more likely that the stem cells (which retain their ability to divide) could develop into a cancer (choice C is a better answer than choice A).

SOLUTIONS TO CHAPTER 12 PRACTICE PASSAGE

1. **C** The passage states that occupational asthma is characterized by restricted air flow through bronchial tubes. Activation of the sympathetic nervous system leads to dilation of these tubes; thus, a sympathetic agonist would be the best choice in this case (choice C is correct, and choice D is wrong). Activation of the parasympathetic system would worsen the air flow, since it leads to bronchial constriction (choice A is wrong). While a parasympathetic antagonist might help, a sympathetic agonist would have a faster and stronger response (choice C is better than choice B).

2. **C** Reduced FEV_1 measurements are typically seen in conditions where air flow is reduced. Item I is false: coal worker's pneumoconiosis is described in the passage as a restrictive disease caused by lung-tissue damage; thus, total lung capacity would be reduced but flow would be normal (choices A and D can be eliminated). Since both remaining answer choices include Item II, Item II must be true and you can focus on Item III. Item III is true: the passage states that obstructive diseases are characterized by reduced air flow (choice B can be eliminated, and choice C is correct). Note that Item II is in fact true: occupational asthma is classified in the passage as an obstructive disease. Note: In Figure 1, the curve for Patient 3 is what would be expected for an obstructive disease; the drop to residual volume is gradual, indicating a reduced flow rate.

3. **B** The passage states that "alveolar hypoxia can lead to pulmonary vasoconstriction," which would increase pulmonary pressures, not decrease them (choice B would not be associated with complicated CWP and is the correct answer choice). The increased pulmonary pressure could lead to a hypertrophy (increase in size) of the right ventricle in order to generate a stronger force with which to move the blood against the higher pressure (choice C could be associated and can be eliminated). Complicated CWP is associated with lung nodules greater than 1 cm in diameter (choice A can be eliminated) and both simple and complicated CWP would have granular blackened areas in the lungs (choice D can be eliminated).

4. **B** This is a two-by-two question, in which two decisions determine the correct answer choice. The passage states that damage to the inspiratory muscles (of which the diaphragm is the primary muscle) can lead to restrictive lung disease characterized by reduced total lung capacity (choices C and D can be eliminated), increased residual volume (choice A can be eliminated), and decreased flow.

5. **A** Most of the cartilage is found near the top of the bronchial tree. After the tertiary bronchial tubes, the cartilage disappears altogether and the tubes are formed out of smooth muscle (choice A is true and the correct answer choice). The conduction zone only participates in ventilation, not gas exchange (choice B is false and can be eliminated). The diaphragm is skeletal muscle and its contraction is predominantly mediated by somatic neurons (and is under voluntary control; choice C is false and can be eliminated). It is true that increased CO_2 would lead to an accumulation of carbonic acid and a decrease in blood pH, but that would cause an increase in ventilation rate in order to remove the excess CO_2 (choice D is false and can be eliminated).

6. **D** Patient 1 is listed on the figure legend as "normal," so choice A can be eliminated first. CWP is a restrictive lung disease caused by damage to the lung tissue, due to chronic inhalation of coal dust. As described in the final paragraph, a patient suffering from this disease would have a reduced total lung capacity (choice C, Patient 3, has an increased total lung capacity and can be eliminated), and a reduced residual volume (choice B, Patient 2, has an increased residual volume and can be eliminated). Note that the x-axis (volume) increases to the left in this figure.

Chapter 13
The Reproductive Systems

13.1 THE MALE REPRODUCTIVE SYSTEM

Anatomy

The principal male reproductive structures that are visible on the outside of the body are the scrotum and the penis. The scrotum is essentially a bag of skin containing the male gonads, which are known as **testes** (testicles). [Does the scrotum have any active role, or is it merely a container?[1]] The testes have two roles: 1) synthesis of sperm (**spermatogenesis**), and 2) secretion of male sex hormones (**androgens**, e.g., testosterone) into the bloodstream. More detail on these topics is given later. Here we will trace the path of a sperm from its origination to its final destination.

The sites of spermatogenesis within the testes are the **seminiferous tubules**. The walls of the seminiferous tubules are formed by cells called **sustentacular cells** (also known as *Sertoli cells*). Sustentacular cells protect and nurture the developing sperm, both physically and chemically; their role will be discussed in more detail below. The tissue between the seminiferous tubules is simply referred to as testicular interstitium.[2] Important cells found in the testicular interstitium are the **interstitial cells** (also known as Leydig cells). They are responsible for androgen (testosterone) synthesis.

The seminiferous tubules empty into the **epididymis**, a long coiled tube located on the posterior (back) of each testicle (Figure 1). The epididymis from each testicle empties into a **ductus deferens** (also called the *vas deferens*), which in turn leads to the **urethra** (the tube inside the penis). To get to the urethra, the ductus deferens leaves the scrotum and follows a peculiar path: it enters the **inguinal canal**, a tunnel that travels along the body wall toward the crest of the hip bone. (There are two inguinal canals, left and right.) From the inguinal canal, the ductus deferens enters the pelvic cavity. Near the back of the urinary bladder, it joins the duct of the seminal vesicle (discussed below) to form the **ejaculatory duct**. The ejaculatory ducts from both sides of the body then join the urethra.

A pair of glands known as **seminal vesicles** is located on the posterior surface of the bladder. They secrete about 60 percent of the total volume of the **semen** into the ejaculatory duct. Semen is a highly nourishing fluid for sperm and is produced by three separate glands: the seminal vesicles, the **prostate**, and the **bulbourethral glands**. These are collectively referred to as the **accessory glands** (see Table 1). The ejaculatory duct empties into the **urethra** as it passes through the prostate gland. One final set of glands, the bulbourethral glands, contributes to the semen near the beginning of the urethra.

Table 1   The Accessory Glands

Gland and secretions	Function of secretions	% of total ejaculate volume
Seminal vesicles—mostly fructose	Nourishment of sperm	60%
Prostate gland—fructose and a coagulant	Nourishment, allows semen to coagulate after ejaculation	35%
Bulbourethral glands—thick, alkaline mucus	Lubricate urethra, neutralize acids in male urethra and in female vagina	3%
Testes—sperm	Male gamete	2%

---

[1] The scrotum is important for temperature regulation. Sperm synthesis in the testes must occur at a few degrees below normal body temperature. This is why the testes are located outside the body. Relaxation of the scrotum facilitates cooling of the testes. When the environment is cold, the scrotum contracts, pulling the testes up against the body, warming them.

[2] *Interstitium* is a term used to describe a thing or a region which is "between" other structures.

The urethra exits the body via the penis. Penile erection facilitates deposition of semen near the opening of the uterus during intercourse. Specialized **erectile tissue** in the penis allows erection. It is composed of modified veins and capillaries surrounded by a connective tissue sheath. Erection occurs when blood accumulates at high pressure in the erectile tissue. Three compartments contain erectile tissue: the **corpora cavernosa** (there are two of these) and the **corpus spongiosum** (only one).

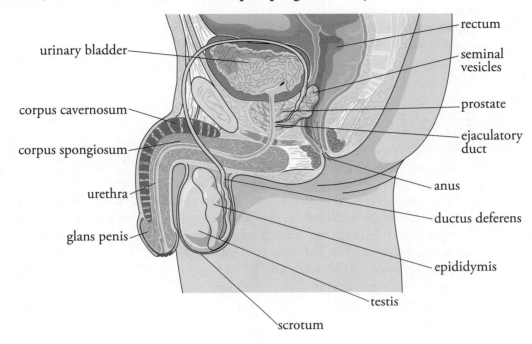

Figure 1   The Male Reproductive System

The Male Sexual Act

The three stages of the male sexual act are arousal, orgasm, and resolution. These events are controlled by an integrating center in the spinal cord, which responds to physical stimulation and input from the brain. The cerebral cortex can activate this integrating center (as in sexual arousal during sleep) or inhibit it (anxiety interferes with sexual function).

Arousal is dependent upon parasympathetic nervous input and can be subdivided into two stages: erection and lubrication. **Erection** involves dilation of arteries supplying the erectile tissue. This causes swelling, which in turn obstructs venous outflow. This causes the erectile tissue to become pressurized with blood. **Lubrication** is also a function of the parasympathetic system. The bulbourethral glands secrete a viscous mucous which serves as a lubricant.

Stimulation by the sympathetic nervous system is required for **orgasm**, which can also be divided into two stages: emission and ejaculation. **Emission** refers to the propulsion of sperm (from the ductus deferens) and semen (from the accessory glands) into the urethra by contractions of the smooth muscle surrounding these organs. Emission is followed by **ejaculation**, in which semen is propelled out of the urethra by rhythmic contractions of muscles surrounding the base of the penis. Ejaculation is actually a reflex reaction caused by the presence of semen in the urethra. Emission and ejaculation together constitute the male orgasm.

Resolution, or a return to a normal, unstimulated state, is also controlled by the sympathetic nervous system. It is caused primarily by a constriction of the erectile arteries. This results in decreased blood flow to the erectile tissue and allows the veins to carry away the trapped blood, returning the penis to a flaccid state. This typically takes 2–3 minutes.

- Name four glands that contribute to semen.[3]
- Which components of the male sexual act can occur if all sympathetic activity is blocked?[4]
- What is the difference between emission and ejaculation?[5]

13.2 SPERMATOGENESIS

What processes in a human being involve meiosis? Only one: **gametogenesis**. This is the process whereby **diploid germ cells** undergo **meiotic division** to produce **haploid gametes**. As discussed in Chapter 7, meiotic cell division fosters genetic diversity in the population (by independent assortment of genes and by recombination). The gametes produced by the male are known as **spermatozoa**, or *sperm*; females produce **ova**, or *eggs*. The role of the sperm is to swim through the female genital tract to reach the egg and fuse with it. This fusion is known as **syngamy**, and it results in a **zygote**. The gametes produced by males and females differ dramatically in structure but contribute equally to the genome of the zygote (except in the special case of the two different sex chromosomes, X and Y, given to male offspring). Although both gametes contribute equally to the genome, the egg provides *every other part of the zygote*, since the only part of the sperm which enters the egg is a haploid genome. The term for this is **maternal inheritance**. For instance, mitochondria are inherited maternally.

Sperm synthesis is called **spermatogenesis** (Figure 2). It begins at puberty and occurs in the testes throughout adult life. [Do females also make gametes throughout adult life?[6]] The seminiferous tubule is the site of spermatogenesis. The entire process of spermatogenesis occurs with the aid of the specialized sustentacular cells found in the wall of the seminiferous tubule. Immature sperm precursors are found in the outer wall of the tubule, and nearly mature spermatozoa are deposited into the lumen; from there they are transported to the epididymis. The cells that give rise to spermatogonia (and to their female counterparts, oogonia) are known as **germ cells**; under the right conditions, they *germ*inate, and give rise to a complete organism.

---

[3] Seminal vesicles, prostate, testes, and bulbourethral glands

[4] Erection and lubrication (arousal only)

[5] Emission is the movement of sperm and semen components into the urethra; ejaculation is the movement of semen from the urethra out of the body.

[6] No. This is discussed later.

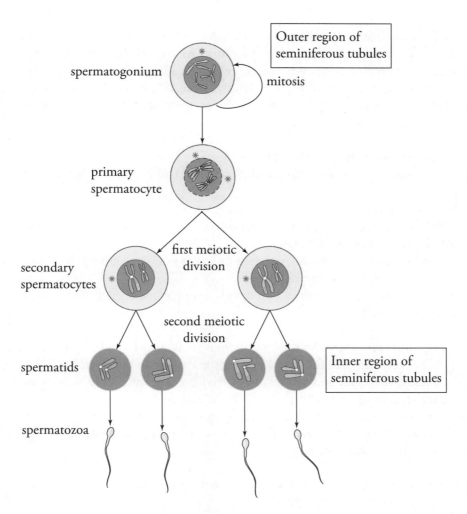

Figure 2   Spermatogenesis

Table 2 below gives the names of the sperm precursors, along with the meiotic role of each stage, and some mnemonic comments. Fill in the female version when you read that section.

Table 2   Gametogenesis

Stage	Jobs	Mnemonic	Female version
spermatogonium	1. Mitotically reproduce prior to meiosis 2. Replicate DNA in S phase of meiosis	The spermatoGONium is GONNA become a sperm.	
primary spermatocyte	Meiosis I	Any gamete precursor (male or female) with "cyte" undergoes a meiotic division.	
secondary spermatocyte	Meiosis II	The *secondary* spermatoCYTE undergoes the *second* meiotic division.	
spermatid	Turn into a spermatozoan	The spermatid's a kid, almost mature	
spermatozoan	Finish maturing: 1. in seminiferous tubule 2. in epididymis	Just remember that a mature sperm is called a spermatozoan.	

As noted in Table 2, the final stages of sperm maturation occur in the epididymis. When they first enter the epididymis, spermatozoa are incapable of motility. Many days later, when they reach the ductus deferens, they are fully capable of motility. But they remain inactive due to the presence of inhibitory substances secreted by the ductus deferens. This inactivity causes sperm to have a very low metabolic rate, which allows them to conserve energy and thus remain fertile during storage in the ductus deferens for as long as a month.

- Do spermatogonia divide by mitosis or by meiosis?[7]
- How many mature sperm result from a single spermatogonium after it becomes committed to meiosis?[8]
- Which of the following statements is/are true?[9]
    - I.   During gametogenesis, sister chromatids remain paired with each other until anaphase of the second meiotic cell division.
    - II. A difference between mitosis and meiosis is that mitosis requires DNA replication prior to cell division but meiosis does not.
    - III. Recombination between sister chromatids during gametogenesis increases the genetic diversity of offspring.

Spermatids develop into spermatozoa in the seminiferous tubules with the aid of sustentacular cells. The DNA condenses, the cytoplasm shrinks, and the cell shape changes so that there is a **head**, containing the haploid nucleus and the acrosome, and a flagellum which forms the **tail**. There is also a **neck** region at the base of the tail, which contains many mitochondria. [Where do these mitochondria get their energy?[10]] The **acrosome** is a compartment on the head of the sperm that contains hydrolytic enzymes required for penetration of the ovum's protective layers. **Bindin** is a protein on the sperm's surface that attaches to receptors on the zona pellucida surrounding the ovum (discussed below).

- Concerning spermatogenesis, which of the following is/are true?[11]
    - I.   Spermatocytes possess a flagellum.
    - II. Flagellar movement of sperm involves rotation of a basal structure embedded in the sperm membrane.
    - III. Spermatids possess a haploid genome.

Hormonal Control of Spermatogenesis

Testosterone plays the essential role of stimulating division of spermatogonia. **Luteinizing hormone (LH)** stimulates the interstitial cells to secrete testosterone. **Follicle stimulating hormone (FSH)** stimulates the sustentacular cells. The hormone **inhibin** is secreted by sustentacular cells; its role is to inhibit

---

[7] Mitosis. Spermatogonia undergo the meiotic S phase (replicate the genome), but the stages which undergo the actual meiotic *divisions* are called spermatocytes. *All* gamete precursors with "cyte" in their name undergo a meiotic division.

[8] Four haploid cells result from the reductive division (meiosis) of one diploid spermatogonium. Compare this to oogenesis.

[9] **Item I: True.** Meiosis I involves the pairing, recombination, and separation of homologous chromosomes. Meiosis II is like mitosis, where sister chromatids separate. Item II: False. Both require DNA replication in a preceding S phase. Item III: False. Sister chromatids don't recombine, homologous chromosomes do. (Even if sister chromatids did recombine, it would make no difference since they are identical.)

[10] From the fructose which the seminal vesicles contribute to the semen and from vaginal secretions.

[11] Item I: False. The flagellum does not begin to form until the spermatid stage. Item II: False. This describes prokaryotic flagella. **Item III: True.** Meiosis is complete by the spermatid stage. Remember, the spermatid's a kid. It's just like a sperm, only immature.

FSH release. [From where, and why?[12]]

- Which of the following is/are true?[13]
    I. Luteinizing hormone reaches its target tissue through the hypothalamic-hypophysial portal system.
    II. The absence of luteinizing hormone does not affect spermatogenesis.
    III. Increased testosterone levels in the blood decrease the production of follicle stimulating hormone.

13.3 DEVELOPMENT OF THE MALE REPRODUCTIVE SYSTEM

The gender of a developing embryo is determined by its sex chromosomes, either XX in females or XY in males. During the early weeks of development, however, male and female embryos are indistinguishable. Early embryos, whether male or female, have undifferentiated gonads, and possess both **Wolffian ducts** that can develop into male internal genitalia (epididymis, seminal vesicles, and ductus deferens) and **Müllerian ducts** that can develop into female internal genitalia (uterine tubes, uterus, and vagina). In the absence of a Y chromosome, Müllerian duct development occurs by default, and female internal genitalia result. Female *external* genitalia (labia, clitoris) are also the default; note that the external genitalia are not derived from the Müllerian ducts. Genetic information on the Y chromosome of XY embryos leads to the development of testes, which cause male internal and external genitalia to develop by producing testosterone and **Müllerian inhibiting factor** (**MIF**).

MIF is produced by the testes and causes regression of the Müllerian ducts; this prevents the development of female internal genitalia. Testosterone secretion by cells which will later give rise to the testes begins around week 7 of gestation. By week 9, testes are formed, and their interstitial cells supply testosterone. The testosterone that is responsible for the development of male external genitalia enters the systemic circulation and must be converted to **dihydrotestosterone** in target tissues in order to exert its effect (Figure 3 on the next page).

- If an XY genotype embryo fails to secrete testosterone, will it have testes or ovaries?[14]

---

[12] FSH and LH are gonadotropins secreted by the anterior pituitary. The reason this occurs is to provide negative feedback.

[13] Item I: False. LH is secreted by the anterior pituitary and reaches its targets via the systemic circulation. GnRH reaches its target via the portal system. Item II: False. LH is necessary because it stimulates the interstitial cells to secrete testosterone, which is necessary for germ cell stimulation. **Item III: True.** Testosterone, estrogen, progesterone, and inhibin are all hormones that exert feedback inhibition upon the anterior pituitary and hypothalamus.

[14] Testosterone is *produced by* the embryonic testes. Their development does not depend on testosterone. Therefore, an XY embryo which didn't secrete testosterone would most likely have testes nonetheless.

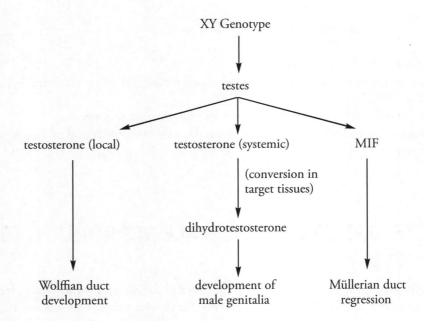

Figure 3 Control of Development of the Male Reproductive System

- Which one of the following would best characterize an embryo with an XY genotype that lacks the receptor for testosterone?[15]
    - A) Testes, ductus deferens, and seminal vesicles are present; external genitalia are female.
    - B) Ovaries, uterine tubes, and uterus are present; external genitalia are female.
    - C) Testes are present; external genitalia are female; neither Müllerian nor Wolffian ducts develop.
    - D) Testes and male external genitalia are present.

The development of the male and female reproductive systems is closely related. As described above, the three main fetal precursors of the reproductive organs are the Wolffian ducts, the Müllerian ducts, and the gonads. While the Wolffian ducts are the precursors of internal male genitalia, they essentially disappear in the female reproductive system. For the Müllerian ducts, this process is reversed; they essentially disappear in the male reproductive system and form the internal genitalia of the female reproductive system. Structures arising from these ducts tend to have the same function (e.g., ductus deferens in males and the uterine tubes in females both carry gametes), but because they arise from different precursors, they are considered to be **analogous structures**.

In both sexes, the gonads go on to form either the testes or the ovaries; because they are derived from the same undeveloped structure, testes and ovaries are considered homologous organs. There are a number of other homologous structures in males and females due to their common origins within the fetus (see Table 3).

---

[15] The XY genotype would lead to the development of testes (choice B is wrong), and the testes would produce MIF and testosterone. MIF would cause the degeneration of the Müllerian ducts, and no female internal genitalia would develop. However, the inability to respond to testosterone (because of the missing receptor) would prevent the development of the Wolffian ducts (choice A is wrong) as well as the male external genitalia (choice D is wrong). The external genitalia would default to female (choice **C** is correct).

Table 3 Homologous Reproductive Structures

Male Organ	Female Organ	Function
Testis	Ovary	Gamete and hormone reproduction
Penis	Clitoris	Erectile tissue, sensation
Bulbourethral glands	Greater vestibular glands	Lubrication
Scrotum	Labia majora	External skin folds

13.4 ANDROGENS AND ESTROGENS

All hormones involved in the development and maintenance of male characteristics are termed **androgens**, while those involved in development and maintenance of female characteristics are termed **estrogens**. The primary androgen produced in the testes is testosterone. It is converted into dihydrotestosterone within the cells of target tissues. The primary estrogen produced in the ovaries is estradiol.

Testosterone is required in the testes for spermatogenesis (Section 13.2). The role of testosterone in the embryonic development of the male internal and external genitalia has already been discussed. After birth the level of testosterone falls to negligible levels until puberty, at which time it increases and remains high for the remainder of adult life. Elevated levels of testosterone are responsible for the development and maintenance of male **secondary sexual characteristics** (maturation of the genitalia, male distribution of facial and body hair, deepening of the voice, and increased muscle mass). The pubertal growth spurt and fusion of the epiphyses (see Chapter 11) also result.

The role of estrogen in the female is analogous to the role of testosterone in the male. Beginning at puberty, estrogen is required to regulate the uterine cycle and for the development and maintenance of female secondary sexual characteristics (maturation of the genitalia, breast development, wider hips, and pubic hair). Estrogen causes the fusion of the epiphyses in females.

- Why are tumors derived from interstitial cells more easily diagnosed in boys than in grown men?[16]
- If testosterone levels are abnormally elevated during childhood, how will the height of the individual be affected?[17]
- How do androgens reach the cytoplasm to bind to cytoplasmic receptors?[18]
- How would an RNA polymerase II inhibitor alter the effects of dihydrotestosterone in target cells?[19]
- Which is the more abundant androgen in the blood: testosterone or dihydrotestosterone?[20]

---

[16] Interstitial cells secrete testosterone. Levels of testosterone are normally very low in boys. An abnormal increase will lead to puberty at an abnormally young age ("precocious puberty"). The results would be less obvious in an adult male.

[17] The child will undergo precocious puberty, involving an early growth spurt, so the child will be unusually tall. But then early fusion of the epiphyses will result in a shorter adult height than expected.

[18] These highly hydrophobic molecules can diffuse through the cell membrane and bind to cytoplasmic receptors.

[19] Once its ligand is bound, the steroid receptor activates transcription of specific mRNA. Messenger RNA is transcribed by RNA pol II. Therefore, we would expect inhibition of pol II to prevent the effects of all steroid hormones.

[20] The concentration of testosterone is higher. Dihydrotestosterone is produced from testosterone inside target cells. It is present in the blood in much lower concentrations than testosterone.

During puberty and adult life, sex steroid production is controlled by the hypothalamus and the anterior pituitary. **Gonadotropin releasing hormone (GnRH)** from the hypothalamus stimulates the pituitary to release the gonadotropins: follicle-stimulating hormone (FSH) and luteinizing hormone (LH). In men, LH acts on interstitial cells to stimulate testosterone production, and FSH stimulates the sustentacular cells. In women FSH stimulates the granulosa cells to secrete estrogen, and LH simulates the formation of the corpus luteum and progesterone secretion. Feedback inhibition by the steroids inhibits the production of GnRH and LH and FSH. Inhibin, produced by sustentacular cells and the granulosa cells, provides further feedback regulation of FSH production (Figure 4).

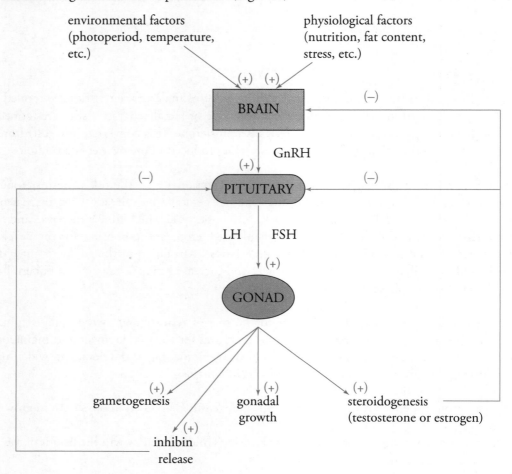

Figure 4   Regulation of Sex Steroid Production

13.5   THE FEMALE REPRODUCTIVE SYSTEM

Anatomy and Development

We mentioned in Section 13.3 that male and female genitalia are derived from a common undifferentiated precursor. Because of this, the structures of the female external genitalia are homologous to those of the male. In the female, the XX genotype leads to the formation of ovaries capable of secreting the female sex hormones (estrogens) instead of testes that secrete androgens. In the male, testosterone causes a pair of skin folds known as **labioscrotal swellings** to grow and fuse, forming the scrotum. In the female, without the influence of testosterone, the labioscrotal swellings form the **labia majora** of the vagina (labia = lips, majora = larger). The structure that gave rise to the penis in the male embryo becomes the **clitoris** in the female, located within the labia majora in the uppermost part of the vulva. Just beneath the clitoris is the **urethral opening**, where urine exits the body. Surrounding the urethral opening is another pair of skin folds called the **labia minora**.

The opening of the **vagina** is also found between the labia minora. The female internal genitalia (vagina, uterine tubes, uterus) are derived from the Müllerian ducts, so there are no homologous structures in the male. The vagina is a tube which would end in the pelvic cavity, except that another hollow organ, the **uterus**, opens into its upper portion. The part of the uterus which opens into the vagina is called the **cervix** ("neck," as in "cervical"). The innermost lining of the uterus (closest to the lumen) is the **endometrium**. It is responsible for nourishing a developing embryo, and in the absence of pregnancy, it is shed each month, producing menstrual bleeding. Surrounding the endometrium is the **myometrium**, which is a thick layer of smooth muscle comprising the wall of the uterus. The uterus ends in two **uterine tubes** (also called *fallopian tubes*), which extend into the pelvis on either side. Each uterine tube ends in a bunch of finger-like structures called **fimbriae**. The fimbriae brush up against the **ovary**, which is the female gonad. [At the time of ovulation, where does the oocyte come from and where does it go?[21]]

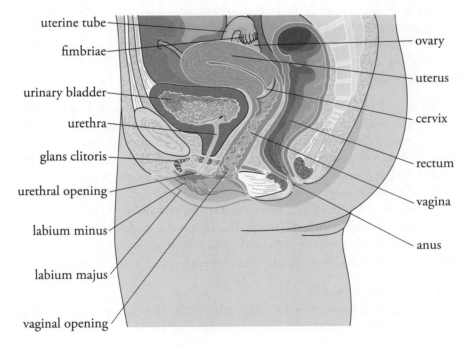

Figure 5   The Female Reproductive System

- What is the fate of the Wolffian ducts and their derivatives in the female?[22]
- Is estrogen production by the ovaries required for the development of the uterine tubes and uterus?[23]

---

[21] It emerges from the ovary (sometimes causing pain in the middle of the menstrual cycle) and must be swept into the uterine tube by a constant flow of fluid into the uterine tube caused by cilia.

[22] In the absence of testosterone, they atrophy.

[23] No, the Müllerian ducts develop into vagina, uterus, and uterine tubes by default as long as MIF is absent.

The Female Sexual Act

The stages are the same as in the male: **arousal**, **orgasm**, and **resolution**. The arousal stage, as in the male, is subdivided into erection and lubrication and is controlled by the parasympathetic nervous system. The clitoris and labia minora contain erectile tissue and become engorged with blood, just as in the male. Lubrication is provided by mucus secreted by **greater vestibular glands** and by the vaginal epithelium. Orgasm in the female is controlled by the sympathetic nervous system and involves muscle contractions, just as in the male, in addition to a widening of the cervix. (These events are thought to facilitate the movement of sperm into the uterus.) The female does not experience ejaculation. Resolution is also the same as in the male, controlled by the sympathetic system, but can take up to 20–30 minutes (compared to 2–3 minutes in the male).

13.6   OOGENESIS AND OVULATION

Oogenesis begins prenatally. In the ovary of a female fetus, germ cells divide mitotically to produce large numbers of **oogonia**. [How is this different from the male scenario?[24]] Oogonia not only undergo mitosis *in utero*, but they also enter the first phase of meiosis and are arrested in prophase I (as primary oocytes). The number of oogonia peaks at about 7 million at mid-gestation (20 weeks into fetal development). At this time mitosis ceases, conversion to primary oocytes begins, and there is a progressive loss of cells so that at birth there are only about 2 million primary oocytes. By puberty this number is further reduced to only about 400,000. Only about 400 oocytes are ever actually **ovulated** (released) in the average woman, and the remaining 99.9 percent will simply degenerate.

The primary oocytes formed in a female fetus can be frozen in prophase I of meiosis for decades, until they re-enter the meiotic cycle. Beginning at puberty and continuing on a monthly basis, hormonal changes in the woman's body stimulate completion of the first meiotic division and ovulation. This meiotic division yields a large secondary oocyte (containing all of the cytoplasm and organelles) and a small **polar body** (containing half the DNA, but no cytoplasm or organelles). The polar body (called the *first* polar body) remains in close proximity to the oocyte. The second meiotic division (i.e., completion of oogenesis) occurs *only if* the secondary oocyte is fertilized by a sperm; this division is also unequal, producing a large ovum and the second polar body. Note that if fertilization does occur, the nuclei from the sperm and egg do not fuse immediately. They must wait for the secondary oocyte to release the second polar body and finish maturing to an ootid and then an ovum. Finally, the two nuclei fuse, and a diploid ($2n$) zygote is formed.

- Is the secondary oocyte haploid?[25]
- When an oogonium undergoes meiosis, three cells result. How many of these are eggs, and why do only three cells result? (Meiosis results in four cells in the male.)[26]

Before we move on to a discussion of the menstrual cycle, you will need more background information on oogenesis. The primary oocyte is not an isolated cell. It is found in a clump of supporting cells called **granulosa cells**, and the entire structure (oocyte plus granulosa cells) is known as a **follicle**. The granulosa cells assist in maturation. [What is the male counterpart of the granulosa cell?[27]] An immature primary oocyte is surrounded by a single layer of granulosa cells, forming a **primordial follicle**.

---

[24] It only happens in *adult* males. Here, we're talking about events in the ovaries of a female while she's still in her mother's womb.

[25] Yes. After the first meiotic division, the cell is haploid; the homologous chromosomes have been separated. (They are, however, still replicated, hence the reason for meiosis II.)

[26] Only one egg results. The three cells which result are two polar bodies plus one ovum. There are only three because the first polar body does not divide. (In meiosis in the male, both cells derived from the first meiotic division go on to divide.)

[27] The cells that support and nurture developing spermatocytes are the sustentacular cells.

As the primordial follicle matures, the granulosa cells proliferate to form several layers around the oocyte, and the oocyte itself forms a protective layer of mucopolysaccharides termed the **zona pellucida**. There may be several follicles in the ovary; they are surrounded and separated by cells termed **thecal cells**. [What is the male counterpart of the thecal cells, and to which hormone do they respond?[28]] Of the several maturing follicles, only one progresses to the point of ovulation each month; all others degenerate. The mature follicle is known as a **Graafian follicle**. During ovulation, the Graafian follicle bursts, releasing the secondary oocyte with its zona pellucida and protective granulosa cells into the fallopian tube. At this point the layer of granulosa cells surrounding the ovum is known as the **corona radiata**. The follicular cells remaining in the ovary after ovulation form a new structure called the **corpus luteum** (Figure 6).

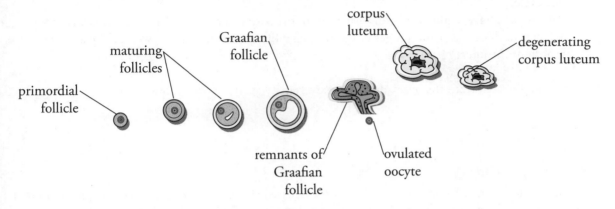

Figure 6   The Fate of a Follicle

Estrogen is made and secreted by the granulosa cells (with help from the thecal cells) during the first half of the menstrual cycle. Both estrogen and progesterone are secreted by the corpus luteum during the second half of the cycle. Estrogen is a steroid hormone that plays an important role in the development of female secondary sexual characteristics, in the menstrual cycle, and during pregnancy. [How does estrogen exert its effect on a cell?[29]] Progesterone is also a steroid hormone involved in the hormonal regulation of the menstrual cycle and pregnancy, but with different effects than estrogen.

13.7   THE MENSTRUAL CYCLE

The menstrual cycle is (on average) a 28-day cycle that includes events occurring in the ovary (discussed above and referred to as the **ovarian cycle**), as well as events occurring in the uterus (the shedding of the old endometrium and preparation of a new endometrium for potential pregnancy), referred to as the **uterine cycle**.

---

[28] They are analogous to the testicular interstitial cells. Both interstitial and thecal cells are stimulated by LH.

[29] A cytoplasmic receptor binds estrogen and binds to specific DNA elements in promoters and enhancers to regulate transcription.

The Ovarian Cycle

The ovarian cycle can be subdivided into three phases (Figure 7):

1) During the **follicular phase**, a primary follicle matures and secretes estrogen. Maturation of the follicle is under the control of follicle stimulating hormone (FSH) from the anterior pituitary. The follicular phase lasts about 13 days.

2) In the **ovulatory phase**, a secondary oocyte is released from the ovary. This is triggered by a surge of luteinizing hormone (LH) from the anterior pituitary. The surge also causes the remnants of the follicle to become the corpus luteum. Ovulation typically occurs on day 14 of the cycle.

3) The **luteal phase** begins with full formation of the corpus luteum in the ovary. This structure secretes both estrogen and progesterone and has a life span of about two weeks. The average length of the luteal phase is about 14 days.

The hormones secreted from the ovary during the ovarian cycle direct the uterine cycle.

The Uterine Cycle

The uterine cycle covers the same 28 days that were discussed above, but the focus is on the preparation of the endometrium for potential implantation of a fertilized egg. The uterine cycle can also be subdivided into three phases (Figure 7):

1) The first phase is **menstruation**, triggered by the degeneration of the corpus luteum and subsequent drop in estrogen and progesterone levels. The sharp decrease in these hormones causes the previous cycle's endometrial lining to slough out of the uterus, producing the bleeding associated with this time period. Menstruation typically lasts about 5 days.

2) During the **proliferative phase** of the menstrual cycle, estrogen produced by the follicle induces the proliferation of a new endometrium. This phase lasts about 9 days.

3) After ovulation the **secretory phase** occurs, in which estrogen and progesterone produced by the corpus luteum further increase development of the endometrium, including secretion of glycogen, lipids, and other material. If pregnancy does not occur, the death of the corpus luteum and decline in the secretion of estrogen and progesterone trigger menstruation once again. The secretory phase typically lasts about 14 days.

The menstrual cycle repeats every 28 days from puberty until menopause (at about age 50–60).

- At what stage of development is the endometrium when ovulation occurs?[30]
- Where is the secondary oocyte during the secretory phase?[31]
- If estrogen and progesterone were given to a woman without cyclic variation, how would this affect menstruation?[32]

---

[30] The endometrium is at the proliferative phase, under the influence of ovarian estrogen.

[31] The secondary oocyte is traveling down the uterine tube toward the uterus. If it fails to implant in the uterus, the secretory phase ends and menstruation begins.

[32] Menstruation occurs because the estrogen and progesterone secreted by the corpus luteum decrease suddenly when the corpus luteum degenerates. If estrogen and progesterone are kept at high levels, such as with a pill (or pregnancy), then menstruation will not occur.

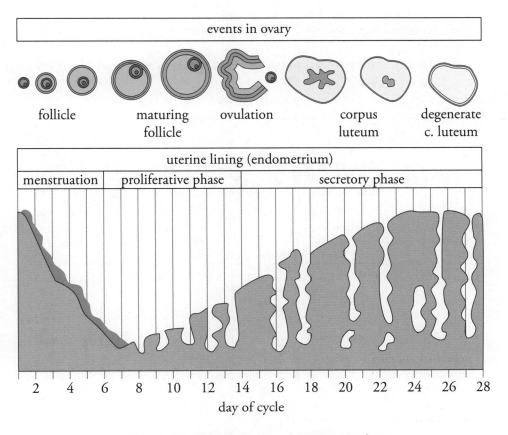

Figure 7   The Ovarian and Uterine Cycles

Focus on the Hormones

The anterior pituitary and the hypothalamus play a role in the menstrual cycle by regulating the secretion of estrogen and progesterone from the ovary (Figure 8, next page). Estrogen and progesterone then regulate the events in the uterus. The following is a summary:

1) GnRH from the hypothalamus stimulates the release of FSH and LH from the anterior pituitary.
2) Under the influence of FSH, the granulosa and thecal cells develop during the follicular phase and secrete estrogen. Secretion of GnRH, FSH, and LH is initially inhibited by estrogen; however, estrogen, which increases throughout the follicular stage, reaches a threshold near the end of this phase and has a positive effect on LH secretion.
3) This sudden surge in LH causes ovulation. After ovulation, LH induces the follicle to become the corpus luteum and to secrete estrogen and progesterone (this marks the beginning of the secretory phase). If pregnancy does not occur, the combined high levels of estrogen and progesterone feedback to strongly inhibit secretion of GnRH, FSH, and LH. When LH secretion drops, the corpus luteum regresses, no longer secretes estrogen or progesterone, and menstruation occurs.

- If LH levels remained high, how would this affect the secretion of estrogen and progesterone?[33]
- What would happen if the estrogen and progesterone levels in a woman's blood were kept artificially high for the entire month?[34]
- What would happen if the artificial hormones were suddenly taken away?[35]

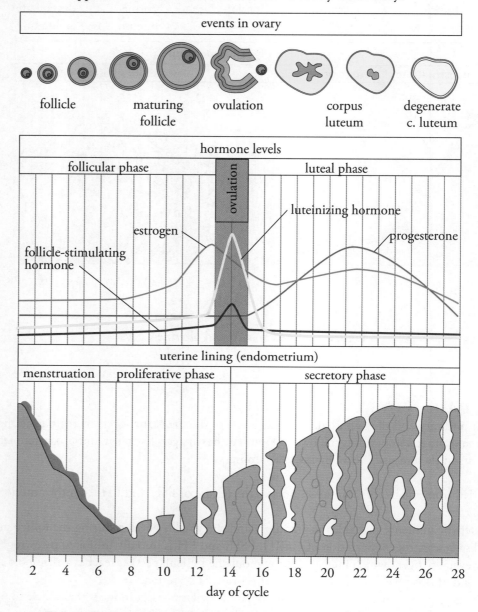

Figure 8 Pituitary and Ovarian Hormones of the Menstrual Cycle

---

[33] If LH levels remained high, the corpus luteum would not regress, and estrogen and progesterone would also remain high, thus maintaining the endometrium so that menstruation would not occur. This is, in effect, what happens if an embryo is fertilized and implants, except the hormone in this case is not LH but hCG, human chorionic gonadotropin, an LH-like hormone (see the next section).

[34] The woman would not ovulate. That's what (most) birth control pills are: estrogen and progesterone.

[35] The endometrium would slough off, and the woman would menstruate. (This is why there are 21 pills of one color and 7 pills of another color. The 7 pills contain no hormones; they are either placebos or sometimes iron supplements. If a woman took the hormone pill every day and never took the 7 placebos, she would never menstruate. Also, the placebos are actually unnecessary; these 7 pills are only present in order to help establish the habit of taking a pill every day.)

13.8 HORMONAL CHANGES DURING PREGNANCY

There are still a couple of points we have not made completely clear: how can pregnancy occur if the uterine lining is lost each month, and why does the body discard the endometrium?

Recall that the physiological reason for endometrial shedding is a decrease in estrogen and progesterone levels, which occurs as the corpus luteum degenerates. Why does the corpus luteum degenerate? Due to a decrease in luteinizing hormone. Why does LH decrease? Due to feedback inhibition from the high levels of estrogen and progesterone secreted by the corpus luteum.

Let's begin with why LH levels decrease. During pregnancy, ovulation should be prevented. The way ovulation is prevented is for the constant high levels of estrogen and progesterone seen during pregnancy to inhibit secretion of LH by the pituitary; no LH surge, no ovulation. Constant high levels of estrogen inhibit LH release. The result is pregnancy without continued ovulation. The *secondary* result is the one we were trying to explain: when the corpus luteum secretes a lot of estrogen and progesterone during the menstrual cycle, LH levels drop, causing the corpus luteum to degenerate. The point is that the corpus luteum degenerates unless fertilization has occurred.

So how can pregnancy occur? If pregnancy is to occur, the endometrium must be maintained, because it is the site of gestation (i.e., where the embryo lives and is nourished). If fertilization takes place, within a few days a developing embryo becomes **implanted** in the endometrium, and a **placenta** begins to develop. The **chorion** is the portion of the placenta that is derived from the zygote. It secretes **human chorionic gonadotropin**, or **hCG**, which can take the place of LH in maintaining the corpus luteum. In the presence of hCG, the corpus luteum does not degenerate, the estrogen and progesterone levels stay elevated, and menstruation does not occur. This answers the question of *how* pregnancy can occur. hCG is the hormone tested for in pregnancy tests because its presence absolutely confirms the presence of an embryo.

- Which of the following occur(s) during the menstrual cycle immediately prior to ovulation?[36]
  I. A surge in luteinizing hormone release from the anterior pituitary
  II. Completion of the second meiotic cell division by the oocyte
  III. Shedding of the endometrium

- As a woman ages, the number of follicles remaining in the ovaries decreases until ovulation ceases. At this point, termed **menopause**, the menstrual cycle no longer occurs. Which of the following occur(s) during menopause?[37]
  I. FSH levels drop dramatically and stay low.
  II. Estrogen levels are abnormally high.
  III. LH levels are very high and stay high.

---

[36] **Item I: True.** The LH surge *causes* ovulation. Item II: False. Meiosis I is completed prior to ovulation. Meiosis II isn't completed until after fertilization. Item III: False. Ovulation occurs around day 14 of the cycle. Menstruation begins at day 1.

[37] In the absence of estrogen and progesterone secretion by follicles, there is no feedback inhibition of LH and FSH, so their levels are very high in postmenopausal women. Thus, only **item III** is true.

- Which of the following statements concerning the menstrual cycle is/are true?[38]
  - I.   The proliferative phase of the endometrium coincides with the maturation of ovarian follicles.
  - II. The secretory phase of the endometrial cycle is dependent on the secretion of estrogen from cells surrounding secondary oocytes.
  - III. Luteinizing hormone levels are highest during the menstrual phase of the endometrial cycle.

13.9   FERTILIZATION AND CLEAVAGE

A secondary oocyte is ovulated and enters the uterine tube. It is surrounded by the **corona radiata** (a protective layer of granulosa cells) and the **zona pellucida** (located just outside the egg cell membrane). The oocyte will remain fertile for about a day. If intercourse occurs, sperm are deposited near the cervix, and are activated, or **capacitated**. Sperm capacitation involves the dilution of inhibitory substances present in semen. The activated sperm will survive for two or three days. They swim through the uterus toward the secondary oocyte.

Fertilization is the fusion of a spermatozoan with the secondary oocyte (Figure 9). It normally occurs in the uterine tube. In order for fertilization to occur, a sperm must penetrate the corona radiata and bind to and penetrate the zona pellucida. It accomplishes this using the **acrosome reaction**. The **acrosome** is a large vesicle in the sperm head containing hydrolytic enzymes which are released by exocytosis. After the corona radiata has been penetrated, an **acrosomal process** containing actin elongates toward the zona pellucida. The acrosomal process has **bindin**, a species-specific protein which binds to receptors in the zona pellucida. Finally, the sperm and egg plasma membranes fuse, and the sperm nucleus enters the secondary oocyte. In about twenty minutes, the secondary oocyte completes meiosis II, giving rise to an ootid and the second polar body. The ootid matures rapidly, becoming an **ovum**. Then the sperm and egg nuclei fuse, and the new diploid cell is known as a **zygote**.

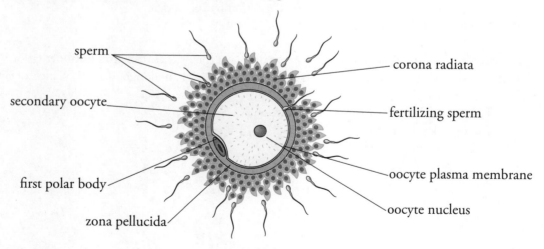

Figure 9   Fertilization

---

[38] **Item I: True.** This is explained in the text. Item II: False. It is secretion of estrogen and progesterone *by the corpus luteum* that drives the secretory phase. The corpus luteum is in the ovary, while the secondary oocyte is out in the uterine tube. Item III: False. The luteinizing hormone level peaks during the proliferative phase, since this is when ovulation occurs.

Penetration of an ovum by more than one sperm is known as **polyspermy**. It is normally prevented by the **fast block to polyspermy** and the **slow block to polyspermy**, which occur upon penetration of the egg by a spermatozoan. The fast block consists of a depolarization of the egg plasma membrane. This depolarization prevents other spermatozoa from fusing with the egg cell membrane. The slow block results from a Ca^{2+} influx caused by the initial depolarization. The slow block is also known as the **cortical reaction**. It has two components: swelling of the space between the zona pellucida and the plasma membrane, and hardening of the zona pellucida. The Ca^{2+} influx has one other noteworthy effect. It causes increased metabolism and protein synthesis, referred to as **egg activation**.

- Because of a particular disease, a man produces sperm without acrosomes. His spermatozoa are abnormal in that they:[39]
    - A) are immotile.
    - B) cannot undergo capacitation.
    - C) are incapable of fertilizing the egg.
    - D) can fertilize the eggs of many species.

- Which one of the following would NOT cause or indicate infertility?[40]
    - A) A lack of progesterone secretion during the latter half of the menstrual cycle
    - B) Failure of mitosis to occur after the male pronucleus fuses with the nucleus of the ovum
    - C) Excessively acidic pH of the vaginal secretions
    - D) A decrease in the concentration of LH after ovulation

13.9

Cleavage

The process of **embryogenesis** begins within hours of fertilization, but proceeds slowly in humans. The first stage is **cleavage**, in which the zygote undergoes many cell divisions to produce a ball of cells known as the **morula**. The first cell division occurs about 36 hours after fertilization. [The morula is the same size as the zygote, which indicates that the dividing cells spend most of their time in what phases of the cell cycle?[41] During cleavage of the zygote, do homologous chromosomes physically interact with each other?[42]]

---

[39] Acrosomal enzymes are necessary for penetration of the corona radiata, and the acrosomal process is necessary for binding to a penetration of the zona pellucida. Sperm that lack an acrosome would be unable to complete these processes, which are necessary for fertilization (choice **C** is correct, and choice D is wrong). The acrosome has nothing to do with motility (motility is the flagella's job; choice A is wrong), and capacitation is the activation of sperm in the female reproductive tract. It has nothing to do with the acrosome (choice B is wrong).

[40] Progesterone is secreted from the corpus luteum, which is formed from the remnants of the Graafian follicle after ovulation. A lack of progesterone might indicate that the corpus luteum did not form, and thus ovulation did not occur (choice A could indicate infertility and can be eliminated). The male pronucleus is just the haploid sperm nucleus. After this fuses with the ovum nucleus, the now diploid zygote must undergo cleavage (rapid mitosis) to form an embryo. If mitosis fails to occur, no embryo would develop (choice B would cause infertility and can be eliminated). Excessively acidic pH in the vagina could be harmful to sperm, which prefer a more alkaline environment. Sperm damaged by acids may not be motile, or may not be able to successfully fertilize an egg (choice C could lead to infertility and can be eliminated). However, LH normally decreases after ovulation. This is expected and not an indicator of infertility (choice **D** is the correct answer choice).

[41] They must spend most of their time during the S (synthesis) and M (mitotic) phases, skipping the G_1 and G_2 (gap or growth) phases.

[42] No. Pairing of homologous chromosomes takes place only during meiosis, which occurs only during gametogenesis.

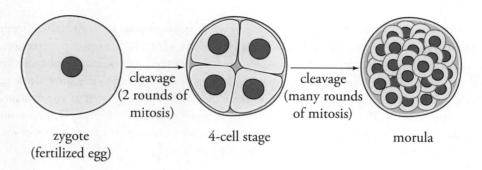

Figure 10   Cleavage

As cell divisions continue, the morula is transformed into a **blastocyst** (Figure 11). This process is known as **blastulation**. The blastocyst consists of a ring of cells called the **trophoblast** surrounding a cavity, and an **inner cell mass** adhering to the inside of the trophoblast at one end of the cavity. The **trophoblast** will give rise to the **chorion** (the zygote's contribution to the placenta). The inner cell mass will become the **embryo**.

- If two inner cell masses form in the blastula, what will the result be?[43]

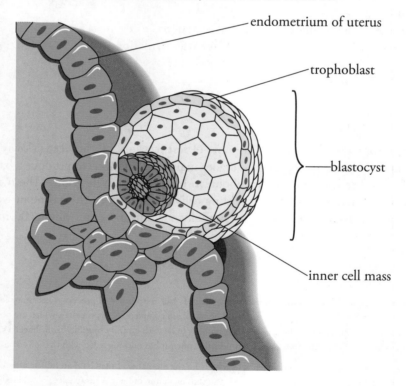

Figure 11   The Blastocyst at the Beginning of Implantation

---

[43] The inner cell mass becomes the embryo. Two inner cell masses derived from a single zygote and enclosed by the same trophoblast will result in a pair of identical twins sharing the same placenta.

13.10 IMPLANTATION AND THE PLACENTA

The developing blastocyst reaches the uterus and burrows into the endometrium, or **implants**, about a week after fertilization (Figure 11). The trophoblast secretes proteases that lyse endometrial cells. The blastocyst then sinks into the endometrium and is surrounded by it, absorbing nutrients through the trophoblast into the inner cell mass. The embryo receives a large part of its nutrition in this manner for the first few weeks of pregnancy. This is why the secretory phase of the endometrial cycle occurs: endometrial cells store glycogen, lipids, and other nutrients so that the early embryo may derive nourishment directly from the endometrium. Later, an organ develops which is specialized to facilitate exchange of nutrients, gases, and even antibodies between the maternal and embryonic bloodstreams: the **placenta**. Because it takes about three months for the placenta to develop, it is during the first trimester (three months) of pregnancy that hCG is essential for maintenance of the endometrium (Section 13.8).

- What happens if the corpus luteum is removed during the first trimester?[44]

During the last six months of pregnancy, the corpus luteum is no longer needed because the placenta itself secretes sufficient estrogen and progesterone for maintenance of the endometrium.

The development of the placenta involves the formation of **placental villi**. These are chorionic projections extending into the endometrium, into which fetal capillaries will grow. Surrounding the villi are sinuses (open spaces) filled with maternal blood. [Does oxygen-containing blood pass from the mother into the developing fetus?[45]]

13.10

The embryo is not the only important structure derived from the inner cell mass. There are three others: amnion, yolk sac, and allantois. The **amnion** surrounds a fluid-filled cavity which contains the developing embryo. Amniotic fluid is the "water" which "breaks" (is expelled) before birth. The **yolk sac** is important in reptiles and birds because it contains the nourishing yolk. Mammals do not store yolk. Our yolk sac is important because it is the first site of red blood cell synthesis in the embryo. Finally, the **allantois** develops from the embryonic gut and forms the blood vessels of the umbilical cord, which transport blood between embryo and placenta.

- Each of the following has the same genome EXCEPT:[46]
    - A) chorion.
    - B) amnion.
    - C) yolk sac.
    - D) endometrium.

[44] The woman menstruates, and the embryo is lost. Remember, the role of hCG is to substitute for LH in stimulating the corpus luteum. The role of the corpus luteum is to make estrogen and progesterone, which maintain the endometrium.

[45] No. The placenta is like a lung in that it facilitates exchange of substances between the two bloodstreams without allowing actual mixing.

[46] The chorion, amnion, and yolk sac are all derived from the inner cell mass of the blastula, and therefore must have the same genome (choices A, B, and C can be eliminated). However, the endometrium is derived from the mother (it is the inner lining of the uterus), and would have a different genome than the embryo (choice **D** is correct).

13.11   POST-IMPLANTATION DEVELOPMENT

We have examined embryogenesis from fertilization through blastulation. The next phase is **gastrulation**. Gastrulation is when the three **primary germ layers** (the **ectoderm**, the **mesoderm**, and the **endoderm**) become distinct.

In primitive organisms, the **blastula** (equivalent to blastocyst) is a hollow ball of cells, and gastrulation involves the **invagination** (involution) of these cells to form layers. Imagine pushing your fist into a big soft round balloon to create an inner layer (contacting your fist) and an outer layer (contacting the air). The inner layer is the endoderm, and the outer layer is the ectoderm. The mesoderm (middle layer) develops from the endoderm. The cavity (where your fist is) is primitive gut, or **archenteron**. The opening (where your wrist is) is the **blastopore**, and will give rise to the anus. The whole structure is the **gastrula**. (Don't be confused: the *gastr*ula has a *blast*opore; the *blast*ula has no opening.)

In humans, things are a little different. The gastrula develops from a double layer of cells called the **embryonic disk**, instead of from a spherical blastula. But the end result is the same: three layers. You need to know what parts of the human body are derived from each layer.

Table 4   Fates of the Primary Germ Layers

Ectoderm	Mesoderm	Endoderm
• Entire nervous system • Pituitary gland (both lobes), adrenal medulla • Cornea and lens • Epidermis of skin and derivatives (hair, nails, sweat glands, sensory receptors) • Nasal, oral, anal epithelium	• All muscle, bone, and connective tissue • Entire cardiovascular and lymphatic system, including blood • Urogenital organs (kidneys, ureters, gonads, reproductive ducts) • Dermis of skin	• GI tract epithelium (except mouth and anus) • GI glands (liver, pancreas, etc.) • Respiratory epithelium • Epithelial lining of urogenital organs and ducts • Urinary bladder

Pay attention to what *types* of thing are derived from each layer, and you'll see that it's relatively easy to memorize. One key thing to note is that **ectoderm** and *epithelium* are not synonymous. Epithelium outside the body (epidermis) is derived from ectoderm, but epithelium inside the body (gut lining) comes from endoderm.

- Which of the following statements is/are true?[47]
  - I. Oxygen must diffuse across the chorionic membrane to reach the fetus from the mother.
  - II. Transplantation of cells from the trophoblast of one embryo to the trophoblast of another embryo will result in an infant with a mixed genetic composition.
  - III. All of the cells of the blastocyst are functionally equivalent.

The next step after gastrulation is **neurulation**, the formation of the nervous system. It begins when a portion of the ectoderm differentiates into the **neural plate**. At the edges of the plate are the **neural crest cells**; these edges thicken and fold upward (the **neural folds**), leaving the bottom of the plate to form the

---

[47] **Item I: True.** The chorion is part of the placenta. Item II: False. The trophoblast is derived from the outer cell mass and gives rise only to the chorion. The embryo is derived entirely from the inner cell mass. Item III: False. The trophoblast and the inner cell mass are both components of the blastocyst, and they have very different roles.

neural tube. The neural tube ultimately develops into the central nervous system (brain and spinal cord). During that process, the neural crest cells separate from the neural tube and the overlying ectoderm (which ultimately becomes the epidermis), then migrate to different parts of the embryo to differentiate into a variety of cell types, including melanocytes, glial cells, the adrenal medulla, some peripheral neurons, and some facial connective tissue (Figure 12). The formation of the neural tube is induced by instructions from the underlying notochord, which is mesodermal in origin. It gives rise to the vertebral column.

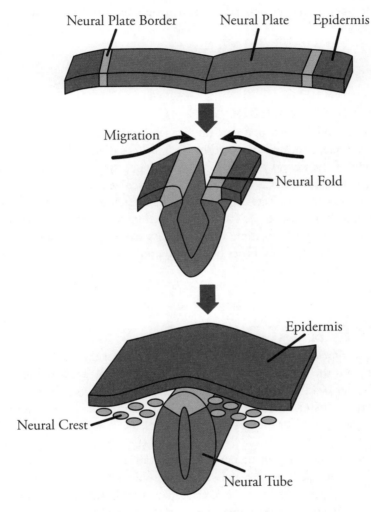

Figure 12 Neural Crest

Neurulation is one component of **organogenesis**, the development of organ systems. By the eighth week of gestation, all major organ systems are present, and the **embryo** is now called a **fetus**. Even though the developmental process has attained staggering complexity, by the end of the first trimester the fetus is still only 5 cm long. [During which trimester is the developing human most sensitive to toxins such as drugs and radiation?[48]]

---

[48] During the first trimester, when the organs are being formed.

- A radioactive dye is detected only in the cells of placental villi. Weeks earlier, it must have been injected into the:[49]
    A) inner cell mass.
    B) trophoblast.
    C) endometrium.
    D) zygote.

- During gastrulation, do tissues derived from the trophoblast move inward to form the lining of the primitive gut?[50]

Environment-Gene Interaction

During this early time period in development, the prenatal environment can play a significant role in gene expression. For example, a lack of folic acid in the mother's diet at this time can lead to significant defects in the formation of the neural tube and central nervous system. Certain illnesses in the mother can lead to issues in the fetus; influenza has been linked to schizophrenia and German measles to deafness, eye abnormalities, and heart defects. Hypoxia in utero, such as might be caused by maternal cigarette smoking (and the resultant vasoconstriction of uterine blood vessels) can lead to a reduction in grey matter development. Fetal alcohol syndrome due to excess maternal alcohol consumption can lead to stunted fetal growth, brain damage, and other behavioral and physical problems.

13.12 DIFFERENTIATION

The specialization of cell types during development is termed **differentiation** because as cells specialize they become different from their parent cells and from each other. By specializing, a cell becomes better able to perform a particular task, while becoming less adept at other tasks. For example, a sensory neuron is the best vehicle for the transmission of a nerve impulse over great distances, but is quite incapable of obtaining nourishment on its own, or even of reproducing itself.

Primitive cells in the zygote and the morula have the potential to become any cell type in the blastocyst, including the trophoblast and the inner cell mass. They are therefore known as **totipotent** cells. Cells of the inner cell mass are more specialized and are referred to as **pluripotent**. They can differentiate into any of the three primary germ layers (ectoderm, mesoderm, or endoderm) and therefore have the capability to become any of the 220 cell types that make up an adult human. However, they cannot contribute to the trophoblast of the blastocyst (i.e., will not become the placenta).

---

[49] The placenta is derived from the chorion, which is derived from the cells of the trophoblast; thus, injecting a dye into the trophoblast would lead to its detection in the placental villi (choice **B** is correct). The inner cell mass ultimately becomes the embryo; thus, dye injected into the inner cells mass would be detected in the embryo, not the placenta (choice A is wrong). The endometrium is derived from the mother and is only the site of implantation and placental development. It does not actually contribute to the placenta; thus, dye injected into the endometrium would not be detected in the placenta (choice C is wrong). The zygote is the precursor to all embryonic and extraembryonic structures. Injecting a dye into the zygote would lead to its detection not only in the placenta, but also in the amnion, chorion, and embryo itself (choice D is wrong).

[50] No. Gastrulation involves only cells derived from the inner cell mass.

13.12

As development continues, cells continue to specialize. After gastrulation, cells from the early embryonic germ layers are each considered **multipotent**. This means they can become many, but not all, cell types. For example, cells of the mesoderm can differentiate into muscle and bone cells, but not into neurons or digestive epithelium.

In other words, totipotent cells differentiate into pluripotent cells, which specialize to become multipotent cells. Most cells in the adult have lost all potency and have become completely specialized mature cells, incapable of changing into other cell types. Adult stem cells are an exception to this, and these cells are discussed in Section A.13 of Appendix I.

Stem cells, because of their ability to become nearly any cell type in the body, are of great interest in research; they remain a potential source for regenerative medicine and tissue replacement after injury or disease. In humans, embryonic stem cells are the only pluripotent cells that have been found. These cells are isolated from the inner cell mass of the blastocyst.

There is a certain point in the development of a cell at which the cell fate becomes fixed; at this point the cell is said to be **determined**. Determination precedes differentiation. This means a cell is determined before it is visibly differentiated. Determination can be **induced** by a cell's environment, such as exposure to diffusible factors or neighboring cells, or it can be preprogrammed.

- During early embryonic development, cells near the developing notochord undergo an irreversible developmental choice to become skeletal muscle later in development, although they do not immediately change their appearance. This is an example of which of the following?[51]
  A) Determination
  B) Differentiation
  C) Totipotency
  D) Induction

13.12

There is such a thing as **dedifferentiation**. This is the process whereby a specialized cell *un*specializes and may become totipotent. If a dedifferentiated cell proliferates in an uncontrolled manner, the result can be cancer. The most important lesson you can learn from the notion of dedifferentiation is that every cell has the same genome. The specialization of cell types is a function of things in the cytoplasm and maybe proteins and RNA in the nucleus, but no genetic changes normally take place during development and differentiation.

- Can you think of two exceptions to this rule, where a particular cell type normally has a unique genome?[52]

---

[51] A cell whose fate is fixed is said to be determined, however, if it has not yet undergone a change in appearance, it has not yet been differentiated (choice **A** is correct, and choice B is wrong). Since the cell is destined to become muscle, it is no longer totipotent (choice C is wrong). Although the cells are found near the notochord, there is no reason to assume the location is the reason for their determination. They could be cytoplasmically determined (choice D is wrong).

[52] One exception is B cells and T cells of the immune system. They undergo gene (DNA!) rearrangements in the process of attaining antigen specificity. The other exception is gametes. They have unique genomes because of 1) reductive division with independent assortment, and 2) recombination.

Table 5 Stem Cells

Term	Definition	Examples
Totipotent	• Can generate trophoblast and inner cell mass	zygote; morula
Pluripotent	• Can differentiate into any of the three primary germ layers • Can generate all adult cell types (over 220 different cells)	inner cell mass of blastocyst (embryonic stem cells); IPS (induced pluripotent stem) cells
Multipotent	• Can produce many (but not all) cell types • More differentiated than pluripotent • Often tissue-specific	three primary germ layers; adult stem cells
Dedifferentiation	• Some cells can go backward and become less specialized • Example: Mature → Multipotent → Pluripotent → Totipotent	iPS cells; cancer cells

13.13 PREGNANCY

The early stages of development already discussed (gastrulation and neurulation) comprise the embryonic stage of development. These eight weeks comprise the majority of the first trimester; during this time all major organ systems appear. The stage of development from eight weeks until birth is known as the fetal stage. This stage covers the second and third trimesters of the pregnancy.

Second Trimester

During this time the organs and organ systems of the fetus continue to develop structurally and functionally. The fetus grows, typically reaching a weight of approximately 0.6 kg, and looks distinctly human.

Third Trimester

This is a stage of rapid fetal growth, including significant deposition of adipose tissue. Most of the organ systems become fully functional. A baby born 1–2 months early has a reasonably good chance of survival.

Mom

The demands placed on the mother's body increase significantly over the course of the pregnancy. Maternal respiratory rate increases to bring in additional oxygen and eliminate additional carbon dioxide. Blood volume in the mother increases by about 50% due to a drop in oxygen levels (because of the metabolic demands of the fetus) and a subsequent release of erythropoietin and renin. This is accompanied by an increase in glomerular filtration rate of a corresponding 50%. The demand for nutrients and vitamins increases by about 30%, the uterus undergoes a very significant increase in size, and the mammary glands increase in size. Additionally, secretory activity begins in the mammary glands, although this is not technically lactation.

13.14 BIRTH AND LACTATION

The technical term for birth is **parturition**. It is dependent on contraction of muscles in the uterine wall. The very high levels of progesterone secreted throughout pregnancy help to repress contractions in uterine muscle, but near the end of pregnancy uterine excitability increases. This increased excitability is likely to be a result of several factors, including a change in the ratio of estrogen to progesterone, the presence of the hormone **oxytocin** secreted by the posterior pituitary, and mechanical stretching of the uterus and cervix.

Weak contractions of the uterus occur throughout pregnancy. As pregnancy reaches full term, however, rhythmic **labor contractions** begin. It is thought that the onset of labor contractions is the result of a positive feedback reflex: the increased pressure on the cervix crosses a threshold that causes the posterior pituitary to increase the secretion of oxytocin. Oxytocin causes the uterine contractions to increase in intensity, creating greater pressure on the cervix that stimulates still more oxytocin release and even stronger contractions.

The first stage of labor is dilation of the cervix. The second stage is the actual birth, involving movement of the baby through the cervix and birth canal, pushed by contraction of uterine (smooth) and abdominal (skeletal) muscle. The third stage is the expulsion of the placenta, after it separates from the wall of the uterus. Contractions of the uterus after birth help to minimize blood loss.

During pregnancy, milk production and secretion would be a waste of energy, but after parturition it is necessary. During puberty, estrogen stimulates the development of breasts in women. The increased levels of estrogen and progesterone secreted by the placenta during pregnancy cause the further development of glandular and adipose breast tissue. But while these hormones stimulate breast development, they inhibit the release of **prolactin** and thus the production of milk. After parturition, the levels of estrogen and progesterone fall and milk production begins. Every time suckling occurs, the pituitary gland is stimulated by the hypothalamus to release a large surge of prolactin, prolonging the ability of the breasts to secrete milk. If the mother stops breast-feeding the infant, prolactin levels fall and milk secretion ceases. The converse is also true: milk secretion can continue for years, as long as nursing continues. The breasts do not leak large amounts of milk when the infant is not nursing. This is because the posterior pituitary hormone **oxytocin** is necessary for **milk let-down** (release). Oxytocin is also released when suckling occurs.

13.14

Chapter 13 Summary

- The primary sex organs produce gametes and hormones. The testes are the male primary sex organ and the ovaries are the female primary sex organ.

- Male internal genitalia are formed from Wolffian ducts and female internal genitalia are formed from Müllerian ducts.

- Spermatogenesis takes place in the seminiferous tubules and results in four haploid sperm from a single spermatogonium. It begins at puberty and continues on a daily basis for the life of the male. FSH stimulates spermatogenesis and LH stimulates testosterone production.

- Sperm travel from the seminiferous tubules to the epididymis, then to the ductus deferens, then to the urethra. Semen is a supportive fluid for sperm, produced by the seminal vesicles, the prostate, and the bulbourethral glands.

- Oogenesis begins prenatally, producing primary oocytes. It occurs again on a monthly basis, beginning at puberty and ending at menopause; this produces one secondary oocyte (which is ovulated) and the first polar body. Oogenesis is only completed if the secondary oocyte is fertilized, in which case an ovum and the second polar body will be produced.

- FSH stimulates follicle development and estrogen secretion during the first half of the menstrual cycle. LH stimulates ovulation and the formation of the corpus luteum, as well as progesterone and estrogen secretion, during the second half of the menstrual cycle.

- Estrogen stimulates growth of the endometrium during the first half of the menstrual cycle; progesterone and estrogen maintain and enhance the endometrium during the second half of the menstrual cycle. If no fertilization takes place, estrogen and progesterone levels fall, and the endometrium is sloughed off.

- Arousal is mediated by the parasympathetic nervous system, while orgasm and resolution are mediated by the sympathetic nervous system.

- Fertilization takes place in the uterine tubes, and cleavage begins 24–36 hours later. The zygote becomes a morula, the morula becomes a blatstula, and the blastula implants in the endometrium.

- The trophoblast becomes the placenta and the inner cell mass becomes the embryo.

- The first eight weeks of development are the embryonic stage, during which gastrulation (formation of the three primary germ layers), neurulation (formation of the nervous system), and organogenesis occur.

- The fetal stage begins at the eighth week of development and ends at the birth of the baby.

- Labor is a positive feedback cycle triggered by mild (initially) uterine contractions that push the baby's head on the cervix. This stimulates the release of oxytocin, which causes a stronger uterine contraction, and a bigger stretch of the cervix. This positive feedback loop will continue until the birth of the baby.

- Prolactin stimulates milk production and oxytocin stimulates milk ejection in a baby-driven cycle.

CHAPTER 13 FREESTANDING PRACTICE QUESTIONS

1. Which of the following structures undergoes mitosis?

A) Spermatid
B) Spermatogonium
C) Primary spermatocyte
D) Secondary spermatocyte

2. Which of the following statements regarding childbirth is true?

A) Release of oxytocin from the anterior pituitary, combined with increased mechanical pressure of the fetal head on the cervix, creates a positive feedback loop that increases uterine contractions.
B) Release of progesterone from the placenta, combined with increased mechanical pressure of the fetal head on the cervix, creates a positive feedback loop that increases uterine contractions.
C) Release of progesterone from the posterior pituitary, combined with increased mechanical pressure of the fetal head on the cervix, creates a negative feedback loop that increases uterine contractions.
D) Release of oxytocin from the posterior pituitary, combined with mechanical pressure of the fetal head on the cervix, creates a positive feedback loop that increases uterine contractions.

3. Which of the following is NOT a difference between spermatogenesis and oogenesis?

A) Spermatogenesis in a male begins at puberty, whereas oogenesis in a female begins when the female is an embryo.
B) Spermatogenesis produces four sperm, whereas oogenesis produces one ovum.
C) Spermatogenesis produces primary spermatocytes for a male's entire life, whereas oogenesis ceases to produce primary oocytes when a female reaches menopause.
D) Spermatogenesis occurs in the testes, whereas oogenesis occurs in the ovaries.

4. Which of the following hormones is NOT elevated during the first trimester of pregnancy?

A) Estrogen
B) Progesterone
C) GnRH
D) hCG

5. Ovulation usually occurs on the 14th day of the ovarian cycle. All of the following occur during ovulation and the days immediately following ovulation EXCEPT:

A) the ovary releases a secondary oocyte.
B) a surge of FSH from the anterior pituitary causes the follicle to become the corpus luteum.
C) the follicle secretes progesterone once it becomes the corpus luteum.
D) a surge of LH can be detected.

6. Ectopic pregnancy, where implantation of the embryo occurs in the fallopian tube rather than the uterus, is possible because:

A) though fertilization takes place in the uterus, implantation does not occur immediately and thus the embryo could migrate back up into the fallopian tubes.
B) fertilization occurs in the fallopian tubes and the embryo may fail to migrate to the uterus.
C) the fimbriae may hold the embryo in the fallopian tube rather than pushing it toward the uterus.
D) fertilization may have occurred in the ovary with subsequent implantation in the fallopian tube.

7. Postpartum women often experience mild to moderate uterine contractions when nursing. These contractions are triggered by the release of:

A) estrogen.
B) oxytocin.
C) progesterone.
D) prolactin.

8. The greater vestibular glands in the female (Bartholin's glands) have a similar function as which of the following male reproductive glands?

A) Bulbourethral glands (Cowper's glands)
B) Seminal vesicles
C) Prostate
D) Testes

CHAPTER 13 PRACTICE PASSAGE

For families struggling with infertility, IVF (in vitro fertilization) can be performed to help couples conceive. In IVF, an egg is harvested from the female partner, sperm are harvested from the male partner, and then egg and sperm are combined in a lab. The embryos are grown and observed in the lab, and then viable embryos are transferred into the uterine cavity. It is estimated that 1–2% of US births annually are via IVF.

Multiple births can develop two ways during IVF. If more than one embryo is transferred into the uterus, both could successfully implant and develop. Alternatively, a single embryo could divide into two. These two mechanisms lead to different types of twins.

Dizygotic or fraternal twins are non-identical and are formed when two genetically different eggs are fertilized by two different sperm. When fraternal twins are delivered, there are typically two placentas. Monozygotic or identical twins are formed when a zygote, morula, or blastocyst splits into two separate embryos. If the cell mass splits before day five, two embryos will develop with separate placentas and separate amniotic sacs; this occurs about 66% of the time. After day five, splitting usually leads to two amniotic sacs but one placenta; this occurs about 33% of the time. The other 1% of identical twins split even later in development.

Five sets of twins are undergoing testing to determine if they are fraternal or identical. Each set share significant physical characteristics. Each set of twins answers a questionnaire (Table 1) and undergoes RFLP genetic testing (Figure 1).

	Gender	Age (years)	Placenta(s)	Amniotic Sac
Twins 1	F/M	2.2	2	2
Twins 2	M/M	14	2	2
Twins 3	F/F	0.5	2	2
Twins 4	F/F	8	1	1
Twins 5	M/M	4	1	2

Table 1 Twin questionnaire results

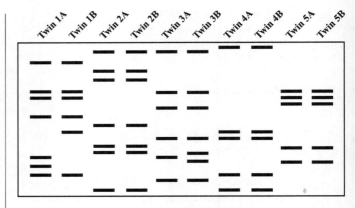

Figure 1 Twin RFLP results

1. Which statement below is NOT supported by the passage?

A) It is common for identical twins to share both a placenta and an amniotic sac.
B) Monozygotic twins have identical genomic sequences and fraternal twins have different genetic information.
C) Most identical twins split before development of the three primary germ layers.
D) Twins with two placentas can be fraternal or identical.

2. A sixth set of twins was supposed to be included in the twin study described in the passage. While their questionnaire responses were appropriate, their RFLP analysis did not work. Which of the following could explain why the RFLP analysis failed?

A) High levels of RNase were detected on the sample collection tools.
B) The tubes that stored the samples were accidentally stored at 32°C for two days.
C) The tubes that stored the samples were contaminated by a DNase.
D) The twins were very young, so their samples were contaminated by proteases.

3. Which of the twins in the passage are monozygotic?

A) Twins 4 and 5
B) Twins 2, 4, 5
C) Twins 2, 3, 4, 5
D) All of the twins

4. How would carrying twins affect maternal hormone levels, compared to a single pregnancy?

A) Human chorionic gonadotropin levels stay high past 6 week of gestation.
B) Significantly more prolactin and oxytocin are made and released from the anterior pituitary.
C) Strong negative feedback inhibits estrogen synthesis and release from the posterior pituitary.
D) Twice as much progesterone is made and released from the corpus luteum and placenta.

5. Which of the following correctly ranks the order from earliest to latest the identical twins from the passage split?

A) 2 – 5 – 4
B) 2/3 – 5 – 4
C) 4 – 5 – 1/2/3
D) 4 – 5 – 2

6. Why do some identical twins have two amniotic sacs but share a placenta?

A) The placenta develops from the inner cell mass, which splits in these twins; the amnion develops from the trophoblast, which is shared in identical twins.
B) All identical twins share a trophoblast, which develops into the amnion, and an inner cell mass, which develops into the placenta.
C) The amnion develops from the inner cell mass, which splits in these twins; the placenta develops from the trophoblast, which is shared in these twins.
D) All identical twins share a trophoblast, which develops into the placenta, and an inner cell mass, which develops into the amnion.

SOLUTIONS TO CHAPTER 13 FREESTANDING PRACTICE QUESTIONS

1. **B** The spermatogonia in the testes periodically undergo mitosis to produce both more spermatogonia and primary spermatocytes, ensuring a continual supply of primary spermatocytes for gametogenesis throughout the male reproductive lifespan. Primary spermatocytes, which are diploid, undergo meiosis I to become haploid secondary spermatocytes, which then undergo meiosis II to become (haploid) spermatids (choices C and D are wrong). Spermatids do not undergo mitosis or meiosis, but develop into mature spermatozoa (choice A is wrong).

2. **D** Labor and delivery is one example of a positive feedback loop, in which the release of oxytocin from the posterior pituitary combined with mechanical pressure of the fetal head work together to increase uterine contractility in an effort to expel the baby from the uterus (choice D is correct, and choice A is wrong). Progesterone, released early in pregnancy from the corpus luteum and later in pregnancy from the placenta itself, decreases uterine contractility (choices B and C are wrong). Levels of progesterone are high early in pregnancy in order to keep the developing fetus inside the uterus, but levels diminish later in pregnancy in anticipation of the upcoming delivery of the baby. Note that this question is a two-by-two elimination; the role of oxytocin in delivery allows the elimination of two answer choices and determining its regulatory mechanism differentiates between the remaining two.

3. **C** Spermatogenesis only begins once a male reaches puberty, and then continues for the rest of his life (choice C is not a difference and is the correct answer choice). Oogenesis begins when a female is an embryo, and the cells are arrested at the primary oocyte phase when she is a fetus (choice A is a difference and can be eliminated). Spermatogenesis produces four sperm from each spermatogonia, whereas oogenesis produces one ovum and two polar bodies per oogonia (choice B is a difference and can be eliminated). The testes are the male gonads and the site of spermatogenesis; the ovaries are the female gonads and the site of oogenesis (choice D is a difference and can be eliminated).

4. **C** The corpus luteum secretes estrogen and progesterone, which help maintain pregnancy (these hormones are elevated in the first trimester; choices A and B can be eliminated). Estrogen and progesterone feedback and inhibit the secretion of GnRH from the hypothalamus (choice C would not be elevated and is the correct answer choice). hCG is a hormone secreted by the embryo that helps to maintain the corpus luteum during the first trimester until the placenta is formed (choice D would be elevated and can be eliminated).

5. **B** During ovulation, the ovary releases a secondary oocyte (choice A is true and can be eliminated). A surge of LH, not FSH from the anterior pituitary, causes the follicle to become the corpus luteum (choice D is true and can be eliminated, and choice B is false and the correct answer choice). Once the follicle becomes the corpus luteum, it produces and secretes progesterone that stabilizes and enhances the endometrium (choice C is true and can be eliminated).

6. **B** Fertilization occurs in the fallopian tube after an egg has been released from the ovary (choices A and D are wrong). The fimbriae sweep the egg from the ovary into the fallopian tube (not the uterus) once it has been ovulated (choice C is wrong). Choice B describes the process accurately, including the correct location of fertilization and the failure to migrate prior to implantation.

7. **B** When suckling occurs, oxytocin is released from the posterior pituitary to trigger milk ejection from the glands toward the nipple. As this hormone is also responsible for stimulating uterine contractions during delivery, it can have a similar but less intense effect when nursing. Prolactin is involved in nursing, but is responsible for stimulating the production of milk and does not have an effect on the uterus (choice D is wrong). Estrogen and progesterone do not play a role in this situation (choices A and C are wrong).

8. **A** The greater vestibular glands are located at the posterior of the vaginal opening, are stimulated on arousal, and secrete an alkaline mucus. This helps neutralize the acidity of the vagina to make it a more hospitable environment for sperm, which can be damaged by acids. The bulbourethral glands in the male are stimulated on arousal and secrete an alkaline mucus into the urethra. This helps neutralize any traces of acid that might remain from earlier passage of urine through that duct, and makes the urethra a more hospitable environment for sperm. The seminal vesicles and the prostate produce semen (a supportive fluid for sperm), and are stimulated at orgasm (choices B and C are wrong), and the testes are the male primary sex organs; they produce sperm and testosterone (choice D is wrong).

SOLUTIONS TO CHAPTER 13 PRACTICE PASSAGE

1. **A** In most pregnancies, the blastocyst has formed by day 5. The passage describes four types of twins:

Twin	Definition	Genome	Extraembryonic Structures
Dizygotic or fraternal twins (non-identical)	Two genetically different eggs are fertilized by two different sperm	Different	Two amnions Two placentas
66% of monozygotic or identical twins	Single fertilization Zygote or morula splits before day 5	Same	Two amnions Two placentas
33% of monozygotic or identical twins	Single fertilization Inner cell mass of blastocyst splits after day 5	Same	Two amnions One placenta
1% of monozygotic or identical twins	Single fertilization Split later in development	Same	One amnion One placenta

Make sure to highlight the word "NOT" and write "A B C D" on the noteboard. Then evaluate each choice, writing a "Y" if it is supported and "N" if it is not. Most identical twins split early and have separate amnions and placentas (write "N" next to "A" on the noteboard). Monozygotic twins have identical genomic sequences and fraternal twins have different genetic information (write "Y" next to "B" on the noteboard). The three primary germ layers develop in gastrulation and most identical twins split before this (write "Y" next to "C" on the noteboard). All fraternal (non-identical) twins and monozygotic or identical twins that split before day 5 develop two placentas and two amnions (write "Y" next to "D" on the noteboard). Since choice A stands out with an "N" instead of a "Y," it is the correct answer choice.

2. **C**   Restriction fragment length polymorphism (RFLP) analysis uses restriction endonucleases to cut stretches of polymorphic DNA into small fragments. The resulting DNA fragments vary in size and are unique to an individual; they are separated via gel electrophoresis and analyzed. RNase enzymes degrade RNA, which is not relevant to RFLP (eliminate choice A). DNA is pretty stable and would likely survive a few days at a high temperature (eliminate choice B). DNase enzymes degrade DNA. This would destroy the samples collected from the twins and would mean no RFLP analysis is possible (choice C is correct). The age of the twins is not relevant to the quality of their DNA sample. In addition, proteases degrade proteins, and this is not relevant to RFLP (eliminate choice D).

3. **B**   Monozygotic twins are identical and have the same genetic information. Twins 1 and 3 have different RFLP patterns, so they do not have the same genome. They must be fraternal (eliminate choices C and D). Also note that twin set 1 has a male and female; these cannot be identical twins. Twin sets 2, 4, and 5 have the same RFLP patterns as each other, so these pairs must have the same genome. They are identical or monozygotic twins (eliminate choice A; choice B is correct).

4. **D**   Human chorionic gonadotropin hormones levels stay high past 6 weeks of gestation in all pregnancies (eliminate choice A). Prolactin is made and released from the anterior pituitary, but oxytocin is made in the hypothalamus and released from the posterior pituitary (eliminate choice B). Estrogen is not made in the brain (eliminate choice C). By process of elimination, the correct answer is choice D. Progesterone is made and released from the corpus luteum and placenta, and it is reasonable progesterone levels would be higher in a woman carrying multiples.

5. **A**   Twin sets 1 and 3 have different RFLP patterns, so they do not have the same genome. They must be fraternal (eliminate choices B and C). Twin sets 2, 4, and 5 have the same RFLP patterns as each other, so these pairs must have the same genome. They are identical or monozygotic twins. Based on the passage, identical twins that split early will develop separate amnions and placenta. Twins that split after day 5 usually have separate amnions and a shared placenta. This means that the small percent of twins that split even later than this (only 1% of identical twins) must share both an amnion and a placenta. Here are the results of the twin study in the passage:

	Gender	Placenta(s)	Amniotic Sac	Results	Split
Twins 1	F/M	2	2	Fraternal	n/a
Twins 2	M/M	2	2	Identical	Before day 5
Twins 3	F/F	2	2	Fraternal	n/a
Twins 4	F/F	1	1	Identical	Long after day 5
Twins 5	M/M	1	2	Identical	Shortly after day 5

This means that twins 2 must have split earliest, then twins 5, and finally twins 4 (eliminate choice D; choice A is correct).

6. **C**   The passage states that if identical twins split after day 5, there will be two amniotic sacs but one placenta. The amnion develops from the inner cell mass (eliminate choices A and B). All twins with two inner cell masses in a blastocyst will develop two separate amnions (eliminate choice D; choice C is correct). The placenta develops from the trophoblast. If a zygote or morula splits, two separate blastocysts will develop, and they will each have their own inner cells mass and trophoblast. This will lead to identical twins with separate amnions and placentas. If the inner cell mass of a blastocyst splits, identical twins will develop their own amnions but will share a placenta because they share a trophoblast.

EFFECTS OF A COMMERCIALLY AVAILABLE BRANCHED-CHAIN AMINO ACID-ALANINE-CARBOHYDRATE-BASED SPORTS SUPPLEMENT ON PERCEIVED EXERTION AND PERFORMANCE IN HIGH INTENSITY ENDURANCE CYCLING TESTS

Marco Gervasi, Davide Sisti, Stefano Amatori, Sabrina Donati Zeppa, Giosuè Annibalini, Giovanni Piccoli, Luciana Vallorani, Piero Benelli, Marco B. L. Rocchi, Elena Barbieri, Anna R. Calavalle, Deborah Agostini, Carmela Fimognari, Vilberto Stocchi & Piero Sestili

Journal of the International Society of Sports Nutrition, volume 17, Article number: 6 (2020)

BACKGROUND

Amino acids are thought to enhance athletic performance in several ways, for example modifying fuel utilization during exercise and preventing mental fatigue and overtraining. A recent (2017) position stand of the International Society of Sports Nutrition states that the three branched-chain amino acids (BCAA), leucine, isoleucine, and valine are unique among the essential amino acids for their roles in protein metabolism, neural function, blood glucose and insulin regulation. It has been suggested that the Recommended Dietary Allowance (RDA) for sedentary individuals (considering that BCAAs occur in nature in a 2:1:1 ratio, leucine: isoleucine: valine) should be 45 mg/kg/day for leucine and 22.5 mg/kg/day for both isoleucine and valine; this RDA is even higher for active individuals. Supplementation with BCAA has been proposed as a possible strategy to limit the development of central fatigue, in particular, in endurance events. Central fatigue, which pertains to the central nervous system (CNS), is a complex phenomenon arising under conditions of low energy availability, ammonia accumulation in blood and tissues, and changes in neurotransmitter synthesis—in particular, an increase in serotonin and a decrease in dopamine—which causes a state of increasing tiredness during exhaustive exercise. The presence of elevated cerebral serotonin levels observed in rats under fatigue, is the basis of a well-accepted theory to account for the onset/increase of central fatigue in humans as well. Indeed, during prolonged sustained exercise, an increased brain uptake of the serotonin precursor Tryptophan (Trp) has been observed in humans. This theory has recently been bolstered by Kavanagh et al., whose study based on paroxetine administration in humans demonstrated the influence of serotonin availability in increasing central fatigue under prolonged maximal contractions. The ability of BCAA to compete with Trp in crossing the blood brain barrier led us to hypothesize that BCAA supplementation could reduce cerebral serotonin synthesis, thus preventing/delaying the onset of central fatigue during prolonged exercise.

Carbohydrates (CHO) also play an important role in supplementation in the course of endurance events, increasing and/or maintaining energetic substrate availability, preventing and/or delaying hypoglycemia and its deleterious effects on brain functions and cognitive performance, and promoting direct anti-fatigue brain responses through the activation of sweet taste oral receptors.

In light of these findings, researchers have turned their attention to the study and development of supplements containing BCAA alone or combined with specific substances (such as CHO), assessing the efficacy of their association. Several recent investigations have shown BCAA supplementation to positively affect prolonged exercise under specific conditions. In particular, BCAA were shown to positively impact the rating of perceived exertion (RPE) and performance. However, due to the great heterogeneity of the experimental protocols and formulations used, the results of these studies are not always unequivocal; hence, the actual efficacy of BCAA – used alone or combined with other components—remains a much debated issue.

This uncertainty may generate confusion and/or false expectations regarding the efficacy of these sport supplements. To shed light on this issue, it is important to perform highly controlled and randomized studies as well as to develop and validate specific and reliable test procedures capable of determining the actual efficacy of supplements intended for use in sports after both short and long term intakes. To this end, a recent study validated a variable high intensity protocol followed by a time to exhaustion (TTE) endurance capacity test (namely high intensity endurance cycling test, HIEC) as a reliable and sensitive method to assess both performance and fatigue, providing a stable platform for the comparative analysis of the effects of different nutritional interventions. HIEC can be performed either at the beginning or at the end of training periods and protocols. In the present study, we applied HIEC to a 9-week program based on High Intensity Interval Training (HIIT), a widely used protocol to improve specific variables of endurance performance. It is worth noting that, to date, to the best of our knowledge, no study has tested the effects of the consumption of a commercially available and established BCAA-alanine-CHO based supplement on HIEC over a medium-long endurance training period.

The first aim of this randomized double-blind placebo-controlled study was to determine whether, the single or prolonged intake of a commercial BCAA, Ala and CHO formula (Friliver® Performance, FP, Dompè Farmaceutici Spa), taken according to the manufacturer's recommendations, affects RPE, performance indexes and relevant serum blood markers in young adults, at the beginning (1d) and at the end (9w) of a 9-week indoor cycling HIIT. The second aim was to verify whether a prolonged supplementation may help participants to comply with the required training load during a 9w HIIT program with progressively increasing volume.

METHODS

Participants

Thirty-two healthy university students (20 males: age 22 ± 1.7 years, height 175.5 ± 6.5 cm, weight 68.2 ± 10.9 kg, BMI 22 ± 2.7 kg/m^2; 12 females: age 21 ± 0.9 years, height 159.5 ± 4.8 cm, weight 52.5 ± 5.3 kg, BMI 21 ± 1.2 kg/m^2) were recruited. The exclusion criteria were: major cardiovascular disease risks, musculoskeletal injuries, upper respiratory infection, smoking and consumption of any medicine or protein/amino acid supplement in the past 3 months. All participants, assessed with a specific questionnaire, performed no more than one 60 min leisure walking or jogging session per week in the 3 months preceding the start of the study; their VO_{2max} values at baseline were in line with—and thus confirmed—their low level of training (see Table 2). The participants were advised to maintain their dietary routine, and to abstain from using additional

dietary supplements during the study period. They were also instructed to refrain from all training activities except for the sessions included in the experimental design. Subjects were asked to refrain from the consumption of alcohol, hypnosedative drugs and beverages containing caffeine on the 2 days prior to the trial.

Study design

This was a randomized double-blind placebo-controlled trial. In order to ensure balance, randomization for permuted blocks ($n = 4$) was used. Stratification was used to ensure equal allocation by gender to each experimental condition. Study design was structured as follows: metabolic/performance (VO_{2max}, W_{peak}, W_{LT1}, W_{LT2} and TTE), biochemical (BCAA, Ala, Trp, CK serum and glucose blood levels) and RPE data were acquired before (1d) and after (9w) the incremental training period.

Supplement and supplementation regimen

FP (Dompè Farmaceutici Spa, Milan, Italy, see Table 1 for the formulation) was taken 1 h before HIEC and each training session according to the manufacturer's recommendations. BCAA and Ala content per single dose is within the range recommended by European Food Safety Authority and comparable to the dosage used in other studies. The PL group ingested a non-caloric placebo that was identical in packaging, appearance and taste to the actual supplement. FP and PL were dissolved in 500 ml of still water and ingested before each training session; neither FP nor PL was taken on rest days. Over the entire study period, the SU group received an average daily dose (total amount of each amino acid in FP/duration in days of the study) of 0.91 g leucine, 0.46 g valine, 0.46 g isoleucine and 0.91 g alanine. Importantly, as verified by the qualified medical specialist (P.B.), none of the participants experienced any side effects or adverse events as a result of the FP or placebo ingestion.

Table 1 Composition of Friliver Performance®

	Per dose	Per 100 g
Energy	71 kcal (304 kJ)	355 kcal (1520 kJ)
Total Carbohydrate	13.2 g	66 g
Sucrose	11.6 g	58 g
Polyalcohol	1.6 g	8 g
L-Leucine	1.6 g	8 g
L-Alanine	1.6 g	8 g
L-Valine	0.8 g	4 g
L-Isoleucine	0.8 g	4 g
Citric Acid	1.06 g	5 g
Orange flavor	0.8 g	4 g

Incremental test

Prior (3 days before) to the pre- and post- training experimental sessions, each subject performed an incremental test to assess individual VO_{2max}, W_{peak}, W_{LT1} and W_{LT2}. Male subjects started cycling on an electronically-braked ergometer at 75 W, and power output was increased by 25 W every 3 min, whereas female subjects started at 50 W, and power output was increased by 20 W every 3 min. All subjects continued increasing power output until volitional exhaustion or cadence dropped below 60 rpm. In the absence of specific literature, intervals were set at 3 min, which represents an appropriate compromise with previous data on incremental exercise test design. Oxygen consumption was monitored breath-by-breath and values of heart rate (HR) were recorded continuously.

Rating of perceived exertion

RPE was determined with the 0–10 OMNI-cycle scale, which combines mode-specific pictorial illustrations with a numerical rating format, using a procedure described in the literature. A standard definition of perceived exertion ("the subjective intensity of effort, strain, discomfort, and fatigue that was felt during exercise") and instructional sets for the OMNI scale were read to the subjects immediately before the exercise test. The initial exercise anchoring procedure was illustrated and performed during the incremental test (see "Incremental Test" section). Participants were asked to point to their RPE on the OMNI-cycle scale, which was in full view at all times during testing.

HIEC test

The HIEC test was performed on a power meter-provided bike. Following a warm up stage (four 5 min continuous progressive increments at a workload corresponding to 50, 60, 65 and 70% W_{peak}), participants performed ten 90 s sprints (SPR) at 90% W_{peak}, separated by 180 s recovery (REC) at 55% W_{peak}. The subjects capable of completing all the 10 SPR recovered for an additional 3 min at 55% W_{peak}, and then performed a final TTE step at 90% W_{peak}. Exhaustion was defined as the inability to maintain power output within 5 W of the target output for 15 s despite verbal encouragement; no feedback on elapsed time was provided. TTE was taken as a performance marker. Subjects were asked to maintain the same predefined cadence throughout the HIEC regardless of the power output variations (from 90 to 55% W_{peak}) introduced by the operator at each REC/SPR change. Subjects were asked to provide their RPE 10 s before the end of each of the warm up, SPR and REC steps.

Design of the 1d and 9w experimental training sessions

The 32 subjects were divided in 4 groups of 8, and they performed the HIEC test on two consecutive days (2 groups per day). On the experimental day, subjects in the first group arrived at the laboratory at 06.00 AM, 2 h before the test, in a fasted state. The second group of the day arrived 2 h later in a fasted state. All subjects had a standardized breakfast consisting of 400 ml of fruit juice and servings of jam tart adjusted according to gender caloric needs (90 g for females and 135 g for males; total breakfast calories: 612–794 kcal, 119.6–150.6 g CHO, 6–8.4 g Protein, 11.4–16.9 g Fat). The design of the experimental session is shown in Fig. 1.

Design of the experimental sessions at 1d and 9w. The experimental sessions were performed in the morning. 1 h after breakfast, participants had their first blood

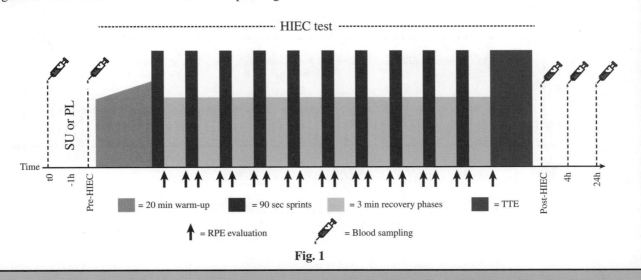

Fig. 1

draw immediately before the consumption of SU or PL; after another 1-h interval, a second blood sampling was performed immediately before the beginning of the HIEC (Pre-HIEC). In the course of the HIEC, RPE was repeatedly evaluated as indicated by the arrows. Further blood samples were collected immediately, at 4 and 24 h after the completion of the HIEC

Blood sampling and analysis

Venous blood samples (5 ml) were obtained from the antecubital vein 1 h after breakfast (immediately before FP or PL ingestion) (T0), 1 h after ingestion (immediately before exercise) (pre-HIEC), immediately post exercise (post-HIEC), after 4 h and 24 h.

Glycemia assessment

Blood glucose was measured by a portable glucometer at the following times: T0 in the fasted state; immediately and 30 min after breakfast; before the intake of FP or PL (1 h after the standardized breakfast); 30 min after intake of SU or PL; and immediately before and after the HIEC test.

Training protocol

Thirty-six indoor cycling training sessions were performed over a 9w period (see Fig. 2). The training sessions were divided into three mesocycles (see Fig. 2).

The 32 subjects were divided in two groups of 16 and trained by two expert instructors with the aim of following the same training program. Each session was choreographed based on conventional principles (warm-up, systematic high intensity interval exercise, and cool-down) widely used in the indoor cycling community. The training program of each session was designed following the same intensity distribution, based on a polarized model, with around 70% of the session time spent in zone 1, 10% spent in zone 2 and 20% spent in zone 3 (see "Incremental Test" section for zone determination). During the training sessions, the HR of each subject (instructor included) was monitored and recorded. HR values were projected onto the wall, as percentage of maximal HR (% HR_{max}), and the subjects were asked to maintain the same intensity as the instructor.

One hour before each training session, the subjects of the SU group ingested a single dose of FP, while the subjects of the PL group ingested the placebo.

Training load analysis

Lucia's TRIMP was used to calculate the Training Load for each session. The concept of Lucia's TRIMP integrates total volume, on the one hand, and total intensity relative to the intensity zones, on the other. Briefly, the score for each zone is calculated by multiplying the accumulated duration in the zone by a multiplier for that particular zone (e.g. 1 min in zone 1 is given a score of 1 TRIMP (1 X 1), 1 min in Zone 2 is given a score of 2 TRIMP (1 X 2), and 1 min in Zone 3 is given a score of 3 TRIMP (1 X 3); the total TRIMP score is then obtained by summing the results of the three zones. Finally, the mean TRIMP scores of each mesocycle performed by the SU and PL groups were compared.

Fig. 2 Structure of training period: nine weeks divided into three mesocycles (three weeks each). The frequency and the duration of the sessions are also indicated. Key: VO_{2max}, maximal oxygen consumption; W_{LT1} and W_{LT2}, power at lactate thresholds; W_{peak}, peak power; HIEC-T, high intensity endurance cycling test.

Diet & Diet Tracking

During the entire training period, subjects' nutrition was monitored daily (by call interviews, always carried out after dinner) and data were collected and processed; macronutrients and total energy intake for experimental and control groups were finally compared in order to exclude differences in nutritional habits.

Statistical analysis

Descriptive statistics were performed using means and standard deviations. Homogeneity between groups was tested using the unpaired t-test. Daily protein, fat, carbohydrate and total caloric intake were compared between groups; the t-test and Cohen's effect size (ES) were used to quantify differences.

RESULTS

Baseline anthropometric, metabolic and biomechanical variables

Anthropometric, metabolic and biomechanical variables of participants were assessed before the beginning of the experimental session as reported in Table 2. No differences were found between the two groups in the tested parameters.

Diet monitoring

Daily caloric intake over the study period was virtually identical for both groups: 1944 ± 876 kcal in the SU group vs. 2043 ± 947 in the PL group, with no significant difference (t-test; $p > 0.05$).

Daily CHO, fat and protein intakes, supplemented vs placebo group were 49.1% vs. 51.1%; 33.4% vs 32.4%; 17.4% vs. 16.9%, respectively. No differences in specific macronutrient intake were found between groups (t-test; $p > 0.05$).

VO_{2max}, W_{peak} and power at lactate thresholds at 1d and 9w

All these variables, namely VO_{2max}, W_{peak}, W_{LT1} and W_{LT2}, were significantly different in pre vs. post 9w training as shown in Table 3. For all variables, p values were <0.001. Results indicate that all post training values were significantly greater than pre-training ones. The effect of SU intake was not significant ($p > 0.05$) for all dependent variables.

Table 2 Anthropometric, metabolic and biomechanical variables of the participants at baseline; Mean, standard deviations and p-values for group are reported

	Supplemented Group ($n=16$)		Placebo Group ($n=16$)		Group (p)
Participants	Males = 10	Females = 6	Males = 10	Females = 6	
Age (yr)	22.1 ± 2.2	20.6 ± 1.0	21.0 ± 1.0	20.5 ± 0.7	0.322
Height (cm)	173.9 ± 6.0	157.2 ± 4.4	177.1 ± 6.8	161.8 ± 4.3	0.072
Weight (kg)	69.2 ± 12.7	50.3 ± 4.8	67.2 ± 6.9	54.6 ± 5.2	0.726
BMI (kg/m^2)	22.8 ± 3.4	20.3 ± 1.2	21.4 ± 1.6	20.8 ± 1.4	0.584
HR_{max} (bpm)	197.3 ± 8.2	197.5 ± 5.0	199.0 ± 7.8	199.7 ± 4.7	0.458
VO_{2max} (ml/kg/min)	42.6 ± 10.4	35.0 ± 8.5	43.9 ± 4.5	28.1 ± 3.1	0.315
W_{peak} (watt)	212.5 ± 33.9	146.7 ± 23.4	230.0 ± 28.4	133.3 ± 23.4	0.844
W_{LT1} (watt)	76.1 ± 11.3	57.7 ± 23.8	73.9 ± 22.3	40.8 ± 14.0	0.312
W_{LT2} (watt)	127.1 ± 23.4	88.2 ± 23.5	138.8 ± 27.6	74.9 ± 16.6	0.928

Table 3 VO_{2max}, W_{peak}, W_{LT1} and W_{LT2}*, in SU and PL groups at 1d and 9w

	Supplemented Group			Placebo Group		
	1d	9w	Δ%	1d	9w	Δ%
VO_{2max}	39.73 ± 10.18	44.58 ± 6.67	+12%	37.95 ± 8.82	42.93 ± 5.54	+13%
W_{peak}	187.81 ± 44.20	231.56 ± 48.91	+23%	193.75 ± 54.79	239.06 ± 56.01	+23%
W_{LT1}	69.21 ± 18.69	103.64 ± 32.95	+50%	64.83 ± 27.12	91.03 ± 26.56	+40%
W_{LT2}	112.50 ± 29.85	155.56 ± 35.34	+38%	114.83 ± 39.59	156.51 ± 40.66	+36%

Perceived exertion during HIEC test

RPE values, measured during the 20 min warm up of the HIEC tests increased progressively, showing a very similar trend in the PL and SU groups in both 1d and 9w periods (Fig. 3a and b, respectively). During the 10 SPR, each of them followed by a REC step, RPE showed an upward trend characterized by a sawtooth pattern in all the conditions tested. As expected, the RPE values reached the maximum at the end of the TTE step (11 points on OMNI cycle scale). Hence, only RPE values starting from 20 min (the end of warm up) to 65 min (prior to TTE phase) were considered for further analyses (data highlighted in grey box).

Perceived exertion at 1d (pre training HIEC test)

The linear regression equation of the curve built on SPR steps showed that intercepts ($p = 0.163$) and slopes ($p = 0.086$) were not significantly different. The linear regression equation of REC steps showed that intercepts were not significantly different ($p = 0.742$), whereas, interestingly, slopes were ($p = 0.001$). This would imply that in REC steps, the SU group showed a lower RPE (Fig. 3c e 3E).

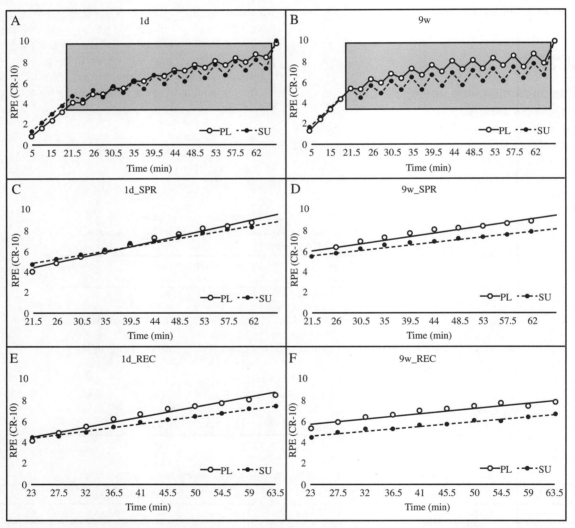

Fig. 3 Perceived exertion rate (RPE) values versus session time; a-b whole RPE time series; c-d RPE values in sprint (SPR) steps at pre-training (1d) and post training (9w) stages, respectively; e-f RPE values in REC steps at 1d and 9w, respectively. Closed circles refer to SU and open circles to the PL group.

Perceived exertion at 9w (post training HIEC test)

The linear regression equation of SPR steps showed that slopes, unlike intercepts ($p = 0.079$), were significantly different ($p = 0.017$), suggesting that in the SPR phase, the SU group showed a lower RPE. The linear regression equation of REC steps showed that slopes were not significantly different ($p = 0.371$), while an extremely significant difference was found between intercepts ($p < 0.001$). This implies that in the REC steps, the SU group showed a systematically lower RPE (Fig. 3d and f).

On the whole, RPE values increased linearly over the execution time of HIEC in both the SU and PL groups (Fig. 3a and b). Notably, the extent of the increment was significantly lower in the SU group than it was in the PL group in all the conditions tested (Fig. 3d, e and f), with the only exception of the 1d pre-training SPR phase (Fig. c); the lowest increment was observed in the 9w post-training REC phase.

Performance during HIEC test: time to exhaustion

TTE values were determined and taken as reliable performance parameters. Analysis of the 1d data failed to reveal significant differences between groups ($371 \pm 147\,s$ for SU; $359 \pm 177\,s$ for PL; $p > 0.05$). On the contrary, with regard to 9w, data showed that the mean TTE was significantly longer for the SU group ($517 \pm 210\,s$) than for the PL group ($321 \pm 214\,s$) ($p = 0.025$).

Training load analysis

TRIMP represents a recognized parameter to express the extent of training load. TRIMP values were compared between groups in the course of the training period, which was divided into three different three-week mesocycles characterized by progressively increasing training loads. During the first mesocycle subjects averaged 98.4 ± 4.9 TRIMP (SU) and 97.9 ± 4.1 (PL) per session; during the second mesocycle, subjects averaged 97.9 ± 5.4 TRIMP (SU) and 96.5 ± 7.1 (PL) per session; no differences in these mesocycles were found between groups ($p > 0.05$). Notably, during the last mesocycle TRIMP values were significantly higher ($p = 0.014$) in the SU group than they were in the PL group, with averages of 109.4 ± 5.7 vs 104.1 ± 6.4 per session, respectively. Data are shown in Fig. 4.

Fig. 4 Training loads in the PL and SU groups as a function of mesocycles and training progression. Bars represent the mean training impulse (TRIMP) associated with the corresponding mesocycle in the PL (white columns) and SU (black columns) groups (standard deviations are reported). Dashed lines (SU) and solid lines (PL) were obtained using a 5-day moving average. $* p < 0.05$ as compared to PL; $\# p < 0.05$ as compared to an earlier time point.

Serum blood levels of BCAA and ratios of free Trp:BCAA

Blood samples were collected immediately before (T0), 1 h after the ingestion (pre-HIEC) of FP or PL, and at the end of the HIEC test (post-HIEC). HPLC analysis of serum blood samples (Fig. 5) showed that total BCAA concentrations ([BCAA] is the total amount of Leu, Isoleu, and Val concentrations) before the ingestion of FP or PL powder at both 1d and 9w were similar, and that at pre-HIEC they increased significantly only in the SU group ($p < 0.05$). [BCAA] measured at post-HIEC decreased significantly in the SU group at 1d and 9w, though to a lesser extent in the latter case.

Fig. 5 Branched chain amino acids [BCAA] serum blood levels. Panels **a** and **b** show analyses performed at 1d and 9w respectively. Values for the SU (black bars) and PL (white bars) groups are reported, with mean and standard deviations. * $p < 0.05$ per group; # $p < 0.05$ per time.

Regarding Trp:BCAA ratios, at pre-HIEC they were consistently higher in the PL group than they were in the SU group (Fig. 6). At 1d, notwithstanding the time-related increase in both groups (pre- vs post-HIEC), the PL group was characterized by a higher ratio than the SU group; interestingly, at 9w a statistically significant increase could be found only in the PL group.

Glycemia

Glycemia was determined prior to breakfast (4.8 ± 0.1 and 5.3 ± 0.2 mM in SU vs PL respectively, $p > 0.05$) and at different time points up to the end of HIEC test. As expected, 30 min after breakfast, glucose levels increased (9.4 ± 1.5 and 8.5 ± 1.8 mM in the SU and PL groups respectively) and decreased thereafter, approaching basal

levels (5.7 ± 0.5 in SU vs 5.6 ± 0.6 mM in PL; $p > 0.05$). No further significant difference between groups was observed post-HIEC (6.1 ± 0.2 vs 5.8 ± 0.6 mM in SU and PL respectively; $p > 0.05$).

DISCUSSION

The effects of FP—an established, commercially available sports nutritional supplement containing BCAA, Ala and CHO—on RPE, performance and the capacity to sustain physical training were investigated in a group of 32 healthy young subjects enrolled in a randomized double-blind placebo-controlled trial. Along with RPE and performance values, a number of relevant nutritional and biological

Fig. 6 Free Trp to BCAA ratios. Trp:BCAA ratios before (pre-HIEC) and after HIEC test (post-HIEC) are shown. Panel **a** shows analyses performed at 1d and panel **b** those performed at 9w. Values for the SU (black bars) and PL (white bars) groups are reported as means with standard deviations. * $p < 0.05$ between groups; # $p < 0.05$ between time points.

parameters were also determined. Notably, to the best of our knowledge, this is the first study adopting a validated and reliable HIEC protocol for these purposes.

The major finding of this study is that a single intake of FP is capable of attenuating RPE, and that its prolonged 9w consumption according to manufacturer's recommendations not only augments RPE-attenuating capacity, but also improves TTE and TRIMP, which both reflect the capacity to sustain training loads. HPLC analysis of blood sampled 1 h after FP ingestion, unlike the sample taken 1 h after PL administration, showed a significant increase in BCAA levels. This finding indicates that BCAA are rapidly absorbed after oral ingestion of FP, and that their increased serum blood concentration is likely related to the above-mentioned effects on RPE, TTE and TRIMP.

Following the first intake, the SU group showed lower RPE values only in the HIEC REC phases, while a significant RPE reduction was found following a chronic (9w) intake also in the high intensity SPR phases. Furthermore, both acute and chronic intake caused a significantly more rapid decrease in RPE observed between the SPR and corresponding REC phases compared to PL. It is worth noting that, unlike previous studies on BCAA and RPE, by virtue of the particular design of the HIEC test, this is the first investigation in which RPE associated with SPR or with REC phases was separately quantitated. This allowed us to determine that FP significantly accelerated the reduction of RPE during the recovery phases compared to PL.

Our results indicate that serum blood circulating Trp:BCAA ratios increase after HIEC in PL, and that FP consumption invariably prevented this effect. Under the conditions we observed in the PL group, namely an increased Trp:BCAA ratio, Trp is supposed to be more available for brain uptake, thus promoting an augmented synthesis of serotonin; on the contrary, a significantly lower Trp:BCAA ratio, which we did observe in the SU group, is thought to antagonize brain Trp uptake, thus limiting serotonin synthesis and availability. According to the widely held belief linking brain serotonin increases with central fatigue development, this sequence of events might have contributed to the lower RPE values we observed upon acute and/or prolonged FP supplementation.

Regarding glycemia, we did not find any variation between the two groups in the glycemic values of pre- and post-HIEC tests, suggesting that the extra CHO of FP do not significantly modify blood glucose prior to or after testing compared to PL. In this regard, it should also be considered that in our setting both groups had ingested a breakfast containing 120–150 g of CHO 1 h before HIEC, that is approximately tenfold the amount of CHO contained in FP. In light of these considerations, the CHO contribution to the functional and metabolic outcomes described thus far is probably limited. Indeed, a recent study by O'Hara et al., using the same experimental setting we adopted in the present investigation, showed that the intake of 40 g of CHO (galactose or glucose) in one liter of water, taken 30 min before HIEC, did not modify the RPE or the TTE compared to the placebo.

Finally, with respect to the possible direct effects of CHO on RPE, only in studies in which CHO were given during —and not prior to (as in our case)—endurance exercise have such effects been observed. On the whole, it can be inferred that in our conditions CHO hardly affect RPE through direct central interactions.

With regard to performance, most of the studies on BCAA-containing supplements have failed to find any significant improvements nor did we find any differences in terms of relevant metabolic parameters (VO_{2max} and Power at Lactate Thresholds) between SU and PL, either upon single (1d) or prolonged (9w) supplementation. However, even though TTE did not improve after the first, acute intake of FP, it did increase significantly following the 9w supplementation. This observation is in line with those of Kephart et al., showing that, although in a different experimental settings, 10-week BCAA supplementation results in increased peak/mean power in well-trained cyclists. Interestingly, the same study also reported a significant increase in serum blood [BCAA] and a consequent improvement in the circulating Trp:BCAA ratio, hence suggesting that performance enhancement could be related to a central fatigue-mediated mechanism. Considering that our SU group did not show any improvement in metabolic parameters or free-fat mass (not shown), we also suggest that the TTE increase might be related to the stable attenuation of RPE rather than to ergogenic or anabolic effects.

With regard to the ability to sustain training loads, our results showed that TRIMP were the same in both groups with work volumes per week <240 min. Interestingly, at higher work volumes (ca. 350 min in the third mesocycle) TRIMP values were significantly higher in the SU than in the PL group. In this regard, it is worth considering that higher TRIMP expresses an increased ability to sustain exercise at high HR values, while lower TRIMP reflects the relative inability to exercise under the same conditions.

On the whole, our data suggest that the higher TRIMP values found in SU subjects at 9w reflect their enhanced capacity to sustain training, whose volume may consequently increase over time leading to better performance than that achieved by PL subjects. Reduction in RPE, which was observed from the very beginning of the test period, is likely to play a pivotal role in the progressively enhanced capacity to sustain higher training volumes. The main limitation of the present study, as well as of similar ones, lies in the use of a multi-ingredient supplement, which makes it difficult to determine the relative impact of each component on the tested markers: as a consequence, ascertaining which of the ingredients had what effect or if there was a synergistic interaction among the ingredients remains an open question. On the other hand, the strength of this study resides in the fact that it details a multi-technique experimental approach that could be applied, in the future, to directly compare the efficacy of formulations containing different constituents (such as caffeine, electrolytes, β-alanine etc.) in attenuating RPE. This would be important because, at present, it is very hard to compare the effects of different sport supplements with different formulations on RPE because they have been studied using non-homogeneous experimental designs and approaches.

CONCLUSIONS

The main findings of this study are that the consumption of FP (a commercially available nutritional supplement containing BCAA, Ala and CHO) according to the producer's suggestions reduces RPE at all the time points tested and that, over a 9w-intake, also improves TTE and TRIMP. Although it was not possible to specifically address mechanistic issues, the effects we observed are in keeping with the theory of RPE sensitivity to serum blood Trp:BCAA ratio, while the contribution of metabolic effects seems negligible. The prolonged intake of FP, which promotes a reduction in RPE and recovery times, can enhance the capacity to sustain higher training loads and ultimately improve endurance performance. Importantly, these effects occur without affecting dietary habits and caloric intake.

Abbreviations

1d : 1 day
9w : 9 weeks
Ala: Alanine
BCAA: Branched-Chain Amino Acids
CHO: Carbohydrate
CK: Creatine Kinase
CNS: Central Nervous System
FP: Friliver Performance
HIEC: High Intensity Endurance Cycling
HIIT: High Intensity Interval Training
HR: Heart Rate
LT: Lactate threshold
PL: Placebo group
RDA: Recommended Dietary Allowance
REC: Recovery phase
RPE: Rating of Perceived Exertion
SPR: Sprint phase
SU: Supplemented group
TRIMP: Training Impulse
Trp: Tryptophan
TTE: Time To Exhaustion
VO_{2max} *:* Maximal oxygen consumption
W: Watt
W_{LT} *:* Power at lactate threshold
W_{peak} *:* Peak power

JOURNAL ARTICLE EXERCISE 3

The science sections on the MCAT include a significant number of passages with experiments. Questions for these passages often ask you to analyze data, read charts and graphs, and come to some reasonable conclusion based on the information they give you. If you don't know how to extract information efficiently and analyze data effectively, you will be at a distinct disadvantage.

There are three "Journal Article Exercises" in this book. In this final exercise, you'll read and extract information from the article, then complete an MCAT passage based on this article. After that, we'll show you the "correct" information to pull out and the answers to the passage.

As before, when analyzing an experiment, you should be able to:

- identify the control group(s)
- extract information from graphs and data tables
- determine how the experimental group(s) change relative to the control
- determine if the results are statistically significant
- come to a reasonable conclusion about WHY the results were observed
- consider potential weaknesses in the study
- determine how to increase the power of the study
- decide what the next most logical experiment or study should be

And, as before, the goal of these exercises is NOT to learn content from the articles, just to get a little more comfortable reading and extracting information from them.

For the (abridged) article on pages 499–508, summarize the purpose of the experiment and the methods in a few sentences. Remember the mnemonic: Oh ouR Car Won't Start (ORCWS).

- O = Organism and Organization
- R = Results
- C = Control and Comparison
- W = Weirdness
- S = Statistics

Try interpreting the data on your own before reading the results/discussion section. When you do read the discussion, consider:

- What are the conclusions of the study?
- How are the conclusions supported by the data?
- What potential weaknesses or flaws do you see in the experimental design? Are these addressed in the discussion section?
- How might this study be potentially biased?
- How might this study be improved?
- What would be the next most logical experiment?

Answer the above questions for the article on pages 499–508.

1. **O = Organism and Organization:**
   - Is the research being conducted on humans or on animals or on bacteria in a petri dish, or something else?

     _____

     _____

   - What is being done to these organisms?

     _____

     _____

   - Are there any unique qualities to these organisms?

     _____

     _____

   - Are there multiple groups?

     _____

     _____

   - Is the study conducted over a long period of time with multiple data points, or is it a short-term study?

     _____

     _____

   - Does it have a large or small n?

     _____

     _____

2. **R = Results:**
   - Where and how are the results presented? Is it a graph? A data table? Figures and images?

     _____

     _____

- What is/are the independent variable(s)?

  _____

  _____

- What is/are the dependent variable(s)?

  _____

  _____

- What are the results of the study?

  _____

  _____

- Do the results show correlation or cause and effect, or both? Describe.

  _____

  _____

3. **C = Control and Comparison:**
   - Is there a control group?

     _____

     _____

   - How does it differ from the experimental group? Is it given a placebo or nothing at all? Is it held under different conditions?

     _____

     _____

   - If there are multiple experimental groups, how do they differ from one another?

     _____

     _____

   - Is it a blinded study? If so, double blind or single blind?

     _____

     _____

4. **W = Weirdness:**
   - Does anything or do any of the results stand out as unexpected?

     _____

     _____

5. **S = Statistics:**
   - Was any sort of statistical analysis done?

     _____

     _____

- How is it presented? Are there error bars on a graph? Standard errors around a mean? Are there *p*-values? Is there an asterisk indicating statistical significance?

  _____

  _____

- Is there any data that is not statistically significant?

  _____

  _____

6. **Interpreting the data:**
   - What are the conclusions of the study?

     _____

     _____

   - How are the conclusions supported by the data?

     _____

     _____

   - What potential weaknesses or flaws do you see in the experimental design? Are these addressed in the discussion section?

     _____

     _____

   - How might this study be potentially biased?

     _____

     _____

   - How might this study be improved?

     _____

     _____

   - What would be the next most logical experiment?

     _____

     _____

7. **Final Summary of Experiment and Results:**

   _____

   _____

   _____

   _____

   _____

   _____

JOURNAL ARTICLE EXERCISE 3 PASSAGE

Thirty young adults who did not participate in regular exercise were recruited for a nine-week study to assess the effect of a sport nutritional supplement containing branched-chain amino acids (BCAA) on the ability to perform sustained cardiovascular activity. The protocol consisted of three, 3-week periods during which 36 indoor cycling training sessions were performed. Training sessions increased in frequency, duration, and intensity over the nine weeks. Half the participants (SU group) ingested a supplement 1 hour before each training session and the other half (PL group) ingested a non-caloric placebo. The 70 kcal supplement consisted of carbohydrates, BCAA (L, V, and I), and alanine. Participants were of similar ages and habitus. Diet was monitored carefully to ensure that calorie intake and macromolecules distribution (daily carbohydrate, protein, and fat intake) were consistent between groups.

At one day and at nine weeks, the groups performed a high-intensity endurance cycling (HIEC) test after consuming a standardized breakfast (between 600–800 kcal) and either the supplement or the placebo. The test consisted of a 20-minute warm-up, followed by ten 90-second sprints at 90% peak power, interspersed with ten 3-minute recovery periods (55% peak power). After the final recovery period, subjects cycled at 90% peak power to exhaustion, defined as the inability to maintain power output within 5 W of the target for 15 seconds. Subjects provided their rate of perceived exertion (RPE) at the end of the warm-up, and after each of the sprint and recovery steps. Results for the sprint steps are shown in Figure 1.

Prolonged exercise can lead to increased brain uptake of tryptophan. Tryptophan is a serotonin precursor, and BCAA can compete with Trp in crossing the blood-brain barrier. Increases in serotonin, as well as decreases in dopamine, lead to *central fatigue*, a complex combination of events that arise under conditions of low energy availability, in which the central nervous system is not able to supply sufficient signal to skeletal muscle. Free Trp:BCAA ratios before and after HIEC are shown in Figure 2.

Figure 2 Free Trp to BCAA ratios before (pre-HIEC) and after HIEC test (post-HIEC) at 1d and at 9w. *$p < 0.05$ between groups; #$p < 0.05$ between time points.

Adapted from Gervasi, M., Sisti, D., Amatori, S. *et al.* Effects of a commercially available branched-chain amino acid-alanine-carbohydrate-based sports supplement on perceived exertion and performance in high intensity endurance cycling tests. *J Int Soc Sports Nutr* 17, 6 (2020).

Figure 1 Sprint RPE vs. time, pre-training (1d) and post training (9w)

1. Which of the following statements is true with regard to the RPE data?

A) The placebo group had a higher RPE at 1d beginning at 39.5 minutes and for all subsequent time points.
B) The supplement group had a lower RPE for all time points measured.
C) The placebo group had a higher RPE for all time points measured at 9w.
D) The supplement group at 9w would have a longer time to exhaustion after the final recovery period.

2. Does the data in Figure 2 support the differences reported in RPE between the two groups?

A) Yes, the placebo group has a significantly higher Trp:BCAA ratio, which is correlated with the reduced RPE reported by this group.
B) Yes, the supplement group has a significantly lower Trp:BCAA ratio, which is correlated with the reduced RPE reported by this group.
C) No, the supplement group has a significantly higher Trp:BCAA ratio post-HIEC, indicating an increase in central fatigue.
D) No, lower Trp:BCAA ratios would lead to increases in serotonin, which is correlated with increases in central fatigue.

3. Which of the following is true of alanine?

A) Its side chain is reactive, so it is often found at the active sites of enzymes.
B) It was included in the experiment because it is a branched chain amino acid.
C) It would travel further up a silica gel plate in TLC than would tyrosine.
D) It can be used in gluconeogenesis because it is a ketogenic amino acid.

4. Researchers concluded that BCAAs reduce RPE and central fatigue. Which of the following casts the most doubt on their conclusion?

A) The supplement contained both carbohydrates and BCAAs.
B) RPEs were not significantly lower for the supplement group in all conditions.
C) Tryptophan was not included in the supplement to help reduce central fatigue.
D) Both groups show higher Trp:BCAA ratios post-HIEC.

SOLUTIONS TO JOURNAL ARTICLE EXERCISE 3

1. **O = Organism and Organization:**
    - Is the research being conducted on humans or on animals or on bacteria in a petri dish, or something else? *Humans.*
    - What is being done to these organisms? *They are subjected to 9 weeks of exercise, half ingest a placebo and half ingest a supplement with carbohydrates and BCAAs (branched chain amino acids).*
    - Are there any unique qualities to these organisms? *All volunteers were young adults that did not regularly participate in exercise prior to the study.*
    - Are there multiple groups? *Not initially, but they were ultimately divided into two groups.*
    - Is the study conducted over a long period of time with multiple data points, or is it a short-term study? *Medium-long time (9 weeks) with data points collected at the beginning and end of the 9 weeks.*
    - Does it have a large or small *n*? *Small n: 32 total subjects.*

2. **R = Results:**
    - Where and how are the results presented? Is it a graph? A data table? Figures and images? *Graphs and data tables.*
    - What is/are the independent variable(s)? *Time and exercise regimen, amount of supplement or placebo ingested.*
    - What is/are the dependent variable(s)? VO_{2max}, *max power, lactate threshold, RPE (rate of perceived exertion), blood BCAA, tryptophan, sugar levels.*
    - What are the results of the study? *Both the placebo and supplement groups showed a similar increase in VO_{2max}, max power, and lactate threshold, however the supplement group showed a significant reduction in RPE during recovery phases (even after a single ingestion) and a reduction in RPE during both recovery and sprint phases, as well as an increase in TTE (time to exhaustion) when consuming the supplement over the 9-week period.*
    - Do the results show correlation or cause and effect, or both? Describe. *Cause and effect. The supplement group showed reduction in RPE and the placebo group did not.*

3. **C = Control and Comparison:**
    - Is there a control group? *Yes.*
    - How does it differ from the experimental group? Is it given a placebo or nothing at all? Is it held under different conditions? *The control group consumed a non-caloric, non-supplemented drink designed to mimic the supplement in the way it looked.*
    - If there are multiple experimental groups, how do they differ from one another? *Only one experimental group.*
    - Is it a blinded study? If so, double blind or single blind? *Double blind; neither the researchers nor the participants knew whether they were ingesting the supplement or the placebo.*

4. **W = Weirdness:**
    - Does anything or do any of the results stand out as unexpected? *The fact that there was no difference in VO_{2max}, max power, and lactate thresholds between the supplement and placebo groups was unexpected. It seems like the supplement only works to reduce perceived effort.*

5. **S = Statistics:**
   - Was any sort of statistical analysis done? *Yes.*
   - How is it presented? Are there error bars on a graph? Standard errors around a mean? Are there *p*-values? Is there an asterisk indicating statistical significance? *P-values, error bars, asterisks.*
   - Is there any data that is not statistically significant? *Yes, initial characteristics of the supplement and placebo groups (age, body weight, etc.), VO_{2max}, max power, and lactate thresholds, dietary intake.*

6. **Interpreting the data:**
   - What are the conclusions of the study? *Ingestion of a BCAA supplement can lower the RPE of high-intensity cycling, allowing participants to work harder for longer with less perceived effort.*
   - How are the conclusions supported by the data? *Data on RPE show significant differences (a reduction of RPE in the supplement group) after both 1 day and 9 weeks. Also, data on Trp:BCAA ratio shows lower levels in the supplement group both after a single ingestion and after 9 weeks of supplementation; since an increased Trp:BCAA ratio is related to increased serotonin levels, and increased serotonin is related to fatigue, a lower Trp:BCAA ratio could account for less perceived exertion.*
   - What potential weaknesses or flaws do you see in the experimental design? Are these addressed in the discussion section? *The possible weakness is that the BCAAs they were testing were consumed in a supplement containing other things as well (carbohydrates, alanine). It may be that these other things could account for the observed effect, or could be acting synergistically with the BCAAs. This was addressed in the discussion section.*
   - How might this study be potentially biased? *It was a small group, and only tested on young adults.*
   - How might this study be improved? *Bigger sample size, more diversity in subjects with regard to age.*
   - What would be the next most logical experiment? *Repeat the experiment with subjects in varying age groups, repeat the experiment with single supplementation (just BCAAs, just carbohydrates, etc.), consider other supplements to test (e.g., caffeine, electrolytes, etc.).*

7. **Final Summary of Experiment and Results:**
   - *In this study a group of approximately 32 young adults were divided into two main groups, one that received a supplement prior to every exercise session over a 9-week period, and one that received a placebo. Both groups were subjected to high intensity interval training sessions that increased in intensity over the 9 weeks. At the beginning and end of the 9 weeks, subjects were asked to rate their perceived exertion during the sprint and recovery sessions of the exercise, and their time to exhaustion was measured. RPE was reduced and TTE was increased in the group receiving supplementation, even though both groups showed similar increases in $VO_{2\,max}$, max power, and lactate thresholds. The conclusion is that supplementation results in a lower RPE, which allows the subjects to work longer and harder, theoretically allowing them to sustain a harder/greater volume training load than the non-supplemented group, and this might ultimately lead to better performance.*

SOLUTIONS TO JOURNAL ARTICLE EXERCISE 3 PASSAGE

1. **C**   In Figure 1, only the data for RPE at 9w is significant, with a *p*-value of 0.01; this data shows that the placebo group had a higher RPE at all 9w time points (choice C is correct). The data for RPE at 1d has a *p*-value of 0.16, indicating that the differences between the placebo and supplement groups are not significant (even if some of the individual data points for the placebo group at 1d appear to be higher; choice A can be eliminated). Similarly, the supplement group does not have a lower RPE for the time points at 1d since the data is not significant (choice B can be eliminated). While it might seem safe to assume that the supplement group would have a longer time to exhaustion than the placebo group, given that their RPE is lower, there is no data shown to support this (choice D can be eliminated).

2. **B**   Figure 2 shows that the supplement group has a significantly lower Trp:BCAA ratio than the placebo group at all time points measured. The passage states that tryptophan is a serotonin precursor, and that increases in serotonin can lead to central fatigue. The reduced Trp:BCAA ratio means that free Trp levels are lower or BCAA levels are higher, and the passage further states that BCAA can compete with Trp in crossing the blood brain barrier. If BCAA levels are higher, less Trp will cross the blood brain barrier, and less Trp means less serotonin (choice D is wrong), which means less central fatigue and a reduced RPE (choice B is correct). Higher Trp:BCAA ratios would mean more Trp, more serotonin, more central fatigue, and a higher RPE, not a reduced RPE; furthermore the placebo group reported higher RPE than the supplement group (choice A is wrong). While choice C is technically correct (the supplement group does have a higher Trp:BCAA ratio post-HIEC at both 1 day and 9 weeks, and likely has an increase in central fatigue because of it), this answer choice does not address the differences in RPE between the groups, which is what this question is asking about (choice C is wrong).

3. **C**   Alanine is a hydrophobic amino acid that would interact more with an organic solvent in TLC than it would with the silica gel plate. Tyrosine is polar and would interact more with the plate than the solvent. Thus, alanine would travel further during TLC than tyrosine (choice C is correct). The side chain of alanine is a methyl group (choice B is wrong) and is unreactive (choice A is wrong). Ketogenic amino acids are not used in gluconeogenesis; they are converted to acetyl-CoA and contribute to ketogenesis (choice D is wrong). Note also that alanine is not ketogenic, but you did not have to know that to eliminate this answer choice.

4. **A**   The fact that the supplement contained both carbohydrates and BCAA means that the reduction in RPE might have been due to the carbohydrates and not the amino acids (choice A is correct). While it is true that the supplement group RPE were not lower than the placebo group RPE for all conditions (day 1, sprint RPE are not statistically different between supplement and placebo groups), they were lower for all other conditions, and most importantly, were lower for both sprint and recovery phases at the end of the nine-week training period. This casts less doubt on the researchers' conclusions than the carbohydrates in the supplement (choice B is wrong). The passage states that tryptophan is a serotonin precursor and that increases in serotonin contribute to central fatigue. Thus, to reduce central fatigue, tryptophan should not have been added to the supplement in order to reduce serotonin levels; in any case, tryptophan is not a branched-chain amino acid, which is what this study examined (choice C is wrong). It is true that both supplement and placebo groups show higher Trp:BCAA ratios post-HIEC, however, the conclusions of the researchers were based on the differences between supplement and placebo groups post-HIEC, not the differences between pre- and post-HIEC. The supplement group had a smaller increase in Trp:BCAA than the placebo group (choice D is wrong).

Appendix I
Some Molecular
Biology Techniques

The material in this section is not *strictly* MCAT material, thus it is presented in this appendix as a reference source; in other words, you don't need to memorize it, but you should read it for familiarity. The MCAT is a test of your ability to deal with new material like this, presented on the exam in passage form. Note also that this is a very general overview. More detail on these processes can be found in *MCAT Biochemistry Review*.

A.1 ENZYME-LINKED IMMUNO-SORBENT ASSAY (ELISA)

As the name suggests, an ELISA is a biochemical technique that utilizes antigen-antibody interactions ("immuno-sorbency") to determine the presence of either

- antigens (like proteins or cytokines), or
- specific immunoglobulins (antibodies)

in a sample (such as cells recovered from a tumor biopsy or a patient's serum). When testing for the presence of a specific antigen, the wells are coated with an antibody specific for that antigen. Then the sample is added, and if the antigen is present, it will bind to the antibodies. The wells are washed and a secondary antibody (specific for the antigen) is added; the secondary antibody is linked to a detection enzyme.

When testing for the presence of a specific antibody in a sample, the *antigen* (for which the antibody is specific) is first allowed to adhere directly to the wells. The sample is added and then mixed with enzyme-linked antibodies.

ELISA can be used to screen patients for viral infections. For example, serum from a patient suspected to be infected with HIV is loaded into wells that are coated with HIV coat proteins. If the serum contains anti-HIV antibodies (indicating infection), the antibodies will adhere to the proteins on the wells, bind enzyme-linked antibodies, and effect a color change.

A.2 RADIOIMMUNOASSAY (RIA)

RIAs are similar to ELISAs but use radiolabeled antigen and antibodies rather than enzyme-linked antibodies. Thus, the presence of target proteins or antibodies is assayed by measuring the amount of radioactivity instead of a color change. RIAs are more extensively used in the medical field to measure the relative amounts of hormones or drugs in patients' sera. A known amount of radiolabeled antigen is mixed with a known amount of antibody and the total amount of radioactivity is measured. Then unlabeled antigen is added in increasing amounts; the unlabeled antigen displaces the radiolabeled antigen so that less radioactivity is measured. This data is used to formulate a standard curve, and the steps are repeated using the patient's serum instead of the unlabeled antigen. The radioactivity is measured and compared to the standard curve to determine the amount of antigen.

A.3 ELECTROPHORESIS

Electrophoresis is a means of separating things by size (for example, nucleic acids or proteins) or by charge (for example, proteins or individual amino acids). A "gel" is made out of either acrylamide or agarose, by solubilizing the acrylamide or agarose, pouring it into a rectangular mold, and then allowing it to cool and solidify. Acrylamide and agarose form "nets" as they solidify; the more acrylamide or agarose used in the initial solution, the smaller the pores in the nets.

The mold used to pour the gel creates wells in the gel into which samples can be loaded. An electrical current is applied such that the end of the gel with the wells is negatively charged and the opposite end is positively charged. This causes the samples to migrate toward the positive pole, according to size; smaller things migrate faster (because they fit more easily through the pores of the gel) and larger things migrate more slowly.

In addition to determining their sizes, fragments of DNA (or RNA) in an electrophoresed gel can be transferred to a more solid and stable membrane in a process called "blotting." There are several types of blots used in biology laboratories.

A.4 BLOTTING

Simply put, blotting is the transfer of DNA or proteins from an electrophoresis gel to a nitrocellulose of PVDF membrane. Once transferred, further experiments can be run to isolate or detect a particular nucleic acid fragment or protein (called "probing"). Blotting is classified by the type of molecule being probed.

Southern blotting allows you detect the presence of specific sequences within a heterogeneous sample of DNA. This process also allows you to isolate and purify target sequences of DNA for further study.

Northern blotting is almost identical to Southern blotting, except that RNA is separated via gel electrophoresis instead of DNA. The rest of the process is the same; once the RNA has been separated on a gel, it is transferred to a nitrocellulose membrane and detected via radiolabeled nucleic acid probe. This technique allows you to determine whether specific gene products (normal or pathologic) are being expressed (if their mRNA is present in a cell, they are probably being translated to protein).

Western blotting allows you to detect the presence of certain proteins within a sample and also serves as a diagnostic tool. You are able to determine, for example, whether cancer cells express certain tumor-promoting growth receptors on their surface.

Several variations of Eastern blotting have been reported, but these tests are not commonly used in molecular biology labs. Eastern blots are used to analyze post-translational modification of peptides, such as the addition of lipids or carbohydrates. The details of this protocol depend on the specifics of the experiment.

A.5 RECOMBINANT DNA

In the past twenty years, a major change has occurred in biology that has allowed it to not only describe the mechanisms of life, but also to manipulate living organisms. The cloning and sequencing of genes, production of recombinant DNA, and the subsequent production of recombinant proteins for use as therapeutic agents in medicine have now become commonplace procedures. A **recombinant protein** is one which has been obtained by transcribing and translating a novel combination of DNA (**recombinant DNA**) from different organisms. For example, the gene for human insulin can be placed in a bacterial plasmid. Bacteria with the plasmid will then produce insulin that can be used to treat diabetes. To a large extent, these advances are due to the development of new technologies for the handling of DNA, such as the discovery of restriction endonucleases that cleave particular DNA sequences.

Restriction endonucleases are bacterial enzymes that recognize specific sequences of DNA and cut the double-stranded molecule in two pieces. A **nuclease** is an enzyme that cuts nucleic acids. An *endonuclease* cuts in the middle of a DNA chain (contrast with *exonucleases*, which nibble nucleotides from the ends of DNA chains). Restriction enzymes have found great use in molecular biology, where they have permitted manipulation of genes to create recombinant DNA.

A.5

Plasmids

Plasmids are small circular ds-DNA molecules found in bacteria that are capable of autonomous replication (replication that is independent of chromosome replication).

Plasmids have been manipulated by recombinant techniques to propagate and express foreign genes in bacteria. They also contain a multiple cloning site, which has restriction sites for dozens of restriction enzymes. This means the plasmid can be digested and any desired sequence with complementary ends can be ligated into the plasmid. Also, plasmids have a drug resistance gene, which helps select and isolate bacteria possessing the plasmid from other bacteria.

Bacterial expression plasmids need extra components. A prokaryotic promoter and start site allow expression of an inserted gene in the bacterial host. The promoter can be either constitutively active or inducible upon addition of a chemical.

Bacterial Transformation

Plasmids can be introduced into bacterial cells via transformation. The bacteria (or other cell types) must usually be coaxed to take up the plasmid. There are several ways to do this; the cells may be cooled in calcium chloride and then heat shocked to facilitate plasmid uptake. In another (called electroporation), an electric field is applied and this pokes holes in the membrane, which allows the plasmid to diffuse into the cell.

Once inside the bacteria, the plasmid will be exposed to the host's replication machinery, which replicates the plasmid. If you are working with an expression plasmid, the DNA is also exposed to bacterial transcription machinery. Newly synthesized mRNA can then access host ribosomes, which translate the encoded protein; on completion of translation, the cells are lysed to release the protein.

If the plasmid remains within the cytosol of the bacterium, the transformation is referred to as transient. In contrast, some plasmids are constructed to integrate within the host's genome. These stable transformations allow the plasmid to be replicated each time the bacterium replicates its own genome.

Complementary DNA

Many applications of DNA technology involve expressing eukaryotic genes in prokaryotic cells such as *E. coli*. This is conceptually simple: all you have to do is get eukaryotic DNA into a plasmid and get the plasmid into a bacterium, and the bacterium should express the gene. However, there are two main problems that need to be overcome. First, prokaryotes lack the equipment necessary for splicing out introns. Second, many eukaryotic genes are extremely long, making them hard to work with. One way to overcome these obstacles is to work with eukaryotic complementary DNA.

Complementary DNA (or cDNA) is produced from fully spliced eukaryotic mRNA. This is accomplished by a special enzyme you have encountered before: reverse transcriptase, obtained from retroviruses. This enzyme reads an RNA template and builds complementary DNA. Therefore, RNA can be isolated from a eukaryotic cell, and converted into cDNA by the addition of reverse transcriptase, some generic primers and dNTP building blocks in buffer. cDNAs carry the complete coding sequences for genes, but lack introns (and thus are smaller than the genomic sequence of the gene). Once a cDNA is ligated into a bacterial plasmid and bacteria are transformed with this plasmid, they can produce the protein encoded by the cDNA.

Artificial Chromosomes

Plasmids can only carry inserts up to a certain size. If large inserts are required, artificial chromosomes can be used. Bacterial artificial chromosomes (BACs) typically carry inserts of 100 to 350 kilobase pairs (kb), while yeast artificial chromosomes (YACs) can carry inserts between 100 and 3000 kb. In other words, BACs can easily carry up to 350,000 base pairs of DNA, and YACs can contain up to 3 million base pair inserts!

Eukaryotic Plasmids

Eukaryotic plasmids also exist. They require many of the same components as bacterial plasmids. Eukaryotes use different selection agents, usually either puromycin or neomycin. They also require different promoters in expression plasmids, as well as a poly-adenylation signal downstream of the inserted gene, to terminate transcription.

Eukaryotic plasmids can be introduced into mammalian host cells via transfection. Similar to transformation, there are several experimental options for transfection. Cells can be chemically transfected, usually using calcium phosphate precipitates, or plasmid packaging in liposomes. These lipid vesicles mask the plasmid, but deliver it to the interior of the cell by fusing with the plasma membrane. Non-chemical options for transfection include electroporation, optical transfection with lasers, or shooting the DNA coupled to a gold nanoparticle into a cell nucleus using a gene gun.

Viruses can also deliver DNA into eukaryotic cells, a process called viral transduction. Transduced cells can express genes carried by the viral vector.

A.6 POLYMERASE CHAIN REACTION

Polymerase chain reaction (PCR) is a very quick and inexpensive method for detecting and amplifying specific DNA sequences, screening hereditary and infectious diseases, cloning genes, and fingerprinting DNA. Designed to generate myriad copies of a single template sequence, PCR allows the amplification and subsequent analysis of very small samples of DNA.

Reverse Transcriptase-Polymerase Chain Reaction (RT-PCR)

This is an extension of classic PCR and is used to detect the relative expression of specific gene products. While RT-PCR does not measure the actual expression or abundance of proteins, the technique provides a gauge of gene transcription by measuring the relative amount of target mRNAs. To conduct an RT-PCR experiment, all of the mRNAs from within a cell population are first isolated, then converted into complementary DNA (cDNA) using the enzyme reverse transcriptase. This "library" of cDNAs is then subjected to PCR, using primers specific for a certain gene of interest. If the gene was actively transcribed at the time of harvest, its mRNA will have yielded a cDNA, which will be amplified by the PCR reaction and visualized on a gel.

Quantitative Polymerase Chain Reaction (qPCR)

In quantitative PCR (qPCR, also called real-time PCR), the PCR product is both detected and quantified, as either an absolute number of copies or as a relative amount normalized to a control. The amplified DNA is detected in "real time," as the reaction progresses. The detection process can either use a dye that is fluorescent and binds DNA, or a fluorescent oligonucleotide probe that hybridizes to the sequence of interest. qPCR can be performed on either DNA or cDNA templates, meaning it can give information on the presence and abundance of a particular DNA sequence in samples (if DNA is the template), or on gene expression (if the template is cDNA).

A.7 DNA SEQUENCING AND GENOMICS

DNA sequencing is a method by which scientists can determine gene sequences. This provides the basis for investigating the genetics of health and disease. Knowing gene sequences is also a critical component of other experimental techniques, for example, when constructing primers for PCR reactions.

The most widely used DNA sequencing method (the Sanger technique) hinges on a simple yet important structural characteristic of DNA molecules. The ringed ribose of a dNTP has various substituents attached to its carbons: a nitrogenous base at the 1' carbon, a hydrogen at the 2' carbon (recall that a hydroxyl group occupies this site in RNA), a hydroxyl group at the 3' carbon, and a string of three phosphates at the 5' carbon. The 3' carbon hydroxyl group serves as the binding site for another dNTP. Without a free 3' carbon hydroxyl group, dNTPs could not be linked together, and DNA synthesis would not be possible. The Sanger technique utilizes a modified dNTP, which lacks the 3' carbon hydroxyl group. These dideoxynucleotide triphosphates (ddNTPs) maintain their 5' carbon triphosphate moiety and can be incorporated normally into a growing DNA molecule, however, because they are lacking the 3' carbon hydroxyl group no further bases can be added to them. Thus, these ddNTPs terminate strand elongation at the point of their insertion. The basic protocol is as follows: a sample of DNA is obtained and denatured into single strands. All of the components necessary for replication, including radiolabeled primers, along with the DNA, are mixed in four separate test tubes. A different dideoxybase is added to each tube. Replication is allowed to proceed, and many fragments of different sizes will be produced in each tube. The fragments are separated via electrophoresis, with each dideoxybase in a separate lane, then transferred to a membrane and visualized with radiosensitive film.

Reading the film from bottom (farthest from the wells) to top (closest to the wells) indicates the sequence (in the 5' to 3' direction) of the strand.

Genomics

The genome of the bacterium *Haemophilus influenzae* was the first to be sequenced and published in 1995. Since then, the genomes of hundreds of organisms have been sequenced and published, including humans and model organisms commonly used in biology laboratories (e.g., *E. coli*, *D. melanogaster*, etc.). Researchers and clinicians have recently started sequencing the genome of many cancers, which allows comparative studies between different types and subtypes of cancer, as well as a better understanding of how the cancer genome is different from a normal one.

Genomic sequencing is generally done in two ways, which can be complementary. The first strategy is to generate a genetic linkage map, with several hundred markers per chromosome. This map is then refined to a physical map by preparing YAC or BAC libraries containing large chromosomal fragments. The library is put in order, then gradually cloned into libraries containing smaller and smaller fragments. Each of these small fragments are eventually sequenced, and assembled into an overall sequence.

The second strategy is a whole-genome shotgun approach, where chromosomes are cut into small fragments, which are cloned and sequenced. This strategy skips generating maps, and because of this, requires much more extensive analysis of sequencing data by computers in order to align fragments.

Genomic data can lead to predictions on how many genes there are in a certain organism, where they are located, how expression is controlled, and how the genome is organized. It also supports larger questions, like how evolution and speciation occur. Finally, genomic data can be used to study genetic variation within and across species. Tools for analysis of genomic data have been developed and are always being refined. Researchers can now submit several different gene or protein sequences and receive a report that predicts how related the sequences are from an evolutionary point of view. There are also tools to multiply align several sequences so we can study how similar and different they are.

A.8 DNA FINGERPRINTING

Much like visualizing subtle differences in the whorl pattern of a thumbprint, DNA fingerprinting allows scientists (and police departments!) to detect sequence variations that make each individual's DNA unique. The ability to appreciate subtle differences within different individuals' DNA comes in handy when matching a DNA sample from a murder suspect to the DNA in a drop of blood found at a crime scene, or when screening for disease-causing genes, or when doing paternity testing. Since the DNA of any two people is more than 99 percent identical, DNA fingerprinting exploits stretches of repetitive and highly variable DNA called **polymorphisms**. These intervening 2–100 base-pair sequences of DNA are structurally variable with respect to their sequence, length, multiplicity, and location within the genome. Two of the several methods of fingerprinting are described below, **restriction fragment length polymorphism** (RFLP) analysis and **short tandem repeat** (STR) analysis.

This method uses restriction endonucleases to cut 10–100 base-pair stretches of polymorphic DNA (called minisatellites) into small fragments. Because of the size variations inherent in this DNA, the resulting DNA fragments (now referred to as RFLPs) also vary in size, and are unique to an individual.

The RFLPs are separated via gel electrophoresis and transferred to a membrane. Southern blotting techniques are used to analyze the sample. The membrane is probed with radiolabeled DNA oligonucleotides that base-pair with specific RFLP sequences, and the membrane is visualized with special film. Polymorphic DNA, even though recovered from the same chromosomal region, will yield unique band distributions for each person. When RFLPs are recovered from DNA sequences within genes, mutations can be detected. For example, sickle cell disease is caused by a single base substitution in the beta chain of hemoglobin. The substituted valine at the sixth position (normally, glutamic acid is present) will introduce a novel restriction site within the gene. When cut with restriction endonucleases, the point mutation generates a different sized RFLP (when compared to the normal gene cut with the same enzymes) and will yield an anomalous banding pattern.

A.8

Short Tandem Repeat (STR) Analysis

Step 1: This method uses PCR to amplify 5–10 base-pair stretches of highly polymorphic and repetitive DNA located within noncoding (introns) regions of the genome. These STRs vary with respect to the sequence and number of repeats found at each locus. To profile an individual, a sample of DNA is obtained and the polymorphic DNA is amplified with PCR.

Step 2: The amplified STRs are separated via electrophoresis and analyzed with Southern blotting.

A.9   ADDITIONAL METHODS TO STUDY THE GENOME

Genomic sequencing is the ultimate study of the genome. However, it is very costly and takes a long time. Depending on the experiment, one of the following methods may be better suited to answering a biological question.

Exome and Targeted Sequencing

Instead of sequencing the entire genome, scientists can target only certain regions of interest. Exome sequencing involves sequencing only the exons of the genome. On a smaller scale, individual genes can be sequenced. These selective techniques involve enriching the DNA of interest (by amplification for example), followed by standard sequencing.

Karyotyping

When generating a karyotype, scientists order all the chromosomes from 1 to 22 plus the sex chromosomes, for a genome-wide view of genetic information. Chromosomes are stained to highlight structural features. Major genetic changes (involving millions of base pairs), aneuploidy (when a cell contains an abnormal number of chromosomes), and some insertions, deletions, or translocations can be revealed.

Fluorescence *in situ* Hybridization

Fluorescence *in situ* hybridization (FISH) uses fluorescently labeled probes to locate the positions of specific DNA sequences on chromosomes. This detects and localizes the presence or absence of specific DNA sequences on chromosomes. Fluorescence microscopy is used to find out where the fluorescent probe is bound to the chromosomes. For example, large chromosomal translocations have been found in several types of cancer. A translocation between chromosomes 2 and 3 is often found in follicular thyroid carcinoma. This translocation produces a fusion gene that contains the promoter from one gene and the coding sequence of another. FISH analysis using chromosome 2 and 3 probes can detect and diagnose this translocation.

A.10

A.10 ANALYZING GENE EXPRESSION

Many of the techniques discussed above give information about gene expression. For example, RT-PCR and qPCR give information on which genes are being transcribed in a given cell population. Western blot analysis can directly test protein expression, and is limited only by the amount of starting lysate and the availability of antibodies specific for the protein being studied. Additional methods have been developed to study gene expression. Each of these techniques can be used to study a certain gene and gather information about its expression and function, or to study certain cells and gain information on which genes they are expressing and how they grow and survive.

Microarrays

Microarrays can be used to study relative RNA amounts between two samples, or to compare RNA levels in one sample to a normal reference. RNA is used as a starting material. The two samples of RNA (either two different experimental samples being compared to each other, or one sample and a control) are reverse-transcribed into cDNA and labeled with fluorescent dyes of different colors, then mixed and applied to an array chip. This chip contains binding sites for every known gene, which act as probes to determine transcript levels in the samples. Microarray data is quantitative, and actual fold-changes can be calculated based on color and intensity.

In situ Hybridization

In situ hybridization (ISH) can be used to determine expression of a gene of interest in a tissue, or in an embryo. A very thin slice (or "section") of a tissue sample is mounted onto a microscope slide. The tissue is fixed to keep transcripts in place, and then permeabilized to open the cell membrane. A labeled probe, which is specific for the transcript of interest, is added to the section and binds to the transcript being studied. An enzyme-linked antibody is added and binds to the probe. When a substrate for the enzyme is added, the target transcript-probe-antibody complex is detected. In this way, it can be determined when and where transcripts are expressed on a multicellular level.

Immunohistochemistry

This technique is similar to ISH, but is specific for proteins instead of nucleic acids. As such, it gives a direct report on protein expression in a tissue. Immunohistochemistry (IHC) requires an antibody against a known protein. This antibody is recognized by a secondary antibody, which is either linked to an enzyme or a fluorescent molecule. IHC is commonly used in the clinic. For example, breast cancer biopsies from women are stained for the estrogen receptor (ER), the progesterone receptor (PR), and a plasma membrane receptor called HER2. Breast tumors are then classified as ER^+ or ER^-, PR^+ or PR^-, and $HER2^+$ or $HER2^-$. These classifications affect which therapy the patient is given.

Flow Cytometry

Flow cytometry again uses many of the same principles already discussed. Here, single cells (either from lab cultures or tissue samples) are stained for certain protein markers using specific antibodies. The antibodies are then linked to a fluorescent tag. Next, the labeled cells are suspended in a fluid stream and passed through a beam of light. Light detectors are found on the other side of, and perpendicular to, the laser. As the labeled cells pass through the light, the beam scatters and the fluorescent tag(s) on the cells can emit light. This combination of scattered and emitted light is measured to give information on cell size, and how many cells in the sample express each of the markers that were labeled. Flow cytometers can have over a dozen different light channels, so many labeled antibodies can be added to one experimental sample. In addition to being analyzed, cells can also be sorted as they go through the machine (a technique called fluorescence-activated cell sorting, or FACS). In this way, a heterogeneous mixture of cells can be sorted based on expression of markers.

A.11

A.11 DETERMINING GENE FUNCTION

Genomic sequencing has revealed thousands of genes with unknown function. There are many ways to discover the function of these genes.

Evolutionary Comparisons

Gene sequences can be compared to all other organisms sequenced. If a human gene of unknown function has much of its sequence in common with a fission yeast protein phosphatase, researchers will test if the unknown human gene may code for a phosphatase.

Protein Domains

Protein domains are conserved patterns in protein sequence and structure. These domains are typically between 25 and 500 amino acids in length and contribute to protein function. Many proteins have several structural domains and one domain can appear in a variety of different peptides from different organisms. Many domains are found in Archaea, Bacteria, and Eukarya. Some domains repeat in tandem and others are found in single copies. For example, zinc fingers are small protein domains which are DNA-binding and commonly found in transcription factors. Pleckstrin homology (PH) domains are approximately 120 amino acids long and function in lipid binding, which targets proteins to appropriate cellular compartments. As such, PH domains occur in a wide range of proteins involved in signaling pathways. Thousands of protein domains have been experimentally determined, and the presence of certain domains can shed light on protein function.

Protein Interactions

Knowing which proteins bind to a protein of interest can shed light on protein function, especially since many proteins function in complexes and pathways. Immunoprecipitations are commonly used to find protein binding partners. In this experiment, cell lysates are collected (as described above) and incubated with an antibody specific for the protein of interest (such as a green protein in Figure 1). A complex forms, including the protein of interest, its binding partners, and an antibody. An antibody binding protein covalently linked to a microscopic bead is added next. The bead can be pulled out of solution (or precipitated) by simple centrifugation (spinning the tube at high speeds). This collects bead complexes at the bottom of the tube. These complexes are then washed and purified from the lysate solution. Proteins that don't bind to the protein of interest are lost. Precipitated proteins can then be identified by Western blot analysis (if you have an idea of what proteins you're looking for), or mass spectrometry (if you have no idea what will be there). Data from these experiments can generate network maps, where protein interactions are used to elucidate functional maps of how proteins are working together in a cell.

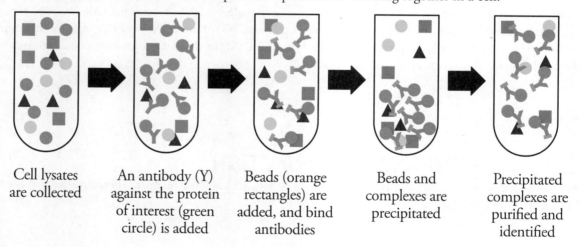

Figure 1   Immunoprecipitation

Cellular Expression

Subcellular location can give information on protein function. To determine the subcellular location of a protein of interest, the gene for this protein can be attached to a reporter system to see where it is expressed. For example, the gene of interest can be cloned into an expression vector, and linked to a fluorescent tag such as GFP (green fluorescent protein). This effectively tags the protein with a fluorescent molecule, meaning cellular location can be determined using a fluorescent microscope. In Figure 2, the first cell (A) is expressing the GFP-tagged protein of interest on the plasma membrane, the second cell (B) expresses it in the cytoplasm, while the last cell (C) expresses it in the nucleus. In this experiment, the nucleus is also stained with a fluorescent dye called DAPI (which shows up blue under the fluorescent microscope). Since the nucleus of cell C has both blue DAPI and green protein, it shows up as a teal circle.

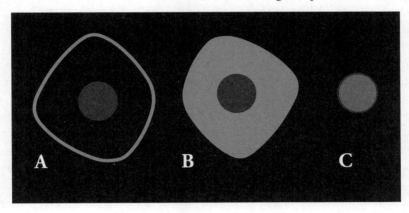

Figure 2   Using GFP-Tagged Proteins to Determine Subcellular Protein Expression

A.11

Altering Expression

Altering gene expression can also be used to help determine gene function. Gene expression can be inhibited or increased, and the subsequent phenotype can shed light on protein function.

Gene expression can be knocked down via RNA interference (or RNAi), which uses microRNA (miRNA) or small interfering RNA (siRNA). These short RNA molecules can bind to mRNAs and decrease their activity, often by promoting degradation of the mRNA transcript. Synthetic RNA has been used in both cell culture and in living organisms as a way to decrease protein expression.

The opposite experiment can also be done, where a protein of interest is over-expressed in a biological system. This can be achieved by attaching the gene of interest to a strong promoter, which will induce high levels of transcription, and therefore gene expression. This genetic construct can be on an expression plasmid or it can be recombined into the genome, either at the endogenous locus (where the gene is normally found), or at another location in the genome. These "knock-in" systems can also be made by increasing gene copy number, or increasing transcript stability (usually by decreasing transcript degradation). No matter how it is done, the cellular and biochemical effects of over-expressing a gene of interest can be investigated.

In vitro mutagenesis is when a gene is cloned, specifically mutated, then returned to a cell. Mutations can alter, destroy, or enhance gene function. These mutated genes can even be put into early multicellular embryos, to study the role of a protein in development and whole-organism function.

A.12   PROTEIN QUANTIFICATION

A good understanding of genomics has led to the field of **proteomics**, the systematic and large-scale study of protein structure and function. This is usually done in a particular context, such as in a certain biochemical pathway, organelle, cell, tissue, or organism. Often, this involves quantitative analysis of proteins. This means measuring amounts of different proteins from a functional standpoint, looking at how the amount, state, or location of a protein changes.

Many different techniques can help with studying proteins quantitatively. Some of these look at proteins in a cell, either alive (FACS, labeling a protein and looking and subcellular location) or not (immunohistochemistry, flow cytometry). Others measure proteins harvested from a cell (ELISA, Western blotting, immunoprecipitation). All these techniques are discussed earlier in this Appendix.

It's common for proteins to be grown in a biological system, then extracted and studied. Often, protein levels in lysates or purified samples must be quantified before an experiment can be started.

The most commonly used quantification method is Bradford Quantification, using UV-Vis spectrophotometers designed for biochemical analysis. This method uses a Bradford reagent containing a blue pigment called Coomassie blue. When proteins bind the pigment, it shifts the absorption peak of the sample. Absorption is measured at 600 nm. This technique is very simple and has good sensitivity.

To perform quantification, first, the negative control sample is put in the spectrophotometer, to set the zero value. Next, the samples with known concentration are applied, and the spectrophotometer generates a concentration curve. This relates absorbance of the sample with protein concentration. A new curve should be made every time proteins are being quantified. Next, the samples are put in the machine one by one. The spectrophotometer applies light in the visible and adjacent (near-UV and near-infrared) ranges. Absorbance is determined and compared to the calibration curve, and the machine usually reports both the absorbance and the subsequent protein concentration.

A.12

Affinity Chromatography

Affinity chromatography is used to separate biochemical mixtures, and it is based on highly specific interactions between macromolecules. While affinity chromatography is most commonly used to purify proteins, it can also be used on other macromolecules (such as nucleic acids). It uses many of the same principles described above: you start with a heterogeneous mixture of molecules (such as cell lysate, growth media, or blood). To isolate a protein of interest, you can either use an antibody or tag the protein with an affinity tag (for example, His-tagged proteins can be purified with nickel-based resins and slightly basic conditions; the bound proteins are eluted by adding imidazole or by lowering the pH). The target molecule is trapped on a stationary phase due to specific binding, and the stationary phase is washed to increase purity. The target protein is then released (or eluted) off the solid phase, in a highly purified state.

A.13   STEM CELLS

Stem cells are undifferentiated cells which can differentiate to become other cell types. Stem cells self-replicate by mitosis.

Embryonic Stem Cells

Embryonic stem cells (ESCs) are found in the inner cell mass of the blastocyst and are the only stem cells in humans which are pluripotent. Pluripotent cells are able to differentiate into any of the three germ layers (endoderm, mesoderm, or ectoderm), and can generate all of the over 220 cells types in the human body. ESCs can replicate indefinitely. While ESCs are the only known pluripotent cells, it's possible that other pluripotent stem cells exist in adults and have not yet been found. In addition, it's possible that multipotent stem cells could dedifferentiate into a pluripotent state, but this has not yet been demonstrated in the lab.

Adult Stem Cells

Adult stem cells are found in various tissues, and function in tissue repair and regeneration. They are multipotent, meaning they can produce many cell types. There are three sources of readily available adult stem cells: bone marrow (to regenerate blood cells), adipose tissue (to regenerate fat tissue), and blood (hematopoietic stem cells that give rise to all other blood cells). Adult stem cells are usually tissue-specific, and differentiate into slightly more differentiated progenitor cells, before completely differentiating. An understanding of this process has led to the discovery of cell hierarchies, where the pattern of maturation is characterized and traced as cells differentiate in a given tissue. It is predicted that both stem cells and progenitor cells can transform into a cancer cell, which may have major implications on the treatment and prevention of cancer.

A.13

Applications of Stem Cells

Stem cells have many important uses in biology. First, therapy using ESCs could revolutionize regenerative medicine and alleviate human suffering. Many diseases could be treated using pluripotent cells, such as blood and immune system genetic disorders, many cancers, spinal cord injuries, Parkinson's disease, juvenile diabetes, and blindness. The basic idea behind these stem cell therapies is to manipulate ESCs to become other cells for use in treatment. For example, ESCs induced to become oligodendrocytes have been used to treat patients with spinal cord injuries.

Many ESCs used in the lab come from embryos that were created for *in vitro* fertilization, but then not required. Because generating human ESC lines requires destroying the blastocyst, work on human ESCs is controversial. In addition to ethical concerns, there are additional risks of host-graft rejection, and formation of tumors from therapeutic ESCs.

Second, ESCs from model organisms (such as mice and rats) can be isolated and manipulated in the lab. These targeted ESCs can then be aggregated with a normal morula or injected into a normal blastocyst. The morula or blastocyst is then injected into the uterus of a pseudopregnant female animal, which carries the embryos to term. Pseudopregnant mice are produced by mating fertile females with vasectomized males.

A few weeks later, chimeric pups are born, which are a mix of targeted stem cells and normal stem cells. Usually animals with different coat colors are used in these experiments. For example, the ESCs used for targeting in the lab could be from a brown mouse, while the normal donor morula or blastocyst could come from an albino strain. Chimeric pups typically have a mix of white and brown fur and are screened to find "founder" animals where the germ line was derived from the targeted ESCs (see Figure 3). In this way, new transgenic lines can be generated and used for study. For example, a knock-in mouse could be made which over-expresses a gene of interest. Models are often made using tissue-specific promoters, so studies can be done on certain tissues without affecting all cells in the animal.

Figure 3   Gene Targeting to Generate Transgenic Mice

Because of the ethical implications of working with human ESCs, there has been a lot of excitement over induced pluripotent stem cells (iPS cells). These cells are made from adult somatic cells by inducing expression of certain genes, usually transcription factors. Induced expression of these proteins causes the somatic cells to regain pluripotency, a characteristic which only ESCs have. iPS cells have many other characteristics in common with ESCs, including morphology and replicative ability. Despite the initial excitement, however, iPS cells have not yet replaced ESCs because they are potentially tumorigenic and have low replication rates.

A.13

A.14 PRACTICAL APPLICATIONS OF DNA TECHNOLOGY

There are dozens of practical uses of DNA technology, some of which (such as forensics and paternity testing) have been already discussed. Many involve transgenic organisms. A transgenic organism is one that carries a foreign gene that has been deliberately inserted into its genome. Many useful transgenic organisms have been developed, but it is important to be aware of the ethical considerations that come with both biotechnology and genetically engineered organisms. This section discusses applications of biotechnology, while the next section discusses some ethical issues to be considered.

Pharmaceuticals

Recombinant bacteria are commonly used by pharmaceutical companies in drug production. An expression plasmid is made that contains a promoter and the gene of interest. The plasmid is transformed into competent bacteria and large cultures of the bacteria are grown in selective media. To harvest the drug of interest, the bacteria are either lysed (if the drug is produced intracellularly), or the growth media is collected and the drug is purified from solution (if the bacteria have been modified so that the drug is secreted from the cell).

Genetic engineering and biotechnology have also been important in the development of vaccines. Here, the gene for a surface protein from a harmful pathogen can be cloned into a harmless virus, which is then used as a vaccine against the pathogenic microbe. This vaccine can be safely administered, since the body will recognize the surface protein as foreign (and will therefore mount an immune response), but will not be infected by the actual pathogen. Without the ability to cut and paste segments of DNA from one source to another (using restriction enzymes, PCR, and plasmids), development of these vaccines would not be possible.

Novel vaccine delivery systems are also being developed. For example, one group has developed transgenic potato plants that express proteins from the cholera bacterium. Ingestion of these potatoes causes production of anti-cholera antibodies, meaning the potato is effectively acting like a cholera vaccine. Although not yet widely available, this could offer a major benefit to impoverished areas, where people must travel long distances to medical clinics to receive vaccination shots.

A.14

Industry

Genetically modified bacteria are also used to produce enzymes required for food processing. For example, the gene for chymosin has been cloned into both prokaryotic and eukaryotic expression plasmids, and bacteria or yeast containing these plasmids produce large amounts of the enzyme chymosin. This enzyme is then purified and used to clot milk in cheese production.

Transgenic cows are being generated to produce milk that has the same characteristics as human breast milk. Additional transgenic animals are being made to produce useful substances (such as goats that excrete silk proteins in their milk, or pigs that produce omega-3 fatty acids).

Both bacteria and plants (such as algae, corn, and poplars) have been genetically modified for use in biofuel production. Biofuel is derived from living organisms and contains energy from geologically recent carbon fixation. Bioethanol (made from carbohydrates via fermentation) and biodiesel (made from animal and plant fats) are common examples of biofuel.

Agriculture

DNA technology has had a great impact on the science of agriculture. Scientists have been able to transfer genes to plants in order to optimize crop yield. For example, some plants express a transgenic enzyme that is harmful to pests, which decreases the need for pesticide use. Others express enzymes making them resistant to diseases or herbicides.

Transgenic plants that are capable of nitrogen fixation are also in production. Most plants need large amounts of nitrate, which is produced from atmospheric nitrogen (a process call nitrogen fixation) by bacteria. Some plants, such as legumes, can fix their own nitrogen. Scientists have identified genes involved in this process and are working to develop transgenic corn and rice strains also capable of nitrogen fixation. Success in this project would mean a decrease in global fertilizer use, which could have a beneficial impact on the environment.

Food has also been modified to increase shelf life and nutritional value. For example, tomatoes have been altered to stay firm during ripening. This means green tomatoes can be picked and transported to grocery shelves without going soft. Golden rice, which contains beta-carotene, has been developed to combat vitamin A deficiency. New rice strains with higher iron content are also being developed.

While genetically modified crops are common, no genetically modified animals have yet been approved for human consumption. However, transgenic fish are in production. One project focuses on transgenic salmon that grow and mature at a faster rate than normal fish.

DNA technology has also been applied to agriculture biotechnology in the form of animal husbandry. DNA fingerprinting has been applied to certain endangered animals (such as the Puerto Rican parrot, orangutans, and some species of African livestock). This allows scientists to identify individual animals, verify their pedigree and ancestors, and track both desirable and undesirable traits. Animals can be registered, and mating pairs can be tracked to make sure the population maintains enough variation to be viable, and that deleterious traits are not passed on to offspring. This is especially important for species that have a small population. These biotechnology-based breeding programs have also been applied to common agriculture livestock species such as cattle and horses.

A.14

Environmental Applications

Bacteria are being engineered to express genes that will help cope with some environmental problems. For example, genetically engineered bacteria have been made to help with sewage treatment, and to degrade harmful compounds. Some bacteria have been made to extract heavy metals from the environment. These metals are then incorporated into different compounds that can be isolated and used to extract the metal. This means bacteria could play a role in the future of both the clean-up of toxic mining waste and the actual mining process.

Phosphorus water pollution promotes algae growth. Genetically modified pigs, which produce the enzyme phytase in their saliva, are able to break down indigestible phosphorus. These pigs may help reduce water pollution, as their manure contains about half the amount of phosphorus as normal pigs.

Genetically modified zebrafish are also being used in environmental biotechnology. For example, transgenic fish have been developed to detect aquatic pollution.

Gene Therapy

Gene therapy is when a genetic disorder is treated by introducing a gene into a cell. This is often to correct or supplement a defective gene. Gene therapy uses genetically modified viruses (such as retroviruses, adenoviruses, or lentiviruses) to deliver genes to somatic human cells. Ideally, the targeted gene will be incorporated into the genome of the cell, but this doesn't always occur. This means treatment efficacy can gradually decreases over time, and repeated treatments may be necessary. Because the targeted cells are somatic, the treatment will only affect the individual patient and will not be passed to later generations. Recent trials in gene therapy have tried to target adult stem cells as a way to increase treatment efficacy and duration.

Gene therapy-based treatments for sickle cell anemia, Parkinson's disease, cystic fibrosis, cancer, HIV, diabetes, muscular dystrophy, and heart disease are currently being developed. While the theory behind this technology is not new, it has been difficult to optimize gene therapy in practice. Because of this, gene therapy is not in widespread practice, but shows promise as a future treatment. Gene therapy of the germ line is also possible in theory, but because of ethical controversy, has not been well developed.

There are some problems associated with gene therapy. Because a foreign particle is being introduced, there is a chance the immune system will respond, and this can reduce treatment efficacy. Current gene therapies are limited to one or two genes, while many disorders are caused by many genes. Finally, there is a small chance of tumor development if the therapy DNA integrates into the genome incorrectly.

Genetic Testing

Biotechnology has also been crucial in developing DNA-based tests. You already learned how RFLP and STR analysis can be used in forensics (to compare crime scene samples to suspects for example), to establish relationships between people, or to study the evolutionary relationship between two species. Genetic testing is another application of these tests. Genetic testing can be done before birth (to look for diseases like hemophilia, cystic fibrosis, and Duchene muscular dystrophy) or after birth (to test for mutations that may lead to increased disease risk).

A.15 SAFETY AND ETHICS OF DNA TECHNOLOGY

Regulatory agencies and governments have started implementing regulations on how biotechnology can be used in industry, medicine, and agriculture. These agencies focus on assessing risk, public education, and mandating policies to protect both scientists and the public. However, with a hot topic like biotechnology, there will always be opponents. Serious considerations of risk and implications are important to mitigate any potential downsides to new technology.

Criticisms of genetically modified crops have received widespread news coverage. Opponents argue introduction of transgenic crops into ecosystems could cause unpredictable results. For example, if pesticide resistance is somehow transferred to the pest, this could cause widespread ecological problems. Biotechnology could therefore inadvertently generate new and hazardous pathogens. Opponents also point out that eating transgenic crops may not be safe, and some critics argue that they're not necessary to solve food availability issues. While there is little data supporting the hypothesis that transgenic foodstuffs are dangerous, it is important to consider that this may be the case.

Concerns over gene therapy are also common. Some are worried about the long-term implications of introducing a foreign gene into a human being. Germ line gene therapy is highly controversial, as development of this technology could lead to eugenics: a deliberate effort to control the genetic makeup of human populations. Some see germ line gene therapy as interfering with evolution. Since genetic variation is important for species survival, some argue that gene therapy is a way of decreasing alleles in a population. While this might seem like a good idea, it is possible that alleles that have a disadvantage in one situation might prove to be advantageous in another situation. If gene targeting or eugenics causes this allele to be lost, the species could suffer. A common example of an allele with multiple effects is the sickle cell allele. In the homozygous form, this allele causes sickle cell disease. However, in the heterozygous form, this allele provides some protection against malaria. What looks like a "bad allele" from one perspective, can actually be a good thing in other situations.

Working with any animal in a laboratory setting raises ethical issues. Agencies have been appointed to ensure lab animals have a good quality of life, are treated humanely, and are used in justified and important experiments. A rigorous peer-reviewed process (usually overseen by veterinarians) ensures researchers justify the use for each and every experimental animal. Despite these attempts, additional concerns exist. For example, in generating experimental animals, many labs also generate normal animals, which are sacrificed simply because they don't have the correct genotype. Also, transgenic animals typically suffer from decreased fertility and may be susceptible to conditions and diseases besides those they are bred to develop and model. Again, close monitoring of animal facilities, usually in conjunction with both local and federal regulations, ensures researchers are acting in a responsible and ethical manner when working with transgenic animals.

A.15

Appendix II
Pedigree Analysis

The AAMC has formally removed pedigree analysis from the list of MCAT topics, but they do still expect you to understand patterns of inheritance (see Section 7.6). One way to learn about and understand patterns of inheritance is by looking at and analyzing data from pedigrees. Thus, although pedigree analysis is no longer required material, we present it here to enhance your understanding of how traits are passed on from generation to generation.

PEDIGREE ANALYSIS

Often it is not possible to perform controlled genetic crosses to ascertain the nature of inheritance of a trait, particularly when people are involved. In these cases, families can be studied to determine the pattern of inheritance. Researchers organize the information learned from families into **pedigrees**, which are charts depicting inheritance of a trait (Figure 1). By studying the pedigree of families, researchers can determine the pattern of inheritance of a gene, whether it is linked to other genes, and whether an individual is likely to pass on a trait to their offspring. Pedigrees follow certain conventions in how they are drawn:

1) Males are represented by squares and females by circles.
2) A cross (mating) between a male and female is represented by a horizontal line connecting them.
3) Offspring from a cross are connected to their parents by a vertical line, and to each other by a horizontal line with vertical branches for each sibling.
4) Offspring of unknown gender (unborn children) are represented by a diamond shape.
5) Individuals afflicted with a trait being studied are shaded in; unaffected or normal individuals are not shaded in.

Many pedigrees make a common assumption: individuals mating into the family (i.e., individuals for which you have no information on their parents or grandparents) are assumed to be homozygous normal unless their phenotype tells you differently. The basis of this assumption is that the traits being studied are usually relatively rare in the human population, and therefore, it is most likely that a non-family member is homozygous for the wild-type allele.

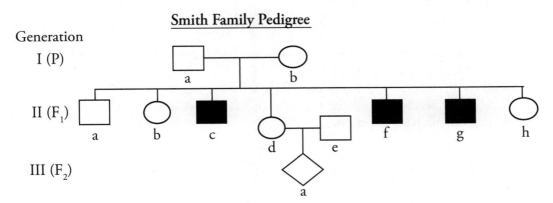

Figure 1 A Pedigree

Once drawn, a pedigree can be analyzed as follows:

Step 1: Is the allele that causes the trait dominant or is it recessive? Recessive traits commonly skip generations (affected individuals can have unaffected parents), but dominant traits do not (affected individuals must have at least one affected parent).

Step 2: Is the gene involved carried on a sex chromosome (sex-linked)? If so, there tends to be an unequal distribution of affected males (more) versus affected females (fewer). If the numbers of affected males and females are approximately equal, the gene is most likely autosomal.

Step 3: If the disease is sex-linked, is it on the X or the Y chromosome? Diseases linked to the Y chromosome will show father-to-son transmission, while diseases linked to the X chromosome will not.

Step 4: Check for mitochondrial inheritance. Affected females will have all affected children, but affected males cannot pass the trait on.

Step 5: Figure out the genotypes and calculate the probabilities of inheritance where necessary. When writing genotypes for sex-linked traits, make sure to include the chromosomes (e.g., $X^A Y$, or $X^A X^a$, etc.). When writing genotypes for autosomal traits, make sure NOT to include the chromosomes (e.g., DD or Dd, etc.).

Step 6: If more than one trait is involved, go through Steps 1–5 for each.

- In the pedigree in Figure 1, the darkened squares represent individuals afflicted with a certain genetic disease. This disease is most likely caused by:[1]
    - A) a dominant allele.
    - B) an autosomal recessive allele.
    - C) an X-linked recessive allele.
    - D) a Y-linked allele.

- In the pedigree in Figure 1, what is the probability that IIIa will have the disease?[2]
    - A) If male, IIIa will have the disease.
    - B) Overall, there is a 1/8 chance that IIIa will have the disease.
    - C) Overall, there is a 1/4 chance that IIIa will have the disease.
    - D) IIIa will not have the disease.

[1] Since the affected individuals have unaffected parents, the disease is most likely recessive (choice A is wrong), and since the affected individuals are all male, it is most likely sex-linked (choice B is wrong). There is no father-to-son transmission (all affected males have an unaffected father), so the disease is X-linked (choice **C** is correct, and choice D is wrong).

[2] The disease is X-linked recessive, and IIe (IIIa's father) is not affected, so IIe cannot pass the allele on. Thus, the probability of IIIa getting the disease depends on the genotype of IId (she would have to be a carrier) and what she passes on to IIIa. It also depends on the gender of IIIa; females would not be affected because they would have to receive the allele from both IId and IIe, and IIe does not carry the disease allele. Bottom line, in order for IIIa to get the disease, IId would have to be a carrier, would have to pass the disease allele on, and IIIa would have to be male. The probability of IId being a carrier is 1/2; we know she received a good X chromosome from her father Ia (all he has is a good X chromosome), and the probability she received the affected X chromosome from her mother (Ib) is 1/2. The probability she passes the bad X chromosome on to IIIa is 1/2; she has one good X and one bad X. The probability that IIIa is male is 1/2. Finally, we can use the rule of multiplication to determine the overall probability: $1/2 \times 1/2 \times 1/2 = 1/8$ overall probability (choice **B** is correct, and choices C and D are wrong). Note that choice A is wrong because being male does not guarantee the disease; IIIa could be male (get the Y chromosome from IIe) and still be unaffected (get the good X chromosome from IId).

Below are example pedigrees for six modes of inheritance (X-linked recessive, X-linked dominant, autosomal recessive, autosomal dominant, mitochondrial, and Y-linked). For each pedigree, determine which mode of inheritance is displayed.

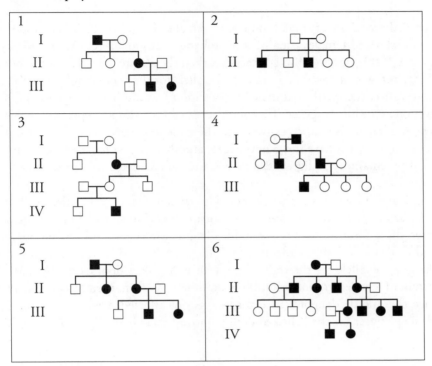

Answers

1) autosomal dominant
2) X-linked recessive
3) autosomal recessive
4) Y-linked
5) X-linked dominant
6) mitochondrial inheritance

Explanations

The easiest inheritance patterns to spot are mitochondrial (passed from mothers to all offspring) and Y-linked (passed from fathers to sons, and females are never affected). Let's start by finding these two. Since Pedigree 6 shows a trait with maternal inheritance, this must be mitochondrial inheritance. The affected father in generation II does not pass the trait to any of his children, but the affected mothers in generations I, II, and III pass the trait onto all their offspring. Pedigree 4 shows a trait with Y-linked inheritance. The trait is passed from father to all sons and does not affect females.

Next, Pedigrees 2 and 3 both show traits that skips generations. That is, there are individuals on the pedigree that are affected by the trait but who have unaffected parents. Therefore, these two pedigrees must be for recessive traits. One is autosomal and the other is X-linked.

Since the trait on Pedigree 2 affects males more than females, it is likely X-linked, and since the trait on Pedigree 3 affects males and females equally, it is probably autosomal. Let's verify this by looking more closely at Pedigree 3. If this trait is X-linked recessive, then the affected female in generation II must have the genotype X^aX^a, and would have had to receive the allele for the trait from both her parents. However, for an X-linked recessive, the unaffected male in generation I would have the genotype X^AY, and would only have X^A to donate to his daughter. Therefore, this pedigree cannot represent an X-linked recessive trait; it must represent an autosomal recessive trait. The male in generation I must have the genotype Aa, the female in generation I must have the genotype Aa, and the affected female in generation II must have the genotype aa. The remaining pedigree, Pedigree 2, must be X-linked recessive.

Finally, Pedigrees 1 and 5 show traits that do not skip generations. That is, affected individuals have affected parents. These are pedigrees for dominant traits; one is X-linked and one is autosomal. The only difference between these two pedigrees is the middle daughter in the second generation; in Pedigree 1 she is unaffected and in Pedigree 5 she is affected. Let's focus on her father (the male in generation I) since this is where she gets the allele for the trait. If the trait is X-linked dominant, the male in generation I would be X^AY; thus all females in generation II would inherit X^A from their father, and all of them would be affected. Since the middle daughter in Pedigree I is not affected, Pedigree 1 must show autosomal dominance and the pedigree for the X-linked dominant trait must be Pedigree 5.

Biology Glossary

After each definition, the section number in the *MCAT Biology* text where the term is discussed is given.

5' cap

A methylated guanine nucleotide added to the 5' end of eukaryotic mRNA. The cap is necessary to initiate translation of the mRNA. [**Sections 4.7 and 4.8**]

A band

The band of the sarcomere that extends the full length of the thick filament. The A band includes regions of thick and thin filament overlap, as well as a region of thick filament only. A bands alternate with I bands to give skeletal and cardiac muscle tissue a striated appearance. The A band does not shorten during muscle contraction. [**Section 11.2**]

A site

Aminoacyl-tRNA site; the site on a ribosome where a new amino acid is added to a growing peptide. [**Section 4.8**]

absolute refractory period

A period of time following an action potential during which no additional action potential can be evoked regardless of the level of stimulation. [**Section 8.1**]

absolute threshold

The minimum stimulus intensity required to activate a sensory receptor 50% of the time. [**Section 8.5**]

accessory glands

The three glands in the male reproductive system that produce semen: the seminal vesicles, the prostate, and the bulbourethral glands. [**Section 13.1**]

accessory organs

1. In the GI tract, organs that play a role in digestion, but are not directly part of the alimentary canal. These include the liver, the gallbladder, the pancreas, and the salivary glands.
2. In the reproductive systems, any organ involved in reproduction that is not a gonad (testis or ovary). [**Section 10.7**]

acetylcholine (ACh)

The neurotransmitter used throughout the parasympathetic nervous system as well as at the neuromuscular junction. [**Section 8.2**]

acetylcholinesterase (AChE)

The enzyme that breaks down acetylcholine in the synaptic cleft. [**Section 8.2**]

acid hydrolases

Enzymes that degrade various macromolecules and that require an acidic pH to function properly. Acid hydrolases are found within the lysosomes of cells. [**Section 6.2**]

acinar cells

Cells that make up exocrine glands, and that secrete their products into ducts. For example, in the pancreas, acinar cells secrete digestive enzymes; in the salivary glands, acinar cells secrete saliva. [**Section 10.5**]

acrosome

A region at the head of a sperm cell that contains digestive enzymes which, when released during the acrosome reaction, can facilitate penetration of the corona radiata of the oocyte and fertilization. [**Sections 13.2 and 13.9**]

actin

A contractile protein. In skeletal and cardiac muscle, actin polymerizes (along with other proteins) to form the thin filaments. Actin is involved in many contractile activities, such as cytokinesis, pseudopod formation, and muscle contraction. [**Sections 6.5 and 11.2**]

action potential

A localized change in a neuron's or muscle cell's membrane potential that can propagate itself away from its point of origin. Action potentials are an all-or-none process mediated by the opening of voltage-gated Na^+ and K^+ channels when the membrane is brought to the threshold potential; opening of the Na^+ channels causes a characteristic depolarization, while opening of the K^+ channels repolarizes the membrane. [**Section 8.1**]

activator proteins

Proteins that bind to enhancer sequences in eukaryotes to increase transcription. [**Section 4.9**]

active transport

The movement of molecules through the plasma membrane against their concentration gradients. Active transport requires input of cellular energy, often in the form of ATP. An example is the Na^+/K^+-ATPase in the plasma membranes of all cells. [**Section 6.4**]

adenine

One of the four aromatic bases found in DNA and RNA; also a component of ATP, NADH, and $FADH_2$. Adenine is a purine; it pairs with thymine (in DNA) and with uracil (in RNA). [**Section 4.1**]

adenohypophysis

See "anterior pituitary gland." [**Section 8.6**]

adipocyte
Fat cell. [Section 9.5]

adrenal medulla
The inner region of the adrenal gland. The adrenal medulla is part of the sympathetic nervous system, and it releases epinephrine (adrenaline) and norepinephrine into the blood when stimulated. These hormones augment and prolong the effects of sympathetic stimulation in the body. [Section 8.4]

adrenergic tone
A constant nervous input to the arteries that keeps them somewhat constricted to maintain a basal level of blood pressure. [Section 9.3]

adrenocorticotropic hormone (ACTH)
A tropic hormone produced by the anterior pituitary gland that targets the adrenal cortex, stimulating it to release cortisol and aldosterone. [Section 8.6]

afferent arteriole
The small artery that carries blood toward the capillaries of the glomerulus. [Section 10.2]

afferent neuron
A neuron that carries information (action potentials) to the central nervous system; a sensory neuron. [Section 8.3]

albumin
A blood protein produced by the liver. Albumin helps to maintain blood osmotic pressure (oncotic pressure). [Section 9.4]

aldosterone
The principal mineralocorticoid secreted by the adrenal cortex. This steroid hormone targets the kidney tubules and increases renal reabsorption of sodium. [Section 10.2]

alimentary canal
Also known as the *gastrointestinal* (GI) *tract* or the *digestive tract*, the alimentary canal is the long muscular "tube" that includes the mouth, esophagus, stomach, small intestine, and large intestine. [Section 10.5]

allele
A version of a gene. For example, the gene may be for eye color, and the alleles include those for brown eyes, those for blue eyes, those for green eyes, etc. At most, diploid organisms can possess only two alleles for a given gene, one on each of the two homologous chromosomes. [Section 7.1]

alveoli
(Singular: *alveolus*) Tiny sacs, with walls only a single cell thick, found at the end of the respiratory bronchiole tree. Alveoli are the sites of gas exchange in the respiratory system. [Section 12.2]

amino acids
The building blocks (monomers) of proteins. There are 20 different amino acids. [Section 3.1]

amino acid acceptor site
The 3' end of a tRNA molecule that binds an amino acid. The nucleotide sequence at this end is CCA. [Section 4.8]

amino acid activation
See "tRNA loading." [Section 4.8]

aminoacyl tRNA
A tRNA with an amino acid attached. This is made by an aminoacyl-tRNA synthetase, an enzyme that is specific to the amino acid being attached. [Section 4.8]

amnion
A sac filled with fluid (amniotic fluid) that surrounds and protects a developing embryo. [Section 13.10]

amylase
An enzyme that digests starch into disaccharides. Amylase is secreted by salivary glands and by the pancreas. [Section 10.6]

anabolism
The process of building complex structures out of simpler precursors (e.g., synthesizing proteins from amino acids). [Section 4.9]

analogous structures
Physical structures in two different organisms that have functional similarity due to their evolution in a common environment, but that have different underlying structure. Analogous structures arise from convergent evolution. [Section 7.10]

anal sphincter
The valve that controls the release of feces from the rectum. It has an internal part made of smooth muscle (thus involuntary) and an external part made of skeletal muscle (thus voluntary). [Section 10.6]

anaphase
The third phase of mitosis. During anaphase, replicated chromosomes are split apart at their centromeres (the sister chromatids are separated from one another) and moved to opposite sides of the cell. [Section 6.6]

anaphase I

The third phase of meiosis I. During anaphase I the replicated homologous chromosomes are separated (the tetrad is split apart) and pulled to opposite sides of the cell. [**Section 7.2**]

anaphase II

The third phase of meiosis II. During anaphase II, the sister chromatids are finally separated at their centromeres and pulled to opposite sides of the cell. Note that anaphase II is identical to mitotic anaphase, except that the number of chromosomes was reduced by half during meiosis I. [**Section 7.2**]

androgens

Male sex hormones. Testosterone is the primary androgen. [**Section 13.4**]

anergic

A term used to describe immune system cells that become unresponsive, but do not go through apoptosis, e.g., B cells and T cells that recognize self-antigens. [**Section 9.8**]

angiotensinogen

A normal blood protein produced by the liver, angiotensinogen is converted to angiotensin I by renin (secreted by the kidney when blood pressure falls). Angiotensin I is further converted to angiotensin II by ACE (angiotensin converting enzyme). Angiotensin II is a powerful systemic vasoconstrictor and stimulator of aldosterone release, both of which result in an increase in blood pressure. [**Section 10.3**]

antagonist

Something that acts to oppose the action of something else. For example, muscles that move a joint in opposite directions are said to be *antagonists*. [**Section 11.2**]

anterior pituitary gland

Also known as the *adenohypophysis*, the anterior pituitary is made of glandular tissue. It makes and secretes six different hormones: FSH, LH, ACTH, TSH, prolactin, and growth hormone. The anterior pituitary is controlled by releasing and inhibiting factors from the hypothalamus. [**Section 8.6**]

antibody (Ab)

Also called *immunoglobulins*, antibodies are proteins secreted by activated B cells (plasma cells) that bind in a highly specific manner to foreign proteins (such as those found on the surface of pathogens or transplanted tissues). The foreign proteins are called *antigens*. Antibodies generally do not destroy antigens directly, rather, they mark them for destruction through other methods, and can inactivate antigens by clumping them together or by covering necessary active sites. [**Section 9.7**]

anticodon

A sequence of three nucleotides (found in the anticodon loop of tRNA) that is complementary to a specific codon in mRNA. The codon to which the anticodon is complementary specifies the amino acid that is carried by that tRNA. [**Section 4.8**]

antidiuretic hormone (ADH)

Also called *vasopressin*, this hormone is produced in the hypothalamus and secreted by the posterior pituitary gland. It targets the kidney tubules, increasing their permeability to water, and thus increasing water retention by the body. [**Section 8.6**]

antigen (Ag)

A molecule (usually a protein) capable of initiating an immune response (antibody production). [**Section 9.7**]

antigen-presenting cell

Cells that possess MHC II (B cells and macrophages), and are able to display bits of ingested antigen on their surface in order to activate T cells. (See also "MHC.") [**Section 9.7**]

antiport

A carrier protein that transports two molecules across the plasma membrane in opposite directions. [**Section 6.4**]

aorta

The largest artery in the body; the aorta carries oxygenated blood away from the left ventricle of the heart. [**Section 9.2**]

apoptosis

Programmed cell death due to external stressors such as toxins or internal signals, such as an increase in the product of a tumor suppressor gene. Apoptosis is mediated by a family of proteins called caspases. [**Section 6.7**]

appendix

A mass of lymphatic tissue at the beginning of the large intestine that helps trap ingested pathogens. [**Section 9.7**]

aqueous humor

A thin, watery fluid found in the anterior segment of the eye (between the lens and the cornea). The aqueous humor is constantly produced and drained, and helps to bring nutrients to the lens and cornea, as well as to remove metabolic wastes. [**Section 8.5**]

arousal

A function in the reproductive system, controlled by the parasympathetic nervous system, that includes erection (via dilation of erectile arteries) and lubrication. [**Section 13.2**]

artery
A blood vessel that carries blood away from the heart chambers. Arteries have muscular walls to regulate blood flow and are typically high-pressure vessels. [**Section 9.2**]

atrioventricular (AV) bundle
Also known as the *bundle of His*, this is the first portion of the cardiac conduction system after the AV node. [**Section 9.2**]

atrioventricular (AV) node
The second major node of the cardiac conduction system (after the SA node). The cardiac impulse is delayed slightly at the AV node, allowing the ventricles to contract just after the atria contract. [**Section 9.2**]

atrioventricular valves
The valves in the heart that separate the atria from the ventricles. The *tricuspid* valve separates the right atrium from the right ventricle, and the *bicuspid* (or *mitral*) valve separates the left atrium from the left ventricle. These valves close at the beginning of systole, preventing the backflow of blood from ventricles to atria, and producing the first heart sound. [**Section 9.2**]

atrium
One of two small chambers in the heart that receive blood and pass it on to the ventricles. The right atrium receives deoxygenated blood from the body through the superior and inferior vena cavae, and the left atrium receives oxygenated blood from the lungs through the pulmonary veins. [**Section 9.2**]

attachment
The first step in viral infection. Attachment of a virus to its host is very specific and is also known as *adsorption*. [**Section 5.1**]

auditory tube
The tube that connects the middle ear cavity with the pharynx; also known as the *Eustachian tube*. Its function is to equalize middle ear pressure with atmospheric pressure so that pressure is equal on both sides of the tympanic membrane. [**Section 8.5**]

autoimmune reaction
An immune reaction directed against normal (necessary) cells. For example, type I diabetes mellitus is an autoimmune reaction directed against the β cells of the pancreas (destroying them and preventing insulin secretion), and against insulin itself. [**Section 9.8**]

autonomic nervous system (ANS)
The division of the peripheral nervous system that innervates and controls the visceral organs (everything but the skeletal muscles). It is also known as the *involuntary nervous system* and can be subdivided into the sympathetic and parasympathetic divisions. [**Section 8.4**]

autotroph
An organism that can makes its own food, typically using CO_2 as a carbon source. [**Section 5.3**]

auxotroph
A bacterium that cannot survive on minimal medium (glucose alone) because it lacks the ability to synthesize a molecule it needs to live (typically an amino acid). Auxotrophs must have the needed substance (the *auxiliary trophic* substance) added to their medium in order to survive. They are typically denoted by the substance they require followed by a "−" sign in superscript. For example, a bacterium that cannot synthesize leucine would be a leucine auxotroph, and would be indicated as Leu⁻. [**Section 5.3**]

avascular
Lacking a blood supply, e.g., cartilage. [**Section 11.8**]

axon
A long projection off the cell body of a neuron down which an action potential can be propagated. [**Section 8.1**]

B cell
A type of lymphocyte that can recognize (bind to) an antigen and secrete an antibody specific for that antigen. When activated by binding an antigen, B cells mature into *plasma cells* (that secrete antibody) and *memory cells* (that patrol the body for future encounters with that antigen). [**Section 9.7**]

bacillus
A bacterium having a rod-like shape (plural = bacilli). [**Section 5.3**]

bacteriophage
A virus that infects a bacterium. [**Section 5.1**]

baroreceptor
A sensory receptor that responds to changes in pressure; for example, there are baroreceptors in the carotid arteries and the aortic arch that monitor blood pressure. [**Section 9.2**]

Bartholin's glands
See "vestibular glands." [**Section 13.5**]

basement membrane
A layer of collagen fibers that separates epithelial tissue from connective tissue. [**Section 10.2**]

basilar membrane

The flexible membrane in the cochlea that supports the organ of Corti (the structure that contains the hearing receptors). The fibers of the basilar membrane are short and stiff near the oval window and long and flexible near the apex of the cochlea. This difference in structure allows the basilar membrane to help transduce pitch. [Section 8.5]

bicarbonate

HCO_3^-. This ion results from the dissociation of carbonic acid and, together with carbonic acid, forms the major blood buffer system. Bicarbonate is also secreted by the pancreas to neutralize stomach acid in the intestines. [Section 9.5]

bicuspid valve

See "atrioventricular valve." [Section 9.2]

bile

A green fluid made from cholesterol and secreted by the liver. It is stored and concentrated in the gallbladder. Bile is an amphipathic molecule that is secreted into the small intestine when fats are present, and it serves to emulsify the fats for better digestion by lipases. [Section 9.5]

binary fission

An asexual method of bacterial reproduction that serves only to increase the size of the population; there is no introduction of genetic diversity. The bacterium simply grows in size until it has doubled its cellular components, then it replicates its genome and splits into two. [Section 5.3]

bipolar cell

A cell in the retina of the eye that receives input from photoreceptors and subsequently synapses on ganglion cells. Bipolar cells belong to a class of neurons called "bipolar neurons" that have a single dendrite and single axon extending from opposite sides of the cell body. [Section 8.5]

blastocyst

A fluid-filled sphere formed about five days after fertilization of an ovum that is made up of an outer ring of cells and an inner cell mass. This is the structure that implants in the endometrium of the uterus. [Section 13.9]

Bohr effect

The tendency of certain factors to stabilize hemoglobin in the tense conformation, thus reducing its affinity for oxygen and enhancing the release of oxygen to the tissues. The factors include increased P_{CO_2}, increased temperature, increased bisphosphoglycerate (BPG), and decreased pH. Note that the Bohr effect shifts the oxy-hemoglobin saturation curve to the right. [Section 9.5]

boiling point elevation

The increase in the boiling point of a solution due to the addition of solute. [Section 6.4]

bone marrow

A non-bony material that fills the hollow spaces inside bones. Red bone marrow is found in regions of spongy bone and is the site of blood cell production. Yellow bone marrow is found in the diaphysis (shaft) of long bones, is mostly fat, and is inactive. [Section 11.7]

bottom-up processing

A tenet of Gestalt psychology wherein the processing of sensory input begins with the sensory receptors and works up to the complex integration of information occurring in the brain. [Section 8.5]

Bowman's capsule

The region of the nephron that surrounds the glomerulus. The capsule collects the plasma that is filtered from the capillaries in the glomerulus. [Section 10.2]

bronchioles

Very small air tubes in the respiratory system (diameter 0.5–1.0 mm). The walls of the bronchioles are made of smooth muscle to help regulate air flow. [Section 12.2]

brush border enzymes

Enzymes secreted by the mucosal cells lining the intestine. The brush border enzymes are disaccharidases and dipeptidases that digest the smallest carbohydrates and peptides into their respective monomers. [Section 10.6]

bulbourethral glands

Small, paired glands found inferior to the prostate in males and at the posterior end of the penile urethra. They secrete an alkaline mucus on sexual arousal that lubricates the urethra and helps to neutralize any traces of acidic urine in the urethra that might be harmful to sperm. [Section 13.1]

Bundle of His

See "atrioventricular (AV) bundle." [Section 9.2]

calcitonin

A hormone produced by the C-cells of the thyroid gland that decreases serum calcium levels. It targets the bones (stimulates osteoblasts) and the kidneys (reduces calcium reabsorption. [Sections 8.6 and 11.9]

calcitriol

A hormone produced from vitamin D that acts to increase serum calcium levels. [Section 11.9]

calmodulin
A cytoplasmic Ca^{2+}-binding protein. Calmodulin is particularly important in smooth muscle cells, where binding of Ca^{2+} allows calmodulin to activate myosin light-chain kinase, the first step in smooth muscle cell contraction. [Section 11.4]

cAMP
See "cyclic AMP." [Section 6.5]

capacitation
An increase in the fragility of the membranes of sperm cells when exposed to the female reproductive tract. Capacitation is required so that the acrosomal enzymes can be released to facilitate fertilization. [Section 13.9]

capillary
The smallest of all blood vessels, typically having a diameter just large enough for blood cells to pass through in single file. Capillaries have extremely thin walls to facilitate the exchange of material between the blood and the tissues. [Section 9.5]

capsid
The outer protein coat of a virus. [Section 5.1]

carbonic anhydrase
An enzyme present in erythrocytes (as well as in other places) that catalyzes the conversion of CO_2 and H_2O into carbonic acid. [Section 9.5]

cardiac conduction system
The specialized cells of the heart that spontaneously initiate action potentials and transmit them to the cardiac muscle cells. The cells of the conduction system are essentially cardiac muscle cells, but lack the contractile fibers of the muscle cells, thus they are able to transmit impulses (action potentials) more quickly and efficiently than cardiac muscle tissue. The cardiac conduction system includes the SA node, the internodal tract, the AV node, the AV bundle, the right and left bundle branches, and the Purkinje fibers. [Section 9.2]

cardiac muscle
The muscle tissue of the heart. Cardiac muscle is striated, uninucleate, and under involuntary control (controlled by the autonomic nervous system). Note also that cardiac muscle is self-stimulatory, and autonomic control serves only to modify the intrinsic rate of contraction. [Section 9.2]

cardiac output
The volume of blood pumped out of the heart in one minute (vol/min); the product of the stroke volume (vol/beat) and the heart rate (beat/min). Cardiac output is directly proportional to blood pressure. [Section 9.2]

cardiac sphincter
See "lower esophageal sphincter." [Section 10.6]

carrier protein
An integral membrane protein that undergoes a conformational change to move a molecule from one side of the membrane to another. See also "uniporter," "antiporter," and "symporter." [Section 6.4]

cartilage
A strong connective tissue with varying degrees of flexibility. Elastic cartilage is the most flexible, forming structures that require support but also need to bend, such as the epiglottis and outer ear. Hyaline cartilage is more rigid than elastic cartilage, and forms the cartilages of the ribs, the respiratory tract, and all joints. Fibrocartilage is the least flexible of them all, and forms very strong connections, such as the pubic symphysis and the intervertebral disks. [Section 11.8]

caspases
A family of proteases that carry out the events of apoptosis. [Section 6.7]

catalase
The primary enzyme in peroxisomes; catalase catalyzes the hydrolysis of hydrogen peroxide (H_2O_2) into water and oxygen. [Section 6.2]

cDNA
Complementary DNA. DNA produced synthetically by reverse transcribing mRNA. Because of eukaryotic mRNA splicing, cDNA contains no introns. [Section A.5]

cecum
The first part of the large intestine. [Section 10.6]

cell surface receptor
An integral membrane protein that binds extracellular signaling molecules, such as hormones and peptides. [Section 6.3]

cell theory
Established by Robert Hooke in 1655, the cell theory asserts that all living organisms are composed of one or more cells and that new cells arise from preexisting, living cells. [Section 5.3]

central canal
The hollow center of an osteon, also known as a *Haversian canal*. The central canal contains blood vessels, lymphatic vessels, and nerves. Bone is laid down around the central canal in concentric rings called *lamellae*. [Section 11.8]

central chemoreceptors
Receptors in the central nervous system that monitor the pH of cerebrospinal fluid to help regulate ventilation rate. [**Section 12.5**]

central nervous system
The subdivision of the nervous system consisting of the brain and spinal cord. [**Section 8.4**]

centriole
A structure composed of a ring of nine microtubule triplets, found in pairs at the MTOC (microtubule organizing center) of a cell. The centrioles duplicate during cell division, and serve as the organizing center for the mitotic spindle. [**Section 6.5**]

centromere
A structure near the middle of eukaryotic chromosomes to which the fibers of the mitotic spindle attach during cell division. [**Section 4.1**]

cerebellum
The region of the brain that coordinates and smooths skeletal muscle activity. [**Section 8.4**]

cerebral cortex
A thin (4 mm) layer of gray matter on the surface of the cerebral hemispheres. The cerebral cortex is the conscious mind, and is functionally divided into four pairs of lobes: the frontal lobes, the parietal lobes, the temporal lobes, and the occipital lobes. [**Section 8.4**]

cerebrospinal fluid (CSF)
A clear fluid that circulates around and through the brain and spinal cord. CSF helps to physically support the brain and acts as a shock absorber. It also exchanges nutrients and wastes with the brain and spinal cord. [**Section 8.4**]

cervix
The opening to the uterus. The cervix is typically plugged with a sticky acidic mucus during non-fertile times (to form a barrier against the entry of pathogens), however, during ovulation, the mucus becomes more watery and alkaline to facilitate sperm entry. [**Section 13.5**]

channel protein
An integral membrane protein that selectively allows molecules across the plasma membrane. See also entries under "ion channel," "voltage-gated channel," and "ligand-gated channel." [**Section 6.3**]

chaperones
A family of proteins that assists in the folding of other proteins. [**Section 4.9**]

chemical synapse
A type of synapse at which a chemical (a neurotransmitter) is released from the axon of a neuron into the synaptic cleft where it binds to receptors on the next structure in sequence, either another neuron or an organ. [**Section 8.2**]

chemoreceptor
A sensory receptor that responds to specific chemicals. Some examples are gustatory (taste) receptors, olfactory (smell) receptors, and central chemoreceptors (respond to pH changes in the cerebrospinal fluid). [**Sections 5.3 and 8.5**]

chemotaxis
Movement that is directed by chemical gradients, such as nutrients or toxins. [**Sections 5.3 and 9.4**]

chemotroph
An organism that relies on a chemical source of energy (such as ATP) instead of using light to make ATP (like phototrophs do). [**Section 5.3**]

chief cells
Pepsinogen-secreting cells found at the bottom of the gastric glands of the stomach. [**Section 10.6**]

cholecystokinin (CCK)
A hormone secreted by the small intestine (duodenum) in response to the presences of fats. It promotes release of bile from the gallbladder and pancreatic juice from the pancreas, and reduces stomach motility. [**Section 10.6**]

cholesterol
A large, ring-shaped lipid found in cell membranes. Cholesterol is the precursor for steroid hormones and is used to manufacture bile salts. [**Sections 3.4 and 6.3**]

chondrocyte
A mature cartilage cell. [**Section 11.6**]

chorion
The portion of the placenta derived from the zygote. The chorionic villi secrete hCG to help maintain the endometrium during the first trimester of a pregnancy. [**Section 13.8**]

choroid
The darkly pigmented middle layer of the eyeball, found between the sclera (outer layer) and the retina (inner layer). [**Section 8.5**]

chromosome
A single piece of double-stranded DNA; part of the genome of an organism. Prokaryotes have circular chromosomes and eukaryotes have linear chromosomes. [**Section 4.1**]

chylomicrons
A type of lipoprotein; the form in which absorbed fats from the intestines are transported to the circulatory system. [**Sections 9.5 and 10.7**]

chyme
Partially digested, semiliquid food mixed with digestive enzymes and acids in the stomach. [**Section 10.6**]

chymotrypsin
One of the main pancreatic proteases; it is activated (from chymotrypsinogen) by trypsin. [**Section 10.7**]

cilia
A hair-like structure on the cell surface composed of microtubules in a "9 + 2" arrangement (nine pairs of microtubules surrounding 2 single microtubules in the center). The microtubules are connected with a contractile protein called *dynein*. Cilia beat in a repetitive sweeping motion, which helps to move substances along the surface of the cell. They are particularly important in the respiratory system, where they sweep mucus out of the trachea and up to the mouth and nose. [**Section 6.5**]

circular smooth muscle
The inner layer of smooth muscle in the wall of the digestive tract. When the circular muscle contracts, the tube diameter is reduced. Certain areas of the circular muscle are thickened to act as valves (sphincters). [**Section 10.5**]

clathrin
A fibrous protein found on the intracellular side of the plasma membrane (also found associated with the Golgi complex) that helps to invaginate the membrane. Typically cell surface receptors are associated with clathrin-coated pits at the plasma membrane, and binding of the ligand to the receptor triggers invagination. [**Section 6.4**]

cleavage
The rapid mitotic divisions of a zygote that begin within 24–36 hours after fertilization. [**Section 13.9**]

coccus
A bacterium having a round shape (plural = cocci). [**Section 5.3**]

cochlea
The curled structure in the inner ear that contains the membranes and hair cells used to transduce sound waves into action potentials. [**Section 8.5**]

codominance
A situation in which a heterozygote displays the phenotype associated with each of the alleles, e.g., human blood type AB. [**Section 7.4**]

codon
A group of three nucleotides that is specific for a particular amino acid, or that specifies "stop translating." [**Section 4.3**]

collagen
A protein fiber with a unique triple-helix structure that gives it great strength. Tissues with a lot of collagen fibers are typically very strong, e.g., bone, tendons, ligaments, etc. [**Section 11.6**]

collecting duct
The portion of the nephron where water reabsorption is regulated via antidiuretic hormone (ADH). Several nephrons empty into each collecting duct, and this is the final region through which urine must pass on its way to the ureter. [**Section 10.2**]

colligative properties
Properties that depend on the number of solute particles in a solution rather than on the type of particle. Colligative properties include boiling point elevation, freezing point depression, and vapor pressure depression. [**Section 6.4**]

colon
See "large intestine." [**Sections 10.1 and 10.6**]

common bile duct
The duct that carries bile from the gallbladder and liver to the small intestine (duodenum). [**Section 10.6**]

compact bone
A dense, hard type of bone constructed from osteons (at the microscopic level). Compact bone forms the diaphysis of the long bones, and the outer shell of the epiphyses and all other bones. [**Section 11.7**]

complement system
A group of blood proteins that bind non-specifically to the surface proteins of foreign cells (such as bacteria), ultimately leading to the destruction of the foreign cell. [**Section 9.7**]

cones
Photoreceptors in the retina of the eye that respond to bright light and provide color vision. [**Section 8.5**]

conjugation
A form of genetic recombination in bacteria in which plasmid and/or genomic DNA is transferred from one bacterium to the other through a conjugation bridge. [**Section 5.3**]

connective tissue
One of the four basic tissue types in the body (epithelial, connective, muscle, and nervous). Connective tissue is a supportive tissue consisting of relatively few cells scattered among a great deal of extracellular material (matrix), and includes adipose tissue (fat), bone, cartilage, the dermis of the skin, tendons, ligaments, and blood. [**Section 11.6**]

convergent evolution
A form of evolution in which different organisms are placed into the same environment and exposed to the same selection pressures. This causes the organisms to evolve along similar lines. As a result, they may share functional, but not structural similarity (because they possessed different starting materials). Convergent evolution produces *analogous structures*. [**Section 7.9**]

cooperativity
A type of substrate binding to a multi-active site enzyme, in which the binding of one substrate molecule facilitates the binding of subsequent substrate molecules. A graph of reaction rate vs. substrate concentration appears sigmoidal. Note that cooperativity can be found in other situations as well, for example, hemoglobin binds oxygen cooperatively. [**Section 9.5**]

copy-number variation
Structural variations in the genome that lead to different copies of certain sections of the DNA, due to duplication of those sections or deletions of those sections. [**Section 4.2**]

cornea
The clear portion of the tough outer layer of the eyeball, found over the iris and pupil. [**Section 8.5**]

corona radiata
The layer of granulosa cells that surround an oocyte after it has been ovulated. [**Section 13.6**]

coronary vessels
The blood vessels that carry blood to and from cardiac muscle. The coronary arteries branch off the aorta and carry oxygenated blood to the cardiac tissue. The coronary veins collect deoxygenated blood from the cardiac tissue, merge to form the coronary sinus, and drain into the right atrium. [**Section 9.2**]

corpus callosum
The largest bundle of white matter (axons) connecting the two cerebral hemispheres. [**Section 8.4**]

corpus luteum
"Yellow body." The remnants of an ovarian follicle after ovulation has occurred. The cells enlarge and begin secreting progesterone, the dominant female hormone during the second half of the menstrual cycle. Some estrogen is also secreted. [**Section 13.6**]

cortex
The outer layer of an organ, e.g., the renal cortex, the ovarian cortex, the adrenal cortex, etc. [**Sections 8.4, 8.5, 8.6, and 10.2**]

cortical reaction
See "slow block to polyspermy." [**Section 13.9**]

corticosteroids
Steroid hormones secreted from the adrenal cortex. The two major classes are the *mineralocorticoids* and *glucocorticoids*. Aldosterone is the principal mineralocorticoid, and cortisol is the principal glucocorticoid. [**Section 8.6**]

cortisol
The principal glucocorticoid secreted from the adrenal cortex. This steroid hormone is released during stress, causing increased blood glucose levels and reducing inflammation. The latter effect has led to a clinical use of cortisol as an anti-inflammatory agent. [**Section 8.6**]

creatine phosphate
An energy storage molecule used by muscle tissue. The phosphate from creatine phosphate can be removed and attached to an ADP to generate ATP quickly. [**Section 11.2**]

cross bridge
The connection of a myosin head group to an actin filament during muscle contraction (the sliding filament theory). [**Section 11.2**]

crossing over
The exchange of DNA between paired homologous chromosomes (tetrads) during prophase I of meiosis. [**Section 7.2**]

cyclic AMP (cAMP)
A cyclic version of adenosine monophosphate, where the phosphate is esterified to both the 5' and the 3' carbons, forming a ring. Cyclic AMP is an important intracellular signaling molecule, often called the "second messenger." It serves to activate cAMP-dependent kinases, which regulate the activity of other enzymes in the cell. Levels of cAMP are in part regulated by adenylyl cyclase, the enzyme that makes cAMP, and the activity of adenylyl cyclase is ultimately controlled by the binding of various ligands to cell surface receptors. [**Section 6.5**]

cytokinesis
The phase of mitosis during which the cell physically splits into two daughter cells. Cytokinesis begins near the end of anaphase, and is completed during telophase. [**Section 6.6**]

cytosine
One of the four aromatic bases found in DNA and RNA. Cytosine is a pyrimidine; it pairs with guanine. [**Section 4.1**]

dendrite
A projection off the cell body of a neuron that receives a nerve impulse from a different neuron and sends the impulse to the cell body. Neurons can have one or several dendrites. [**Section 8.1**]

dense connective tissue
Connective tissue with large amounts of either collagen fibers or elastic fibers, or both. Dense tissues are typically strong (e.g., bone, cartilage, tendons, etc.). [**Section 11.6**]

depolarization
The movement of the membrane potential of a cell away from rest potential in a more positive direction. [**Section 8.1**]

dermis
A layer of connective tissue underneath the epidermis of the skin. The dermis contains blood vessels, lymphatic vessels, nerves, sensory receptors, and glands. [**Section 12.6**]

desmosome
A general cell junction, used primarily for adhesion. [**Section 6.5**]

determination
The point during cellular development at which a cell becomes committed to a particular fate. Note that the cell is not differentiated at this point; determination comes before differentiation. Determination can be due to cytoplasmic effects or to induction by neighboring cells. [**Section 13.12**]

diaphragm
The primary muscle of inspiration. The diaphragm is stimulated to contract at regular intervals by the respiratory center in the medulla oblongata (via the phrenic nerve). Although it is made of skeletal muscle (and can therefore be voluntarily controlled), these stimulations occur autonomously. [**Section 12.3**]

diaphysis
The shaft of a long bone. The diaphysis is hollow and is made entirely from compact bone. [**Section 11.7**]

diastole
The period of time during which the ventricles of the heart are relaxed. [**Section 9.2**]

diastolic pressure
The pressure measured in the arteries while the ventricles are relaxed (during diastole). [**Section 9.3**]

diencephalon
The portion of the forebrain that includes the thalamus and hypothalamus. [**Section 8.4**]

difference threshold
The minimum noticeable difference between any two sensory stimuli, 50% of the time. [**Section 8.5**]

differentiation
The specialization of cell types, especially during embryonic and fetal development. [**Section 13.12**]

diffusion
The movement of a particle (the solute) from its region of high concentration to its region of low concentration (or *down its concentration gradient*). [**Section 6.4**]

diploid organism
An organism that has two copies of its genome in each cell. The paired genomes are said to be homologous. [**Section 7.1**]

distal convoluted tubule
The portion of the nephron tubule after the loop of Henle, but before the collecting duct. Selective reabsorption and secretion occur here; most notably regulated reabsorption of water and sodium. [**Section 10.2**]

divergent evolution
A form of evolution in which the same organism is placed into different environments with different selection pressures. This causes the organisms to evolve differently; to diverge from their common ancestor. The resulting (new) species may share structural (but not necessarily functional) similarity; divergent evolution produces *homologous structures*. [**Section 7.9**]

DNA ligase
See "ligase." [**Section 4.4**]

DNA polymerase
Also called DNA pol, this is the enzyme that replicates DNA. Eukaryotes and prokaryotes have different versions of this enzyme. [**Section 4.4**]

domain Archaea/extremophiles
One of the three main taxonomic domains, Archaea live in the world's most extreme environments (hot springs, hypersaline environments, etc.). They possess characteristics of both prokaryotes and eukaryotes. [**Section 5.3**]

dominant

1. The allele in a heterozygous genotype that is expressed.

2. The phenotype resulting from either a heterozygous genotype or a homozygous dominant genotype. [Section 7.1]

dorsal root ganglion

A group of sensory neuron cell bodies found just posterior to the spinal cord on either side. A pair of root ganglia exists for each spinal nerve that extends from the spinal cord. The ganglia are part of the peripheral nervous system (PNS). [Section 8.4]

downstream

Toward the 3' end of an RNA transcript (the 3' end of the DNA coding strand). Stop codons and (in eukaryotes) the poly-A tail are found "downstream." [Section 4.7]

ductus deferens

A thick, muscular tube that connects the epididymis of the testes to the urethra. Muscular contractions of the vas deferens during ejaculation help propel the sperm outward. Severing of the vas deferens (vasectomy) results in sterility of the male. [Section 13.1]

duodenum

The first part (approximately 5 percent) of the small intestine. [Section 10.6]

dynein

A contractile protein connecting microtubules in the "9 + 2" arrangement of cilia and eukaryotic flagella. The contraction of dynein produces the characteristic movements of these structures. [Section 6.5]

ectoderm

One of the three primary (embryonic) germ layers formed during gastrulation. Ectoderm ultimately forms external structures such as the skin, hair, nails, and inner linings of the mouth and anus, as well as the entire nervous system. [Section 13.11]

edema

Swelling. [Section 9.5]

efferent arteriole

The small artery that carries blood away from the capillaries of the glomerulus. [Section 10.2]

efferent neuron

A neuron that carries information (action potentials) away from the central nervous system; a motor neuron. [Section 8.3]

ejaculation

A subphase of male orgasm, a reflex reaction triggered by the presence of semen in the urethra. Ejaculation is a series of rhythmic contractions of muscles near the base of the penis that increase pressure in the urethra, forcing the semen out. [Section 13.1]

ejection fraction

The fraction of the end-diastolic volume ejected from the ventricles in a single contraction of the heart. The ejection fraction is normally around 60 percent of the end-diastolic volume. [Section 11.3]

elastin

A fibrous, connective-tissue protein that has the ability to recoil to its original shape after being stretched. Elastin is found in great amounts in lung tissue, arterial tissue, skin, and the epiglottis. [Section 11.6]

electrical synapse

A type of synapse in which the cells are connected by gap junctions, allowing ions (and therefore an action potential) to spread easily from cell to cell. [Section 8.2]

electron transport chain

A series of enzyme complexes found along the inner mitochondrial membrane. NADH and $FADH_2$ are oxidized by these enzymes; the electrons are shuttled down the chain and are ultimately passed to oxygen to produce water. The electron energy is used to pump H^+ out of the mitochondrial matrix; the resulting H^+ gradient is subsequently used to drive the production of ATP. [Sections 2.5, 5.1, and 6.2]

elongation factors

Proteins that assist with peptide bond formation during eukaryotic translation. [Section 4.8]

embryonic stage

The period of human development from implantation through eight weeks of gestation. Gastrulation, neurulation, and organogenesis occur during this time period. The developing baby is known as an *embryo* during this time period. [Section 13.13]

emission

A subphase of male orgasm. Emission is the movement of sperm (via the ductus deferens) and semen (via the accessory glands) into the urethra in preparation for ejaculation. [Section 13.1]

endocrine gland

A ductless gland that secretes a hormone into the blood. [Section 8.6]

endocrine system
A system of ductless glands that secrete chemical messengers (hormones) into the blood. [**Section 8.6**]

endocytosis
The uptake of material into a cell, usually by invagination. See also "phagocytosis," "pinocytosis," and "receptor-mediated endocytosis." [**Sections 5.1 and 6.4**]

endoderm
One of the three primary (embryonic) germ layers formed during gastrulation. Endoderm ultimately forms internal structures, such as the inner lining of the GI tract and some glandular organs. [**Section 13.11**]

endometrial cycle
The 28 days of the menstrual cycle as they apply to the events in the uterus. The endometrial cycle is also known as the *uterine cycle*, and has three subphases: menstruation, the proliferative phase, and the secretory phase. [**Section 13.8**]

endometrium
The inner epithelial lining of the uterus that thickens and develops during the menstrual cycle, into which a fertilized ovum can implant, and which sloughs off during menstruation if a pregnancy does not occur. [**Section 13.5**]

endospore
A bacterial structure formed in unfavorable growth conditions. Endospores have very tough outer shells made of peptidoglycan and can survive harsh conditions. The bacterium inside the endospore is essentially dormant and can become active (called germination) when conditions again become favorable. [**Section 5.3**]

endosymbiotic theory
The theory that mitochondria and chloroplasts originated as independent unicellular organisms living in symbiosis with larger cells. [**Section 6.2**]

endothelial cells
Cells that form the inner linings of arteries and veins and the walls of capillaries. Endothelial cells are involved in a number of important vascular functions. [**Section 9.1**]

endotoxin
A normal component of the outer membrane of Gram-negative bacteria. Endotoxins produce extreme immune reactions (septic shock), particularly when many of them enter the circulation at once. [**Section 5.3**]

end plate potential
The depolarization of the motor end plate on a muscle cell. [**Section 11.2**]

enteric nervous system
The nervous system of the gastrointestinal tract. It controls secretion and motility within the GI tract, and is linked to the central nervous system. [**Section 10.5**]

enterogastrone
A hormone secreted by the small intestine (duodenum) in response to the presence of food. It decreases the rate at which chyme leaves the stomach and enters the small intestine. [**Section 10.6**]

enterokinase
A duodenal enzyme that activates trypsinogen (from the pancreas) to trypsin. [**Section 10.6**]

envelope
A lipid bilayer that surrounds the capsid of an animal virus. The envelope is acquired as the virus buds out through the plasma membrane of its host cell. Not all animal viruses possess an envelope. [**Section 5.1**]

epidermis
The outermost layer of the skin. The epidermis is made of epithelial tissue that is constantly dividing at the bottom; the cells migrate to the surface (dying along the way) to be sloughed off at the surface. [**Section 12.6**]

epididymis
A long, coiled duct on the outside of the testis in which sperm mature. [**Section 13.1**]

epigenetics
Changes in gene expression that are not due to mutations, but are long-term and heritable (e.g., DNA methylation, chromatin remodeling, and RNA interference). [**Section 4.9**]

epiglottis
A flexible piece of cartilage in the larynx that flips downward to seal the trachea during swallowing. [**Sections 10.6 and 12.2**]

epinephrine
A hormone produced and secreted by the adrenal medulla that prolongs and increases the effects of the sympathetic nervous system. [**Section 8.4**]

epiphyseal plate
A band of cartilage (hyaline) found between the diaphysis and the epiphyses of long bones that allows bone growth during childhood. [**Section 11.9**]

epiphysis
One of the two ends of a long bone (pl: epiphyses). The epiphyses have an outer shell made of compact bone and an inner core of spongy bone. The spongy bone is filled with red bone marrow, the site of blood cell formation. [**Section 11.7**]

epistasis
A situation in which the expression of one gene prevents expression of all allelic forms of another gene, e.g., the gene for male pattern baldness is epistatic to the hair color gene. [**Section 7.4**]

epithelial tissue
One of the four basic tissue types in the body (epithelial, connective, muscle, and nervous). Epithelial tissue is a lining and covering tissue (e.g., skin, the lining of the stomach and intestines, the lining of the urinary tract, etc.) or a glandular tissue (e.g., the liver, the pancreas, the ovaries, etc.). [**Section 12.7**]

epitope
The specific site on an antigenic molecule that binds to a T cell receptor or to an antibody. [**Section 9.7**]

EPSP
Excitatory postsynaptic potential; a slight depolarization of a postsynaptic cell, bringing the membrane potential of that cell closer to the threshold for an action potential. [**Section 8.2**]

equilibrium potential
The membrane potential at which there is no driving force on an ion, and there is no net movement of ions across the membrane. [**Section 8.1**]

erectile tissue
Specialized tissue with a lot of space that can fill with blood upon proper stimulation, causing the tissue to become firm. Erectile tissue is found in the penis, the clitoris, the labia, and the nipples. [**Section 13.1**]

erythrocyte
A red blood cell; they are filled with hemoglobin, and the function of the erythrocytes is to carry oxygen in the blood. [**Section 9.4**]

erythropoietin
A hormone produced and released by the kidney that stimulates the production of red blood cells by the bone marrow. [**Section 10.4**]

estrogen
The primary female sex hormone. Estrogen stimulates the development of female secondary sex characteristics during puberty, maintains those characteristics during adulthood, stimulates the development of a new uterine lining after menstruation, and stimulates mammary gland development during pregnancy. [**Section 13.4**]

eukaryotic
A cell characterized by the presence of a nucleus and other membrane-bound organelles. Eukaryotes can be unicellular (protists) or multicellular (fungi, plants, and animals). [**Section 6.1**]

excision
The removal (and usually the activation) of a viral genome from its host's genome. [**Section 5.1**]

excitation-contraction coupling
The mechanism that ensures that skeletal muscle contraction does not occur without neural stimulation (excitation). At rest, cytosolic $[Ca^{2+}]$ is low, and the troponin-tropomyosin complex covers the myosin-binding sites on actin. When the muscle is stimulated by a neuron, Ca^{2+} is released from the sarcoplasmic reticulum into the cytosol of the muscle cell. Ca^{2+} binds to troponin, causing a conformation change in the troponin-tropomyosin complex that shifts it away from the myosin-binding sites. This allows myosin and actin to interact according to the sliding filament theory. [**Section 11.2**]

excretion
The elimination of waste products from the body. [**Section 10.1**]

exocrine gland
A gland that secretes its product into a duct, which ultimately carries the product to the surface of the body or into a body cavity. Some examples of exocrine glands and their products are sweat glands (sweat), gastric glands (acid, mucus, protease), the liver (bile), sebaceous glands (oil), and lacrimal glands (tears). [**Section 8.6**]

exocytosis
The secretion of a cellular product to the extracellular medium through a secretory vesicle. [**Section 6.4**]

exon
A nucleotide sequence in RNA that contains protein-coding information. Exons are typically separated by introns (intervening sequences) that are spliced out prior to translation. [**Section 4.7**]

exotoxin
A toxin secreted by a bacterium into its surrounding medium that help the bacterium compete with other species. Some exotoxins cause serious diseases in humans (botulism, tetanus, diphtheria, toxic shock syndrome). [**Section 5.3**]

expiration
The movement of air out of the respiratory tract. Expiration can be passive (caused by relaxation of the diaphragm and elastic recoil of the lungs) or active (caused by contraction of the abdominal muscles, which increases intraabdominal pressure and forces the diaphragm up past its normal relaxed position). [**Section 12.3**]

facilitated diffusion
Movement of a hydrophilic molecule across the plasma membrane of a cell, down its concentration gradient, through a channel, pore, or carrier molecule in the membrane. Because of the hydrophilic nature of the molecule, it requires a special path through the lipid bilayer. [**Section 6.4**]

facultative anaerobe
An organism that will use oxygen to produce energy (aerobic metabolism) if it is available, and that can ferment (anaerobic metabolism) if it is not. [**Section 5.3**]

fallopian tubes
See "uterine tubes." [**Section 13.5**]

fascicle
A bundle of skeletal muscle cells. Fascicles group together to form skeletal muscles. [**Section 11.2**]

fast block to polyspermy
The depolarization of the egg plasma membrane upon fertilization, designed to prevent the entry of more than one sperm into the egg. [**Section 13.9**]

fertilization
The fusion of a sperm with an ovum during sexual reproduction. In humans, fertilization typically occurs in the uterine tubes and requires capacitation of the sperm and release of the acrosomal enzymes. Fertilization is a species-specific process, requiring binding of a sperm protein to an egg receptor. [**Section 13.9**]

F (fertility) factor
A bacterial plasmid that allows the bacterium to initiate conjugation. Bacteria that possess the F factor are known as F+ "males." [**Section 5.3**]

fetal stage
The period of human development beginning at eight weeks of gestation and lasting until birth (38–42 weeks of gestation). During this stage the organs formed in the embryonic stage grow and mature. The developing baby is known as a *fetus* during this time period. [**Section 13.13**]

fibrinogen
A blood protein essential to blood clotting. The conversion of fibrinogen to its active form (fibrin) is among the final steps in clot formation, and is triggered by thrombin. [**Section 9.4**]

fibroblast
A generic connective tissue cell that produces fibers; the progenitor of all other connective tissue cell types. [**Section 11.6**]

filtration
The movement of a substance across a membrane via pressure. In the kidney, filtration refers specifically to the movement of plasma across the capillary walls of the glomerulus, into the capsule and tubule of the nephron. Filtration at the glomerulus is driven by blood pressure. [**Section 10.1**]

fimbriae
Fingerlike projections of the uterine (fallopian) tubes that drape over the ovary. [**Section 13.5**]

flagella
A long, whip-like filament that helps in cell motility. Many bacteria are flagellated, and sperm are flagellated. [**Section 5.3**]

fluid mosaic model
The current understanding of membrane structure, in which the membrane is composed of a mix of lipids and proteins (a mosaic) that are free to move fluidly among themselves. [**Section 6.3**]

follicle
A developing oocyte and all of its surrounding (supporting) cells. [**Section 13.6**]

follicle stimulating hormone (FSH)
A tropic hormone produced by the anterior pituitary gland that targets the gonads. In females, FSH stimulates the ovaries to develop follicles (oogenesis) and secrete estrogen; in males, FSH stimulates spermatogenesis. [**Section 13.2**]

follicular phase
The first phase of the ovarian cycle, during which a follicle (an oocyte and its surrounding cells) enlarges and matures. This phase is under the control of FSH from the anterior pituitary, and typically lasts from day 1 to day 14 of the menstrual cycle. The follicle secretes estrogen during this time period. [**Section 13.7**]

F_1 generation
The first generation of offspring from a given genetic cross. [Section 7.3]

formylmethionine (fMet)
A modified methionine used as the first amino acid in all prokaryotic proteins. [Section 4.8]

frameshift mutation
A mutation caused by an insertion or deletion of base pairs in a gene sequence in DNA such that the reading frame of the gene (and thus the amino acid sequence of the protein) is altered. [Section 4.5]

Frank-Starling mechanism
A mechanism by which the stroke volume of the heart is increased by increasing the venous return to the heart (thus stretching the ventricular muscle). [Section 9.2]

freezing-point depression
The decrease in the freezing point of a solution due to the addition of solute. [Section 6.4]

functional syncytium
A tissue in which the cytoplasms of the cells are connected by gap junctions, allowing the cells to function as a unit. Cardiac and smooth muscle tissues are examples of functional syncytiums. [Section 9.2]

gallbladder
A digestive accessory organ near the liver. The gallbladder stores and concentrates bile produced by the liver, and is stimulated to contract by cholecystokinin (CCK). [Section 10.6]

ganglion
A clump of gray matter (unmyelinated neuron cell bodies) found in the peripheral nervous system. [Section 8.4]

gap junction
A junction formed between cells, consisting of a protein channel called a *connexon* on each of the two cells, that connect to form a single channel between the cytoplasms of both cells. Gap junctions allow small molecules to flow between the cells, and are important in cell-to-cell communication, for example, in relaying the action potential between cardiac muscle cells, and relaying nutrients between osteocytes. [Sections 6.5 and 9.2]

gap phase
A phase in the cycle between mitosis and S phase (G_1) or between S phase and mitosis (G_2). During gap phases the cell undergoes normal activity and growth; G_1 may include preparation for DNA replication and G_2 includes preparation for mitosis. Note that non-dividing cells remain permanently in G_1, known as G_0 for these cells. [Section 6.6]

gastrin
A hormone released by the G cells of the stomach in the presence of food. Gastrin promotes muscular activity of the stomach as well as secretion of hydrochloric acid, pepsinogen, and mucus. [Section 10.6]

gastrulation
The division of the inner cell mass of a blastocyst (developing embryo) into the three primary germ layers. Gastrulation occurs during weeks 2–4 of gestation. [Section 13.11]

gene
A portion of DNA that codes for some product, usually a protein, including all regulatory sequences. Some genes code for rRNA and tRNA, which are not translated. [Sections 4.3 and 7.1]

gene pool
The sum of all genetic information in a population. [Section 7.7]

genetic code
The "language" of molecular biology that specifies which amino acid corresponds to which three-nucleotide group (a codon). [Section 4.3]

genome
All the genetic information in an organism; all of an organism's chromosomes. [Section 4.1]

genotype
The combination of alleles an organism carries. In a homozygous genotype, both alleles are the same, whereas in a heterozygous genotype the alleles are different. [Section 7.1]

glial cells
Specialized non-neuronal cells that provide structural and metabolic support to neurons; for example, the Schwann cell. [Section 8.1]

glomerulus
The ball of capillaries at the beginning of the nephron where blood filtration takes place. [Section 10.2]

glucagon
A peptide hormone produced and secreted by the α cells of the pancreas. It targets primarily the liver, stimulating the breakdown of glycogen, thus increasing blood glucose levels. [**Section 10.7**]

glycolipid
A membrane lipid consisting of a glycerol molecule esterified to two fatty acid chains and a sugar molecule. [**Section 6.3**]

goblet cells
Unicellular exocrine glands found along the respiratory and digestive tracts that secrete mucus. [**Section 10.5**]

Golgi apparatus
A stack of membranes found near the rough ER in eukaryotic cells that is involved in the secretory pathway. The Golgi apparatus is involved in protein glycosylation (and other protein modification) as well as sorting and packaging proteins. [**Section 6.2**]

gonadotropin releasing hormone (GnRH)
A hormone released from the hypothalamus that triggers the anterior pituitary to secrete FSH and LH. [**Section 13.4**]

gonadotropins
Anterior pituitary tropic hormones FSH (follicle stimulating hormone) and LH (luteinizing hormone) that stimulate the gonads (testes and ovaries) to produce gametes and to secrete sex steroids. [**Section 13.4**]

G-protein-linked receptor
A cell surface receptor associated with an intracellular protein that binds and hydrolyzes GTP. When GTP is bound, the protein is active, and can regulate the activity of adenylyl cyclase; this modifies the intracellular levels of the second messenger cAMP. When the GTP is hydrolyzed to GDP, the protein becomes inactive again. [**Section 6.5**]

Graafian follicle
A large, mature, ovarian follicle with a well-developed antrum and a secondary oocyte. Ovulation of the oocyte occurs from this type of follicle. [**Section 13.6**]

Gram-negative bacteria
Bacteria that have a thin peptidoglycan cell wall covered by an outer plasma membrane. They stain very lightly (pink) in Gram stain. Gram-negative bacteria are typically more resistant to antibiotics than Gram-positive bacteria. [**Section 5.3**]

Gram-positive bacteria
Bacteria that have a thick peptidoglycan cell wall, and no outer membrane. They stain very darkly (purple) in Gram stain. [**Section 5.3**]

granulosa cells
The majority of the cells surrounding an oocyte in a follicle. Granulosa cells secrete estrogen during the follicular phase of the ovarian cycle. [**Section 13.6**]

gray matter
Unmyelinated neuron cell bodies and short unmyelinated axons. [**Section 8.4**]

growth hormone
A hormone released by the anterior pituitary that targets all cells in the body. Growth hormone stimulates whole body growth in children and adolescents, and increases cell turnover rate in adults. [**Section 8.6**]

guanine
One of the four aromatic bases found in DNA and RNA. Guanine is a purine; it pairs with cytosine. [**Section 4.1**]

gustatory receptors
Chemoreceptors on the tongue that respond to chemicals in food. [**Section 8.5**]

gyrase (DNA gyrase)
A prokaryotic enzyme used to twist the single circular chromosome of prokaryotes upon itself to form supercoils. Supercoiling helps to compact prokaryotic DNA and make it sturdier. [**Section 4.1**]

H zone
The region at the center of an A band of a sarcomere that is made up of myosin only. The H zone gets shorter (and may disappear) during muscle contraction. [**Section 11.2**]

hair cells
Sensory receptors found in the inner ear. Cochlear hair cells respond to vibrations in the cochlea caused by sound waves and vestibular hair cells respond to changes in position and acceleration (used for balance). [**Section 8.5**]

haploid organism
An organism that has only a single copy of its genome in each of its cells. Haploid organisms possess no homologous chromosomes. [**Section 7.1**]

Hardy-Weinberg law

A law of population genetics that states that the frequencies of alleles in a given gene pool do not change over time. There are five assumptions required for this law to hold true: there must be no mutation, there must be no natural selection, there must be no migration, there must be random mating between individuals in the population, and the population must be large. A population meeting all of these conditions, in which the allele frequency is not changing, is said to be in *Hardy-Weinberg equilibrium*. [**Section 7.7**]

hCG

Human chorionic gonadotropin; a hormone secreted by the trophoblast cells of a blastocyst (i.e., a developing embryo) that prolongs the life of the corpus luteum, and thus increases the duration and amount of secreted progesterone. This helps to maintain the uterine lining so that menstruation does not occur. The presence of hCG in the blood or urine of a woman is used as a positive indicator of pregnancy. [**Section 13.8**]

helicase

An enzyme that unwinds the double helix of DNA and separates the DNA strands in preparation for DNA replication. [**Section 4.4**]

hematocrit

The percentage of whole blood made up of erythrocytes. The typical hematocrit value is between 40–45 percent. [**Section 9.4**]

hematopoiesis

The synthesis of blood cells (occurs in the red bone marrow). [**Section 11.5**]

hemizygous gene

A gene appearing in a single copy in diploid organisms, e.g., X-linked genes in human males. [**Section 4.5**]

hemoglobin

A four-subunit protein found in red blood cells that binds oxygen. Each subunit contains a heme group, a large multi-ring molecule with an iron atom at its center. One hemoglobin molecule can bind four oxygen molecules in a cooperative manner. [**Section 9.4**]

hemophilia

A group of X-linked recessive disorders in which blood fails to clot properly, leading to excessive bleeding if injured. [**Section 9.4**]

hemostasis

The stoppage of bleeding; blood clotting. [**Section 9.4**]

Henry's Law

Henry's Law states that the amount of gas that will dissolve into liquid is dependent on the partial pressure of that gas as well as the solubility of that gas in the liquid. [**Section 12.4**]

hepatic portal vein

A vein connecting the capillary bed of the intestines with the capillary bed of the liver. This allows amino acids and glucose absorbed from the intestines to be delivered first to the liver for processing before being transported throughout the circulatory system. [**Section 9.5**]

Hershey-Chase experiments

Experiments with phage and bacteria that definitively determined DNA to be the genetic information of the cell. [**Section 7.1**]

heterochromatin

Densely packed, tightly coiled DNA, generally inactive (i.e., not being transcribed). [**Section 4.1**]

heterotroph

An organism that cannot make its own food, and thus must ingest other organisms. [**Section 5.3**]

heterozygous

A genotype in which two different alleles are possessed for a given gene. [**Section 7.3**]

Hfr bacterium

High frequency of recombination bacterium. An F+ bacterium that has the fertility factor integrated into its chromosome. When conjugation takes place, it is able to transfer not only the F factor, but also its genomic DNA. [**Section 5.3**]

hnRNA

Heterogeneous nuclear RNA; the primary transcript made in eukaryotes before splicing. [**Section 4.7**]

homeostasis

The maintenance of relatively constant internal conditions (such as temperature, pressure, ion balance, pH, etc.) regardless of external conditions. [**Sections 8.6 and 10.1**]

homologous chromosomes

A pair of similar chromosomes that have the same genes in the same order, but may have different versions (alleles) of those genes. One of the pair of chromosomes came from Mom in an ovum, and the other came from Dad in a sperm. Humans have 23 pairs of homologous chromosomes. [**Section 7.1**]

homologous structures
Physical structures in two different organisms that have structural similarity due to a common ancestor, but may have different functions. Homologous structures arise from divergent evolution. [**Section 7.9**]

homozygous
A genotype in which two identical alleles are possessed for a given gene. The alleles can both be dominant (homozygous dominant) or both be recessive (homozygous recessive). [**Section 7.3**]

humoral immunity
Specific defense of the body by antibodies, secreted into the blood by B cells. [**Section 9.7**]

hydroxyapatite
Hard crystals consisting of calcium and phosphate that form the bone matrix. [**Section 11.7**]

hyperpolarization
The movement of the membrane potential of a cell away from rest potential in a more negative direction. [**Section 8.2**]

hypodermis
Also called subcutaneous layer, this is a layer of fat located under the dermis of the skin. The hypodermis helps to insulate the body and protects underlying muscles and other structures. [**Section 12.6**]

hypophysis
The pituitary gland. [**Section 8.6**]

hypothalamic-pituitary portal system
A set of veins that connect a capillary bed in the hypothalamus (the primary capillary plexus) with a capillary bed in the anterior pituitary gland (the secondary capillary plexus). Releasing and inhibiting factors from the hypothalamus travel along the veins to directly affect cells in the anterior pituitary. [**Section 8.6**]

hypothalamus
The portion of the diencephalon involved in maintaining body homeostasis. The hypothalamus also controls the release of hormones from the pituitary gland. [**Section 8.6**]

I band
The region of a sarcomere made up only of thin filaments. The I band is bisected by a Z line. I bands alternate with A bands to give skeletal and cardiac muscle a striated appearance. I bands get shorter (and may disappear completely) during muscle contraction. [**Section 11.2**]

ileocecal valve
The sphincter that separates the final part of the small intestine (the ileum) from the first part of the large intestine (the cecum). It is typically kept contracted (closed) so that chyme can remain in the small intestine as long as possible. The ileocecal valve is stimulated to relax by the presence of food in the stomach. [**Section 10.6**]

ileum
The 55 percent (approximately) of the small intestine. [**Section 10.6**]

immunoglobulins
See "antibody." [**Section 9.4**]

implantation
The burrowing of a blastocyst (a developing embryo) into the endometrium of the uterus, typically occurring about a week after fertilization. [**Section 13.10**]

imprinting
Physical change to a gene on DNA, such as methylation or histone binding, that renders it inactive, so that only one allele of the gene is expressed. [**Section 4.9**]

incomplete dominance
A situation in which a heterozygote displays a blended version of the phenotypes associated with each allele, e.g., pure-breeding white-flowered plants crossed with pure-breeding red-flowered plants produces heterozygous offspring plants with pink flowers. [**Section 7.4**]

inducible system
A system (set of genes) where the expression of those genes is stimulated by an abundance of substrate (e.g., the lac operon). [**Section 4.9**]

inflammation
An irritation of a tissue caused by infection or injury. Inflammation is characterized by four cardinal symptoms: redness (rubor), swelling (tumor), heat (calor), and pain (dolor). [**Section 9.5**]

inhibin
A protein hormone secreted by the sustentacular cells of the testes or the granulosa cells of the ovaries that acts to inhibit the release of FSH from the anterior pituitary. [**Section 13.2**]

initiation factors
Eukaryotic proteins that assemble in a complex to begin translation. [**Section 4.8**]

innate immunity

General, nonspecific protection to the body, including the skin (barrier), gastric acid, phagocytes, lysozyme, and complement. [**Section 9.7**]

inner cell mass

The mass of cells in the blastocyst that ultimately give rise to the embryo and other embryonic structures (the amnion, the umbilical vessels, etc.). [**Section 13.9**]

inspiration

The movement of air into the respiratory tract. Inspiration is an active process, requiring contraction of the diaphragm. [**Section 12.3**]

insulin

A peptide hormone produced and secreted by the β cells of the pancreas. Insulin targets all cells in the body, especially the liver and muscle, and allows them to take glucose out of the blood (thus lowering blood glucose levels). [**Section 10.7**]

integral membrane protein

A protein embedded in the lipid bilayer of a cell. These are typically cell surface receptors, channels, or pumps. [**Section 6.2**]

intercalated discs

The divisions between neighboring cardiac muscle cells. Intercalated disks include gap junctions, which allow the cells to function as a unit. [**Section 9.2**]

interleukin

A chemical secreted by a T cell (usually the helper Ts) that stimulates activation and proliferation of other immune system cells. [**Section 9.7**]

intermediate filaments

Cytoskeletal filaments with a diameter in between that of the microtubule and the microfilament. Intermediate filaments are composed of many different proteins and tend to play structural roles in cells. [**Section 6.5**]

interneuron

A neuron found completely within the central nervous system. Interneurons typically connect sensory and motor neurons, especially in reflex arcs. [**Section 8.3**]

internodal tract

The portion of the cardiac conduction system between the SA node and the AV node. [**Section 9.2**]

interphase

All of the cell cycle except for mitosis. Interphase includes G_1, S phase, and G_2. [**Section 6.6**]

interstitial cell

Also called *Leydig cells*, these are cells within the testes that produce and secrete testosterone. They are stimulated by luteinizing hormone (LH). [**Section 13.1**]

intron

A nucleotide sequence that intervenes between protein-coding sequences. In DNA, these intervening sequences typically contain regulatory sequences, however, in RNA, they are simple spliced out to form the mature (translated) transcript. [**Section 4.7**]

ion channel

A protein channel in a cell plasma membrane that is specific for a particular ion, such as Na^+ or K^+. Ion channels may be constitutively open (leak channels), or regulated (voltage-gated or ligand-gated). [**Section 6.4**]

IPSP

Inhibitory postsynaptic potential; a slight hyperpolarization of a postsynaptic cell, moving the membrane potential of that cell further from threshold. [**Section 8.2**]

iris

A pigmented membrane found just in front of the lens of the eye. In the center of the iris is the *pupil*, a hole through which light enters the eyeball. The iris regulates the diameter of the pupil in response to the brightness of the light. [**Section 8.5**]

islets of Langerhans

Also called simply "islet cells," these are the endocrine cells in the pancreas. Different cell types within the islets secrete insulin, glucagon, and somatostatin. [**Section 10.5**]

juxtaglomerular apparatus (JGA)

A contact point between the afferent arteriole of the glomerulus and the distal convoluted tubule of the nephron. It is involved in regulating blood pressure. [**Section 10.3**]

juxtaglomerular cells

The cells of the afferent arteriole at the juxtaglomerular apparatus. They are baroreceptors that secrete renin upon sensing a decrease in blood pressure. [**Section 10.3**]

keratin

A protein-based substance secreted by cells of the epidermis as they migrate outward. The keratin makes the cells tougher (better able to withstand abrasion) and helps make the skin waterproof. [**Sections 6.5 and 12.6**]

kinetochores

Multiprotein complexes that attach the spindle fibers to the centromere of a chromosome. [**Section 4.1**]

labia
The folds of skin that enclose the vaginal and urethral openings in females. [**Section 13.5**]

labor contractions
Strong contractions of the uterus (stimulated by oxytocin) that force a baby out of the mother's body during childbirth. Labor contractions are part of a positive feedback cycle, during which the baby's head stretches the cervix, that stimulates stretch receptors that activate the hypothalamus, that stimulates the posterior pituitary to release oxytocin, that stimulates strong uterine contractions (labor contractions) that cause the baby's head to stretch the cervix. The cycle is broken once the baby is delivered. [**Section 13.14**]

lac operon
A set of genes for the enzymes necessary to import and digest lactose, under the control of a single promoter, whose expression is stimulated by the presence of lactose (this is an inducible system). [**Section 4.9**]

lacteals
Specialized lymphatic capillaries in the intestines that take up lipids as well as lymph. [**Sections 9.5 and 10.6**]

lacunae
Small cavities in bone or cartilage that hold individual bone or cartilage cells. [**Section 11.7**]

lagging strand
The newly forming daughter strand of DNA that is replicated in a discontinuous fashion, via Okazaki fragments that will ultimately be ligated together; the daughter strand that is replicated in the opposite direction that the parental DNA is unwinding. [**Section 4.4**]

lag phase
A short period of time prior to exponential growth of a bacterial population during which no, or very limited, cell division occurs. [**Section 5.3**]

large intestine
The final part of the digestive tract, also called the colon. The primary function of the large intestine is to reabsorb water and to store feces. [**Section 10.6**]

larynx
A rigid structure at the top of the trachea made completely out of cartilage. The larynx has three main functions: (1) its rigidness ensures that the trachea is held open (provides an open airway), (2) the epiglottis folds down to seal the trachea during swallowing, thus directing food to the esophagus, and (3) this is where the vocal cords are found (voice production). [**Section 12.2**]

lawn
A dense growth of bacteria that covers the surface of a Petri dish. [**Section 5.3**]

Law of Independent Assortment
Mendel's second law, which states that genes found on different chromosomes, or genes found very far apart on the same chromosome (i.e., unlinked genes) sort independently of one another during gamete formation (meiosis). [**Section 7.3**]

Law of Segregation
Mendel's first law, also called the *Principle of Segregation*, states that the two alleles of a given gene will be separated from one another during gamete formation (meiosis). [**Section 7.3**]

leading strand
The newly forming daughter strand of DNA that is replicated in a continuous fashion; the daughter strand that is replicated in the same direction that the parental DNA is unwinding. [**Section 4.4**]

leak channel
An ion channel that is constitutively open, allowing the movement of the ion across the plasma membrane according to its concentration gradient. [**Section 6.4**]

length-tension relationship
The relationship of muscle length to its ability to generate strong contractions. Maximum tension (contraction strength) is achieved at sarcomere lengths between 2.0 and 2.2 microns. Tension decreases outside of this range. [**Section 11.2**]

leukocyte
A white blood cell; leukocytes are involved in disease defense. [**Section 9.4**]

Leydig cell
See "interstitial cell." [**Section 13.1**]

ligament
A strong band of connective tissue that connects bones to one another. [**Section 11.8**]

ligand
The specific molecule that binds to a receptor. [Section 6.5]

ligand-gated ion channel
An ion channel that is opened or closed based on the binding of a specific ligand to the channel. Once opened, the channel allows the ion to cross the plasma membrane according to its concentration gradient. [Section 6.4]

ligase
An enzyme that connects two fragments of DNA to make a single fragment; also called *DNA ligase*. This enzyme is used during DNA replication and is also used in recombinant DNA research. [Section 4.4]

linkage
The failure of two separate genes to obey the Law of Independent Assortment, as might occur if the genes were found close together on the same chromosome. [Section 7.5]

lipoproteins
Large conglomerations of protein, fats, and cholesterol that transport lipids in the bloodstream. [Sections 3.4 and 9.4]

liver
The largest organ in the abdominal cavity. The liver has many roles, including processing of carbohydrates and fats, synthesis of urea, production of blood proteins, production of bile, recycling of heme, and storage of vitamins. [Section 9.5]

local autoregulation
The ability of tissues to regulate their own blood flow in the absence of neural stimulation. This is generally accomplished via metabolic wastes (such as CO_2) that act as vasodilators. [Section 9.3]

log phase
The period of exponential growth of a bacterial population. [Section 5.3]

long bone
The most common class of bone in the body, long bones have a well-defined shaft (the diaphysis) and two well-defined ends (the epiphyses). [Section 11.7]

longitudinal muscle
The outer layer of smooth muscle in the wall of the digestive tract. When the longitudinal muscle contracts, the tube shortens. [Section 10.5]

loop of Henle
The loop of the nephron tubule that dips downward into the renal medulla. The loop of Henle sets up a concentration gradient in the kidney, so that from the cortex to the renal pelvis osmolarity increases. This gradient is ultimately used to concentrate urine at the collecting duct. [Section 10.2]

loose connective tissue
Connective tissue that lacks great amount of collagen or elastic fibers, e.g., adipose tissue and areolar (general connective) tissue. [Section 11.6]

lower esophageal sphincter
Formerly called the *cardiac sphincter*, this sphincter marks the entrance to the stomach. Its function is to prevent reflux of acidic stomach contents into the esophagus; note that it does not regulate entry into the stomach. [Section 10.6]

lumen
The inside of a hollow organ (e.g., the stomach, intestines, bladder, etc.) or a tube (e.g., blood vessels, ureters, etc.). [Sections 6.2 and 10.5]

luteal phase
The third phase of the ovarian cycle, during which a corpus luteum is formed from the remnants of the follicle that has ovulated its oocyte. The corpus luteum secretes progesterone and estrogen during this time period, which typically lasts from day 15 to day 28 of the menstrual cycle. Formation of the corpus luteum is triggered by the same LH surge that triggers ovulation. [Section 13.7]

luteinizing hormone (LH)
A tropic hormone produced by the anterior pituitary gland that targets the gonads. In females LH triggers ovulation and the development of a corpus luteum during the menstrual cycle; in males, LH stimulates the production and release of testosterone. [Section 13.2]

lymphatic system
A set of vessels in the body that runs alongside the vessels of the circulatory system. It is a one-way system, with lymphatic capillaries beginning at the tissues and ultimately emptying into the large veins near the heart. It serves to return excess tissue fluid (lymph) to the circulatory system, and filters that fluid through millions of white blood cells on its way back to the heart. [Section 9.6]

lymph node
A concentrated region of white blood cells found along the vessels of the lymphatic system. [Section 9.6]

lymphocyte
The second most common of the five classes of leukocytes. Lymphocytes are involved in specific immunity and include two cell types, B cells and T cells. B cells produce and secrete antibodies and T cells are involved in cellular immunity. [Section 9.4]

lymphokine
A chemical secreted by a T cell (usually the helper Ts) that stimulates activation and proliferation of other immune system cells. [Section 9.7]

lysogenic cycle
A viral life cycle in which the viral genome is incorporated into the host genome where it can remain dormant for an unspecified period of time. Upon activation, the viral genome is excised from the host genome and typically enters the lytic cycle. [Section 5.1]

lysosome
A eukaryotic organelle filled with digestive enzymes (acid hydrolases) that is involved in digestion of macromolecules such as worn organelles or material ingested by phagocytosis. [Section 6.2]

lysozyme
An enzyme that lyses bacteria by creating holes in their cell walls. Lysozyme is produced in the end stages of the lytic cycle so that new viral particles can escape their host; it is also found in human tears and human saliva. [Section 5.1]

lytic cycle
A viral life cycle in which the host is turned into a "virus factory" and ultimately lysed to release the new viral particles. [Section 5.1]

macrophage
A large, nonspecific, phagocytic cell of the immune system. Macrophages frequently leave the bloodstream to crawl around in the tissues and perform "clean up" duties, such as ingesting dead cells or cellular debris at an injury site, or pathogens. [Sections 6.2 and 9.4]

macula densa
The cells of the distal tubule at the juxtaglomerular apparatus. They are receptors that monitor filtrate osmolarity as a means of regulating filtration rate. If a drop is osmolarity is sensed, the macula densa dilates the afferent arteriole (to increase blood pressure in the glomerulus and thus increase filtration) and stimulates the juxtaglomerular cells to secrete renin (to raise systemic blood pressure). [Section 10.3]

maternal inheritance
Genes that are inherited only from the mother, such as mitochondrial genes (all of a zygote's organelles come only from the ovum). [Section 6.2]

mechanoreceptor
A sensory receptor that responds to mechanical disturbances, such as shape changes (being squashed, bent, pulled, etc.). Mechanoreceptors include touch receptors in the skin, hair cells in the ear, muscle spindles, and others. [Section 8.5]

medium
The environment in which or upon which bacteria grow. It typically contains a sugar source and any other nutrients that bacteria may require. "Minimal medium" contains nothing but glucose. [Section 5.3]

medulla
The inner region of an organ, e.g., the renal medulla, the ovarian medulla, the adrenal medulla, etc. [Sections 8.4 and 10.2]

medulla oblongata
The portion of the hindbrain that controls respiratory rate and blood pressure, and specialized digestive and respiratory functions such as vomiting, sneezing, and coughing. [Section 8.4]

meiosis
A type of cell division (in diploid cells) that reduces the number of chromosomes by half. Meiosis usually produces haploid gametes in organisms that undergo sexual reproduction. It consists of a single interphase (G_1, S, and G_2) followed by two sets of chromosomal divisions, meiosis I and meiosis II. Meiosis I and II can both be subdivided into four phases similar to those in mitosis. [Section 7.2]

melanin
A pigment produced by melanocytes in the bottom cell layer of the epidermis. Melanin production is increased on exposure to UV radiation (commonly called "tanning" and helps prevent cellular damage due to UV radiation. [Section 12.6]

memory cell
A cell produced when a B cell is activated by antigen. Memory cells do not actively fight the current infection, but patrol the body in case of future infection with the same antigen. If the antigen should appear again in the future, memory cells are like "preactivated" B cells, and can initiate a much faster immune response (the secondary immune response). [Section 9.7]

meninges
The protective, connective tissue wrappings of the central nervous system (the dura mater, arachnoid mater, and pia mater). [Section 8.4]

menopause
The period of time in a woman's life when ovulation and menstruation cease. Menopause typically begins in the late 40s. [Section 13.8]

menstruation
The first phase of the uterine (endometrial) cycle, during which the unused endometrium from the previous cycle is shed off. Estrogen and progesterone levels are low during this time period. Menstruation typically lasts from day 1 to day 5 of the cycle. [Section 13.7]

mesoderm
One of the three primary (embryonic) germ layers formed during gastrulation. Mesoderm ultimately forms "middle" structures such as the bones, muscles, blood vessels, heart, kidneys, etc. [Section 13.11]

metaphase
The second phase of mitosis. During metaphase, replicated chromosomes align at the center of the cell (the metaphase plate). [Section 6.6]

metaphase I
The second phase of meiosis I. During metaphase I the paired homologous chromosomes (tetrads) align at the center of the cell (the metaphase plate). [Section 7.2]

metaphase II
The second phase of meiosis II. Metaphase II is identical to mitotic metaphase, except that the number of chromosomes was reduced by half during meiosis I. [Section 7.2]

MHC
Major histocompatibility complex, a set of proteins found on the plasma membranes of cells that help display antigen to T cells. MHC I is found on all cells and displays bits of proteins from within the cell; this allows T cells to monitor cell contents and if abnormal peptides are displayed on the surface, the cell is destroyed by killer T cells. MHC II is found only on macrophages and B cells. This class of MHC allows these cells (known as antigen presenting cells) to display bits of "eaten" (phagocytosed or internalized) proteins on their surface, allowing the activation of helper Ts. [Section 9.7]

microfilament
The cytoskeleton filaments with the smallest diameter. Microfilaments are composed of the contractile protein actin. They are dynamic filaments, constantly being made and broken down as needed, and are responsible for events such as pseudopod formation and cytokinesis during mitosis. [Section 6.5]

microtubule
The largest of the cytoplasmic filaments. Microtubules are composed of two types of protein, α tubulin and β tubulin. They are dynamic fibers, constantly being built up and broken down, according to cellular needs. Microtubules form the mitotic spindle during cell division, form the base of cilia and flagella, and are used for intracellular structure and transport. [Section 6.5]

microvilli
Microscopic outward folds of the cells lining the small intestine; microvilli serve to increase the surface area of the small intestine for absorption. [Section 10.5]

midbrain
The portion of the brain responsible for visual and auditory startle reflexes. [Section 8.4]

milk let-down
The release of milk from the mammary glands via contraction of ducts within the glands. Contraction is stimulated by oxytocin, which is released from the posterior pituitary when the baby begins nursing. [Section 13.14]

missense mutation
A point mutation in which a codon that specifies an amino acid is mutated into a codon that specifies a different amino acid. [Section 4.5]

mitochondrion
An organelle surrounded by a double-membrane (two lipid bilayers) where ATP production takes place. The interior (matrix) is where PDC and the Krebs cycle occur, and the inner membrane contains the enzymes of the electron transport chain and ATP synthase. [Section 6.2]

mitosis
The phase of the cell cycle during which the replicated genome is divided. Mitosis has four phases (prophase, metaphase, anaphase, telophase) and includes cytokinesis (the physical splitting of the cell into two new cells). [Section 6.6]

mitral valve
See "atrioventricular valve." [Section 9.2]

monocistronic mRNA
mRNA that codes for a single type of protein, such as is found in eukaryotic cells. [Section 4.7]

morula
A solid clump of cells resulting from cleavage in the early embryo. Because there is very little growth of these cells during cleavage, the morula is only about as large as the original zygote. [Section 13.9]

motor end plate
The portion of the muscle cell membrane at the neuromuscular junction; essentially the postsynaptic membrane at this synapse. [Section 11.2]

motor unit
A motor neuron and all the skeletal muscle cells it innervates. Large motor units are typically found in large muscles (e.g., the thighs and buttocks) and produce gross movements. Small motor units are found in smaller muscles (e.g., the rectus muscles that control movements of the eyeball, the fingers) and produce more precise movements. [Section 11.2]

motor unit recruitment
A mechanism for increasing tension (contractile strength) in a muscle by activating more motor units. [Section 11.2]

mRNA
Messenger RNA; the type of RNA that is read by a ribosome to synthesize protein. [Section 4.3]

mRNA surveillance
The monitoring of mRNA transcripts to eliminate those that are defective (e.g., have no stop codon, have premature stop codons, or that have somehow stalled in translation). [Section 4.9]

mucociliary escalator
The layer of ciliated, mucus-covered cells in the respiratory tract. The cilia continually beat, sweeping contaminated mucus upward toward the pharynx. [Sections 6.5 and 12.1]

mucosa
The layer of epithelial tissue that lines body cavities in contact with the outside environment (respiratory, digestive, urinary, and reproductive tracts). [Section 10.6]

Müllerian ducts
Early embryonic ducts that can develop into female internal genitalia in the absence of testosterone. [Section 13.3]

Müllerian inhibiting factor (MIF)
A substance secreted by embryonic testes that causes the regression of the Müllerian ducts. [Section 13.3]

multipolar neuron
A neuron with a single axon and multiple dendrites; the most common type of neuron in the nervous system. [Section 8.1]

myelin
An insulating layer of membranes wrapped around the axons of almost all neurons in the body. Myelin is essentially the plasma membranes of specialized cells; *Schwann cells* in the peripheral nervous system, and *oligodendrocytes* in the central nervous system. [Section 8.1]

myofiber
A skeletal muscle cell, also known as a muscle fiber. Skeletal muscle cells are formed from the fusion of many smaller cells (during development), consequently they are very long and are multinucleate. [Section 11.2]

myofibril
A string of sarcomeres within a skeletal muscle cell. Each muscle cell contains hundreds of myofibrils. [Section 11.2]

myoglobin
A globular protein found in muscle tissue that has the ability to bind oxygen. Myoglobin helps to store oxygen in the muscle for use in aerobic respiration. Muscles that participate in endurance activities (including cardiac muscle) have abundant supplies of myoglobin. [Section 11.2]

myometrium
The muscular layer of the uterus. The myometrium is made of smooth muscle that retains its ability to divide in order to accommodate the massive size increases that occur during pregnancy. The myometrium is stimulated to contract during labor by the hormone oxytocin. [Section 13.5]

myosin
One of the contractile proteins in muscle tissue. In skeletal and cardiac muscle, myosin forms the thick filaments. Myosin has intrinsic ATPase activity and can exist in two conformations, either high energy or low energy. [Section 11.2]

myosin light-chain kinase (MLCK)
A kinase in smooth muscle cells activated by calmodulin in the presence of Ca^{2+}. As its name implies, this kinase phosphorylates myosin, activating it so that muscle contraction can occur. [Section 11.4]

Na$^+$/K$^+$ ATPase
A protein found in the plasma membranes of all cells in the body that uses the energy of an ATP (hydrolyzes ATP) to move three Na$^+$ ions out of the cell and two K$^+$ ions into the cell, thus establishing concentration gradients for these ions across the cell membrane. [Section 6.4]

natural selection
The mechanism described by Charles Darwin that drives evolution. Through mutation, some organisms possess genes that make them better adapted to their environment. These organisms survive and reproduce more than those that do not possess the beneficial genes, thus these genes are passed on to offspring, making the offspring better adapted. Over time, these genes (and the organisms that possess them) become more abundant, and the less beneficial genes (and the organisms that possess them) become less abundant. [Section 7.7]

ncRNA (non-coding RNA)
RNA that is not translated into protein, including tRNA, rRNA, snRNA, miRNA, etc. [Section 4.7]

negative feedback
A form of regulation in which the end result of a series of events inhibits the trigger for that series. Hormones are generally regulated via negative feedback. For example, insulin is released when blood glucose levels rise. It causes the cells of the body to take glucose out of the blood, leading to a drop in glucose levels. The fall in glucose levels stops insulin release. [Section 8.6]

nephron
The functional unit of the kidney. Each kidney has about a million nephrons; this is where blood filtration and subsequent modification of the filtrate occurs. The nephron empties into collecting ducts, which empty into the ureter. [Section 10.2]

Nernst equation
The equation that can predict the equilibrium potential for any ion based on the electrochemical gradients for that ion across the membrane. [Section 8.1]

neurohypophysis
See "posterior pituitary gland." [Section 8.6]

neuromuscular junction (NMJ)
The synapse between a motor neuron and a muscle cell. At the NMJ, the muscle cell membrane is invaginated and the axon terminus is elongated so that a greater area of membrane can be depolarized at one time. [Sections 8.2 and 11.2]

neuron
The basic functional and structural unit of the nervous system. The neuron is a highly specialized cell, designed to transmit action potentials. [Section 8.1]

neurotransmitter
A chemical released by the axon of a neuron in response to an action potential that binds to receptors on a postsynaptic cell and causes that cell to either depolarize slightly (EPSP) or hyperpolarize slightly (IPSP). Examples are acetylcholine, norepinephrine, GABA, dopamine, and others. [Section 8.2]

neurulation
The formation of the nervous system during weeks 5–8 of gestation. Neurulation begins when a section of the ectoderm invaginates and pinches off to form the neural groove, which ultimately forms the neural tube, from which the brain and spinal cord develop. [Section 13.11]

nociceptors
Pain receptors. Nociceptors are found everywhere in the body except for the brain. [Section 8.5]

nodes of Ranvier
Gaps in the myelin sheath of the axons of peripheral neurons. Action potentials can "jump" from node to node, thus increasing the speed of conduction (saltatory conduction). [Section 8.1]

nondisjunction
The failure of homologous chromosomes or sister chromatids to separate properly during cell division. This could occur during anaphase I of meiosis (homologous chromosomes), or during anaphase II of meiosis or anaphase of mitosis (sister chromatids). [Section 7.2]

nonsense mutation
A point mutation in which a codon that specifies an amino acid is mutated into a stop (nonsense) codon. [Section 4.5]

norepinephrine (NE)
The neurotransmitter used by the sympathetic division of the ANS at the postganglionic (organ-level) synapse. [Section 8.2]

nuclear envelope
The double lipid bilayer that surrounds the DNA in eukaryotic cells. [Section 6.2]

nuclear localization sequence
A sequence of amino acids that directs a protein to the nuclear envelope, where it is imported by a specific transport mechanism. [Section 6.2]

nuclear pore
A protein channel in the nuclear envelope that allows the free passage of molecules smaller than 60 kD. [Section 6.2]

nucleolus
A region within the nucleus where rRNA is transcribed and ribosomes are partially assembled. [Section 6.2]

nucleoside
A structure composed of a ribose molecule linked to one of the aromatic bases. In a deoxynucleoside, the ribose is replaced with deoxyribose. [Section 4.1]

nucleosome
A structure composed of two coils of DNA wrapped around an octet of histone proteins. The nucleosome is the primary form of packaging of eukaryotic DNA. [Section 4.1]

nucleotide
A nucleoside with one or more phosphate groups attached. Nucleoside triphosphates (NTPs) are the building blocks of RNA and are also used as energy molecules, especially ATP. Deoxynucleoside triphosphates (dNTPs) are the building blocks of DNA; in these molecules, the ribose is replaced with deoxyribose. [**Section 4.1**]

nucleus
An organelle bounded by a double membrane (double lipid bilayer) called the nuclear envelope. The nucleus contains the genome and is the site of replication and transcription. [**Section 6.2**]

obligate aerobe
An organism that requires oxygen to survive (aerobic metabolism only). [**Section 5.3**]

obligate anaerobe
An organism that can only survive in the absence of oxygen (anaerobic metabolism); oxygen is toxic to obligate anaerobes. [**Section 5.3**]

Okazaki fragments
Small fragments of DNA produced on the lagging strand during DNA replication, joined later by DNA ligase to form a complete strand. [**Section 4.4**]

olfactory receptors
Chemoreceptors in the upper nasal cavity that respond to odor chemicals. [**Section 8.5**]

oncogenes/protooncogenes
Mutated genes that cause cancer. Protooncogenes are the normal version of these genes before their mutations. [**Section 6.7**]

oncotic pressure
The osmotic pressure in the blood vessels due only to plasma proteins (primarily albumin). [**Section 9.4**]

oogonium
A precursor cell that undergoes mitosis during fetal development to produce more oogonium. These cells are then activated to produce primary oocytes, which remain dormant until stimulated to undergo meiosis I during some future menstrual cycle. [**Section 13.6**]

operator
A specific DNA nucleotide sequence where transcriptional regulatory proteins can bind. [**Section 4.9**]

operon
A nucleotide sequence on DNA that contains three elements: a coding sequence for one or more enzymes, a coding sequence for a regulatory protein, and upstream regulatory sequences where the regulatory protein can bind. An example is the lac operon found in prokaryotes. [**Section 4.9**]

optic disk
The "blind spot" of the eye, this is where the axons of the ganglion cells exit the retina to form the optic nerve. There are no photoreceptors in the optic disk. [**Section 8.5**]

optic nerve
The nerve extending from the back of the eyeball to the brain that carries visual information. The optic nerve is made up of the axons of the ganglion cells of the retina. [**Section 8.5**]

organ of Corti
The structure in the cochlea of the inner ear made up of the basilar membrane, the auditory hair cells, and the tectorial membrane. The organ of Corti is the site where auditory sensation is detected and transduced to action potentials. [**Section 8.5**]

organogenesis
The stage of human development during which the organs are formed. Organogenesis begins after gastrulation and is completed by the 8th week of gestation. [**Section 13.11**]

orgasm
A function of the reproductive system controlled by the sympathetic nervous system. In males, orgasm includes emission and ejaculation; in females it is mainly a series of rhythmic contractions of the pelvic floor muscles and the uterus. [**Section 13.1**]

origin of replication
The specific location on a DNA strand where replication begins. Prokaryotes typically have a single origin of replication, while eukaryotes have several per chromosome. [**Section 4.4**]

osmosis
The movement of water (the solvent) from its region of high concentration to its region of low concentration. Note that the water concentration gradient is opposite to the solute concentration gradient, since where solutes are concentrated, water is scarce. [**Section 6.4**]

osmotic pressure

The force required to resist the movement of water by osmosis. Osmotic pressure is essentially a measure of the concentration of a solution. A solution that is highly concentrated has a strong tendency to draw water into itself, so the pressure required to resist that movement would be high. Thus, highly concentrated solutions are said to have high osmotic pressures. [Section 6.4]

ossicles

The three small bones found in the middle ear (the *malleus*, the *incus*, and the *stapes*) that help to amplify the vibrations from sound waves. The malleus is attached to the tympanic membrane and the stapes is attached to the oval window of the cochlea. [Section 8.5]

osteoblast

A cell that produces bone. [Section 11.9]

osteoclast

A phagocytic-like bone cell that breaks down bone matrix to release calcium and phosphate into the bloodstream. [Section 11.9]

osteocyte

A mature, dormant osteoblast. [Section 11.6]

osteon

The unit of compact bone, formerly called a *Haversian system*. Osteons are essentially long cylinders of bone; the hollow center is called the *central canal*, and is where blood vessels, nerves, and lymphatic vessels are found. Compact bone is laid down around the central canal in rings (lamellae). [Section 11.7]

outer ear

The portion of the ear consisting of the pinna and the external auditory canal. The outer ear is separated from the middle ear by the tympanic membrane (the eardrum). [Section 8.5]

oval window

The membrane that separates the middle ear from the inner ear. [Section 8.5]

ovarian cycle

The 28 days of the menstrual cycle as they apply to events in the ovary. The ovarian cycle has three subphases: the follicular phase, ovulation, and the luteal phase. [Section 13.7]

ovary

The female primary sex organ. The ovary produces female gametes (ova) and secretes estrogen and progesterone. [Section 13.5]

ovulation

The release of a secondary oocyte (along with some granulosa cells) from the ovary at the approximate midpoint of the menstrual cycle (typically around day 14). Ovulation is triggered by a surge in LH. [Section 13.6]

oxytocin

A hormone released by the posterior pituitary that stimulates uterine contractions during childbirth and milk ejection during breastfeeding. [Sections 8.6 and 13.14]

P site

Peptidyl-tRNA site; the site on a ribosome where the growing peptide (attached to a tRNA) is found during translation. [Section 4.8]

pacemaker potential

A self-initiating action potential that occurs in the conduction system of the heart and triggers action potentials (and thus contraction) in the cardiac muscle cells. The pacemaker potential is triggered by the regular, spontaneous depolarization of the cells of the conduction system, due to a slow inward leak of positive ions (Na^+ and Ca^{2+}). [Section 9.2]

pancreas

An organ in the abdominal cavity with two roles. The first is an exocrine role: to produce digestive enzymes and bicarbonate, which are delivered to the small intestine via the pancreatic duct. The second is an endocrine role: to secrete insulin and glucagon into the bloodstream to help regulate blood glucose levels. [Section 10.7]

pancreatic duct

The main duct of the pancreas. The pancreatic duct carries the exocrine secretions of the pancreas (enzymes and bicarbonate) to the small intestine (duodenum). [Section 10.6]

parasite

An organism that requires the aid of a host organism to survive, and that harms the host in the process. [Section 5.1]

parasympathetic nervous system

The division of the autonomic nervous system known as the "resting and digesting" system. It causes a general decrease in body activities such as heart rate, respiratory rate, and blood pressure, an increase in blood flow to the GI tract, and an increase in digestive function. Because the preganglionic neurons all originate from either the brain or the sacrum, it is also known as the *craniosacral* system. [Section 9.3]

parathyroid hormone (PTH)
A hormone produced and secreted by the parathyroid glands that increases serum calcium levels. It targets the bones (stimulates osteoclasts), the kidneys (increases calcium reabsorption), and the small intestine (increases calcium absorption). [**Section 11.9**]

parietal cells
Cells found in gastric glands that secrete hydrochloric acid (for hydrolysis of ingested food) and gastric intrinsic factor (for absorption of vitamin B_{12}). [**Section 10.6**]

partial pressure
The contribution of an individual gas to the total pressure of a mixture of gases. Partial pressures are used to describe the amounts of the various gases carried in the bloodstream. [**Section 12.4**]

passive transport
Movement across the membrane of a cell that does not require energy input from the cell. Passive transport relies on concentration gradients to provide the driving force for movement, and includes both simple and facilitated diffusion. [**Section 6.4**]

penetrance
The percentage of individuals with a particular genotype that actually display the phenotype associated with that genotype. [**Section 7.4**]

penetration
The second step in viral infection, the injection of the viral genome into the host cell. [**Section 5.1**]

pepsin
A protein-digesting enzyme secreted by the chief cells of the gastric glands. Pepsin is secreted in its inactive form (pepsinogen) and is activated by gastric acid. It is unusual in that its pH optimum is around 1–2; most of the enzymes in the body function best at neutral pHs. [**Section 10.6**]

peptide hormone
A hormone made of amino acids (in some cases just a single, modified amino acid). Peptide hormones are generally hydrophilic and cannot cross the plasma membranes of cells, thus receptors for peptide hormones must be found on the cell surface. Binding of a peptide hormone to its receptor usually triggers a second messenger system within the cell. [**Section 8.6**]

peptidoglycan
A complex polymer of sugars and amino acids; the substance from which bacterial cell walls are made. [**Section 5.3**]

peptidyl transferase
The enzymatic activity of the ribosome that catalyzes the formation of a peptide bond between amino acids. It is thought that the rRNA of the ribosome possesses the peptidyl transferase activity. [**Section 4.8**]

perfusion
The flow of blood through a tissue. [**Section 9.1**]

peripheral chemoreceptors
Receptors in the carotid arteries and the aorta that monitor blood pH to help regulate ventilation rate. [**Section 12.5**]

peripheral membrane protein
A protein that is associated with the plasma membrane of a cell, but that is not embedded in the lipid bilayer. Peripheral proteins typically associate with embedded proteins through hydrogen bonding or electrostatic interactions. [**Section 6.3**]

peripheral nervous system
All parts of the nervous system except for the brain and spinal cord. [**Section 8.4**]

peripheral resistance
The resistance to blood flow in the systemic circulation. Peripheral resistance increases if arteries constrict (diameter decreases), and an increase in peripheral resistance leads to an increase in blood pressure. [**Section 9.3**]

periplasmic space
The space between the inner and outer cell membranes in Gram-negative bacteria. The peptidoglycan cell wall is found in the periplasmic space, and this space sometimes contains enzymes to degrade antibiotics. [**Section 5.3**]

peristalsis
A wave of contraction that sweeps along a muscular tube, pushing substances along the tube (e.g., food through the digestive tract, urine through the ureters, etc.). [**Section 10.5**]

peroxisome
Small organelles that contain hydrogen peroxide produced as a byproduct of lipid metabolism. Peroxisomes convert hydrogen peroxide to water and oxygen by way of the enzyme catalase. [**Section 6.2**]

phagocytosis
The nonspecific uptake of solid material by a cell accomplished by engulfing the particle with plasma membrane and drawing it into the cell. [**Section 6.2**]

pharynx
A passageway leading from behind the nasal cavity to the trachea. The pharynx is divided into three regions, named for their location. The *nasopharynx* is behind the nasal cavity, the *oropharynx* is behind the oral cavity, and the *laryngopharynx* is behind the larynx. [**Sections 10.6 and 12.2**]

phenotype
The physical characteristics resulting from the genotype. Phenotypes are usually described as dominant or recessive. [**Section 7.1**]

pheromones
Chemical signals released from one organism that result in a social response in members of the same species. [**Section 8.5**]

phospholipid
The primary membrane lipid. Phospholipids consist of a glycerol molecule esterified to two fatty acid chains and a phosphate molecule. Additional, highly hydrophilic groups are attached to the phosphate, making this molecule extremely amphipathic. [**Sections 3.4 and 6.3**]

photoreceptor
A receptor that responds to light. [**Section 8.5**]

phototroph
An organism that utilizes light as its primary energy source. [**Section 5.3**]

pilus
A long projection on a bacterial surface involved in attachment, e.g., the sex pilus attaches F⁺ and F⁻ bacteria during conjugation. [**Section 5.3**]

pinocytosis
The nonspecific uptake of liquid particles into a cell by invagination of the plasma membrane and subsequent "pinching off" of a small bit of the extracellular fluid. [**Section 6.4**]

placenta
An organ that develops during pregnancy, derived in part from the mother and in part from the zygote. The placenta is the site of exchange of nutrients and gases between the mother's blood and the fetus's blood. The placenta is formed during the first three months of pregnancy. [**Section 13.10**]

placental villi
Zygote-derived projections that extend into the endometrium of the uterus during pregnancy. Fetal capillaries grow into the placental villi, which are surrounded by a pool of maternal blood. This facilitates nutrient and gas exchange between the mother and the fetus, without actually allowing the bloods to mix. [**Section 13.10**]

plaque
A clear area in a lawn of bacteria. Plaques represent an area where bacteria are lysing (dying) and a usually caused by lytic viruses. [**Section 5.3**]

plasma
The liquid portion of blood; plasma contains water, ions, buffers, sugars, proteins, etc. Anything that dissolves in blood dissolves in the plasma portion. [**Section 9.4**]

plasma cell
An activated B cell that is secreting antibody. [**Section 9.7**]

plasmid
A small, extrachromosomal (outside the genome), circular DNA molecule found in prokaryotes. [**Sections 5.3 and A.5**]

platelets
Extremely small pseudo-cells in the blood, important for clotting. They are not true cells, but are broken-off bits of a larger cell (a megakaryocyte). [**Section 9.4**]

pleura
The membranes that line the surface of the lungs (visceral pleura) and the inside wall of the chest cavity (parietal pleura). [**Section 12.3**]

pleural pressure
The pressure in the (theoretical) space between the lung surface and the inner wall of the chest cavity. Pleural pressure is negative with respect to atmospheric pressure; this keeps the lungs stuck to the chest cavity wall. [**Section 12.3**]

point mutation
A type of mutation in DNA where a single base is substituted for another. [**Section 4.5**]

polar body
A small cell with extremely little cytoplasm that results from the unequal cytoplasmic division of the primary (produces the first polar body) and secondary (produces the second polar body) oocytes during meiosis (oogenesis). The polar bodies degenerate. [**Section 13.6**]

poly-A tail
A string of several hundred adenine nucleotides added to the 3' end of eukaryotic mRNA. [**Section 4.7**]

polycistronic mRNA
mRNA that codes for several different proteins by utilizing different reading frames, nested genes, etc. Polycistronic mRNA is a characteristic of prokaryotes. [**Section 4.7**]

polymerase chain reaction (PCR)
A very quick and inexpensive method for detecting and amplifying specific DNA sequences. [**Section A.6**]

polyspermy
The fertilization of an oocyte by more than one sperm. This occurs in some animals, but in humans, blocks to polyspermy exist (the fast block and the slow block) so that only a single sperm can penetrate the oocyte. [**Section 13.9**]

population
A subset of a species consisting of members that mate and reproduce with one another. [**Section 7.7**]

pore
A pathway through a plasma membrane that restricts passage based only on the size of the molecule. Pores are made from porin proteins. [**Section 6.4**]

portal system
A system of blood vessels where the blood passes from arteries to capillaries to veins, then through a second set of capillaries, and then through a final set of veins. There are two portal systems in the body, the hepatic portal system and the hypothalamic portal system. [**Section 10.7**]

posterior pituitary gland
Also known as the *neurohypophysis*, the posterior pituitary is made of nervous tissue (i.e., neurons) and stores and secretes two hormones made by the hypothalamus: oxytocin and ADH. The posterior pituitary is controlled by action potentials from the hypothalamus. [**Section 8.6**]

postganglionic neuron
In the autonomic division of the PNS, a neuron that has its cell body located in an autonomic ganglion (where a preganglionic neuron synapses with it), and whose axon synapses with the target organ. [**Section 8.4**]

potassium leak channel
An ion channel specific for potassium found in the plasma membrane of all cells in the body. Leak channels are constitutively open and allow their specific ion to move across the membrane according to its gradient. Potassium leak channels allow potassium to leave the cell. [**Section 6.4**]

power stroke
The step in the sliding filament theory during which myosin undergoes a conformational change to its low energy state, in the process dragging the thin filaments (and the attached Z lines) toward the center of the sarcomere. Note that the power stroke requires ATP only indirectly: to set the myosin molecule in its high-energy conformation during a different step of the sliding filament theory. [**Section 11.2**]

preganglionic neuron
In the autonomic division of the PNS, a neuron that has its cell body located in the CNS, and whose axon extends into the PNS to synapse with a second neuron at an autonomic ganglion. (The second neuron's axon synapses with the target organ.) [**Section 8.4**]

primary active transport
Active transport that relies directly on the hydrolysis of ATP. [**Section 6.4**]

primary bronchi
The first branches off the trachea. There are two primary bronchi, one for each lung. [**Section 12.2**]

primary immune response
The first encounter with an antigen, resulting in activated B cells (for antibody secretion) and T cells (for cellular lysis and lymphocyte proliferation). The primary immune response takes approximately ten days, which is long enough for symptoms of the infection to appear. [**Section 9.7**]

primary oocytes
Diploid cells resulting from the activation of an oogonium; primary oocytes are ready to enter meiosis I. [**Section 13.6**]

primary spermatocytes
Diploid cells resulting from the activation of a spermatogonium; primary spermatocytes are ready to enter meiosis I. [**Section 13.2**]

primase
An RNA polymerase that creates a primer (made of RNA) to initiate DNA replication. DNA pol binds to the primer and elongates it. [**Section 4.4**]

prions
Misfolded, self-replicating proteins responsible for a class of diseases known as transmissible spongiform encephalopathies (TSEs) that cause degeneration of CNS tissues. [**Section 5.2**]

productive cycle
A life cycle of animal viruses in which the mature viral particles bud from the host cell, acquiring an envelope (a coating of lipid bilayer) in the process. [**Section 5.1**]

progesterone
A steroid hormone produced by the corpus luteum in the ovary during the second half of the menstrual cycle. Progesterone maintains and enhances the uterine lining for the possible implantation of a fertilized ovum. It is the primary hormone secreted during pregnancy. [**Section 13.6**]

prokaryote
An organism that lacks a nucleus or any other membrane-bound organelles. All prokaryotes belong to either Domain Bacteria or Domain Archaea (formerly Kingdom Monera). [**Section 5.3**]

prolactin
A hormone secreted by the anterior pituitary that targets the mammary glands, stimulating them to produce breast milk. [**Section 13.14**]

proliferative phase
The second phase of the uterine (endometrial) cycle, during which the endometrium (shed off during menstruation) is rebuilt. This phase of the cycle is under the control of estrogen, secreted from the follicle developing in the ovary during this time period. The proliferative phase typically lasts from day 6 to day 14 of the menstrual cycle. [**Section 13.7**]

promoter
The sequence of nucleotides on a chromosome that activates RNA polymerase so that transcription can take place. The promoter is found upstream of the *start site*, the location where transcription actually begins. [**Section 4.7**]

prophase
The first phase of mitosis. During prophase the replicated chromosomes condense, the spindle is formed, and the nuclear envelope breaks apart into vesicles. [**Section 6.6**]

prophase I
The first phase of meiosis I. During prophase I the replicated chromosomes condense, homologous chromosomes pair up, crossing over occurs between homologous chromosomes, the spindle is formed, and the nuclear envelope breaks apart into vesicles. Prophase I is the longest phase of meiosis. [**Section 7.2**]

prophase II
The first phase of meiosis II. Prophase II is identical to mitotic prophase, except that the number of chromosomes was reduced by half during meiosis I. [**Section 7.2**]

proprioceptor
A receptor that responds to changes in body position, such as stretch on a tendon, or contraction of a muscle. These receptors allow us to be consciously aware of the position of our body parts. [**Section 8.5**]

prostate
A small gland encircling the male urethra just inferior to the bladder. Its secretions contain nutrients and enzymes and account for approximately 35 percent of the ejaculate volume. [**Section 13.1**]

prosthetic group
A non-protein, but organic, molecule (such as a vitamin) that is covalently bound to an enzyme as part of the active site. [**Sections 10.5 and 10.9**]

proximal convoluted tubule
The first portion of the nephron tubule after the glomerulus. The PCT is the site of most reabsorption; all filtered nutrients are reabsorbed here as well as most of the filtered water. [**Section 10.2**]

ptyalin
Salivary amylase (see "amylase"). [**Section 10.6**]

pulmonary artery
The blood vessel that carries deoxygenated blood from the right ventricle of the heart to the lungs. [**Section 9.2**]

pulmonary circulation
The flow of blood from the heart, through the lungs, and back to the heart. [**Section 9.1**]

pulmonary edema
A collection of fluid in the alveoli of the lungs, particularly dangerous because it impedes gas exchange. Common causes of pulmonary edema are increased pulmonary blood pressure or infection in the respiratory system. [**Section 12.4**]

pulmonary vein
One of several vessels that carry oxygenated blood from the lungs to the left atrium of the heart. [**Section 9.2**]

pupil
A hole in the center of the iris of the eye that allows light to enter the eyeball. The diameter of the pupil is controlled by the iris in response to the brightness of the light. [**Section 8.5**]

purine bases
Aromatic bases found in DNA and RNA that are derived from purine. They have a double-ring structure and include adenine and guanine. [**Section 4.1**]

Purkinje fibers
The smallest (and final) fibers in the cardiac conduction system. The Purkinje fibers transmit the cardiac impulse to the ventricular muscle. [**Section 9.2**]

pyloric sphincter
The valve that regulates the passage of chyme from the stomach into the small intestine. [**Section 10.6**]

pyrimidine bases
Aromatic bases found in DNA and RNA that have a single-ring structure. They include cytosine, thymine, and uracil. [**Section 4.1**]

receptor-mediated endocytosis
A highly specific cellular uptake mechanism. The molecule to be taken up must bind to a cell surface receptor found in a clathrin-coated pit. [**Section 6.4**]

recessive
The allele in a heterozygous genotype that is not expressed; the phenotype resulting from possession of two recessive alleles (homozygous recessive). [**Section 7.1**]

recombination frequency (RF)
The RF value; the percentage of recombinant offspring resulting from a given genetic cross. The recombination frequency is proportional to the physical distance between two genes on the same chromosome. If the recombination frequency is low, the genes under consideration may be linked. [**Section 7.5**]

rectum
The final portion of the large intestine. [**Section 10.6**]

reflex arc
A relatively direct connection between a sensory neuron and a motor neuron that allows an extremely rapid response to a stimulus, often without conscious brain involvement. [**Section 8.3**]

relative refractory period
The period of time following an action potential when it is possible, but difficult, for the neuron to fire a second action potential, due to the fact that the membrane is further from threshold potential (hyperpolarized). [**Section 8.1**]

release factor
A cytoplasmic protein that binds to a stop codon when it appears in the A site of the ribosome. Release factors modify the peptidyl transferase activity of the ribosome, such that a water molecule is added to the end of the completed protein. This releases the finished protein from the final tRNA, and allows the ribosome subunits and mRNA to dissociate. [**Section 4.8**]

renal reabsorption
The movement of a substance from the filtrate (in the renal tubule) back into the bloodstream. Reabsorption reduces the amount of a substance in the urine. [**Section 10.1**]

renal tubule
The portion of the nephron after the glomerulus and capsule; the region of the nephron where the filtrate is modified along its path to becoming urine. [**Section 10.1**]

renin
An enzyme secreted by the juxtaglomerular cells when blood pressure decreases. Renin converts angiotensinogen to angiotensin I. [**Section 10.3**]

replication
The duplication of DNA. [**Section 4.4**]

replication bubbles
Multiple sites of replication found on large, linear eukaryotic chromosomes. [**Section 4.4**]

replication fork(s)
The site(s) where the parental DNA double helix unwinds during replication. [**Section 4.4**]

repolarization
The return of membrane potential to normal resting values after a depolarization or hyperpolarization. [**Section 8.1**]

repressible system
A system (set of genes) where the expression of those genes is inhibited by the gene product (e.g., the trp operon). [**Section 4.9**]

repressor
A regulatory protein that binds DNA at a specific nucleotide sequence (sometimes known as the operator) to prevent transcription of downstream genes. [**Section 4.9**]

residual volume
The volume of air remaining in the lungs after a maximal forced exhalation, typically about 1200 mL. [**Section 12.3**]

resolution
A function of the reproductive system (controlled by the sympathetic nervous system) that returns the body to its normal resting state after sexual arousal and orgasm. [**Section 13.1**]

respiratory acidosis
A drop in blood pH due to hypoventilation (too little breathing) and a resulting accumulation of CO_2. [**Section 12.1**]

respiratory alkalosis
A rise in blood pH due to hyperventilation (excessive breathing) and a resulting decrease in CO_2. [**Section 12.1**]

resting membrane potential

An electrical potential established across the plasma membrane of all cells by the Na$^+$/K$^+$-ATPase and the K$^+$ leak channels. In most cells, the resting membrane potential is approximately –70 mV with respect to the outside of the cell. [Section 6.4]

restriction endonuclease

A bacterial enzyme that recognizes a specific DNA nucleotide sequence and that cuts the double helix at a specific site within that sequence. [Section A.5]

retina

The innermost layer of the eyeball. The retina is made up of a layer of photoreceptors, a layer of bipolar cells, and a layer of ganglion cells. [Section 8.5]

retinal

A chemical derived from vitamin A found in the pigment proteins of the rod photoreceptors of the retina. Retinal changes conformation when it absorbs light, triggering a series of reactions that ultimately result in an action potential being sent to the brain. [Section 8.5]

retrovirus

A virus with an RNA genome (e.g., HIV) that undergoes a lysogenic life cycle in a host with a double-stranded DNA genome. In order to integrate its genome with the host cell genome, the virus must first reverse-transcribe its RNA genome to DNA. [Section 5.1]

reverse transcriptase

An enzyme that polymerizes a strand of DNA by reading an RNA template (an RNA dependent DNA polymerase); used by retroviruses in order to integrate their genome with the host cell genome. [Section 5.1]

ribosome

A structure made of two protein subunits and rRNA; this is the site of protein synthesis (translation) in a cell. Prokaryotic ribosomes (also known as 70S ribosomes) are smaller than eukaryotic ribosomes (80S ribosomes). The S value refers to the sedimentation rate during centrifugation. [Section 4.3]

RNA-dependent RNA polymerase

A viral enzyme that makes a strand of RNA by reading a strand of RNA. All prokaryotic and eukaryotic RNA polymerases are DNA dependent; they make a strand of RNA by reading a strand of DNA. [Section 5.1]

RNA interference (RNAi)

Small non-coding RNAs that bind to mRNAs, these double-stranded RNAs are then degraded and gene expression is reduced. [Section 4.7]

RNA polymerase

An enzyme that transcribes RNA. Prokaryotes have a single RNA pol, while eukaryotes have three; in eukaryotes, RNA pol I transcribes rRNA, RNA pol II transcribes mRNA, and RNA pol III transcribes tRNA. [Section 4.7]

RNA translocation

The movement of new mRNA transcripts to particular locations within the cell prior to their translation. [Section 4.9]

rods

Photoreceptors in the retina of the eye that respond to dim light and provide us with black and white vision. [Section 8.5]

rough endoplasmic reticulum

A large system of folded membranes within a eukaryotic cell that has ribosomes bound to it, giving it a rough appearance. These ribosomes synthesize proteins that will ultimately be secreted from the cell, incorporated into the plasma membrane, or transported to the Golgi apparatus or lysosomes. [Section 6.2]

rRNA

Ribosomal RNA; the type of RNA that associates with ribosomal proteins to make a functional ribosome. It is thought that the rRNA has the peptidyl transferase activity. [Section 4.7]

rule of addition

A statistical rule stating that the probability of either of two independent (and mutually exclusive) events occurring is the *sum* of their individual probabilities. [Section 7.3]

rule of multiplication

A statistical rule stating that the probability of two independent events occurring together is the *product* of their individual probabilities. [Section 7.3]

saltatory conduction

A rapid form of action potential conduction along the axon of a neuron in which the action potential appears to jump from node of Ranvier to node of Ranvier. [Section 8.1]

sarcolemma

The plasma membrane of a muscle cell. [Section 11.2]

sarcomere

The unit of muscle contraction. Sarcomeres are bounded by Z lines, to which thin filaments attach. Thick filaments are found in the center of the sarcomere, overlapped by thin filaments. Sliding of the filaments over one another during contraction reduces the distance between Z lines, shortening the sarcomere. [Section 11.2]

sarcoplasmic reticulum (SR)
The smooth ER of a muscle cell, enlarged and specialized to act as a Ca^{2+} reservoir. The SR winds around each myofibril in the muscle cell. [Section 11.2]

Schwann cell
One of the two peripheral nervous system supporting (glial) cells. Schwann cells form the myelin sheath on axons of peripheral neurons. [Section 8.1]

sclera
The white portion of the tough outer layer of the eyeball. [Section 8.5]

sebaceous glands
Oil-forming glands found all over the body, especially on the face and neck. The product (sebum) is released to the skin surface through hair follicles. [Section 12.6]

secondary active transport
Active transport that relies on an established concentration gradient, typically set up by a primary active transporter. Secondary active transport relies on ATP indirectly. [Section 6.4]

secondary immune response
A subsequent immune response to previously encountered antigen that results in antibody production and T cell activation. The secondary immune response is mediated by memory cells (produced during the primary immune response) and is much faster and stronger than the primary response, typically taking only a day or less. This is not long enough for the infection to become established; symptoms do not appear, thus the person is said to be "immune" to that particular antigen. [Section 9.7]

secondary oocyte
A haploid cell resulting from the first meiotic division of oogenesis. Note that the cytoplasmic division in this case is unequal, producing one large cell with almost all of the cytoplasm (the secondary oocyte) and one smaller cell with virtually no cytoplasm (the first polar body). The secondary oocyte, along with some follicular cells, is released from the ovary during ovulation. [Section 13.6]

secondary sexual characteristics
The set of adult characteristics that develop during puberty under the control of the sex steroids. In males, the secondary sex characteristics include enlargement and maturation of the genitalia, growth of facial, body, and pubic hair, increased muscle mass, and lowering of the voice. In females, the characteristics include the onset of menstruation and the menstrual cycle, enlargement of the breasts, widening of the pelvis, and growth of pubic hair. [Section 13.4]

secondary spermatocytes
Haploid cells resulting from the first meiotic division of spermatogenesis. Secondary spermatocytes are ready to enter meiosis II. [Section 13.2]

second messenger
An intracellular chemical signal (such as cAMP) that relays instructions from the cell surface to enzymes in the cytosol. [Section 6.5]

secretin
A hormone secreted by the small intestine (duodenum) in response to low pH (e.g., from stomach acid). It promotes the release of bicarbonate from the pancreas to act as a buffer. [Section 10.6]

secretion
1. The secretion of useful substances from a cell, either into the blood (endocrine secretion) or into a cavity or onto the body surface (exocrine secretion).

2. In the nephron, the movement of substances from the blood to the filtrate along the tubule. Secretion increases the rate at which substances can be removed from the body. [Sections 10.2 and 10.5]

secretory phase
The third phase of the uterine (endometrial) cycle, during which the rebuilt endometrium is enhanced with glycogen and lipid stores. The secretory phase is primarily under the control of progesterone and estrogen (secreted from the corpus luteum during this time period), and typically lasts from day 15 to day 28 of the menstrual cycle. [Section 13.7]

semen
An alkaline, fructose-rich fluid produced by three different glands in the male reproductive tract and released during ejaculation. Semen is very nourishing for sperm. [Section 13.1]

semicircular canals
Three loop-like structures in the inner ear that contain sensory receptors to monitor balance. [Section 8.5]

semiconservative replication
DNA replication. Each of the parental strands is read to make a complementary daughter strand, thus each new DNA molecule is composed of half the parental molecule paired with a newly synthesized strand. [Section 4.4]

semilunar valves

The valves in the heart that separate the ventricles from the arteries. The pulmonary semilunar valve separates the right ventricle from the pulmonary artery, and the aortic semilunar valve separates the left ventricle from the aorta. These valves close at the end of systole, preventing the backflow of blood from arteries to ventricles, and producing the second heart sound. [Section 9.2]

seminal vesicles

Paired glands found on the posterior external wall of the bladder in males. Their secretions contain an alkaline mucus and fructose, among other things, and make up approximately 60 percent of the ejaculate volume. [Section 13.1]

seminiferous tubules

Small convoluted tubules in the testes where spermatogenesis takes place. [Section 13.1]

senescence

The process of biological aging at the cellular (and organismal) level. [Section 6.7]

Sertoli cells

See "sustentacular cells." [Section 13.1]

serum

Plasma with the clotting factors removed. Serum is often used in diagnostic tests since it does not clot. [Section 9.4]

sex-linked trait

A trait determined by a gene on either the X or the Y chromosomes (the sex chromosomes). [Section 7.4]

Shine-Dalgarno sequence

The prokaryotic ribosome-binding site on mRNA, found 10 nucleotides 5' to the start codon. [Section 4.8]

signal recognition particle (SRP)

A cytoplasmic protein that recognizes the signal sequences of proteins destined to be translated at the rough ER. It binds first to the ribosome translating the protein with the signal sequence, then to an SRP receptor on the rough ER. [Section 6.2]

signal sequence

A short sequence of amino acids, usually found at the N-terminus of a protein being translated, that directs the ribosome and its associated mRNA to the membranes of the rough ER where translation will be completed. Signal sequences are found on membrane-bound proteins, secreted proteins, and proteins destined for other organelles. [Section 6.2]

signal transduction

The intracellular process triggered by the binding of a ligand to its receptor on the cell surface. Typically this activates second messenger pathways. [Section 6.5]

silent mutation

A point mutation in which a codon that specifies an amino acid is mutated into a new codon that specifies the same amino acid. [Section 4.5]

simple diffusion

The movement of a hydrophobic molecule across the plasma membrane of cell, down its concentration gradient. Since the molecule can easily interact with the lipid bilayer, no additional help (such as a channel or pore) is required. [Section 6.4]

single nucleotide polymorphisms (SNPs)

Variations in a single nucleotide from one person's DNA gene sequence to another's. These minor mutations can produce changes in phenotype. [Section 4.2]

single strand binding proteins

Proteins that bind to and stabilize the single strands of DNA exposed when helicase unwinds the double helix in preparation for replication. [Section 4.4]

sinoatrial (SA) node

A region of specialized cardiac muscle cells in the right atrium of the heart that initiate the impulse for heart contraction; for this reason the SA node is known as the "pacemaker" of the heart. [Section 9.2]

sister chromatid

Identical copies of a chromosome, produced during DNA replication and held together at the centromere. Sister chromatids are separated during anaphase of mitosis. [Section 6.6]

skeletal muscle

Muscle tissue that is attached to the bones. Skeletal muscle is striated, multinucleate, and under voluntary control. [Section 11.2]

sliding filament model

The mechanism of contraction in skeletal and cardiac muscle cells. It is a series of four repeated steps: (1) myosin binds actin, (2) myosin pulls actin toward the center of the sarcomere, (3) myosin releases actin, and (4) myosin resets to its high-energy conformation. [Section 11.2]

slow block to polyspermy
Also known as the *cortical reaction*, the slow block occurs after a sperm penetrates an oocyte (fertilization). It involves an increase in intracellular $[Ca^{2+}]$ in the egg, which causes the release of cortical granules near the egg plasma membrane. This results in the hardening of the zona pellucida and its separation from the surface of the egg, preventing the further entry of more sperm into the egg. [**Section 13.9**]

slow twitch fibers
Skeletal muscle cells that contract slowly but are fatigue resistant due to a high concentration of myoglobin and a good blood supply. [**Section 11.2**]

small intestine
The region of the digestive tract where virtually all digestion and absorption occur. It is subdivided into three regions: the duodenum, the jejunum, and the ileum. [**Section 10.6**]

smooth endoplasmic reticulum
A network of membranes inside eukaryotic cells involved in lipid synthesis (steroids in gonads), detoxification (in liver cells), and/or Ca^{2+} storage (muscle cells). [**Section 6.2**]

smooth muscle
Muscle tissue found in the walls of hollow organs, e.g., blood vessels, the digestive tract, the uterus, etc. Smooth muscle is nonstriated, uninucleate, and under involuntary control (controlled by the autonomic nervous system). [**Section 11.4**]

soma
The cell body of a neuron. [**Section 8.1**]

somatic nervous system
The division of the peripheral nervous system that innervates and controls the skeletal muscles; also known as the *voluntary nervous system*. [**Section 8.3**]

spatial summation
Integration by a postsynaptic neuron of inputs (EPSPs and IPSPs) from multiple sources. [**Section 8.2**]

spermatid
A haploid but immature cell resulting from the second meiotic division of spermatogenesis. Spermatids undergo significant physical changes to become mature sperm (spermatozoa). [**Section 13.2**]

spermatogenesis
Sperm production; occurs in human males on a daily basis from puberty until death. Spermatogenesis results in the production of four mature gametes (sperm) from a single precursor cell (spermatogonium). For maximum sperm viability, spermatogenesis requires cooler temperatures and adequate testosterone. [**Section 13.2**]

spermatogonium
A diploid cell that can undergo mitosis to form more spermatogonium, and can also be triggered to undergo meiosis to form sperm. [**Section 13.2**]

S (synthesis) phase
The phase of the cell cycle during which the genome is replicated. [**Sections 4.4 and 6.6**]

sphincter of Oddi
The valve controlling release of bile and pancreatic juice into the duodenum. [**Section 10.6**]

sphygmomanometer
A blood pressure cuff. [**Section 9.3**]

spirochete
A bacterium having a spiral shape (plural = spirochetes). [**Section 5.3**]

spleen
An abdominal organ that is considered part of the immune system. The spleen has four functions: (1) it filters antigen from the blood, (2) it is the site of B cell maturation, (3) it stores blood, and (4) it destroys old red blood cells. [**Section 9.7**]

spliceosome
A complex made of many proteins and several small nuclear RNAs (snRNAs) that assembles around an intron to be spliced out of the primary transcript. [**Section 4.7**]

splicing
One type of eukaryotic mRNA processing in which introns are removed from the primary transcript and exons are ligated together. Splicing of transcripts can be different in different tissues. [**Section 4.7**]

spongy bone
A looser, more porous type of bone tissue found at the inner core of the epiphyses in long bones and all other bone types. Spongy bone is filled with red bone marrow, important in blood cell formation. [**Section 11.7**]

start site
The location on a chromosome where transcription begins. [**Section 4.7**]

steroid hormone
A hormone derived from cholesterol. Steroids are generally hydrophobic and can easily cross the plasma membranes of cells, thus receptors for steroids are found intracellularly. Once the steroid binds to its receptor, the receptor-steroid complex acts to regulate transcription in the nucleus. [**Section 8.6**]

stomach

The portion of the digestive tract that stores and grinds food. Limited digestion occurs in the stomach, and it has the lowest pH in the body (pH 1–2). [Section 10.6]

stop codon

A group of three nucleotides that does not specify a particular amino acid, but instead serves to notify the ribosome that the protein being translated is complete. The stop codons are UAA, UGA, and UAG. They are also known as *nonsense codons*. [Section 4.3]

striated muscle

See "skeletal muscle." [Section 11.2]

stroke volume

The volume of blood pumped out of the heart in a single beat (contraction). [Section 9.2]

submucosa

The layer of connective tissue directly under the mucosa of an open body cavity. [Section 10.5]

submucosal plexus

A network of neurons found in the submucosa of the gut; it helps to regulate enzyme secretion, gut blood flow, and ion and water flow in the lumen. Part of the enteric nervous system. [Section 10.5]

sudoriferous gland

A sweat gland located in the dermis of the skin. Sweat consists of water and ions (including Na^+ and urea) and is secreted when temperatures rise. [Section 12.6]

summation

1. The integration of input (EPSPs and IPSPs) from many presynaptic neurons by a single postsynaptic neuron, either temporally or spatially. Summation of all input can either stimulate the postsynaptic neuron and possibly lead to an action potential, or it can inhibit the neuron, reducing the likelihood of an action potential.

2. The integration of single muscle twitches into a sustained contraction (tetany). [Sections 8.2 and 11.2]

surfactant

An amphipathic molecule secreted by cells in the alveoli (type 2 alveolar cells) that reduces surface tension on the inside of the alveolar walls. This prevents the alveoli from collapsing upon exhale and sticking together, thus reducing the effort required for inspiration. [Section 12.2]

sustentacular cells

Cells that form the walls of the seminiferous tubules and help in spermatogenesis. Sustentacular cells are also called *Sertoli cells*, and respond to FSH. [Section 13.1]

symbiotic bacteria

Bacteria that coexist with a host, where both the bacteria and the host derive a benefit. [Section 5.3]

sympathetic nervous system

The division of the autonomic nervous system known as the "fight or flight" system. It causes a general increase in body activities such as heart rate, respiratory rate, and blood pressure, and an increase in blood flow to skeletal muscle. It causes a general decrease in digestive activity. Because all of its preganglionic neurons originate from the thoracic or lumbar regions of the spinal cord, it is also known as the *thoracolumbar* system. [Section 8.4]

symport

A carrier protein that transports two molecules across the plasma membrane in the same direction. For example, the Na^+-glucose cotransporter in intestinal cells is a symporter. [Section 6.4]

synapse

A neuron-to-neuron, neuron-to-organ, or muscle cell-to-muscle cell junction. [Section 8.2]

synapsis

Pairing of homologous chromosomes in a diploid cell, as occurs during prophase I of meiosis. [Section 7.2]

synaptic cleft

A microscopic space between the axon of one neuron and the cell body or dendrites of a second neuron, or between the axon of a neuron and an organ. [Section 8.1]

synaptonemal complex

A structure that forms in early prophase I that mediates synapsis (pairing of homologous chromosomes). [Section 7.2]

syncytium

A large multinucleate cell, typically formed by the fusion of many smaller cells during development (e.g., a skeletal muscle cell), or formed by nuclear division in the absence of cellular division. [Sections 10.5 and 11.3]

synergist

Something that works together with another thing to augment the second thing's activity. For example, a muscle that assists another muscle is said to be a synergist. An enzyme that helps another enzyme is a synergist. [Section 11.2]

synovial fluid

A lubricating, nourishing fluid found in joint capsules. [Section 11.8]

systemic circulation
The flow of blood from the heart, through the body (not including the lungs), and back to the heart. [**Section 9.1**]

systole
The period of time during which the ventricles of the heart are contracted. [**Section 9.2**]

systolic pressure
The pressure measured in the arteries during contraction of the ventricles (during systole). [**Section 9.3**]

T cell
A type of lymphocyte. The major subtypes of T cells are the helper T cells (CD4) and the killer T cells (CD8, or cytotoxic T cells). Helper T cells secrete chemicals that help killer Ts and B cells proliferate. Killer T cells destroy abnormal self-cells (e.g., cancer cells) or infected cells. [**Sections 9.4 and 9.7**]

tandem repeats
Regions of the genome where short sequences of nucleotides are repeated one after the other, anywhere from three to 100 times. [**Section 4.2**]

telencephalon
The cerebral hemispheres. [**Section 8.4**]

telomere
A specialized region at the ends of eukaryotic chromosomes that contains several repeats of a particular DNA sequence. These ends are maintained (in some cells) with the help of a special DNA polymerase called *telomerase*. In cells that lack telomerase, the telomeres slowly degrade with each round of DNA replication; this is thought to contribute to the eventual death of the cell. [**Sections 4.1, 4.4, and 6.7**]

telophase
The fourth (and final) phase of mitosis. During telophase the nuclear envelope reforms, chromosomes decondense, and the mitotic spindle is disassembled. [**Section 6.6**]

telophase I
The fourth phase of meiosis I. Telophase I is identical to mitotic telophase, except that the number of chromosomes is now reduced by half. After this phase the cell is considered to be haploid. Note, however, that the chromosomes are still replicated, and the sister chromatids must still be separated during meiosis II. [**Section 7.2**]

telophase II
The fourth and final phase of meiosis II. Telophase II is identical to mitotic telophase, except that the number of chromosomes was reduced by half during meiosis I. [**Section 7.2**]

temporal summation
Summation by a postsynaptic cell of input (EPSPs or IPSPs) from a single source over time. [**Section 8.2**]

tendon
Strong bands of connective tissue that connect skeletal muscle to bone. [**Section 11.2**]

testcross
A genetic cross between an organism displaying a recessive phenotype (homozygous recessive) and an organism displaying a dominant phenotype (for which the genotype is unknown), done to determine the unknown genotype. [**Section 7.3**]

testes
The primary male sex organ. The testes are suspended outside the body cavity in the scrotum and have two functions: (1) produce sperm, and (2) secrete testosterone. [**Section 13.1**]

testosterone
The primary androgen (male sex steroid). Testosterone is a steroid hormone produced and secreted by the interstitial cells of the testes. It triggers the development of secondary male sex characteristics during puberty (including spermatogenesis) and maintains those characteristics during adulthood. [**Section 13.2**]

tetanus
A smooth sustained muscle contraction, such as occurs in skeletal muscle when stimulation frequency is high enough (this is the normal type of contraction exhibited by skeletal muscle). [**Section 11.2**]

tetrad
A pair of replicated homologous chromosomes. Tetrads form during prophase I of meiosis so that homologous chromosomes can exchange DNA in a process known as "crossing over." [**Section 7.2**]

thalamus
The central structure of the diencephalon of the brain. The thalamus acts as a relay station and major integrating area for sensory impulses. [**Section 8.4**]

thecal cells
A layer of cells surrounding the granulosa cells of the follicles in an ovary. Thecal cells help produce the estrogen secreted from the follicle during the first phase of the ovarian cycle. [**Section 13.6**]

thermoreceptor
A receptor that responds to changes in temperature. [**Section 8.5**]

theta replication
DNA replication in prokaryotes, so named because as replication proceeds around the single, circular chromosome, it takes on the appearance of the Greek letter theta. [**Section 4.4**]

thick filament
In skeletal and cardiac muscle tissue, a filament composed of bundles of myosin molecules. The myosin head groups attach to the thin filaments during muscle contraction and pull them toward the center of the sarcomere. [**Section 11.2**]

thin filament
In skeletal and cardiac muscle tissue, a filament composed of actin, tropomyosin, and troponin. Thin filaments are attached to the Z lines of the sarcomeres and slide over thick filaments during muscle contraction. [**Section 11.2**]

thrombus
A blood clot that forms in an unbroken blood vessel. Thrombi are dangerous because they can break free and begin traveling in the bloodstream (become an *embolus*). Emboli ultimately become stuck in a small vessel and prevent adequate blood delivery to tissues beyond the sticking point, leading to tissue death. A brain embolism can lead to stroke, a heart embolism to a heart attack, and a pulmonary embolism to respiratory failure. [**Section 9.4**]

thymine
One of the four aromatic bases found in DNA. Thymine is a pyrimidine; it pairs with adenine. [**Section 4.1**]

thymus
An immune organ located near the heart. The thymus is the site of T cell maturation and is larger in children and adolescents. [**Section 9.7**]

thyroid stimulating hormone (TSH)
A tropic hormone produced by the anterior pituitary gland that targets the thyroid gland, stimulating it to produce and release thyroid hormone. [**Section 8.6**]

thyroxine
Also called *thyroid hormone*, thyroxine is produced and secreted by follicle cells in the thyroid gland. It targets all cells in the body and increases overall body metabolism. [**Section 8.6**]

tidal volume
The volume of air inhaled and exhaled in a normal, resting breath, typically about 500 mL. [**Section 12.3**]

tight junction
Also called *occluding junctions*, tight junctions form a seal between cells that prevents the movement of substances across the cell layer, except by diffusion through the cell membranes themselves. Tight junctions are found between the epithelial cells lining the intestines and between the cells forming the capillaries in the brain (the blood-brain barrier). [**Section 6.5**]

tolerance
The unresponsiveness of the immune system to normal proteins. [**Section 9.8**]

tolerant anaerobe
An organism that can survive in the presence of oxygen (oxygen is not toxic), but that does not use oxygen during metabolism (anaerobic metabolism only). [**Section 5.3**]

top-down processing
A tenet of Gestalt psychology where the brain applies experience and expectations to interpret sensory information. [**Section 8.5**]

topoisomerase
An enzyme that cuts one or both strands of DNA to relieve the excess tension caused by the unwinding of the helix by helicase during replication. [**Section 4.4**]

total lung capacity
The maximum volume of air that the lungs can contain. Total lung capacity is the sum of the vital capacity and the residual volume, and is typically about 6000 mL (6 L). [**Section 12.3**]

totipotent
Having the ability to become anything, e.g., a zygote is totipotent. [**Section 13.12**]

trachea
The main air tube leading into the respiratory system. The trachea is made of alternating rings of cartilage and connective tissue. [**Sections 10.6 and 12.2**]

transcription
The enzymatic process of reading a strand of DNA to produce a complementary strand of RNA. [**Sections 4.3 and 4.7**]

transduction
The transfer by a lysogenic virus of a portion of a host cell genome to a new host. [**Section 5.1**]

transition mutation
A point mutation in which a pyrimidine is substituted for a pyrimidine, or a purine is substituted for a purine. [**Section 4.5**]

translation
The process of reading a strand of mRNA to synthesize protein. Protein translation takes place on a ribosome. [**Sections 4.3 and 4.7**]

transmembrane domain
The portion of an integral membrane protein that passes through the lipid bilayer. [**Section 6.2**]

transposons
Segments of the genome that can "jump" from one location to another. Can lead to mutations depending on the final location of the transposon. [**Section 4.5**]

transverse tubule
See "T tubules." [**Section 11.2**]

transversion mutation
A point mutation in which a pyrimidine is substituted for a purine, or vice versa. [**Section 4.5**]

tricuspid valve
See "atrioventricular valve." [**Section 9.2**]

tRNA
Transfer RNA; the type of RNA that carries an amino acid from the cytoplasm to the ribosome for incorporation into a growing protein. [**Section 4.7**]

tRNA loading
The attachment of an amino acid to a tRNA (note that this is a specific interaction). tRNA loading requires two high-energy phosphate bonds. [**Section 4.8**]

trophoblast
The outer ring of cells of a blastocyst. The trophoblast takes part in formation of a placenta. [**Section 13.9**]

tropic hormone
A hormone that controls the release of another hormone. [**Section 8.6**]

tropomyosin
A helical protein that winds around actin helices in skeletal and cardiac muscle cells to form the thin filament of the sarcomere. In the absence of Ca^{2+}, tropomyosin covers the myosin-binding sites on actin and prevents muscle contraction. When calcium is present, a conformational change in tropomyosin occurs so that the myosin-binding sites are exposed and muscle contraction can occur. [**Section 11.2**]

troponin
A globular protein that associates with tropomyosin as part of the thin filament of the sarcomere. Troponin is the protein that binds Ca^{2+}, which causes the conformational change in tropomyosin required to expose the myosin-binding sites on actin and initiate muscle contraction. [**Section 11.2**]

trp operon
A set of genes for the enzymes necessary to synthesize tryptophan, under the control of a single promoter, the expression of which is inhibited by the presence of tryptophan (this is a repressible system). [**Section 4.9**]

trypsin
The main protease secreted by the pancreas; trypsin is activated (from trypsinogen) by enterokinase, and subsequently activates the other pancreatic enzymes. [**Section 10.7**]

T-tubules
Also called *transverse tubules*, these are deep invaginations of the plasma membrane found in skeletal and cardiac muscle cells. These invaginations allow depolarization of the membrane to quickly penetrate to the interior of the cell. [**Section 11.2**]

tumor suppressor genes
Genes that produce proteins that are the inherent defense system in cells to prevent the conversion of the cell into a cancer cell. p53 is a well-known tumor suppressor gene. [**Section 6.7**]

tympanic membrane
The membrane that separates the outer ear from the middle ear. The tympanic membrane is also known as the *eardrum*. [**Section 8.5**]

type I fibers
Also known as red slow twitch or red oxidative fibers, these are skeletal muscle cells that contract slowly and are extremely resistant to fatigue. [**Section 11.2**]

type IIA fibers
Also known as fast twitch oxidative fibers, these are skeletal muscle cells that contract quickly and are somewhat resistant to fatigue. [**Section 11.2**]

type IIB fibers
Also known as white fast twitch fibers, these are skeletal muscle cells that contract quickly and fatigue quickly. [**Section 11.2**]

umbilical cord
The cord that connects the embryo of a developing mammal to the placenta in the uterus of the mother. The umbilical cord contains fetal arteries (carry blood toward the placenta) and veins (carry blood away from the placenta). The umbilical vessels derive from the *allantois*, a structure that develops from the embryonic gut. [**Section 13.10**]

uniport
A carrier protein that transports a single molecule across the plasma membrane. [**Section 6.4**]

universal acceptor (recipient)
A person with blood type AB⁺. Because this person's red blood cells possess all of the typical blood surface proteins, they will not display an immune reaction if transfused with any of the other blood types. [**Section 9.4**]

universal donor
A person with blood type O⁻. Because this person's red blood cells possess none of the typical blood surface proteins, they cannot initiate an immune reaction in a recipient. [**Section 9.4**]

upstream
Toward the 5' end of an RNA transcript (the 5' end of the DNA coding strand). The promoter and start sites are "upstream." [**Section 4.7**]

uracil
One of four aromatic bases found in RNA. Uracil is pyrimidine; it pairs with adenine. [**Section 4.7**]

urea
A waste product of protein breakdown, produced by the liver and released into the bloodstream to be eliminated by the kidney. [**Sections 9.4 and 10.1**]

ureters
The tubes that carry urine from the kidneys to the bladder. [**Section 13.11**]

urethra
The tube that carries urine from the bladder to the outside of the body. In males it also carries semen and sperm during ejaculation. [**Section 13.1**]

urinary sphincter
The valve that controls the release of urine from the bladder. It has an internal part made of smooth muscle (thus involuntary) and an external part made of skeletal muscle (thus voluntary). [**Section 10.6**]

uterine cycle
The shedding of the old endometrium and preparation of a new endometrium for potential pregnancy. [**Section 13.7**]

uterine tubes
Also called *fallopian tubes*, these tubes extend laterally from either side of the uterus and serve as a passageway for the oocyte to travel from the ovary to the uterus. This is also the normal site of fertilization. Severing of the uterine tubes (tubal ligation) results in sterility of the female. [**Section 13.5**]

uterus
The muscular female organ in which a baby develops during pregnancy. [**Section 13.5**]

vaccination
The deliberate exposure of a person to an antigen in order to provoke the primary immune response and memory cell production. Typically the antigens are those normally associated with pathogens, thus if the live pathogen is encountered in the future, the secondary immune response can be initiated, preventing infection and symptoms. [**Section 9.7**]

vagal tone
The constant inhibition provided to the heart by the vagus nerve. Vagal tone reduces the intrinsic firing rate of the SA node from 120 beats/minute to around 80 beats/minute. [**Section 9.2**]

vagina
The birth canal; the stretchy, muscular passageway through which a baby exits the uterus during childbirth. [**Section 13.5**]

vagus nerves
Cranial nerve pair X. The vagus nerves are very large mixed nerves (they carry both sensory input and motor output) that innervate virtually every visceral organ. They are especially important in transmitting parasympathetic input to the heart and digestive smooth muscle. [**Section 8.4**]

van't Hoff factor
The van't Hoff factor (or ionizability factor, i) tells us how many ions one unit of a substance will produce in a solution. For example, glucose is non-ionic (does not dissociate) so $i = 1$, however NaCl dissociates into Na⁺ and Cl⁻, therefore $i = 2$. [**Section 6.4**]

vasa recta
The capillaries that surround the tubules of the nephron. The vasa recta reclaims reabsorbed substances, such as water and sodium ions. [**Section 10.2**]

vas deferens
See "ductus deferens." [**Section 13.1**]

vein
A blood vessel that carries blood toward the heart chambers. Veins do not have muscular walls, have valves to ensure that blood flows in one direction only, and are typically low-pressure vessels. [Section 9.1]

vena cava
One of two large vessels (superior and inferior) that return deoxygenated blood to the right atrium of the heart. [Section 9.2]

venous return
The amount of blood returned to the heart by the vena cavae. [Section 9.2]

ventricle
One of two large chambers in the heart. The ventricles receive blood from the atria and pump it out of the heart. The right ventricle has thin walls and pumps deoxygenated blood to the lungs through the pulmonary artery. The left ventricle has thick walls and pumps oxygenated blood to the body through the aorta. [Section 9.2]

vestibular glands
Paired glands near the posterior of the vaginal opening that secrete an alkaline mucus upon sexual arousal. The mucus helps to reduce the acidity of the vagina (which could be harmful to sperm) and lubricates the vagina to facilitate penetration. [Section 13.5]

villi
(Singular: *villus*.) Folds of the intestinal mucosa that project into the lumen of the intestine; villi serve to increase the surface area of the intestine for absorption. [Section 10.6]

viroids
Short pieces of circular single-stranded RNA that do not code for proteins but interfere with normal gene expression. Mostly they cause diseases in plants; the only human disease linked to viroids is hepatitis D. [Section 5.2]

virus
A nonliving, intracellular parasite. Viruses are typically just pieces of nucleic acid surrounded by a protein coat. [Section 5.1]

vital capacity
The maximum amount of air that can be forcibly exhaled from the lungs after filling them to their maximum level, typically about 4500 mL. [Section 12.3]

vitamin
One of several different nutrients that must be consumed in the diet, and generally not synthesized in the body. Vitamins can be hydrophobic (fat-soluble) or hydrophilic (water-soluble). [Section 10.9]

vitreous humor
A thick, gelatinous fluid found in the posterior segment of the eye (between the lens and the retina). The vitreous humor is only produced during fetal development and helps maintain intraocular pressure (the pressure inside the eyeball). [Section 8.5]

voltage-gated ion channel
An ion channel that is opened or closed based on the electrical potential across the plasma membrane. Once opened, the channel allows ions to cross the membrane according to their concentration gradients. [Section 6.4]

Weber's law
Weber's law states that two stimuli must differ by a constant proportion in order for their difference to be perceptible. [Section 8.5]

white matter
Myelinated axons. [Section 8.4]

Wolffian ducts
Early embryonic ducts that can develop into male internal genitalia under the proper stimulation (testosterone). [Section 13.3]

X-chromosome inactivation
The silencing of one of the two X chromosomes in female cells, so that only one is active. [Section 4.7]

yolk sac
An embryonic structure particularly important in egg-laying animals because it contains the yolk, the only source of nutrients for the embryo developing inside the egg. In humans, the yolk sac is very small (since mammals get their nutrients via the placenta) and is the site of synthesis of the first red blood cells. [Section 13.10]

Z lines
The ends of a sarcomere. [Section 11.2]

zona pellucida
A thick, transparent coating rich in glycoproteins that surrounds an oocyte. [Section 13.6]

zygote
A diploid cell formed by the fusion of two gametes during sexual reproduction. [Section 13.9]

zymogen
An inactive precursor of an enzyme, activated by various methods (acid hydrolysis, cleavage by another enzyme, etc.). [Sections 4.9 and 10.6]

NOTES

NOTES

NOTES

NOTES

NOTES

NOTES

NOTES

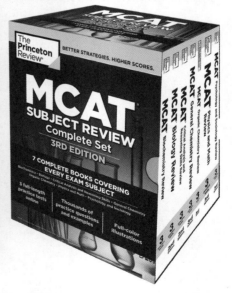